CARDIAC ALLOGRAFT REJECTION

CARDIAC ALLOGRAFT REJECTION

edited by

William Dec, M.D.
Heart Failure & Transplantation Service
Harvard Medical School
Boston, Massachusetts

Jagat Narula, M.D., Ph.D.
Heart Failure/Transplantation Center
Hahnemann University School of Medicine
Philadelphia, Pennsylvania

Manel Ballester, M.D.
Department of Cardiology
Hospital Universitari Arnau de Vilanova
Universitat de Lleida
Lleida, Spain

Ignasi Carrio, M.D.
Department of Nuclear Medicine
Hospital de Sant Pau
Barcelona, Spain

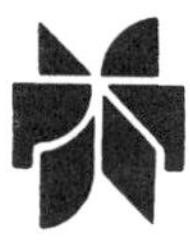

KLUWER ACADEMIC PUBLISHERS
BOSTON / DORDRECHT / LONDON

Distributors for North, Central and South America:
Kluwer Academic Publishers
101 Philip Drive
Assinippi Park
Norwell, Massachusetts 02061 USA
Telephone (781) 871-6600
Fax (781) 681-9045
E-Mail <kluwer@wkap.com>

Distributors for all other countries:
Kluwer Academic Publishers Group
Distribution Centre
Post Office Box 322
3300 AH Dordrecht, THE NETHERLANDS
Telephone 31 78 6392 392
Fax 31 78 6392 254
E-Mail <services@wkap.nl>

Electronic Services <http://www.wkap.nl>

Library of Congress Cataloging-in-Publication Data

Cardiac allograft rejection / edited by William Dec . . . [et al.].
p.; cm.
Includes bibliographical references and index.
ISBN 0-7923-7329-4 (hardback : alk. paper)
1. Heart—Transplantation—Complications. 2. Graft rejection. I. Dec, William, 1952–
[DNLM: 1. Graft Rejection. 2. Heart Transplantation. 3. Transplantation, Homologous.
WG 169 C2655 2001]
RD598.35.T7 C346 2001
617.4'120592—dc21 2001029221

Printed on acid-free paper.

Printed in the United States of America

The Publisher offers discounts on this book for course use and bulk purchases. For further information, send email to <Kluwer@wkap.com>.

TABLE OF CONTENTS

Section IV. Radionuclide Imaging for Surveillance of Cardiac Allograft Rejection

CONTRIBUTING AUTHORS

A ftab A Ansari, MD, Department of Pathology and Laboratory Medicine, Room 4107 B Winship Cancer Center, Emory University School of Medicine, 1365 B Clifton Road, NE, Atlanta, GA 30322

Barbara Czerska, MD, Heart Failure and Transplantation Section, Henry Ford Hospital, 2799 West Grand Boulevard, K-2, Detroit, Michigan 48202

Dale G Renlund, MD, Division of Cardiology, LDS Hospital, 8th Avenue and C Street, Salt Lake City, Utah 84143

Deirdre Cunningham, MD, Imutran LtD (a Novartis Pharma AG Co), PO Box 399, Cambridge, CB2 2YP, UNITED KINGDOM

Edward F Philbin, MD, Chairmen, Division of Cardiology, Department of Medicine, The Albany Medical College, Mail Code 44, 47 New Scotland Avenue, Albany, NY 12208

Edward K Kaspar, MD, Director, Cardiomyopathy and Heart Transplant Service, Division of Cardiology, Johns Hopkins Hospital, 600 North Wolfe Street/Carneigie 568, Baltimore, MD 21287

Elizabeth H. Hammond, MD, Chairman, Department of Pathology, LDS Hospital, 8th Avenue and C Street, Salt Lake City, Utah 84143

Francis G, Blankenberg, MD, Division of Nuclear Medicine, Stanford University School of Medicine, 300 Pasteur Drive, Rm H-0101, Stanford, California 94305

G William Dec, MD, Heart Failure and Transplant Unit, Massachusetts General Hospital, Bigelow 645, 55 Fruit Street, Boston, MA 02114

Hannah A Valantine, MD, Stanford University School of Medicine, Division of Cardiology, Falk Building, 300 Pasteur Drive, Stanford, CA 94305

H. William Strauss, MD, Director, Division of Nuclear Medicine, Stanford University School of Medicine, 300 Pasteur Drive, Rm H-0101, Stanford, California 94305

Ignasi Carrio, MD, Director, Nuclear Medicine Department, Autonomous University of Barcelona, Hospital Sant Pau, Pare Claret 167, 08025 Barcelona SPAIN

Ilan S Wittstein, MD, Division of Cardiology, Johns Hopkins Hospital, 600 North Wolfe Street, Baltimore, MD 21287

Jagat Narula, MD, PhD, Director, Center for Heart Failure and Transplantation Center, Hahnemann University Hospital, Broad and Vine Streets, Mail Stop 115, Philadelphia, Pennsylvania 19102

James Frost, MD, Division of Nuclear Medicine, Johns Hopkins Hospital, 601 North Caroline Street, Baltimore, MD 21287

Jan F Gummert, MD, PhD, Herzzentrum Leipzig, University Leipzig, Russenstrasse 19, 04289 Leipzig, GERMANY

Jay B Sundstrom, PhD, Department of Pathology and Laboratory Medicine, Room 4107 B Winship Cancer Center, Emory University School of Medicine, 1365 B Clifton Road, NE, Atlanta, GA 30322

Jeffrey D Hosenpud, MD, Chairman, Division of Cardiovascular Medicine, Medical College of Wisconsin, 9200 W Wisconsin Avenue, Milwaukee, WI 53226

Johnathan F Tait, MD, PhD, Division of Nuclear Medicine, Stanford University School of Medicine, 300 Pasteur Drive, Rm H-0101, Stanford, California 94305

Joren C Madsen, MD, DPhil, Division of Cardiovascular Surgery, Massachusetts General Hospital, Edwards Building, 55 Fruit Street, Boston, MA 02114

Joseph Kurtz, PhD, Transplantation Biology Research Center, Massachusetts General Hospital, 13th Street MG East Building 149-5102, Boston, MA 02129

Jussi Tikkanen, MD, Transplantation Laboratory, University of Helsinki, Helsinki University Central Hospital, POB 21, FIN-00014, University of Finland FINLAND

Karl Lemström, MD, PhD, Transplantation Laboratory, University of Helsinki, Helsinki University Central Hospital, POB 21, FIN-00014, University of Finland FINLAND

Ke Lin, MD, Division of Nuclear Medicine, Johns Hopkins Hospital, 601 North Caroline Street, Baltimore, MD 21287

Kimberley C Jallow, MD, PhD, Department of Pathology and Laboratory Medicine, Emory University School of Medicine, Emory University Hospital, H wing, Atlanta, GA 30322

Kwabena Mawulawde, MD, Cardiothoracic Surgical Associates of Augusta, 820 St Sebastian Way, Suite 2-D, Augusta, GA 30901

Manel Ballester, MD, Chairman, Department of Cardiology, Hospital Universitari, Arnau de Vilanova Universitat de Lleida Alcalde Rovita, Roure 80, 25198 Lleida, Spain

Marlene L Rose, PhD, MRCPath, Imperial College School of Medicine, NHLI Heart Science Centre, Harefield Hospital, Harefield, Middlesex UB9 6JH, UNITED KINGDOM

Mary E Keohane, MD, Department of Pathology, Henry Ford Hospital, 2799 West Grand Blvd, K-6, Detroit, Michigan 48202

Megan Sykes, MD, PhD, BMT Section, Transplantation Biology Research Center, Massachusetts General Hospital, 13th Street MG East Building 149-5102, Boston, MA 02129

Mireia Puig, MD, Center for Heart Failure and Transplantation Research, Hahnemann University Hospital, Broad and Vine Streets, Mail Stop 115, Philadelphia, Pennsylvania 19102

Mitsuaki Isobe, MD, PhD, Chairman, Department of Cardiovascular Medicine, Graduate School of Medicine, Tokyo Medical and Dental University, 1-5-45 Yushima, Bunkyo-ku, Yokyo 113-8516, JAPAN

Nadia S Giannetti, MD, McGill University Health Centre, 687 Pine Avenue West, Montreal, Que, H3a-1A1, CANADA

Navneet Narula, MD, Department of Pathology, Hahnemann University Hospital, Broad and Vine Streets, Mail Stop 115, Philadelphia, Pennsylvania 19102

Pekka Häyry, MD, PhD, Transplantation Laboratory, University of Helsinki, Helsinki University Central Hospital, POB 21, FIN-00014, University of Finland FINLAND

Petri K Koskinen, MD, PhD, Transplantation Laboratory, University of Helsinki, Helsinki University Central Hospital, POB 21, FIN-00014, University of Finland, FINLAND

Randall E Morris, MD, Director, Transplantation Immunology, Falk Cardiovascular Research Center, 300 Pasteur Drive, Stanford, CA 94305

Robert C Robbins, MD, Division of Cardiovascular Surgery, Stanford University School of Medicine, 300 Pasteur Drive, Stanford, California 94305

Robert L Yowell, MD, PhD, Department of Pathology, LDS Hospital, 8th Avenue and C Street, Salt Lake City, Utah 84143

Rohit Srivastava, MBBS, MD, Division of Cardiovascular Medicine, Medical College of Wisconsin, 9200 W Wisconsin Avenue, Milwaukee, Wi 53226

Roope Sihvola, MD, Transplantation Laboratory, University of Helsinki, Helsinki University Central Hospital, POB 21, FIN-00014, University of Finland FINLAND

Shiv Pillai, MD, PhD, Cancer Center, Massachusetts General Hospital, 13th Street MG East Building 149, Boston, MA 02129

Sudhir Kushwaha, MD, Division of Cardiovascular Medicine, Mayo School of Medicine, 200 First Street, SW, Rochester, Minnesota 55905

Thomas DiSalvo, MD, MPH, Heart Failure and Transplant Unit, Massachusetts General Hospital, Bigelow 645, 55 Fruit Street, Boston, MA 02114

Thomas Wekerle, MD, Vienna General Hospital, University of Vienna, Waehringer Guertel 18, A-1090 Vienna, AUSTRIA

Todd Koelling, MD, Division of Cardiology, University of Michigan Medical Center, 1500 East Medical Center Drive, Ann Arbor, Michigan 48109

Tujia Ikoren, MD, PhD, Senior Lecturer, Department of Surgery, Helsinki University Central Hospital, PB 340, 00029 Helsinki, FINLAND

PREFACE

Heart transplantation remains one of the major scientific achievements of twentieth century medicine. During the past four decades, it has evolved from an unproved experimental surgical technique to the most effective form of therapy for refractory end-stage heart disease. It has captured the public's imagination and expanded our understanding of fundamental immunologic mechanisms that are responsible for cellular and humorally-mediated immunity. Despite its successes, many clinical and scientific problems remain. One or more bouts of acute cellular or humoral (vascular) rejection will occur in over 75% of transplant recipients despite current immunosuppressive strategies. Further, rejection directly results in approximately 20% of post-transplant deaths and is believed to play a major role in the development of late allograft dysfunction and coronary vasculopathy.

This book by international experts in the fields of transplantation medicine, immunobiology, and cardiac imaging provides the reader with an up-to-date, concise summary of the latest developments in the diagnosis and treatment of acute cardiac rejection. It is axiomatic that a more complete understanding of the pathogenic processes involved in rejection will ultimately lead to its prevention. Thus, recent experimental animal transplant models have been frequently summarized throughout the text in order of focus on the evolving role of histocompatability antigens, antibody mediated immunity, cytokines, and myocardial apoptosis in the rejection process.

Endomyocardial biopsy, despite its shortcomings, remains the standard methodology for establishing the diagnosis of rejection. Important limitations include its invasive nature, high cost, and modest sampling error. Transplant centers throughout the world have focused efforts on the development and validation of highly sensitive and specific noninvasive methods for the detection of clinically relevant allograft rejection. A host of modalities including echocardiography, magnetic resonance imaging, electrocardiographic, and serologic markers have been prospectively examined and their utility are reviewed in this text. Radionuclide imaging techniques are particularly appealing for routine surveillance of rejection. Potential targets for rejection-specific radionuclide imaging include necrotic myocytes, activated infiltrating lymphocytes, apoptotic myocytes, and upregulated accessory HLA antigens on cardiac myocytes. The exciting possibility exists that one or more of these novel imaging strategies may soon substantially decrease the need for routine surveillance endomyocardial biopsy while providing a more accurate evaluation of the rejection process.

A more complete scientific understanding of the immunobiology of the rejection process has led us to the next frontier of heart transplantation—establishment of organ-specific tolerance. Genetic manipulation of donor and recipient combined with improved immunosuppressive strategies may soon replace nonspecific immunosuppression with individualized protocols designed to achieve long-term cardiac tolerance. Ultimately, these improvements in clinical management will pave the way for successful human xenotransplantation. The authors hope that this book provides an accurate and timely summary of the mechanisms, diagnosis, and treatment of acute cardiac rejection. We believe it will be useful to transplant cardiologists, cardiovascular surgeons, cardiac pathologists, and transplant scientists who seek to prolong the lifespan and improve the quality of life of their transplant recipients.

To Donna, Navneet, Eulalia and Rosa.

Antoni Tàpies. Spanish Modern Artist (1923-)

Born on the 13th of December 1923 in Barcelona, Spain, in 1944 he studied law and later art in Barcelona. Strongly influenced two Spanish innovators, painter Joan Miró and architect Antoni Gaudí, in the mid-1950's Tàpies gave up pure oil painting for a new medium: oil or latex paint mixed with sand or grit, which he would spread over a canvas and then either incise with markings resembling heiroglyphs, or mold into clothlike textures, creating extremely thick surfaces. He is considered one of the most successful Spanish artists of the 20th Century.

Now, at the age of 78, he paints and lives at his home, in Catalonia, Spain. Antoni Tàpies kindly agreed to paint his vision of cardiac rejection, which illustrates the book cover. The editors would like to express their gratitude to the Catalan painter for this contribution.

CARDIAC ALLOGRAFT REJECTION

Section 1: Immunopathology of Cardiac Allograft Rejection

1. HISTOCOMPATIBILITY ANTIGENS AND TRANSPLANT REJECTION

Shiv Pillai M.B.B.S., Ph.D.
Cancer Center, Massachusetts General Hospital and Harvard Medical School

The specific or adaptive immune system is characterized by the generation and activation of immune cells with an enormous repertoire for the recognition of foreign shapes and by the phenomenon of memory. This sophisticated system of host defense is not found in invertebrates, protochordates, or in some primitive jawless fish. The vertebrate immune system evolved about 450 million years ago in cartilaginous fish, ancestors of present day skates and sharks.[1]

Host defense in invertebrates is provided largely by pre-formed agglutinins, phagocytic cells, and the complement system. These entitites make up the innate immune sytem and have been retained over evolutionary time, in both invertebrates and vertebrates, serving in the latter as part of a first line of defense against pathogens.[2] As we shall see in the course of this chapter, some of the components of specific immunity in vertebrates also participate in innate immunity.

B lymphocytes are activated by antigen and differentiate into antibody secreting plasma cells. Although antibodies are extremely diverse and can neutralize and destroy pathogens in a number of ways, they are incapable of targeting certain intracellular pathogens because they cannot scan the inside of cells to see if it they are potentially infected. Moreover, even if virally infected host cells were to express a viral envelope protein on the cell surface, antibodies and complement may not effectively target such cells for destruction. Circulating antibodies may well be "distracted" by the vast cloud of recently discharged viral particles that they would encounter in the vicinity of infected cells, and thereby fail to recognize the virus-production factory as a target.

T cells co-evolved with B cells. They have the ability to look "into" and destroy other host cells if the latter are infected. The basic design of T cell recognition depends on an intrinsic ability to ignore free or soluble antigens. T cell receptors can only recognize antigenic peptides that are appropriately exhibited on cell surfaces. The molecules that bring these peptides to the cell surface, and then exhibit them so that they may be scanned by passing T cells, are known as *Major Histocompatibility Complex* (MHC) proteins (Figure 1). These are the most polymorphic proteins known, encoded in most vertebrate species by a very large number of alleles.

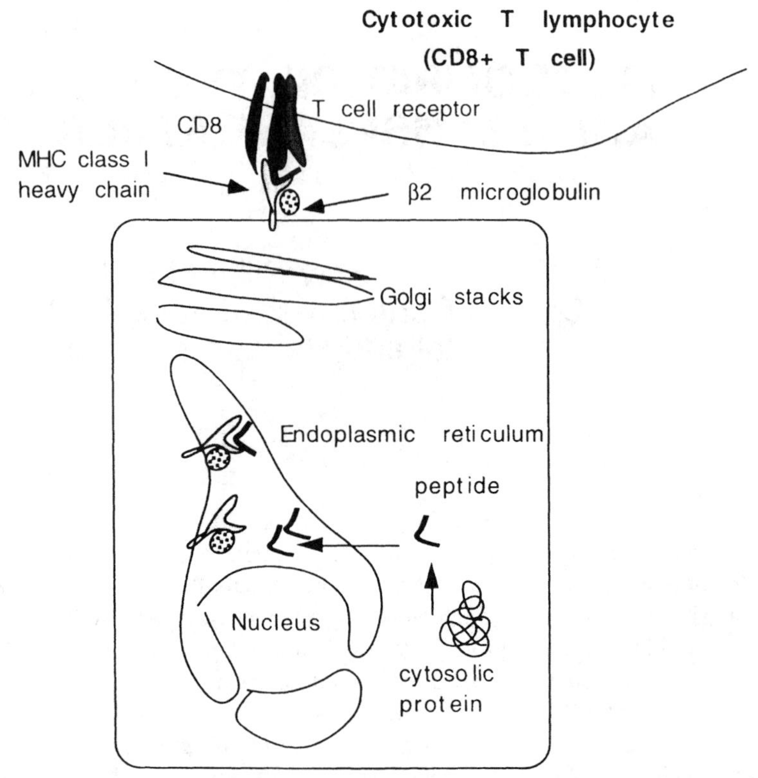

Figure 1. T cells see MHC-peptide complexes. T cell receptors on cytotoxic (CD8) T cells recognize peptides derived from the cytosol of the host cell which are presented by MHC class I molecules. MHC class II molecules, in contrast, generally present peptides from extracellularly derived proteins which have been degraded in a post-endocytic acidic compartment. Peptides presented by MHC class II molecules are recognized by helper (or CD4) T cells.

The antigen receptor on T cells is made up of two transmembrane polypeptides of the immmunoglobulin superfamily, the T cell receptor (TCR) α and β chains.[3,4] Receptor diversity is generated by the rearrangement, in developing thymocytes, of gene segments that encode these polypeptides. The variable domains of the TCR α and β chains contribute to the antigen binding site. TCRs recognize cell surface MHC molecules which are complexed with peptides of either exogenous or endogenous origin (Figure 2). It is now believed that all TCRs initially generated in the thymus are capable of recognizing MHC like shapes. We will return to this issue when we discuss why a relatively large proportion of T cells in any one individual have the potential to be alloreactive. The antigen recognizing TCR α and β chains associate with proteins of the CD3 complex, (CD3 γ, δ, ε, and ζ) which are required for the initiation of signaling from the antigen receptor.

MHC proteins evolved at the same time as B and T cells, to provide a mechanism for T cell receptors to focus exclusively on antigenic fragments that are held on the cell surface. Since T cell receptors recognize only MHC-peptide complexes,

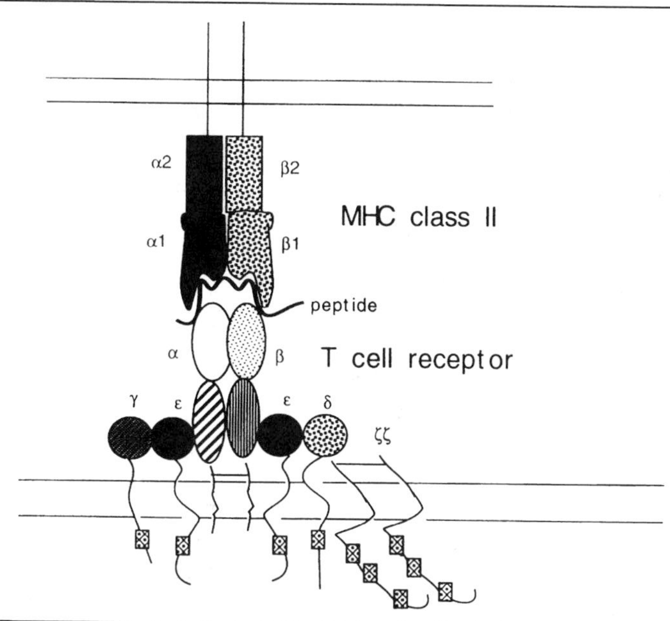

Figure 2. A schematic view of a T cell receptor on a T cell making contact with an MHC class II molecule on an antigen presenting cell. The structure of the MHC class II molecule is described in the legend to Figure 4. The T cell receptor is made up of two antigen recognizing chains (TCRα and β) complexed with CD3 proteins (γ, δ, ε, and ζ) which participate in signal transduction.

free viruses or viral antigens are totally ignored by T lymphocytes. Although the physiological function of MHC molecules relates to antigen recognition by T cells, they acquired their name because they were discovered in the context of transplant rejection. They were originally referred to as *Major* Histocompatibility Complex Antigens because they were identified as the most prominent antigens involved in experimental graft rejection. Elegant genetic studies, which helped create the field of immunogenetics, established that these antigens map to a single chromosome in the mouse, to a set of genes that came to be known as the H-2 locus. The corresponding locus in man is on chromosome 6 and is referred to as the *Human Leukocyte Antigen* or *HLA* locus. MHC molecules in man are called HLA molecules and in this chapter the terms MHC and HLA will be used interchangeably. HLA molecules are found on leukocytes but their expression is not restricted to white cells. MHC class I molecules are expressed on all nucleated cells and are recognized by T cell receptors on cytotoxic or $CD8^+$ T cells (Cytotoxic T Lymphocytes or CTLs). They generally present peptides derived from proteins synthesized "endogenously" in the cell expressing the MHC class I molecule of interest. MHC class II molecules are primarily expressed on B cells and other professional antigen presenting cells (mainly macrophages and dendritic cells). Their expression may be induced on endothelial and epithelial cells exposed to cytokines such as γ-interferon. The induction of MHC class II expression on many cell types may be of protective significance in the context of certain infections, and this could be of relevance from

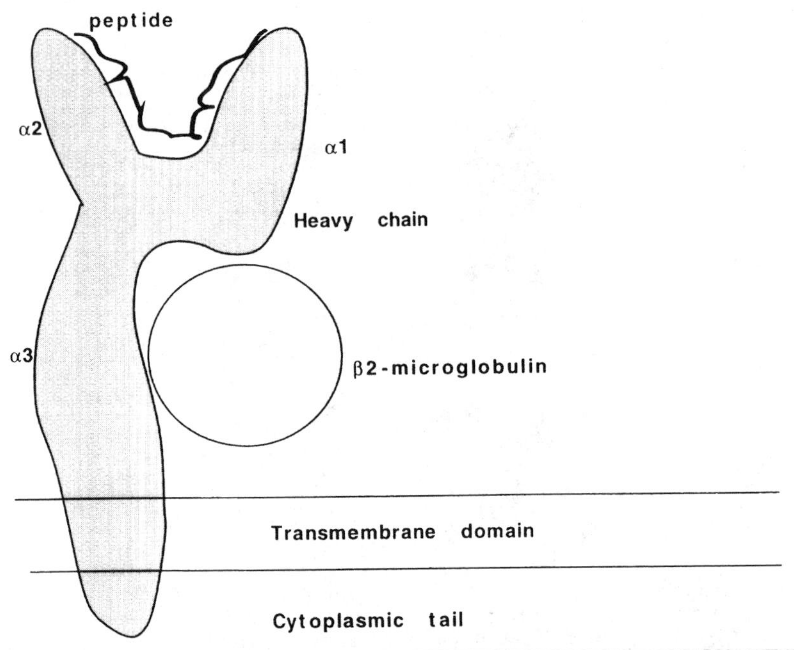

Figure 3. A schematic view of the structure of MHC class I molecules. Peptides rest in a groove between two a-helical ridges in the α1 and α2 domains of the MHC class I heavy chain. β2 microglobulin is a non-anchored chain that associates with the α3 domain of the MHC class I heavy chain.

the standpoint of clinical transplantation in the context of the "direct" pathway for alloreactive immune responses. MHC class II molecules generally present peptides derived from exogenous proteins which must be internalized by the antigen presenting cell. These proteins are "processed" into peptides intracellularly. MHC class II-peptide complexes are recognized by antigen receptors on helper or $CD4^+$ T cells.

THE STRUCTURE OF MHC PROTEINS

MHC molecules are cell surface glycoproteins which contain two membrane-proximal immunoglobulin like domains as well as two more distal specialized domains which together form a peptide binding groove embedded between two α-helical ridges. MHC class I molecules are made up of two polypeptide chains and a tightly associated peptide moiety (Figure 3). The MHC class I heavy chain is a transmembrane glycoprotein of about 40–45 kDa which associates tightly with a small non-anchored 12 kDa immunoglobulin superfamily protein known as β2 microglobulin. MHC class II molecules are heterodimers which consist of an α and a β chain, both of which are transmembrane glycoproteins (Figure 4).

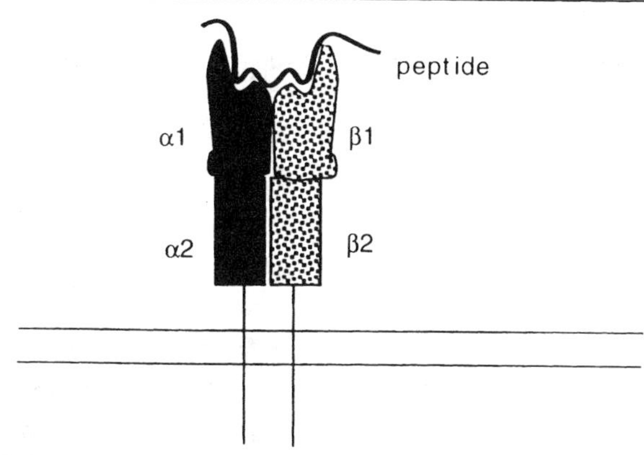

Figure 4. A schematic view of an MHC class II molecule. This molecule is made up of two transmembrane polypeptides, the a chain and the b chain. The α1 and β1 domains contribute to the peptide binding groove. The α2 and β2 domains are immunoglobulin like in structure.

Our current understanding of MHC function owes a great deal to the knowledge of the structure of MHC molecules obtained by x-ray crystallography. Crystal structures are available for a range of HLA class I and class II molecules complexed with specific peptides and also, more recently for HLA class I -peptide -T cell receptor complexes.[5–8] The MHC class I heavy chain is made up of three domains. The α1 and α2 domains combine to contribute to two α-helical ridges which surround a long, narrow, groove whose floor has a β-pleated structure. This groove is where specific peptides are snugly bound and presented to appropriate T cell receptors. The surface contains distinct crevices into which specific side-chains of a highly specific peptide may fit. Peptides that are presented by MHC class I molecules are usually 8 or 9 amino acids in length. For a particular MHC class I molecule, the specific crevices in the groove dictate that certain invariant amino acid side-chains must be present in peptides that bind specifically to it. These residues on the peptide are referred to as anchor residues since they are critical for the tight binding of a set of peptides to individual class I heavy chains.

The α3 domain of the MHC class I heavy chain has a typical immunoglobulin fold structure, consisting of a β sandwich where adjacent β sheets are held together by a disulfide bridge. This domain interacts with β2 microglobulin, a non-anchored protein which also has a similar immunoglobulin domain like structure. The α3 domain is also involved in the interaction of MHC class-I molecules with the CD8 molecule on cytotoxic T cells.

The antigen binding groove on MHC class II molecules broadly resembles that found in MHC class I molecules. This groove is contributed to by the α1 domain of the α chain and the β1 domain of the β chain. The MHC class I groove is approximately 25A° long and is closed at both ends; it can therefore only accommodate relatively short peptides. The MHC class II groove is open-ended and can accommodate larger peptides. Non-polymorphic portions of the α2 and β2 immunoglobulin like domains contribute to the interaction with CD4 on T cells.

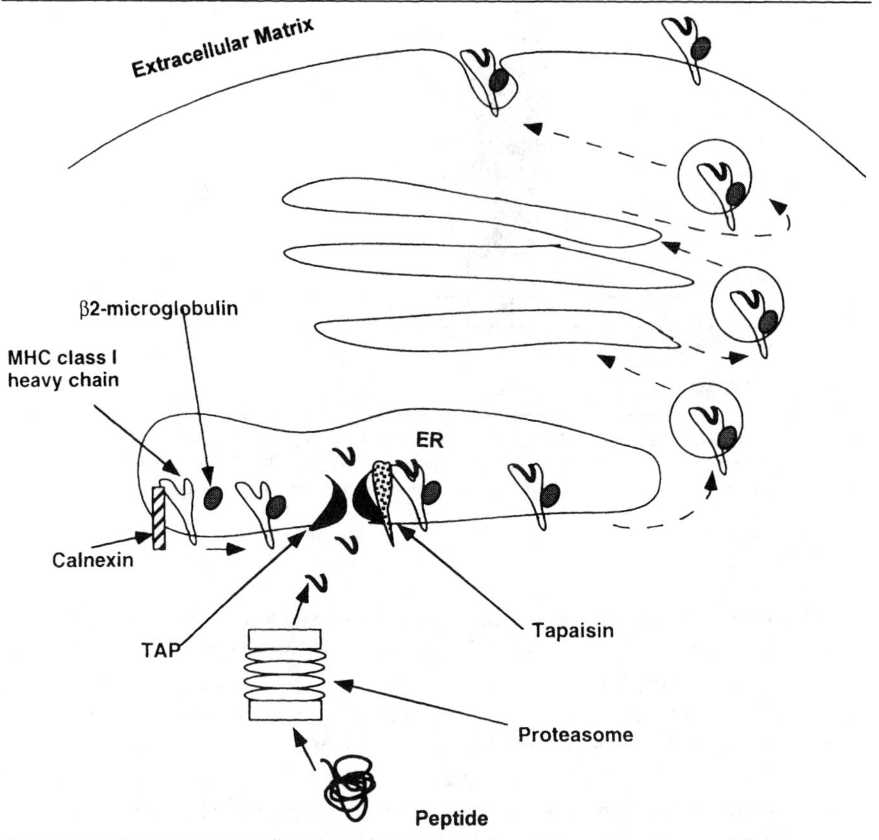

Figure 5. An overview of the MHC class I or "Endogenous" pathway. Cytosolic proteins synthesized by the presenting or target cell are ubiquitinated and degraded in 26S proteasomes into peptides which are 8 or 9 amino acids long. These peptides are translocated into the ER lumen through the TAP1/2 transporter. Nascent class I molecules are held in proximity to TAP by a transmembrane chaperone known as Tapaisin where they await the entry of peptide. Peptide-MHC complexes are transported out of the ER by vesicular transport, via the Golgi stacks to the cell surface.

THE MHC CLASS I PATHWAY

MHC class I molecules are designed to complete their folding and assembly processes in the endoplasmic reticulum (ER).[9,10] Egress from the ER and subsequent transport to the cell surface requires that the complete trimolecular complex of heavy chain, β2 microglobulin, and peptide be properly assembled (Figure 5). The MHC class I heavy chain is translocated into the ER by a classic signal peptide dependent mechanism through the Sec 61 channel. Sec 61 is an ER protein whose subunits form a channel through which polypeptide chains that contain signal peptides are translocated into the ER. The MHC class I heavy chain protein is anchored in the ER membrane and folds partially in conjunction with a resident transmembrane ER chaperone known as calnexin. In this compartment it associates with the β2 microglobulin component, which is also translocated into the lumen of the ER in a signal-peptide dependent manner. β2-microglobulin is not an integral membrane protein; it is initially translocated into the lumen of the ER, and can be secreted. The heavy chain-β2 microglobulin heterodimer remains associated in a complex with a protein known as tapaisin until it receives a peptide which is either 8 or 9 amino acids in length and which can fit into its specific groove. Tapaisin forms a bridge between MHC class I molecules and the TAP (Transporter associated with Antigen Processing) heterodimers which pump peptides into the ER from the cytosol. The TAP transporter is a pump made up of two transmembrane ATPases, TAP1 and TAP2, that form a peptide-translocation channel in the ER membrane. TAP1 and TAP2 are encoded by genes that are a part of the MHC complex (discussed below).

Cellular proteins which lack signal peptides are generally destined for the cytosol and the nucleus. Most of these proteins are degraded in the cytosol in proteasomes.[11,12] As a prelude to being degraded in proteasomes, many proteins are covalently tagged in the cell with tandem repeats of a peptide known as ubiquitin. Proteasomes are highly organized cylindrical protein-degradation machines made up of 4 circular segments of 7α, 7β, 7β, and 7α protein subunits respectively, which together make up the 20S proteasome. The 20S proteasome core contains a number of proteolytic activities. At either end of the core is a "cap" structure which combines with the 20S proteasome to generate the 26S proteasome. The cap contains proteins that can contribute to the unfolding and deubiquitination of target proteins. Three subunits of the proteasome, LMP-2, LMP-7, and MECL-1 may be induced by interferon-γ. LMP-2 and LMP-7, like TAP-1 and TAP-2, are encoded within the class II region of the HLA complex on chromosome 6.

Although proteins that are targeted to proteasomes are primarily cytosolic or nuclear polypeptides, proteins retained within the ER as well as cleaved signal peptides may be translocated out of the ER lumen via the Sec 61 channel. Translocated proteins are ubiquitinated and targeted for proteasomal degradation. Proteins from the secretory pathway, including misfolded ER retained MHC molecules, may also therefore be targeted to the cytosol and to the MHC class I antigen presentation pathway.[13,14]

THE MHC CLASS II PATHWAY

Unlike the MHC class I pathway which is designed to eventually present cytosolically derived peptides to CD8 cytotoxic T cells, the MHC class II pathway is explicitly designed to present peptides derived from proteins that are sampled from the environment by professional antigen presenting cells (Figure 6). Even though MHC class II molecules are synthesized on ER bound ribosomes and assemble initially in the ER, they are designed NOT to sample peptides in the ER lumen itself (these peptides must be presented by MHC class I molecules). The α and β chains of MHC class II molecules assemble in the ER membrane and associate immediately with a third component known as the invariant chain (Ii). The invariant chain is a Type II transmembrane protein (in Type II proteins the carboxy-terminus protrudes into the lumen of the ER whereas in Type I proteins the N-terminus is exposed to the lumen). The C-terminus of the invariant chain folds into and occludes the antigen binding

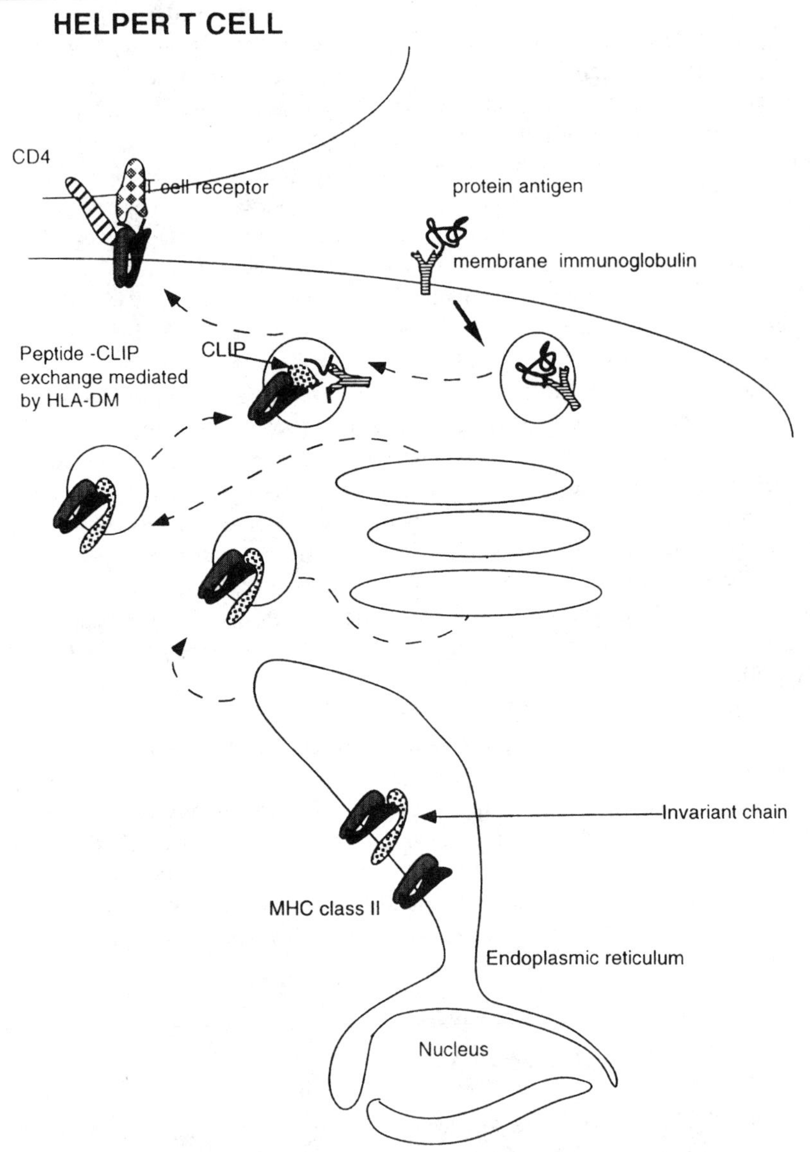

Figure 6. The MHC class II or "Exogenous pathway". Shown here is a B lymphocyte. the antigen receptor internalizes specific protein antigen by endocytosis and targets them to the pre-lysosomal MIIc compartment where they are processed into peptides. Newly synthesized MHC class II proteins are targetd to the MIIc compartment by the associated invariant chain, which also protects the groove of MHC class II molecules from being occupied by endogenous peptides in the ER. The inavariant chain is cleaved to yield a peptide known as CLIP which is displaced from the groove by endogenous peptides. This peptide exchange is catalysed by the H-2 M protein.

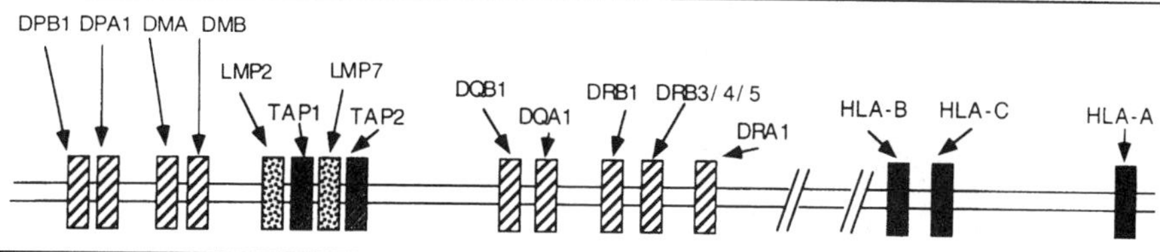

Figure 7. A simplified view of the HLA locus on chromosome 6. The TAP and LMP genes are encoded within the class II region. The class II region between the class II and Class I regions is not shown.

groove of the MHC class II molecule. Occupancy of the peptide-binding groove by the invariant chain prevents endogenous peptides that enter the ER from occupying the groove. This permits the efficient loading of MHC class II grooves with exogenously derived peptides in a post-Golgi compartment. The N terminus of Ii protrudes into the cytosol and provides targeting signals to direct $(\alpha\beta\text{Ii})_3$ nonamers through the Golgi stacks to a specialized acidic late endosomal/lysosomal compartment known as the MIIc compartment. The invariant chain is proteolytically cleaved to yield a peptide called CLIP which remains tightly bound to the MHC class II groove.

Proteins from outside the cell are sampled and internalized by endocytic receptors on the antigen presenting cell. In the case of a B lymphocyte the antigen receptor functions as the endocytic receptor as shown in Figure 6. Internalized proteins are cleaved into peptides by proteases such as cathepsin-L and cathepsin-S. A distinct type of HLA molecule, a heterodimer known as HLA-DM, performs a unique function in the MIIc compartment. This molecule serves as a peptide-exchanger, displacing CLIP from the MHC groove and permitting exogenously derived peptides to slide into the groove.[15,16] MHC class II- peptide complexes are then transported to the cell surface. In general, peptides that bind the class II groove tend to be longer than those that bind to the corresponding groove in class I molecules—the average length of MHC class II binding peptides ranges from 14 to 18 amino acids, but since peptides can spill out of both ends of the non-occluded MHC class II groove they can even be considerably longer.

HLA GENES AND HLA POLYMORPHISM

The arrangement of the HLA locus on chromosome 6 is depicted in a simplified fashion in Figure 7. This locus occupies a 2–3 centimorgan region (corresponding roughly to 4×10^6 base pairs) and contains at least 50 different genes. The locus may be arbitrarily divided into three broad gene clusters. The HLA class II gene cluster includes genes encoding the various HLA class II chains discussed below as well as the genes for the α and β chains of HLA-DM, TAP1, TAP2, LMP2, and LMP7. The HLA class III gene cluster lies between the HLA class II and HLA class I gene clusters and includes a number of genes of immunological importance most of which have nothing to do with MHC function. Included in this cluster are genes for complement components C2 and C4 and for tumor necrosis factor α and β. There are three classical HLA class I loci, HLA-A, HLA-B, and HLA-C. Individuals inherit and co-dominantly express two HLA-A, two HLA-B, and two HLA-C genes, one from each parent. Each class I locus is characterized by an enormous number of alleles in the population (probably about a thousand—only about a tenth of these are typed by serological methods), and MHC genes are the most polymorphic genes in nature. The β2 microglobulin genes is minimally polymorphic and is located on chromosome 15 rather than on chromosome 6.

Each HLA class II molecule is encoded by two genes, one for the α chain and the other for the β chain. Every individual inherits two DP β genes, two DQ β genes, and from two to four DR β genes (each chromosome 6 includes a DRB1 locus and may include an additional DRB 3, 4, or 5 locus as well). Each individual also inherits two DPα genes, two DQα genes, and two DRα genes. In general the HLA class II β gene loci are more polymorphic than the α gene loci. Thus, each person may express at least six distinct HLA class II heterodimers. Certain combinations of genes on chromosome 6 are inherited more frequently than would be expected. This phenomenon of linkage disequilibrium occurs because certains stretches of the geneome are less prone to meiotic recombination. Linkage disequilibrium is of particular relevance when we attempt to correlate HLA polymorphisms with disease, since inheritance of a particular allele may be causally related to the co-inheritance of an allele of a more distant gene which is in linkage disequlibrium.

The exons of MHC genes which encode the peptide-binding groove regions are extraordinarily polymorphic. Human HLA alleles are now numbered in the hundreds. Why are MHC genes so polymorphic? The teleological explanation often given is that the tremendous diversity of MHC genes protects a species at a population rather than an individual level. A rare virus which might be lethal to some members will never prove lethal to all. This tremendous polymorphism is probably of immense value for the survival of all vertebrate species but makes transplantation a somewhat more difficult endeavor.

MHC MOLECULES PARTICIPATE IN POSITIVE AND NEGATIVE SELECTION OF T CELLS

During T cell development in the thymus $CD4^{+}CD8^{+}$ double positive (DP) T cells go through a process known as thymic education. DP T cells which bear T cell receptors which can recognize MHC molecules with moderate avidity receive trophic and differentiation signals. Cells bearing receptors that recognize MHC class II — peptide complexes with moderate avidity are positively selected and differentiate into $CD4^{+}$ T cells. Cells bearing receptors that recognize MHC class I-peptide complexes in the thymic cortex with moderate avidity are positively selected and commit to the CD8 lineage. DP positive T cells that recognize MHC-peptide complexes with high avidity receive signals that induce their death by apoptosis. This process of clonal deletion is often called negative selection. As a result of these selection processes, T cells with high affinity for self are eliminated, and positive selection helps identify T cells whose receptors can recognize self MHC molecules, albeit weakly, when the latter present self peptides. Some of these T cells will obviously recognize these very same MHC molecules with high affinity during an immune response if they happen to harbor an appropriate non-self peptide in their antigen binding grooves. The majority of T cell receptors that are made have an inbuilt bias towards the recognition of MHC like structures. T cells bearing antigen receptors that do not recognize self-MHC structures with any affinity whatsoever are probabaly never generated; if they ever were, they would receive no trophic signals and would "die by neglect".

From the viewpoint of transplantation, it should be borne in mind that a TCR which recognizes (self MHC + self peptide) moderately well, may recognize some (foreign MHC + self peptide) or (foreign MHC + foreign peptide) combinations with relatively high affinity. Each person's T cells are educated so that they can form part of a repertoire that is capable of recognizing many foreign peptides in a self-MHC context. This recognition of self-MHC "restricted" antigen constitutes the phenomenon of MHC restriction. However this process always creates a T cell repertoire capable of recognizing a large number of foreign MHC molecules rather well. This inherent ability of most TCRs to recognize some allogeneic MHC molecules with high affinity explains why massive *alloreactive* repsonses are generated in the transplant context. This is also the primary reason why these very polymorphic MHC molecules were initially discovered during the course of experimental studies on transplantation.

MHC CLASS I MOLECULES AND NATURAL KILLER CELLS

Although Natural Killer (NK) cells are probably not critical in considerations of solid-organ transplantation, donor NK cells have on occassion been suggested to exert "veto" activity against recipient anti-donor CTLs. The biology of NK cells is intimately linked to MHC class I molecules and they will be therefore briefly discussed in this chapter.

NK cells are now recognized to be cells of lymphoid origin that participate in innate immunity and which are designed to attack cells that do not express self MHC class I molecules. They recognize and eliminate cells that are considered to be "missing self". Many viruses attempt to subvert $CD8^+$ CTL activation by down-regulating MHC class I molecules. NK cells represent a first line of defense against viruses by targeting virally infected cells because the latter express low levels of MHC class I, or because viral peptides displace self-peptides and make MHC class I molecules on infected host cells look sufficiently "different". NK cells do not lyse MHC class I expressing host cells. This is because these killer cells express inhibitory receptors which bind to MHC class I molecules on potential target cells and are thus induced to generate signals that antagonize the induction of cytolytic activity.

Two types of MHC class I recognizing inhibitory receptors on human NK cells have been described. One category of receptors known as Killer Inhibitory Receptors (or KIRs) recognize classical MHC class I molecules and a second category, receptors of the CD94/NKG2 type, recognize MHC class I molecules in a very unusual way. KIRs are members of the immunoglobulin superfamily and their extracellular immunoglobulin-like domains recognize HLA-B and HLA-C molecules. These receptors generate negative signals by activating a specific tyrosine phosphatase in NK cells. The HLA-B and HLA-C molecules recognized by KIRs are typical tri-molecular complexes composed of heavy chain, β2 microglobulin, and peptide.[17]

The CD94/NKG2 heterodimer recognizes an interesting non-classical MHC class I molecule called HLA-E. HLA-E has an unusual peptide binding groove which accommodates hydrophobic signal peptides which are cleaved in the ER from the N-termini of classical HLA class I heavy chains (HLA-A, HLA-B, and HLA-C) as well as from the signal peptide of another non-classical HLA class I molecule called HLA-G.[18] HLA-E is designed to inform NK cells that the potential target the killer might be considering is "clean" because it expresses HLA class I molecules and should therefore be spared. CD94 and NKG2 possess extracellular C-type lectin domains which recognize trimolecular HLA-E complexes. The NKG2 subunit delivers a negative signal to the NK cell in the same way that KIRs do. HLA-G molecules are non-polymorphic MHC class I like proteins that are expressed in fetal trophoblastic cells. The fetal trophoblast down-regulates conventional HLA class I molecules and thus presumably avoids provoking maternal CTLs. By expressing HLA-G, which provides a signal peptide that can fit in the groove of HLA-E, fetal trophoblast cells may protect the fetus from maternal NK activity which could potentially see fetal cells as cells with "missing self".

MINOR HISTOCOMPATIBILITY ANTIGENS

Self peptides that are either generated by proteolysis within the cell or which are cleaved after internalization by an antigen presenting cell, are presented by MHC molecules. The proteins that yield these peptides may often be present in the species in polymorphic forms. While the HLA A-2 molecule, for instance, inherited by one individual, may present a specific peptide X derived from some cellular protein, the identical HLA A-2 molecule of another individual may present a slightly different polymorphic peptide X1. T cells from each of these individuals would not be tolerized against the peptide-MHC complex presented by cells of the other individual. Polymorphisms in non-MHC proteins that yield different MHC binding peptides contribute to transplant rejection, although generally not with the same potency as differences in MHC molecules themselves. These polymorphic peptides constitute minor histocompatibility antigens.[19]

"NON-CLASSICAL" MHC MOLECULES

The major histocompatibilty complex molecules that are considered "classical" are HLA-A, HLA-B and HLA-C (MHC class I) and HLA DP, HLA-DQ, and HLA-DR (MHC class II). Many other molecules have been discovered that structurally resemble HLA molecules but which are not categorized as "classical" MHC molecules and which are generally non-polymorphic. Some of these MHC like molecules are encoded by genes within the MHC locus while others are products of genes on other chromosomes. Some of these "non-classical" molecules actually present antigens, some help in antigen presentation without actually presenting antigen themselves, and others have nothing to do with antigen presentation whatsoever.[20]

Several "non-classical" MHC molecules have been encountered earlier in this chapter. The HLA-DM molecule was discussed in a previous section. This is structurally an MHC class II protein, is encoded within the MHC class II region on chromosome 6, and participates in the peptide exchange process necessary for the loading of conventional MHC class II antigen binding grooves. HLA-DO is also MHC encoded, is MHC class II-like in structure, and may be an inhibitor of HLA-DM function during the CLIP-peptide exchange process.

There are a large number of interesting non-polymorphic MHC class I like molecules, known as MHC class IB proteins, that are the products of genes that lie within the MHC class I region on chromosome 6. They are all made up of heavy chains associated with β-2 microglobulin, but not all present peptides. Two such molecules have already been described in the section on NK cells. HLA-E presents signal peptides derived from the classical HLA-A, B, and C heavy chain proteins and from the HLA-G class IB heavy chain protein. HLA-G is expressed in fetal trophoblast cells and may particpate in the inactivation of maternal NK cells as discussed above.

CD1 molecules are non-polymorphic MHC class I like molecules that are not encoded within the MHC. There are five different CD1 isotypes in man, CD1a, CD1b, CD1c, CD1d, and CD1e. CD1 molecules associate with β-2 microglobulin and fold like MHC class I proteins but are targeted within the cell like MHC class II proteins to the MIIc compartment. CD1b proteins are capable of binding to and presenting glycolipids from mycobacteria. CD1d molecules in man are restriction elements for a subset of unusual T cells which may participate in immune regulation and some of which express an NK cell marker, NK1.1. Although CD1 restricted T cells might one day prove important for transplant rejection, at present there is no evidence to suggets that this is true.

An MHC class I like molecule encoded within the HLA class I region on chromosome 6 and which was once named HLA-H is now called HFE. HFE is a regulator of iron absorption in the gut and is mutated in patients with hereditary hemochromatosis. While this molecule folds like an MHC class I heavy chain and associates with β-2 microglobulin, it does not contain a functional peptide binding groove. Another MHC class I like protein which lacks a typical groove structure but which participates in a transport related function is the FcRn protein. This molecule is involved in the transcytotic transport (across the placental or gut epithelium) of maternal IgG during fetal development and in neonates. HFE and FcRn are not of direct relevance to transplantation immunology.

MHC AND DISEASE

While specific polymoprphic alleles of HLA class I and class II molecules have been linked to certain diseases for decades, an understanding of the pathogenetic meaning of these linkages has only recently begun to emerge.[21,22] The advent of DNA based typing of HLA molecules (particularly for HLA class II) permits accurate and meaningful analysis of every known allelic form in patients and controls, thus permitting valid conclusions to be drawn regarding the linkage of specific HLA class II alleles either to disease susceptibility or to resistance. Linkage of an allelic form of an MHC gene to a disease could potentially reflect linkage disequilibrium. With

DNA typing it is now possible to rule in or rule out linkage disequilibrium to other MHC class II genes.

In chronic inflammatory diseases that may eventually require organ transplantation as a therapeutic modality, the following potential mechanisms of HLA and disease linkage should be considered.

For susceptibility alleles:

1. A specific MHC allele may confer susceptibility because it specifically binds to and presents a disease-related peptide (which may be of self or non-self origin) to pathogenic T cells.
2. A specific MHC allele may confer susceptibility because it facilitates the deletion of potentially protective T cells during negative selection in the thymus thus creating a "hole in the repertoire".
3. A specific MHC allele may confer susceptibility because it competes with a resistance generating allele for a specific peptide, thus preventing the formation of a protective MHC-peptide complex that could have activated T cells that would have benefitted the host.

In a similar vein, the following scenarios may explain why the inheritance of a specific allele may confer protection or resistance:

1. A specific MHC allele may be protective because it presents a peptide that plays a dominant role in invoking the activity of protective T cells (that could potentially contribute to the elimination of a pathogen for instance).
2. A specific MHC allele may confer resistance because it provokes the deletion of certain self-reactive T cells during thymic education that could otherwise contribute to pathogenetic processes. A useful "hole in the repertoire" might be generated by the inheritance of a specific allele.
3. A specific MHC allele may prove protective because it can compete for peptides with a susceptibility allele and thus prevent the generation of disease-provoking pro-inflammatory MHC-peptide complexes.

TISSUE TYPING- THE ADVENT OF NEW TECHNOLOGIES

Until very recently HLA typing for transplantation depended largely on serological approaches. Panels of sera from multiparous women who have developed antibodies against paternally derived HLA molecules have been carefully characterized and are used in typing. Typically lymphocytes from patients and prospective donors are incubated in individual wells of microtiter plates and incubated with a battery of antisera in the presence of complement. Complement mediated lysis in a particular well indicates the presence of a relevant antigen. Some HLA-D region alleles have also historically been typed by using a mixed lymphocyte culture approach. While these methods have been remarkably reproducible and have proved fairly useful from a limited clinical context over the last few decades, they are incomplete in their scope. For HLA class II alleles serological typing is gradually being replaced in most centers by more specific DNA typing approaches. For example, the HLA-DR4 "allele" could be the product of at least 11 different DRB1 alleles (DRB1*0401 to DRB1*0411) that may be distinguished by DNA typing. HLA class II typing is currently performed in most modern centers by a polymerase chain reaction (PCR)—sequence specific oligonucleotide approach.[23] This involves amplifying specific segments of genomic DNA by PCR and hybridizing this amplified segment with a battery of specific short DNA probes.

DNA typing of HLA class I alleles is making its way to the clinic more slowly because of the tremendous number of HLA class I alleles that have been discovered by DNA sequencing. While automated sequencing strategies have been widely used in research laboratories, DNA based strategies for HLA class I allele identification are only now being adapted for wider clinical use. Only about a 100 HLA class I alleles can be serologically typed, although several hundred HLA class I alleles may be distinguished by more sophisticated typing. As a result serological typing is ALWAYS equivocal.[24] Terms such as "split antigens" and "cross-reactive" antigen groups reflect the inadequacy of currently used serological methods to actually distinguish between "true" alleles. A recent large study has demonstrated that the use of a DNA typing approach dramatically improves the success rate in bone-marrow transplantation.[25]

MHC ANTIGENS AND TRANSPLANTATION

The pace of progress in the understanding of modern immunology has been driven, in part, by the challenges presented by human organ transplantation. Histocompatibility antigens were discovered in the artificial context of experimental organ transplantation. Their extreme polymorphism ensures that donor antigens will be distinct from recipient "self" and this is why they play such a major role in rejection.

There are two broad pathways by which MHC molecules may contribute to transplant rejection. These are commonly referred to as the "direct" pathway and the "indirect" pathway (Figure 8).[26–29] In the direct pathway recipient T cells "directly" recognize donor MHC molecules which may be loaded with recipient or donor peptides. In the indirect pathway, antigen presenting cells of the recipient present fragments of donor MHC proteins which can complex with newly synthesized recipient MHC molecules. These complexes of recipient MHC antigens complexed with donor MHC peptides activate recipient T cells that are specific for these complexes. Although this pathway has historically been described as the "indirect" pathway, it represents the normal way the immune system presents foreign antigens, usually, but not exclusively, in an MHC class II context to CD4 T cells.

An understanding of the critical role played by MHC antigens in inducing alloreactive T cell repsonses in a transplant setting has led to a number of studies attempting to harness this information for therapeutic purposes. Experimental studies have attempted to suppress transplant rejection by the therapeutic use of peptides derived from both the non-polymorphic and polymorphic regions of the MHC. While there have been varying degrees of success in animal models, (and a clinical trial is in progress), this remains an evolving modality for immunomodulation.

Non-polymorphic MHC derived peptides have been used in a number of experimental protocols and have been shown on occassion to suppress immune responses.

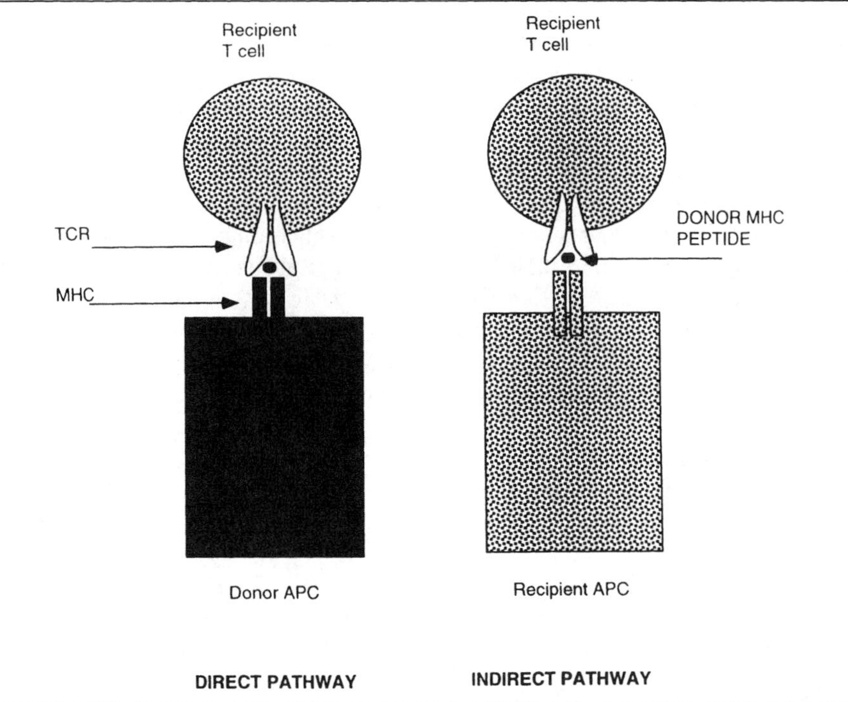

Figure 8. MHC antigens trigger alloreactive T cells by the direct and indirect pathways. In the direct pathway a donor APC presents donor peptides to host T cells. In the indirect pathway, host APCs present donor peptides to host T cells.

How exactly these peptides work remains very poorly understood. In a number of studies[30] in which cardiac allograft rejection was examined in a rat model, the HLA-B7.75–84 peptide administered orally or intravenously in conjunction with low doses of cyclosporine was found to prevent chronic rejection.

Polymorphic MHC peptides have been used to induce specific tolerance in studies aiming to suppress the indirect pathway of rejection (see Chapter 8). In these animal studies various therapeutic protocols have been attempted. It is of some interest to note that in an important human study,[31] the indirect pathway has been demonstrated to be important for acute cardiac allograft rejection. Indirect immune responses were detected against immunodominant donor peptides bound to a specific recipient HLA-DR class II molecule. the absence of indirect alloreactivity correlated with the absence of rejection. Unfortunately this study also demonstrated the phenomenon of intramolecular antigenic spreading. Immunodominance is often a temporally restricted phenomenon, and the therapeutic use of peptides may be far more complicated than initially assumed.

It is becoming increasingly clear that HLA matching plays an extremely important role in the success of organ transplantation. Practically all the published data on HLA mismatches and transplant rejection is inherently flawed. Of necessity, these very important studies have been based on HLA typing performed using available, but clearly limited, serological approaches. Tissue matches determined by serological means are often not matches at all. Just as much of the data on MHC and disease was virtually uninterpretable before the advent of accurate and properly performed DNA typing, most available data on HLA Class I mismatches and clinical outcome after transplantation has been based on serological typing. Most studies on HLA Class II typing have also relied on serological methods which should now be considered unacceptable.

In a recently published study, Sasazuki and colleagues have noted a dramatic improvement in the outcome of bone marrow transplantation when donors and recipients were matched using DNA typing approaches for both HLA class I and HLA class II genes.[25] Even though most, if not all, studies on clinical solid organ transplantion have depended on less specific HLA typing approaches, it is clear from a number of studies[32–34] that graft survival in heart transplantation is influenced by the extent of HLA compatibility.

CONCLUSIONS AND A LOOK AT THE FUTURE

Over the past 15 years dramatic advances have been made in the HLA field. The structure of HLA class I and class II molecules have been elucidated, the fact that these molecules present peptides has been established, and the pathways by which they acquire these peptides from endogenous and exogenous proteins have been dissected in minute detail. While many of these advances have been of conceptual importance in immunology and cell biology, the impact of this knowledge is beginning to be felt in the arena of clinical organ transplantation as well. It is expected that in the years to come, the growing availability of molecular typing at the DNA level of both HLA class I and HLA class II genes will dramatically improve survival after cardiac transplantation. Strategies for the generation of immunological tolerance are being currently explored and these have received a great impetus from the improved understanding of the structure and function of HLA molecules.

REFERENCES

1. Rast, JP, Anderson, MK, Strong, SJ, Luer, C, Litman, RT, and Litman, GW (1997). alpha, beta, gamma, and delta T cell antigen receptor genes arose early in vertebrate phylogeny. Immunity *6*, 1–11.
2. Janeway, CAJ (1998). The road less travelled by: the role of innate immunity in the adaptive immune response. J. Immunol. *161*, 539–544.
3. Matis, LA (1990). The molecular basis of T cell specificity. Annu. Rev. Immunol *8*, 65–82.
4. Davis, MM, Boniface, JJ, Reich, Z, Lyons, D, Hampl, J, Arden, B, and Chien, Y-h (1998). Ligand recognition by alpha-beta T cell receptors. Annu. Rev. Immunol. *16*, 523–544.
5. Bjorkman, PJ, Saper, MA, Samraoui, B, Bennett, WS, Strominger, JL, and Wiley, DC (1987). Structure of the human class I histocompatibility antigen, HLA-A2. Nature *329*, 506–512.
6. Stern, LJ, Brown, JH, Jardetzky, TS, Gorga, JC, Urban, RG, Strominger, JL, and Wiley, DC (1994). Crystal structure of the human class II MHC protein HLA DR1 complexed with an influenza virus peptide. Nature *368*, 215–221.
7. Garcia, KC, Degano, M, Pease, LR, Huang, M, Peterson, PA, Teyton, L, and Wilson, IA (1998). Structural basis of plasticity in T cell receptor recognition of a self-peptide-MHC antigen. Science *279*, 1166–1172.
8. Madden, D (1995). The three dimensional structure of peptide-MHC complexes. Annu. Rev. Immunol. *13*, 587–622.

9. Germain, RH, and Margulies, DH (1993). The biochemistry and cell biology of antigen processing and presentation. Annu. Rev. Immunol. *11*, 403–450.
10. Pamer, E, and Cresswell, P (1998). Mechanisms of MHC class I restricted antigen presentation. Annu. Rev. Immunol. *16*, 323–358.
11. Brown, MG, Driscoll, J, and Monaco, JJ (1991). Structural and serological similarity of MHc linked LMP and proteasome (multicatalytic proteinase) complexes. Nature *353*, 355–357.
12. Monaco, JJ, and Nandi, D (1995). The genetics of proteasomes and antigen processing. Annu. Rev. Genetics *29*, 729–754.
13. Wiertz, EJHJ, Tortorella, D, Bogyo, M, Yu, J, Mothes, W, Jones, TR, Rapoport, TA, and Ploegh, HL (1996). Sec61-mediated transfer of a membrane protein from the endoplasmic reticulum to the proteasome for destruction. Nature *384*, 432–438.
14. Ploegh, HL (1998). Viral strategies of immune evasion. Science *280*, 248–253.
15. Denzin, LK, and Cresswell, P (1995). HLA-DM induces CLIP dissociation from MHC class II alpha beta dimers and facilitates peptide loading. Cell *82*, 155–165.
16. Roche, PA (1995). HLA DM: An In vivo facilitator of MHC class II peptide loading. Immunity *3*, 259–262.
17. Lanier, LL (1998). Follow the leader: NK cell receptors for classical and non-classical MHC class I. Cell *92*, 705–707.
18. Braud, VM, Allan, DSJ, O'Callaghan, CA, Soderstrom, K, D'Andrea, A, Ogg, GS, Lazetic, S, Young, NT, Bell, JI, Philips, JH, Lanier, L, and McMichael, AJ (1998). HLA-E binds to natural killer cell receptors CD94/NKG2A, B and C. Nature *391*, 795–798.
19. Simpson, E, and Roopenian, D (1997). Minor histocompatibility antigens. Curr. Opin. in Immunol. *9*, 655–661.
20. Wilson, IA, and Bjorkman, PJ (1998). Unusual MHC-like molecules: CD1, Fc receptor, the hemochromatosis gene product and viral homologs. Curr. Opin. Immunol. *10*, 67–73.
21. Wucherpfennig, KW, and Strominger, JC (1995). Molecular mimicry in T cell mediated autoimmunity: viral peptides activate human T cell clones specific for myelin basic protein. Cell *80*, 695–705.
22. Gilbert, SC, Plebanski, M, Gupta, S, Morris, J, Cox, M, Aidoo, M, Kwiatowski, D, Greenwood, BM, Whittle, HC, and Hill, AVS (1998). Association of malaria parasite population structure, HLA, and immunological antagonism. Science *279*, 1173–1177.
23. Kimura, A, Sasazuki, T. Eleventh International Histocompatibility Workshop protocol for the HLA DNA typing technique. In: Tsuji K, Aizawa M, Sasazuki T eds. *HLA 1991. Proceedings of the Eleventh International Histocompatibility Workshop and Conference. Volume 1.* New York and Oxford; 1992:397–418.
24. van Rood, JJ, and Oudshoorn, M (1998). An HLA matched donor! An HLA matched donor? What do you mean by HLA matched donor. Bone Marrow Transplant *22*, Suppl 1: S83.
25. Sasazuki, T, Juji, T, and Morishima, Y et al. (1998). Effect of matching HLA class I alleles on clinical outcome after transplantation of hematopoietic stem cells from an unrelated donor. N. Eng. J. Med. *339*, 1177–1185.
26. Parham, P, Clayberger, C, Zom, SL, Ludwig, DS, Schoolnik, GK, and Krensky, AM (1987). Inhibition of alloreactive cytotoxic T cells by peptides from the a2 domain of HLA-A2. Nature *325*, 625–628.
27. Chicz, RM, Urban, RG, Lane, WS, Gorga, JC, Stern, LJ, Vignali, DA, and Strominger, JL (1992). Predominant naturally processed peptides bound to HLA DR1 are derived from MHC related molecules and are heterogeneous in size. Nature *358*, 764–768.
28. Shoskes, DA, and Wood, KJ (1994). Indirect presentation of MHC antigens in transplantation. Immunology Today *15*, 32–38.
29. Sayegh, MH, Watschinger, B, and Carpenter, CB (1994). Mechanisms of T cell recognition of alloantigen. The role of peptides. Transplantation *57*, 1295–1302.
30. Magee, CC, and Sayegh, MH (1997). Peptide-mediated immunosuppression. Curr. Opin. in Immunol. *9*, 669–675.
31. Liu, Z, Colovai, AI, Tugulea, S, Reed, EF, Fischer, PE, Mancini, D, Rose, EA, Cortesini, R, Michler, RE, and Suciu-Foca, N (1996). Indirect recognition of donor HLA-DR peptides in organ allograft rejection. J. Clin. Invest. *98*, 1150–1157.
32. Opelz, G, and Wujciak, T (1994). The influence of HLA compatibility on graft survival after heart transplantation. N.Eng. J. Med. *330*, 816–819.
33. Jarcho, J, Naftel, DC, Shroyer TW et al. (1994). Influence of HLA mismatch on rejection after heart transplantation: a multiinstitutional study. J. Heart. Lung. Transplant. *13*, 583–596.
34. Hosenpud, JD, Edwards, EB, Lin, H-M, and Daily, P (1996). Influence of HLA matching on thoracic transplant outcomes. Ana analysis from the UNOS/ISHLT thoracic registry. Circulation *94*, 170–174.

2. IMMUNOLOGY OF CELLULAR AND HUMORAL REJECTION AFTER CARDIAC TRANSPLANTATION

Marlene L. Rose, Sudhir Kushwaha and Deirdre Cunningham
National Heart and Lung Institute, Imperial College School of Medicine, Harefield and Brompton Hospital, Harefield, Middlesex, UB9 6JH, UK

INTRODUCTION

The major complication following cardiac transplantation remains acute and chronic allograft rejection. Rejection is mediated both by cells and antibody, the different components of the immune response predominating at different times. It is interesting to note that, in the early days of human cardiac transplantation, detection of antibodies was considered to be the most obvious way to monitor the recipient's immune response. In a report published during that time,[1] it was found using an indirect immunofluorescent staining technique in a study of 5 patients surviving for more than 7 days after cardiac transplantation that serum samples from these patients contained antibodies directed against components of cardiac myofibres. These antibodies were detected early (4 or 5 days) after transplantation and their presence appeared to correlate with clinical signs of rejection.

In spite of this early indication that humoral immune mechanisms might be implicated in the rejection process, the possible role of antibody-mediated mechanisms in damaging the transplanted heart has been subsequently largely neglected. This is due to the development of techniques for routine endomyocardial biopsy and the relative ease with which acute rejection can be diagnosed by the presence within the biopsy of a mononuclear cellular infiltrate.

1. CELLULAR REJECTION

The introduction of routine surveillance endomyocardial biopsies regimes has made available to research teams pieces of transplanted donor tissue. Detection of antigens in situ by monoclonal antibodies (MoAbs) and immunocytochemical techniques is a powerful method that gives clues to the role of certain cells or antigens in normal or pathological responses. Particularly useful are longitudinal studies where examination of sequential biopsies can reveal the temporal pattern of expression of antigens and their correlation with rejection episodes. It is clear that important changes to donor endothelial cells and MHC antigens occur after transplantation and these can be described immunocytochemically. This chapter describes the immunocytochemical detection of:

1) Cells within the infiltrate
2) MHC antigens
3) Endothelial antigens and adhesions molecules
4) Cytokines and nitric oxide

NATURE OF THE INFILTRATE

The type of immunosuppressive drug that the patient receives can affect the appearance of the infiltrate. Rose et al.[2] in an immunoperoxidase study of 17 biopsies from patients receiving azathioprine and steroids reported a ten-fold increase in numbers of CD3 cells in biopsies showing histological signs of rejection, compared to control biopsies taken from donor heart prior to transplantation. Approximately 85% of the T cells were of the CD8 subset. In contrast, a clear accumulation of CD8 cells was not characteristic of rejection in patients taking cyclosporine, where large numbers of infiltrating cells were found regardless of whether the biopsy was diagnosed as rejection. Hoshinaga et al.[3] in a study of 22 patients, 13 taking azathioprine and steroids and 9 receiving cyclosporine, reported a similar magnitude of influx of T cells into the biopsy during rejection and found 2–3 times as many CD8 cells as CD4. In addition, they demonstrated macrophages within the infiltrate (using OKM1), increasing in number with the severity of rejection. Using the MoAbs RFD7, it has been confirmed that macrophages can be a large component of the infiltrate during rejection.[4]

The explanation for the difficulty in detecting a predominantly CD8 infiltrate in biopsies from patients taking cyclosporine is probably because of the unusually cellular appearance of some of these biopsies. The introduction of cyclosporine has produced a curious endocardial infiltrate called the "Quilty" effect.[5] In the absence of myocytolysis, this infiltrate is not generally considered to be diagnostic of rejection, although a recent study has shown it to be more frequently found in biopsies showing rejection than in rejection-free biopsies.[6] Immunocytochemical staining has shown the infiltrate predominantly to consist of T cells[6] as well as macrophages and endothelial cells (unpublished results). The suggestion, that Epstein Barr virus is associated with this condition and that the infiltrate resembles an EBV induced lymphoma, was made on the finding of EBV genomic sequences by in-situ hybridization in 10 out of 18 biopsies.[7] However, this finding was not confirmed in a larger study.[8] Indeed, the immunocytochemical findings of predominant T cells and not B cells would also not support this hypothesis.

The clinical use of monitoring T cells in endomyocardial biopsies was addressed in a longitudinal study of 111 biopsies from 8 patients followed for the first two years.[9] These authors concluded that counting numbers of CD8 cells/unit area was useful adjunct to diagnosis of rejection, and anything above 3 cells/field (using 400 X magnification) identified acute rejection. They emphasize the importance of identifying T cells using MoAbs and immunoperoxidase and not relying on morphological discrimination by eye.

PRESENCE OF ACTIVATED CELLS IN BIOPSIES

With increasing knowledge of T cell activation and the molecular mechanisms whereby lymphoid cells damage tissues, it should be possible to devise tests to look for infiltrating cells that may be actively involved in tissue destruction. Granzyme A and perforin are two proteins found in the intracellular granules of cytotoxic T cells and NK cells and are thought to be released specifically at the killer cell target interface in vitro. Perforin is a cytolytic molecule which, in the presence of calcium, can polymerize to form 16 mm pores through the membrane of the target cell.[10] Granzyme A is a serine esterase and its precise role in killing is unknown. The majority of T cells expressing perforin and Granzyme A in vivo will be of the CD8 phenotype.

An experimental study[11] has demonstrated infiltrating cells containing mRNA for serine esterase (Granzyme A) in murine cardiac allografts several days before rejection. In a study of 29 endomyocardial biopsies from heart transplant patients, lymphocytes expressing mRNA for both Granzyme A and perforin were found in all biopsies showing histological signs of rejection and in 50% of biopsies not thought to be showing rejection.[12] This elegant study using in-situ hybridization with antisense probes for mRNA suggested the presence of these lymphocytes precedes histological damage. It is, however, important to follow-up these studies with a demonstration of cells expressing the protein products of the mRNA in endomyocardial biopsies. The presence of message does not necessarily mean the cells are expressing the active proteins. It is conceivable that, in patients taking immunosuppressive drugs, protein translation may be inhibited. Perforin has been demonstrated immunocytochemically within the cardiac infiltrate of a mouse model of myocariditis,[13] but none of these cells were T lymphocytes, they were all NK cells.

Activated CD4 T cells express receptors for Interleukin-2. It has been difficult to demonstrate T cells expressing IL-2R immunocytochemically in clinical biopsies and our own studies have only found these cells in biopsies showing moderate to severe rejection.[14] Salmon et al.[15] also found very few activated cells (IL-2R, Ki-67 or PCNA positive) in biopsies showing grade 1 or 2 rejection.

MHC ANTIGENS

MHC antigens are the major target of the immune response following allograft rejection. Two facts about expression of MHC antigens account for the current interest in understanding their precise distribution in organs: first, expression is not a constant feature of a cell, it can be upregulated by cytokines and downregulated by substances that counteract or inhibit cytokine production,[16] second, quantitative changes in expression alters the magnitude of the immune response.

The advent of MoAbs, the use of frozen sections and advances in immunocytochemical techniques have revolutionized knowledge about the normal distribution of MHC antigens in different tissues. Although constitutively present on many nucleated cells, MHC Class I (HLA-A, B, C) antigens are only weakly expressed or absent on endocrine cells, hepatocytes, smooth muscle[17,18,19] normal skeletal[20] and cardiac muscle.[21] Class II (HLA-DR, DP and DQ) antigens, originally thought to be restricted to macrophages, dendritic cells, monocytes and activated T cells have also been described on human endothelial and epithelial cells.[19,22]

Upregulation of Class I and Class II antigens has been extensively described in donor organs following allotransplantation and in skin and gut during Graft versus Host disease. Altered MHC antigen expression has also been described in a number of disease models and human diseases including autoimmune disorders, inflammatory states and malignancies.

CLASS I MHC IN THE NORMAL AND TRANSPLANTED HEART

Table 1 summarizes the distribution of MHC antigens in normal and transplanted heart. In normal heart taken prior to transplantation, all the interstitial structures are Class I positive (Figure 1). The interstitial cells have been identified as microvascular endothelial cells and leukocytes of the monocyte/dendritic series (as described below). In contrast, the myocardial plasma membrane is negative for MHC antigens.[21] Faint staining of the intercalating discs also has been reported.[18] After transplantation, there is a dramatic upregulation of MHC Class I on the myocardial plasma membrane and intercalating discs (Figure 2).[21,22,23,24] This is almost always accompanied by an infiltrate and, in biopsies taken within the first year after transplantation, the Class I induction is usually focal and close to an infiltrate. Class I is

Table 1. Distribution of HLA Class I and Class II Antigens in Normal and Rejecting Hearts

	Normal		Rejection	
	Class I	Class II	Class I	Class II
Myocardial Plasma Membrane	–	–	++	–
Intercalating Discs	+–	–	++	–
Capillaries	+	+	+	++?
Venules	+	+–	+	+
Arterioles	+	+–	+	+
Endocardium	+	–	+	+
Coronary Endothelium	+	+	+	+

1. Using MoAb W6/32
2. Using MoAb L243
– negative staining
+– weak positive staining
+ medium positive staining
++ strong positive staining

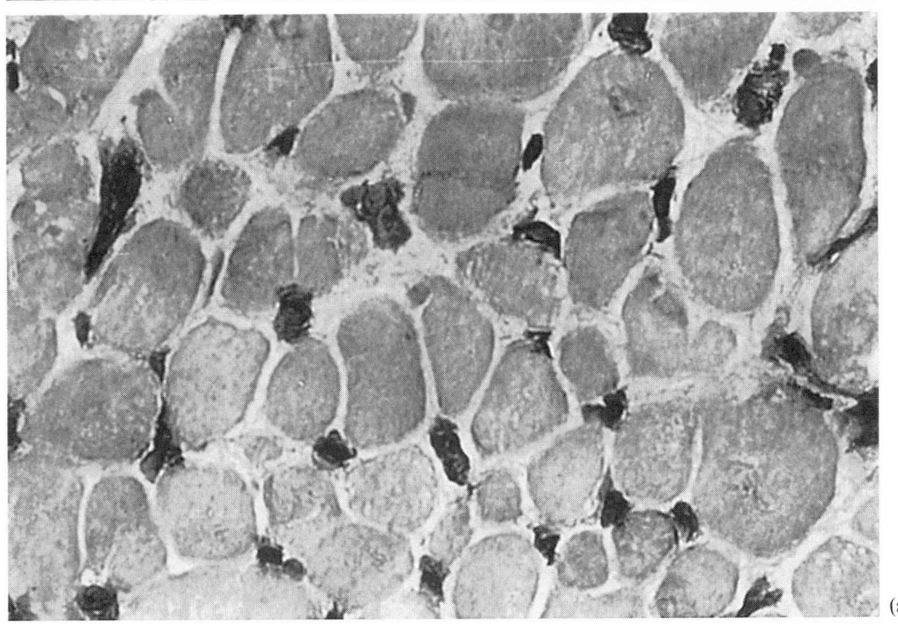
(a)

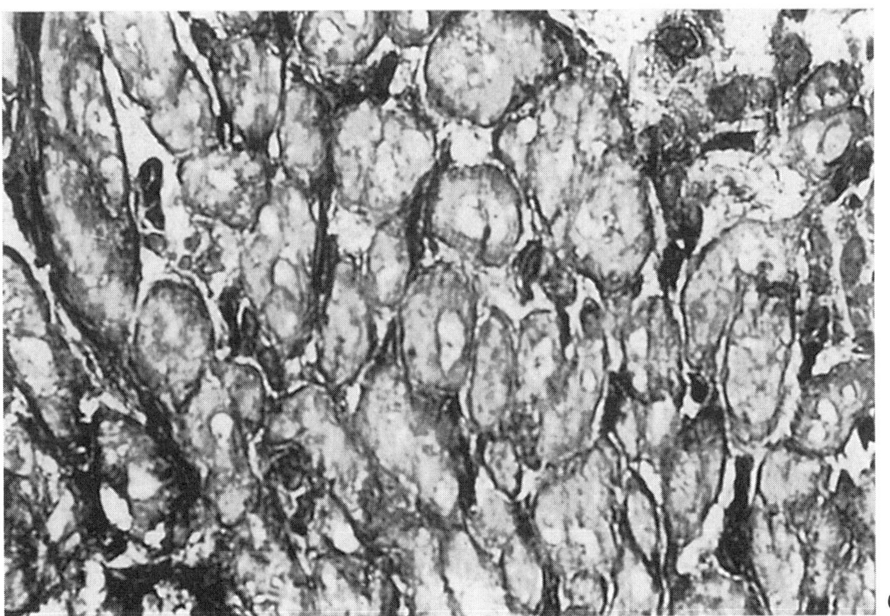
(b)

Figure 1. Photomicrograph of normal endomyocardial biopsy taken from donor heart prior to implantation (a) and endomyocardial biopsy with mild rejection (b) stained with the monoclonal antibody W6/32 directed against MHC class I determinants. All the interstitial structures are positive; the myocardium is negative in the pre-transplant biopsy but becomes positive during rejection. [Immunoperoxidase staining. Cryostat sections, 6 micrometers, counterstained with Hemtoxylin; Reproduced with permission from Rose ML, Yacoub MH. Immunochemical analysis of transplanted heart and lung. In: Immunology of Heart and Lung Transplantation, eds Rose ML, Yacoub HM, Arnold E, London, 1993]

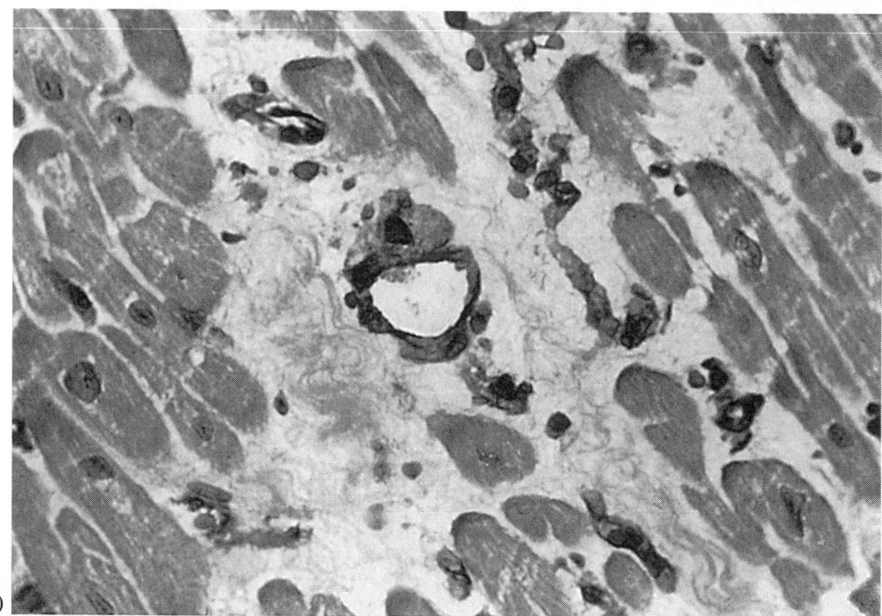

(a)

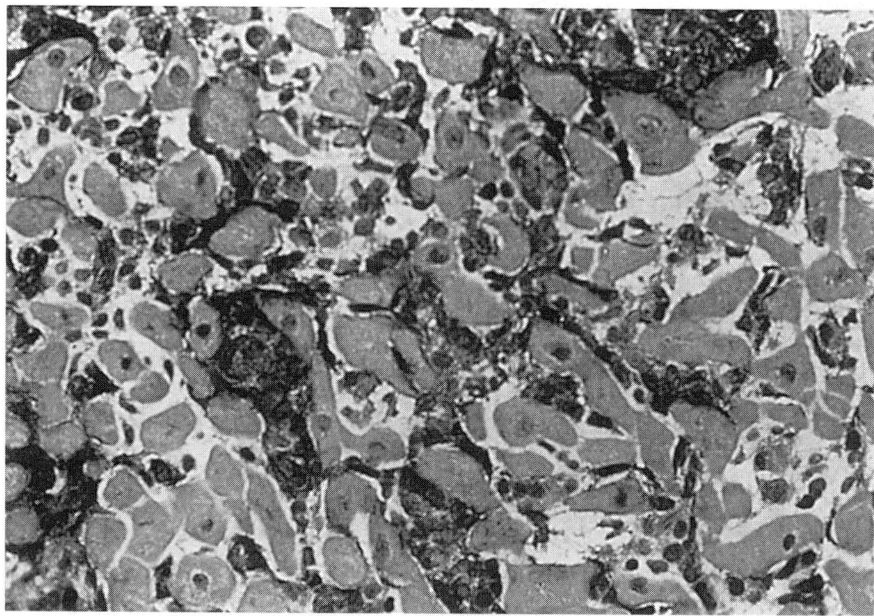

(b)

Figure 2. Photomicrograph of donor endomyocardial biopsy taken prior to transplantation (a) and biopsy showing signs of rejection (b), stained with the monoclonal antibody L243 against HLA-DR determinants. The majority of the interstitial structures are positive in the normal heart (a). The infiltrating cells but not the myocardium are positive during rejection (b). [Immunoperoxidase staining. Cryostat sections, 6 micrometers, counterstained with Hemtoxylin; Reproduced with permission from Rose ML, Yacoub MH. Immunochemical analysis of transplanted heart and lung. In: Immunology of Heart and Lung Transplantation, eds Rose ML, Yacoub HM, Arnold E, London, 1993]

not induced on the myocardium of donor hearts during the four hour (maximum) ischemic time prior to transplantation. A sequential study of 114 biopsies from 11 patients studied within the first year of transplantation showed that upregulation of Class I on the myocardium was associated with rejection episodes, diagnosed by histologic assessment of endomyocardial biopsy.[22] Alpha and beta interferons are produced from leukocytes and fibroblasts respectively, and gamma interferon is produced by activated T cells: all are able to upregulate MHC Class I antigens. It is reasonable to assume that Class I induction in cardiac biopsies from transplant patients is caused by locally produced interferons from activated macrophages or T cells. However, the precise lymphokines that caused induction within the graft is not known. Technically, it has proven difficult to visualize cytokines immunocytochemically, but much progress has been made using polymerase chain reaction technology to amplify RNA message for cytokines (see section below). The correlation between induction of MHC Class I on the heart and clinical rejection is not absolute.[22,23,24] One hundred percent of first rejection episodes and 79% of subsequent rejection episodes coincided with Class I expression.[22] Steinhoff[24] reported that 57 out of 78 rejection episodes were characterized by induction of Class I on the myocardium. Class I induction takes 3–4 weeks to disappear following treatment.[22] This explains why, after the first rejection episode, only 31% of biopsies with induced Class I are diagnosed as rejection.

Experimental studies in rats have shown massive induction of donor-specific Class I on myocardium during rejection of allografted heart.[25]

The molecular mechanisms of damage to the myocardium are not known. Although T cells of both phenotype (CD4 and CD8) and macrophages are found in histologically damaged biopsies, it is not known which cell/cells damage the myocytes. Should cytotoxic T cells be involved, induction of MHC Class I antigens on the myocardium would be a prerequisite for damage. However, it is equally possible that damage is mediated directly by cytokines and macrophages and, in some cases, antibody. Certain cytokines (tumor necrosis factor and IL-1) have been shown to have negative inotropic effects on cardiac myocytes[26,27] due to upregulation of iNOS.

CLASS II MHC IN NORMAL HEART AND IDENTIFICATION OF CLASS II POSITIVE STRUCTURES

In normal heart, the majority of interstitial structures bind MoAbs against common determinant of Class II, DR and DP subdeterminants (Table 1, Figure 3). Identification of these cells with various MoAbs revealed the large majority to be microvascular and venule endothelial cells, and only a small number to be cells of the monocyte/macrophage/dendritic series. Arterioles are Class II negative. Thus, MoAbs that bind to endothelial cells (anti-CD31 MoAbs) show a pattern of staining identical to that found with MoAbs against common determinant or DR Class II. These immunocytochemical observations have been confirmed by quantitating the numbers of cells binding different MoAbs.[4] Labarrere and colleagues independently concluded that the majority of Class II positive cells in cardiac biopsies were endothelial cells.[28] This is a contrasting situation to rat heart where endothelial cells

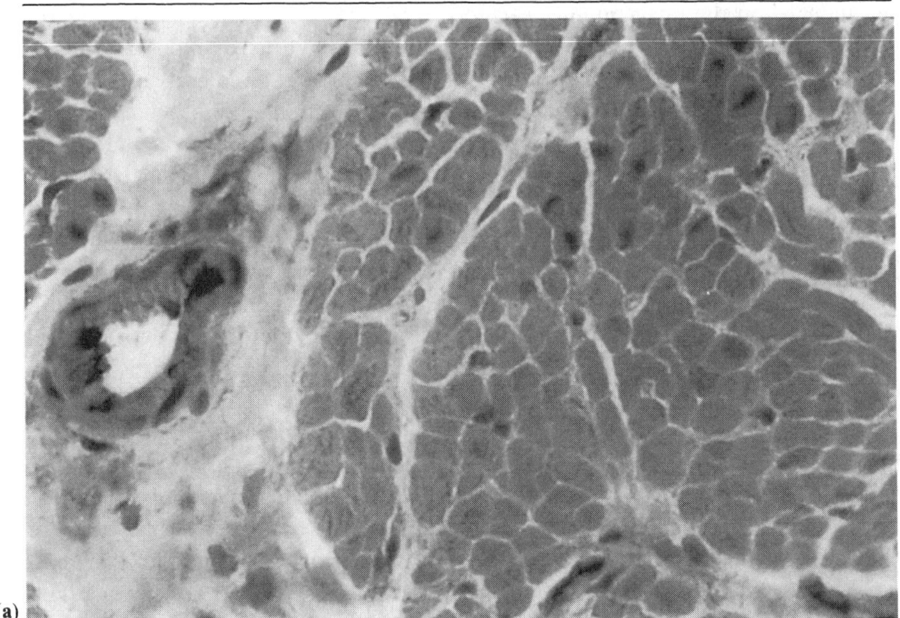

(a)

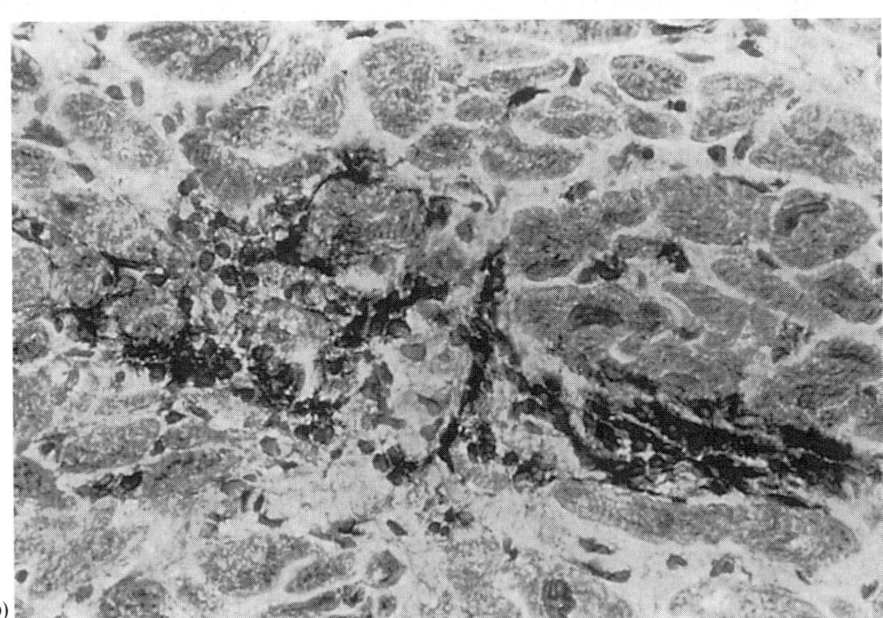

(b)

Figure 3. Photomicrograph of donor endomyocardial biopsy taken prior to transplantation (a) and showing histological signs of rejection (b), stained with the monoclonal antibody CD 106, against VCAM-1. There is localized up-regulation of VCAM-1 within the area of the infiltrate. [Immunoperoxidase staining. Cryostat sections, 6 micrometers, counterstained with Hemtoxylin; Reproduced with permission from Rose ML, Yacoub MH. Immunochemical analysis of transplanted heart and lung. In: Immunology of Heart and Lung Transplantation, eds Rose ML, Yacoub HM, Arnold E, London, 1993]

do not constitutively express Class II and the majority of Class II positive cells are dendritic cells.[29] Some have reported that the endothelial cells in normal human heart are not normally Class II positive.[30] However, these authors used antibody against von Willebrand's Factor (vWF) to identify endothelial cells. Our studies have shown only about 30% of endothelial cells are vWF positive in the heart[31] and, moreover, it is the larger vessels which are more likely to be vWF positive and the larger vessels tend to be Class II negative.[32] Fuggle[33] also reported that endothelial cells in the larger vessels tend to be negative for Class II antigens whereas the microvascular endothelial cells are positive. Using MoAbs specific for the subdeterminants of Class II,[22,24,28] it was shown that DR and DP are strongly expressed on the endothelial cells of normal heart, but DQ was barely visible.

CLASS II ANTIGENS IN TRANSPLANTED HEART

In biopsies from transplant patients showing rejection, there is upregulation of Class II expression on interstitial structures (Figure 4). The close apposition of the normally Class II positive microvascular endothelial cells and Class II positive infiltrating cells makes it difficult to determine whether there is upregulation of Class II on the microvascular endothelial cells when immunoperoxidase staining is used. Indeed, the major increase in Class II is clearly on infiltrating cells. However, studies using fluorescent antibody either against vWF to identify the larger endothelial cells[30] or against the DR determinant[34] have reported more vascular cells becoming Class II positive during rejection. Our own studies have shown that the normally negative endocardium becomes Class II positive following transplantation.[35] Using MoAbs against DQ determinants which are normally scarcely expressed on endothelial cells, clear upregulation is observed associated with rejection episodes.[22,24,28] Intriguingly, studies have reported upregulation of DR and ICAM-1 on arterioles in biopsies from patients who are developing accelerated coronary artery disease.[36]

Endothelial Antigens and Adhesion Molecules

Endothelial cells are numerous in the heart and, as described above, they constitutively express MHC Class I, DR and DP antigens. This means they can be recognized by the recipient's immune system. The endothelium forms the major barrier between the graft and the host's immune cells and, in fact, endothelial cells may participate in allograft rejection in three ways:

1. They allow adhesion and extravasation of circulating leukocytes.
2. They may present alloantigen to recipient lymphocytes.
3. They may be the primary target during allograft rejection.

Adhesion Molecules

A number of adhesion or accessory molecules have been described[37] that may facilitate leukocyte/endothelial adhesion. Such adhesive interactions may also be the

(a)

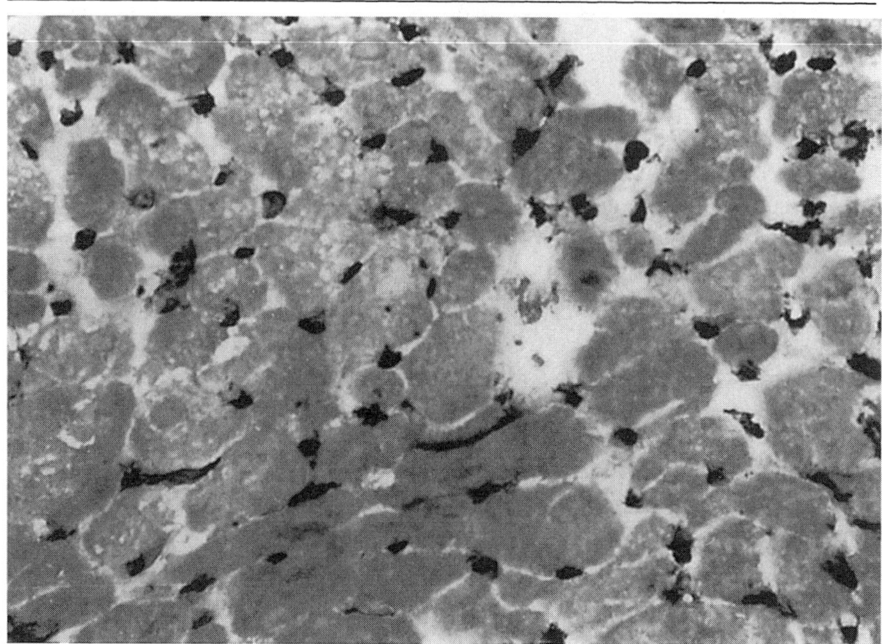

(b)

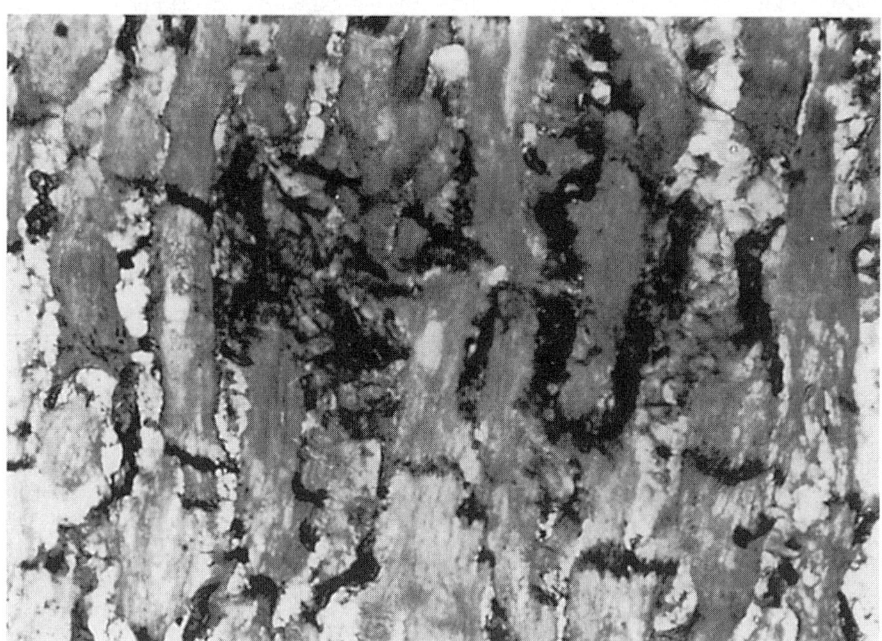

Figure 4. Photomicrograph of endomyocardial biopsy taken prior to transplantation (a) and showing histological signs of rejection (b), stained with a monoclonal antibody directed against ICAM-1. ICAM-1 is constitutively expressed on endothelial cells in the normal biopsy (a). There is up-regulation fo ICAM-1 around myocardial membranes and intercalating discs within the area of cellular infiltration during rejection (b). [Immunoperoxidase technique. Cryostat sections, 6 micron, counterstained with Hematoxylin]

Table 2. Distribution of Adhesion Molecules in Normal and Transplanted Heart during Rejection

MoAb	Capillaries Normal/Rejection	Venules	Arterioles	Endocardium
PECAM	+/+	+/+	+/+	+/+
VCAM	–/++	+–/+	+–/+	–/+
ICAM	+/+	+/+	+/+	+–/+
ELAM	–/++	+/+	–/–	–/–

– = negative staining
+– = weakly or occasionally positive staining
\+ = positive staining
++ = strong positive staining

first step in cellular interactions leading to lymphocyte activation and cytotoxic responses. Some of these molecules such as intercellular adhesion molecule-1 (ICAM-1, CD54) and platelet endothelial cellular molecule (PECAM, CD31) are present constitutively on cultured umbilical vein cells and others such as vascular cell adhesion molecule-1 (VCAM-1, CD106) and endothelial leukocyte adhesion molecule-1 (ELAM-1 or E-selectin) are inducible after cytokine activation. Fifteen biopsies from normal donor heart and fifteen endomyocardial biopsies showing histological signs of rejection were investigated for expression of ICAM-1, PECAM, ELAM, and VCAM.[35] PECAM was found to be present on all endothelial cells but ELAM and VCAM, not constitutively expressed by endothelial cells, were discretely upregulated during rejection (Table 2). Two large longitudinal studies would agree that VCAM-1 upregulation is significantly associated with the degree of rejection and the presence of a CD3+ infiltrate.[38,39] These studies have suggested that persistent expression of VCAM-1 is indicative of persistent rejection and its disappearance is a sign of successful anti-rejection therapy. There is less agreement about the utility of ICAM-1 and E-selectin as diagnostic markers.

Several important points from these findings are as follows:

1. VCAM-1 is not expressed on normal capillaries but there is a localized induction on capillaries, arterioles and venules in biopsies showing signs of rejection (Figure 3). Moreover, there is always an accumulation of lymphocytes within the vessels showing VCAM induction. The discrete pattern of induction and the fact that the ligand for VCAM-1 is found only on lymphocytes and eosinophils[40] suggests a role for VCAM in allowing egress of mononuclear cells into the allografted heart.
2. ICAM-1 is constitutively expressed in the microvasculature of the heart and other organs.[4] Others report increased intensity of staining on the vasculature during rejection.[38,39] However, we find a dramatic and focal induction of ICAM-1 on intercalating discs and the myocardial plasma membrane during rejection.
3. E-selectin is weakly expressed in normal biopsies.[35,39,42] Although there is reported upregulation during rejection,[39] our own studies[35] and those of others[41] suggest it is not sufficient to be of clinical utility.

Thus, the constitutive expression of selectins may facilitate leukocytes rolling, but the upregulation VCAM-1 and ICAM-1 may aid firm adhesions and transendothelial migration.

In the murine model, the blockage of the ICAM-1:LFA-1 interaction using antisense oligonucleotides to ICAM-1[41] or a combination of anti-ICAM-1 and LFA-1 monoclonal antibodies resulted in the induction of specific tolerance.[42] However, the failure to reproduce this result in the rat cardiac allograft model[43] and the fact that ICAM-1 knock-out animals reject their grafts at rates similar to that of the wild-type[44] is disappointing and suggests other interactions come into play in the absence of ICAM-1.

PRESENTATION OF ALLOANTIGENS TO RECIPIENT LYMPHOCYTES

In rats and mice, the only Class II positive cells in grafted hearts and kidneys are dendritic cells.[29] Dendritic cells are very potent stimulators of the alloimmune response, moreover, they are of bone marrow origin and eventually become replaced by host cells. It has been demonstrated that, after they leave the graft, they may survive indefinitely.[45] It has thus been suggested that one approach to immunosuppression would be to render human organs non-immunogenic by perfusing them with antibody against dendritic cells or the common leukocyte antigen. However, the observation, that in humans endothelial cells in the graft express donor MHC antigens, raises the important questions about the immunogenicity of human endothelial cells. It has now been shown that human endothelial cells can cause direct allostimulation of resting CD4+ and CD8+ T cells.[46,47,48] which means they have to be considered as an important and permanent immunogenic component of the graft.

COSTIMULATORY PATHWAYS

In addition to the engagement of the T cell receptor by antigen-MHC, the activation and sustained proliferation of T lymphocytes requires a second costimulatory signal provided by cell surface molecules on the surface of antigen presenting cells. Examples of costimulatory signals include the interaction of the B7 family with the CD28/CTLA4 ligand[49] or CD40 with the CD40 ligand (CD40L).[50] The absence of a second signal results in antigen-specific unresponsiveness or anergy.[51,52] The requirement for a second signal has been exploited for the induction of tolerance in rodent models. CTLA4-Ig is a fusion protein that has been shown to block CD28 costimulation and, in a murine cardiac allograft model, a 12 day course of CTLA4-Ig prolonged graft survival.[53] Similarly, blockade of the CD40:CD40L interaction using an antibody to CD40L also results in the prolongation of cardiac allograft survival.[54] However, the simultaneous blockade of both the CD28 and CD40 pathways appears to be necessary for long-term graft acceptance.[55] CD40 is and its ligand CD40L are coexpressed by human microvascular endothelial cells in cardiac biopsies[56] and by arterial endothelial cells and smooth muscle cells in atherosclerotic plaques.[57]

ENDOTHELIAL MARKERS VWF AND PAL-E DEMONSTRATE INVOLVEMENT OF ENDOTHELIAL CELLS IN ALLOGRAFT REJECTION

Factor VIII related antigen or von Willebrand's Factor (vWF) is a large molecular weight glycoprotein which is synthesized by endothelial cells.[58] We found antibody against vWF to bind to only about 30% of endothelial cells in the normal heart and, moreover, these tended to be the larger vessels (venules and arterioles) and the staining was very granular, typical of Weibel Palade bodies. During rejection, there was increased expression of vWF and Pal-E manifested by increased numbers of positive cells as well as enhanced intensity of staining of swollen endothelial cells.

These results demonstrate involvement of endothelial cells early in the rejection process. They do not discriminate between cell mediated or humoral rejection and it is highly likely that endothelial cells are involved (although mechanistically the responses may be different) regardless of the effector mechanisms. Immunocytochemical observations by Labarrere and colleagues[59] showing disappearance of endothelial thrombomodulin and antithrombin III from endomyocardial biopsies during rejection episodes would support this hypothesis.

DETECTION OF CYTOKINES

Cytokines play a central role in the inflammatory and allospecific components of allograft rejection and in the migration of cells into graft tissue. They are effectors of differentiation and activation, tissue destruction and regulation of the immune response. They are involved in the activation and clonal expansion of CD4+ and CD8+ T lymphocytes (IL-2, IFNγ), B lymphocytes (IL-2, IL-4), and in upregulation of MHC Class I and Class II antigens (IFNγ, TNFα) and adhesions molecules (IFNγ, TNFα, IL-4) expression. Thus, they increase the immune response of the recipient and enhance the immunogenicity of the allograft. IL2 participates in the activation and proliferation of both the cytotoxic CD8+ T cell and the large granular lymphocyte (which gives rise to the cytotoxic NK cell) and thus may trigger cell damage or necrosis. In addition to their indirect activities via upregulation of cytotoxic cells, some cytokines may also have direct cytotoxic effects (e.g. TNFα, IFNγ).[60] It has proved technically difficult to demonstrate cytokines directly (i.e. the proteins) in organ allografts due to the fact the cytokines are produced in very small quantities and, unless they are receptor bound, they are probably washed away during tissue processing. However, when abundant, cytokines can be detected immunocytochemically. Thus IL2, IFNγ and TNFα have been detected in the rejection of cardiac and renal allografts.[61–63]

In order to avoid the technical problems associated with protein detection, many workers have measured cytokine mRNA transcripts—the most common method being use of polymerase chain reaction to amplify the transcripts. In a sequential study of biopsies collected from 12 patients during the first four months post transplant, Cunningham et al.[64] found the cytokines IL-2, IL-4, and IL-10 to be most commonly associated with histopathological evidence of rejection. In contrast, IL-1β, TNFα and TNFβ were found in both rejecting and nonrejecting biopsies. This clinical study is in broad agreement with the results obtained using an experimental murine model of cardiac allograft rejection.[65]

Further analysis of biopsies from the Cunningham study[69] showed that IL-2 was statistically correlated with mild and moderate rejection, while IL-4 and IL-10 correlated with mild rejection. That IL-2 is associated with early rejection was shown by Wu et al.[65] using heterotopic transplant of hearts into cynomolgus monkeys. Thus, it is established that IL-2 seems to be exclusively expressed in allogeneic grafts appearing early in the rejection process. IL-10 may have an autoregulatory function, possibly preventing the progression of mild rejection to severe rejection, was also suggested by the findings of Azzawi et al.[67] Using in-situ hybridization, they demonstrated that IL-10 was more prominent in mild than moderate rejection.

It has been suggested that the Th1 subset of CD4+ T cells (which secrete IL2 and IFNγ) may be instrumental in the initiation of the acute rejection cascade, while the Th2 subset (secreting predominantly IL4, IL5, and IL10), may be more important in establishing and maintaining tolerance (the Th1/Th2 paradigm).[68] The role of the Th2 cell products IL4 and IL10 in acute rejection may be the limitation of Th1 cytokine production locally in the graft or these cytokines may also stimulate antibody production, as there is evidence that elevated titers of anti-heart antibodies are generally associated with more frequent or severe episodes of acute rejection (see below).

Other cytokines which may be of importance in transplantation include IL12 which is important in the development of the Th1 cell and IL15 which utilizes the same β and γ receptors as IL2 but has its own α chain.[69,70] Thus, by triggering the same signal transduction pathway as IL2, IL15 may act as an IL2 substitute, particularly in the immunosuppressed individual. Consequently, proliferation of alloreactive T cells may also be sustained by IL15 which is insensitive to the immunosuppressive effects of cyclosporine. Both IL12 and IL15 are products of activated macrophages. It has recently been shown that other macrophage-associated products are upregulated in animal models of chronic cardiac rejection.[71] It has recently been shown that IL15 is upregulated in human renal allograft rejection[72] while, in the human cardiac allograft, IL15 is ubiquitously present.[73]

ROLE OF NITRIC OXIDE

Recent studies have demonstrated a role for nitric oxide (NO) in alloimmune responses and during cardiac allograft rejection. NO, which can be produced in large amounts by inducible NO synthase (iNOS), has the potential to be negatively inotropic and may be cytotoxic to cardiac myocytes[73] and appears to play an integral role in cardiac allograft rejection. Using a rat model of heterotopic abdominal cardiac transplantation, Yang demonstrated that iNOS mRNA, protein activity and iNOS protein was present in macrophages infiltrating the myocardium and in endothelial cells and cardiac myocytes in the rejecting hearts.[74] The authors concluded that synthesis of NO by iNOS may contribute to myocyte necrosis and ventricular failure during cardiac allograft rejection. These results were confirmed by Worrall who further demonstrated that selective iNOS inhibition prolonged survival, improved performance and reduced the pathological changes in the cardiac allografts.[75] In the same rat cardiac transplant model, Worrall also demonstrated that corticosteroids resulted in inhibition of iNOS expression during cardiac allograft rejection.[76] Similarly, immunosuppressive therapy with FK506 and cyclosporine A reduce iNOS expression in rejecting cardiac allografts.[77]

In addition, NO produced by iNOS in cytokine-treated macrophages has been demonstrated to induce apoptosis of these macrophages.[78] Therefore, it is likely that NO may be cytotoxic through an apoptotic mechanism. Szabolcs and co-workers have demonstrated apoptosis of cardiac myocytes during cardiac transplant rejection in a heterotopic rat model of cardiac transplantation.[79] The expression of iNOS mRNA, protein and enzyme paralleled the increase of apoptotic cardiac myocytes until maximal rejection of the graft.

These findings have been confirmed in humans by the same group.[80] Right ventricular endomyocardial biopsies obtained from 30 cardiac allograft recipients with significant cardiac rejection (ISHLT grade 3A/B) were compared with 12 biopsies with no rejection (ISHLT grade 0). Immunohistochemical studies for iNOS demonstrated strong cytoplasmic reactivity in macrophages and cardiac myocytes in only the rejecting grafts. Biopsies with rejection showed a 30-fold increase of apoptotic cells compared with controls and most of these cells were found to be in proximity to macrophage-rich inflammatory infiltrates.

2. ANTIBODY MEDIATED REJECTION

The destructive effects of pre-existing antibody against donor antigens in clinical renal transplantation[81] and experimental xenotransplantation[82] have been recognized for many years. Hyperacute rejection provides clear evidence of antibody mediated damage to the graft. A more difficult question is defining the role of antibody in chronic graft survival. The multiplicity of mechanisms of antibody damage, the fact that many antibodies produced after transplantation are harmless and some may actually be beneficial has made evaluation of damaging antibodies in the clinic difficult. It is extremely likely that each time recipient T cells are stimulated by an allograft, B lymphocytes are stimulated to make antibody. The antibody response will include many specificities, some against alloantigens but some against "autoantigens", that is antigens not normally seen by the immune system but released as a result of T cell damage. Thus, the speed and severity of antibody mediated damage will vary across a clinical spectrum and include hyperacute rejection, acute rejection and chronic rejection. Although most attention has focused on donor-reactive or anti-HLA antibodies in the past, it is becoming increasingly clear that antibodies against endothelial cells and other non-HLA antigens are of clinical importance.

HYPERACUTE REJECTION

Hyperacute rejection results in failure of the allografted organ within 24 hours. Histologically, it is associated with the presence of a large infiltrate of polymorphonuclear granulocytes. Damage to the vascular endothelium occurs[83] and deposits of IgG, IgM, and the complement components C1 and C3 have been detected by direct immunofluorescence on the endothelium of both small and large vessels.[84,85]

INVOLVEMENT OF LYMPHOCYTOTOXIC ANTIBODIES

Hyperacute rejection of the cardiac allograft is a rare event. Kemnitz et al.[85] reported 2 cases out of a review of 524 patients, and our own experience of approximately 1500 cases would confirm an incidence of about 0.5% (unpublished). In the early 1980's, a number of anecdotal case reports demonstrated that hyperacute rejection of cardiac allografts was associated with the presence, before transplantation, of cytotoxic antibodies directed against donor lymphocytes.[86,87] However, large studies have shown that positive donor reactive crossmatches do not necessarily, or indeed usually, result in hyperacute rejection. Multiple studies[88–91] have shown that about 10% of patients will have a positive crossmatch with donor cells (defined as killing between 10–50% of donor cells). Early data from this institute demonstrated that patients transplanted against a positive crossmatch do not usually have hyperacute rejection but long-term actuarial graft survival is significantly pooer.[88,89] These results were confirmed in a much larger study[90] of 636 cardiac transplant patients. One year actuarial survival for a negative crossmatch (n = 580) was 73% compared to 56% for the positive crossmatch recipients (n = 56). More recently, using antibody-coated magnetic beads to separate donor T or B cells has enabled one to distinguish between a donor reactive T or B cell crossmatch. The Dynabead crossmatch was performed on 289 cardiac transplants.[90] One year survival for a negative crossmatch was 73%; for a B cell positive crossmatch recipients, 62%; and for T cell positive crossmatch, 28% (Figure 5). Moreover, the T cell positive crossmatch (all IgG responses) was found to be a predictor of very early graft failure. Thus in our hands, a donor reactive crossmatch, in particular an IgG T cell crossmatch, is highly predictive of early graft failure. Although our studies did not prove the response to be against MHC Class I antigens on donor T cells, our results suggest that the heart, like the kidney,[92] undergoes rapid rejection in the presence of IgG antibodies against Class I antigens of the donor.

An alternative method to determine the pretransplant antibody status of patients is to test their serum against a panel of at least 40 HLA-typed lymphocytes representing all the common HLA antigens in a complement-dependent lymphocytotoxic assay. These reactivities are known as "Panel Reactive Antibodies" (PRAs). Some authors report no significant effect of lymphocytotoxic antibody status on graft survival,[89] while others have found a PRA in excess of 10% to be a risk factor for acute and chronic rejection events.[91]

In a study of 699 cardiac transplants, 261 were PRA negative (i.e. <11% PRA frequency), 57 patients had PRA frequencies of 11–50% and 21 patients had PRA frequencies of 51–100%.[93] There was found a marked, though not significant, reduction in graft survival associated with highly sensitized recipients (PRA > 50%) where one year survival was 52% compared to 72% for PRA negative recipients and 75% for transplant recipients with PRA 11–50%. In order to determine how predictive the PRA status is of positive crossmatch, the PRA was analyzed in 636 cardiac transplant patients where donor crossmatching was performed. It was found that, for 570

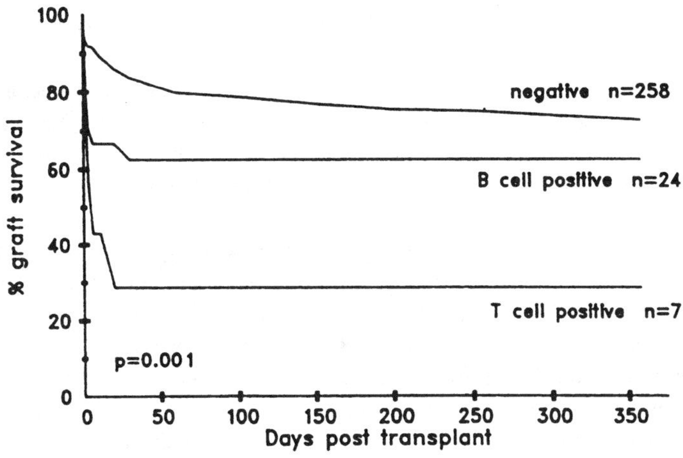

Figure 5. Effect of the donor reactive T and B lymphocyte crossmatch result on graft survival from 289 cardiac transplant operations performed between 1989 and 1992. [Reproduced with permission from: Smith JD, Danskine AJ, Laylor RM, et al. Transplant Immunology 1993;1:60–65]

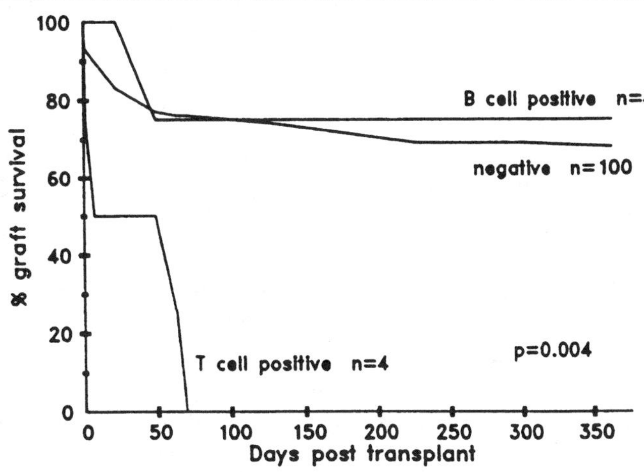

Figure 6. Effect of the donor reactive T and B lymphocyte crossmatch result on graft survival from 108 heart-lung transplants performed between 1989 and 1992. [Reproduced with permission from: Smith JD, Danskine AJ, Laylor RM, et al. Transplant Immunology 1993;1:60–65]

patients with a PRA frequency <11% (PRA negative), 26 positive crossmatches were found (4.5%) whilst for 50 recipients with a PRA between 11% and 50%, 18 positive crossmatches were found (35%) and for 16 patients, who were considered highly sensitized (PRA > 50%), 12 positive crossmatches were found (75%). Thus, it appears that the PRA test is predictive of a positive crossmatch. We believe the major effect of PRA status on graft survival (Figure 6) is due to presence of a positive crossmatch in those patients with medium to high PRAs.

HYPERACUTE REJECTION AND NON-LYMPHOCYTOTOXIC ANTIBODIES

Conversely, hyperacute rejection may occur in patients who had a negative prospective lymphocytotoxic crossmatch.[83,84,91] In a review of 463 heart transplant patients, 15 patients died of "hyperacute" rejection.[91] Only two of these were found to have had a positive retrospective crossmatch against donor lymphocytes and these were weakly positive. Brasile et al.[83] reported four cases of hyperacute rejection in patients with negative crossmatches against their donor lymphocytes. All patients were found to have cytotoxic antibodies against a panel of cultured endothelial cells. Similarly, evidence for anti-endothelial antibodies was reported in a group of 11 cardiac transplant patients who underwent hyperacute rejection in the presence of negative crossmatches.[84] The above studies describe immunohistology of the rejected heart as containing IgG, IgM and complement deposits on blood vessels. The presence of immune components on the vessels does not mean the antigens are not HLA; it is known that human cardiac endothelial cells strongly express MHC Class I and Class II antigens.[21] However, there is also a tissue-specific antigen system on the surface of vascular endothelial cells which is shared by peripheral blood monocytes but not lymphocytes.[93] The endothelial cell-monocyte antigen system has been implicated in rapid rejection of HLA identical renal grafts and it may be playing a part in the cases of hyperacute cardiac rejection described above.

ACUTE REJECTION

ANTI-HEART ANTIBODIES DETECTED BY IMMUNOFLUORESCENCE

Despite the early attempts to monitor rejection by immunofluorescent detection of antibody within cardiac biopsies,[1] it soon became clear that a much more precise method of monitoring rejection was by the presence of a mononuclear infiltrate within the biopsy. As a consequence, detailed cellular criteria for the histopathological diagnosis and grading of rejection in endomyocardial biopsy samples have been established[94] and remain the gold standard of cardiac rejection. Nevertheless, there has been a recent resurgence of interest in the role of antibody in acute rejection. Schuuman et al.[95,96] investigated 221 endomyocardial biopsies from 21 patients after cardiac transplantation by direct immunofluorescence for deposits of immunoglobulin (IgG, IgM, IgA) and complement components (C1q, C4, C3c, C5). These data were correlated with histological grading of biopsies according to the Billingham criteria[94] and cytoimmunologic monitoring of blood samples.[97] Deposits of IgG associated with both blood capillaries and myocyte membranes were observed in nearly all of the biopsies examined. Similar deposits of fixed IgG have also been found in a high proportion of donor biopsy specimens collected prior to transplantation.[95] This can, therefore, be interpreted as the "normal" pattern of direct immunofluorescent staining, thereby increasing the difficulty of interpretation of both direct and indirect immunofluorescent staining patterns after transplantation. Following transplantation, the authors reported deposits of IgM and immune complexes around myocyte fibrils which were significantly more prevalent in biopsies with confirmed histopathological features of rejection. Others have reported that this histological picture of immunoglobulin and complement deposition within the heart is associated with decreased survival rates compared with typical cellular rejection.[98]

These studies confirm early findings of Maisch[99] and Harkiss[100] who demonstrated by indirect immunofluorescence that many cardiac transplant recipients develop circulating IgG and IgM antibodies after cardiac transplantation.

Many cardiac biopsies contain immunoglobulin deposits but their significance is not clear. There is considerable difficulty in interpreting immunofluorescence on the heart, especially when looking for IgG deposits. Excessive background due to the binding of "normal" serum to "normal" heart tissue[101] has been described. Hammond has called the phenomenon of vascular deposits of Ig and complement "vascular rejection" and suggests it is associated with poor survival.[98] However, Cherry et al.[102] investigated 46 biopsies for presence of linear deposits of immunoglobulin in the capillaries. He found that 39 of the 46 biopsies had vascular deposits of Ig and there was no significant correlation with anti-HLA antibodies in the circulation. Neither was there any correlation between these biopsies and the patient showing cardiac hemodynamic instability. The situation is further complicated by studies of Laberrere and colleagues[103] who suggest that the presence of IgM within biopsies, far from being a sign of rejection, is a sign of clinical stability.

Estimation of vascular damage is an important issue following cardiac transplantation, whether or not antibodies mediate the damage. Page-Faulk and colleages[104] suggest it can be estimated directly by looking for indices of vascular function concerned with hemostasis and coagulation. Using MoAbs against thrombomodulin, antithrombin III and fibrin and immunocytochemical techniques, they find clinical instability is associated with the presence of fibrin in the biopsies and down-regulation of endothelial reactivity for thrombomodulin and antithrombin III. Our labs found immunocytochemical evidence of endothelial activation/damage as assessed by increased expression of endothelial molecules, von-Willebrand's factor and Pal-E.[31]

ANTI-HEART ANTIBODIES DETECTED BY WESTERN BLOTTING

We have found results obtained using this technique to be easier to interpret than those generated by immunofluorescent analysis. The endogenous IgG and IgM can be clearly seen on the blots and distinguished from other bands of reactivity, which are directed against cardiac components. The sensitivity of the method can be increased further using an enhanced chemiluminescent (ECL) detection system.[105]

Using this methodology, a group of 22 patients who had undergone orthotopic heart transplantation were investigated for the first three months following transplantation.[106] Relatively few (2 of 22) patients had strong IgM and IgG circulating anti-heart antibodies prior to transplantation, but their presence was associated with unusually severe or frequent rejection episodes requiring more intensive immunosuppressive therapy during the first 3 postoperative months. The majority of patients (20 of 22) were found to produce anti-heart antibodies during the early post-transplant period. In 10 patients, there was an increased IgM response only; the other 10 demonstrated increases in IgM and IgG reactivity. In these patients there was no difference in the frequency of rejection episodes or the amount of methylprednisolone required. However, there was a difference in the severity of rejection episodes as assessed by the need for ATG or OKT3 therapy. Results of the studies using both immunofluorescent and Western blotting techniques show that the majority of patients make circulating antibodies that react with the myocardium in the early period following transplantation. The precise role of these circulating antibodies remains to be established.

ANTIBODIES DETECTED USING LYMPHOCYTOTOXIC ASSAYS

Panel Reactive Antibodies (PRAs)

It is now apparent that, as in the case of anti-heart antibodies detected by Western blotting or immunofluorescence of cardiac biopsies, the majority of patients produce lymphocytotoxic or Panel Reactive Antibodies during the initial 6 months following transplantation.[106–109] These antibodies have multiple specificities and are not necessarily related to the donor HLA typing. Unfortunately, in most cases the specificities remain unknown. Smith et al.[108] could only assign an HLA specificity in 50% of patients producing PRAs after transplantation; in none of these cases was the HLA specificity the same as the donor. The stimulus which elicits the production of these antibodies has not been established, although it has been suggested that they may be produced in response to HLA-determinants expressed by donors of blood used for pre- or perioperative transfusions.[110,111] Again, the situation concerning the relevance of these antibodies to rejection and graft survival is unclear. One group has reported a positive association of post-transplant PRA with frequency of rejection episodes[107] while Smith and colleagues[108] found no such correlation either with rejection frequency or 12-month graft survival.

An interesting question arising from these studies regards the longevity or persistence of these antibodies. The majority of studies are cross-sectional and not longitudinal. In the longitudinal study of Smith et al.,[108] 70% of patients were PRA positive at 2 months but only 15% were still positive at 12 months post-transplant. A short-lived response (lasting only months) might be expected if the stimulus is transient (e.g. blood transfusions) but a long-lived response might persist in the face of persistent alloantigen, such as expressed on the graft. A short-lived response would also be expected to be less clinically damaging than one characterized by continuous production of antibody. The kinetics of panel reactive antibody production suggest that they are short-lived and provide an interesting contrast with formation of anti-endothelial antibodies (see Chronic Rejection, below) which can appear early post-transplant and persist for a number of years.

Donor Specific Responses

Unlike panel reactive antibodies, the formation of donor reactive antibodies after transplantation has been associated with an increase in the severity of rejection episodes as diagnosed by the presence of resistance to steroid treatment.[108] The association was particularly noticeable when IgG antibodies were detected against donor HLA antigens. The HLA specificity of the response was confirmed by blocking studies that showed that 75% of these donor reactive responses could be blocked with monoclonal antibody against MHC determinants. Other studies have suggested that the occurrence of anti-HLA antibodies is underestimated using traditional tests because of blocking of antibodies by soluble HLA antigens or anti-idiotypic antibodies.[109] Using 421 serological samples from 65 cardiac transplant recipients, Suciu-Foca et al. increased the detection on anti-HLA antibodies from 23% to 42% by passing patients' sera through immunoabsorbant columns containing anti-MHC antibodies. The frequency of sera showing anti-HLA antibodies in the 21 patients who rejected their grafts during the first 36 months was 53% to 73% compared to 15% to 18% of sera from patients with functioning allografts. The same authors emphasized the apparent paradox that sera from 15%–18% of long-term patients also contained anti-HLA antibodies including anti-idiotypic antibodies in some stable patients. They suggest that formation of anti-idiotypic antibodies may be a method of blocking anti-HLA antibodies and might also explain the apparent cyclical variation in the appearance of these antibodies.

CHRONIC REJECTION

The integrity of the endothelium is recognized as being a crucial factor in maintaining normal vessel function. The "response to injury" hypothesis, first suggested by Ross[112] as an explanation for spontaneous coronary artery disease is also attractive as a hypothesis to explain transplant vaculopathy. In spontaneous CAD, it is postulated that mechanical forces (e.g. sheer stress) produce the initial endothelial injury, whereas in transplant vasculopathy an immunological injury to the endothelium would produce the initial insult. Thus, the damaged endothelium would allow egress of inflammatory cells, plasma proteins and lipids which would result in cytokine release and activation/proliferation of intimal cells. Following the initial immunological endothelial insult, a second stage may accelerate the process by non-immunological risk factors, such as high LDL cholesterol by mechanism not dissimilar to that in spontaneous CAD.

Stratification of transplant vasculopathy into early (within 2 years) and late (3–14 years) disease has revealed an association between acute rejection episodes and early but not late disease.[113] This evidence suggests the early more aggressive disease may have a different pathology involving more of an immunological component that late transplant vasculopathy. It is now recognized that direct recognition of MHC molecules presented by dendritic cells or endothelial cells is responsible for the rapid cellular events leading to acute rejection.[48] Recent evidence[114] suggests that indirect presentation (i. e. processing and presenting) of major and minor transplantation antigens (i.e. key cytosolic proteins) is extremely important in eliciting chronic graft rejection.

We have applied the technique of SDS-PAGE and Western blotting to demonstrate the occurrence of peptide-specific anti-endothelial antibodies in heart transplant recipients with accelerated coronary artery disease.[115] Circulating anti-endothelial cell antibodies were detected in the serum of 20 of 21 patients with angiographically-proven transplant vasculopathy within 2 years of transplantation compared with 9 of 20 cases without disease. A number of bands of reactivity were found; the bands most commonly associated with transplant vasculopathy were a doublet of endothelial cell proteins at 56 and 58 kDaltons. These bands were found in 15 of 21 patients with transplant vasculopathy. In contrast, only one sample from patients free of transplant vasculopathy demonstrated these polypeptides. Antibodies against 56 and 58 kDa, which are generally of the IgM type, were present in only three patients prior to transplantation.

Longitudinal studies of individual patients who developed transplant vasculopathy have shown that anti-endothelial antibodies are produced early after surgery and persist until the time of diagnosis.[116] Interestingly, among patients free of disease at 2 years, weak activity against endothelial cells was occasionally observed but did not persist.[116] The endothelial antigen of 56/58 kDa have been identified as the intermediate filament vimentin.[117] Vimentin is the intermediate filament characteristic of endothelial cells, smooth muscle cells and fibroblasts. An ELISA to detect anti-vimentin antibodies has been developed and is now being used for monitoring after transplantation. The formation of antibodies directed against vimentin may be found to reflect disease activity within the coronary arteries. Further understanding of the precise role of antibodies directed against endothelial cells in the pathogenesis of transplant vasculopathy awaits their further identification and characterization.

ACKNOWLEDGEMENTS

The work from the authors' laboratories described in this article is supported by the British Heart Foundation. I would like to thank Drs. Mike Dunn, Samantha Crisp, and John Smith for providing the illustrations.

REFERENCES

1. Ellis RJ, Lillehei CW, Fischetti VA, et al. Heart-reactive antibody: an index of cardiac rejection in human heart transplantation. Circulation 1970;42 (Supplement II) II-91–II-97.
2. Rose ML, Gracie JA, Fraser A, Chisholm P, Yacoub MH. Use of monoclonal antibodies to quantitate T lymphocyte subpopulations in human cardiac allografts. Transplantation 1984;38: 230–4.
3. Hoshinaga K, Mohanakumar T, Goldman MH, et al. Clinical significance of in situ detection of T lymphocyte subsets and monocyte/macrophage lineages in heart allografts. Transplantation 1984;38:634–7.
4. Rose ML, Page C, Hengstenberg C, Yacoub MH. Identification if antigen presenting cells in normal and transplanted human heart: Importance of endothelial cells. Human Immunology 1990;28: 179–85.
5. Imakita M, Cohnert TR, Billingham ME. Endocardial infiltrates: the "Quilty" effect. J Heart Transplant 1988;7:57–61.
6. Pardo-Mindan FJ, Lozano MD. "Quilty effect" in heart transplantation: Is it related to acute rejection? J Heart Transplant 1991;10:937–91.
7. Kemnitz J, Cohnert TR. Lymphoma-like lesion in human orthotopic cardiac allografts. Am J Clin Path 1988;89:430 (Abstract).
8. Nakhleh RE, Copenhaver CM, Werdin K, McDonald K, Kubo S, Strickler JG. Lack of evidence for involvement of Epstein-Barr virus in the development of the "Quilty" lesion of transplanted hearts: an in situ hybridization study. J Heart Transplant 1991:10:504–7.
9. DeLourdes P, Higuchi M, Campas de Assis RV, et al. Usefulness of T cell phenotype characteris-

tics in endomyocardial biopsy fragments from human cardiac allografts. J Heart Lung Transplant 1991;10:235–42.
10. Podack ER, Young JD, Cohn ZA. Isolation and biochemical and functional characterization of perforin 1 from cytolytic T cell granules. Proc Natl Acad Science 1985;82:8629–33.
11. Mueller C, Shelby J, Weissman IL, Peinat-Frey T, Eichwald EJ. Expression of the protease gene HF as a marker in rejecting allogeneic murine heart transplants. Transplantation 1991;51:514–7.
12. Griffiths GM, Namikawa R, Mueller C, Liu CC, Young JE, Billingham M, Weissman I. Granzyme A and perforin as markers of rejection in cardiac transplantation. Eur J Immunology 1991;21: 687–92.
13. Yoshinori S, Shinkai Y, Kawasaki A, Yagita H, Okumura K, Takaku F, Yazaki Y. Expression of perforin in infiltrating cells in murine hearts with acute myocarditis caused by Coxsackievirus B3. Circulation 1991;84:788–95.
14. Suitters AJ, Rose ML, Dominguez MJ, Yacoub MH. Selection of donor specific cytotoxic T cells within the allografted human heart. Transplantation 1990;49:1105–9.
15. Salmon RN, Maguire JA, Esmore D, Hancock WH. Analysis of proliferating cell nuclear antigen expression aids histologic diagnosis and is predictive of progression of human cardiac allograft rejection. Am J Path 1994;145:876–82.
16. Halloran PF, Madrenas J. The regulation of MHC transcription. Transplantation 1990;50:725–38.
17. Fleming KA, McMichael A, Morton JA, Woods J, McGee J. Distribution of HLA class I antigens in normal human tissue and in mammary cancer. J Clin Pathol 1981;34:779–84.
18. Daar AS, Fuggle SV, Fabre JW, Ting A, Morris PJ. The detailed distribution of HLA-A, B, C antigens in normal human organs. Transplantation 1984;38:287–92.
19. Natali PG, Bigotti A, Nicotra MR, Viora M, Manfredi D, Ferrone S. Distribution of human class I (HLA-A,B, C) histocompatibility antigens in normal and malignant tissues of non-lymphoid origin. Cancer Research 1984;44:4679–87.
20. Appleyard ST, Dunn MJ, Rose ML, Dubowitz V. Increased expression of HLA ABC class I antigens by muscle fibers in Duchenne dystrophy, inflammatory myopathy and other neuromuscular disorders. Lancet 1985;1:361–3.
21. Rose ML, Coles MI, Griffin RJ, Pomerance A, Yacoub MH. Expression of class I and class II major histocompatibility antigens in normal and transplanted human heart. Transplantation 1986;41: 776–80.
22. Suitters AJ, Rose ML, Higgins A, Yacoub MH. MHC antigen expression in sequential biopsies from transplant patients-correlation with rejection. Clin Experimental Immunology 1987;69: 575–83.
23. Ahmed-Ansari A, Tadros TS, Knopf WD, Murphy DA, Hertzler G, Feighan J, Letherby A, Sell KW. Histocompatibility complex class I and class II expression by myocytes in cardiac biopsies post-transplantation. Transplantation 1988;45:972–8.
24. Steinhoff G, Wonigeit K, Schafers HJ, Haverich A. Sequential analysis of monomorphic and polymorphic major histocompatibility complex antigen expression in human heart allograft biopsy specimens. J Heart Transplant 1989;8:360–7.
25. Milton AD, Fabre JW. Massive induction of donor type class I and class II major histocompatibility complex antigens during heart allograft rejection in the rat. J Experimental Medicine 1985; 161:98–112.
26. Ungureanu-Longrois D, Balligand JL, Simmons WW, Okada I, Kobzik L, Lowenstein CJ, Kunkel SL, Michel T, kelly RA, Smith TW. Induction of nitric oxide synthase activity by cytokines in venticular myocytes is necessary but not sufficient to decrease contractile responses to beta-adrenergic agonists. Circulation Research 1995;77:494–502.
27. Matsumori A, Yamada T, Suzuki H, Matoba Y, Sasayama S. Increased circulating cytokines in patients with myocarditis and cardiomyopathy. British Heart J 1994;72:561–6.
28. Labarrere CA, McIntyre JA, Halbrook H, Faulk WP. Major histocompatibility antigens in transplanted human hearts for perfusion. J Heart Lung Transplant 1991;10:409–15.
29. Hart DNJ, Fabre JW. Demonstration and characterization of Ia-positive dendritic cells in the interstial connective tissues of rat hearts and other tissues but not brain. J Exper Medicine 1981; 153:347–61.
30. Carforio ALP, Botazzo GF, Counihan PJ, Burke M, Poloniecki J, Davies MJ, Pepper JR. Class II major histocompatibility complex antigens on cardiac endothelium: an early marker of rejection in the transplanted human heart. Transpl Proceedings 1990;22:1830–3.
31. Hengstenberg C, Rose ML, Page C, Taylor PM, Yacoub MH. Immunocytochemical changes suggestive of damage to endothelial cells during rejection of human cardiac allografts. Transplantation 1990;49:895–9.
32. Page C, Rose ML, Piggott R, Yacoub MH. Heterogeneity of vascular endothelial cells. Am J Pathol 1993;141:673–83.

33. Fuggle SV, Errasti P, Daar AS, Fabre JW, Ting A, Morris PJ. Localization of major histocompatibility complex antigens (HLA-ABC and DR) antigens in 46 kidneys. Transplantation 1983; 35:385–90.
34. Carlquist JF, Hammond ME, Yowell RL, O'Connell J, Anderson JL. Correlation between class II antigen (DR) expression and interleukin-2 induced lymphocyte proliferation during acute cardiac allograft rejection. Transplantation 1990;50:582–8.
35. Taylor PM, Rose ML, Yacoub MH, Pigott R. Induction of vascular adhesion molecules during rejection of human cardiac allografts. Transplantation 1992;54:451–7.
36. Labarrere CA, Pitts D, Nelson DR, Faulk WP. Coronary artery disease in cardiac allografts; association with arteriolar endothelial HLA-DR and ICAM-1 antigens. Transplant Proc 1995;27: 1939–40.
37. Springer TA. Traffic signals for lymphocyte recirculation and leukocyte emigration: the multistep paradigm. Cell 1994;76:301–14.
38. Herskovitz A, Mayne AE, Willoughby SB, Kanter K, Ansari AA. Patterns of myocardial cell adhesion molecule expression in human endomyocardial biopsies after cardiac transplantation. Am J Path 1994;145:1082–94.
39. Briscoe DM, Yeung AC, Schoen EL, Allred EN, Stravrakis G, Ganz P, Cotran RS, Pober JS. Predictive value of inducible endothelial cell adhesion molecule expression for acute rejection of human cardiac allografts. Transplantation 1995;59:204–11.
40. Elices MJ, Osborn L, Takada Y, et al. VCAM-1 on activated endothelium interacts with leukocyte antigen VLA-4 at a site distinct from the VLA-4 fibronectin binding site. Cell 1990;60:577–82.
41. Stepkowski SM, Tu Y, Condon TP, Bennett CF. Blocking of heart allograft rejection by intercellular adhesion molecule-1 antisense oligonucleotides alone or in combination with other immunosuppressive modalities. J Immunol 1994:153:5336–46 [published erratum appears in J Immunol 1995;1:154:1521].
42. Isobe M, Suzuki J, Yamazaki S, Sekiguchi M. Acceptance of primary skin graft after treatment with anti-inter cellular adhesion molecule-1and anti-leukocyte function-associated antigen-1 monoclonal antibodies in mice. Transplantation 1996;62:411–13.
43. Brandt M, Steinmann J, Steinhoff G, Haverich A. Treatment with monoclonal antibodies to ICAM-1 and LFA-1 in rat heart allograft rejection. Transpant Int 1997;10:141–4.
44. Schowengerdt KO, Zhu JY, Stepkowski SM, Tu Y, Entman ML, Ballantyne CM. Cardiac allograft survival in mice deficient in intercellular adhesion molecule-1. Circulation 1995;92:82–7.
45. Lechler RJ, Batchelor JR. Restoration of immunogenecity to passenger cells depleted kidney allografts by the addition of donor strain dendritic cells. J Exper Med 1982;155:31–41.
46. Savage COS, hughes CWC, McIntyre BW, Picard JK, Pober JS. Human CD4+ T cells proliferate to HLA-DR+ allogeneic vascular endothelium. Identification of accessory interactions. Transplantation 1993;56:128–34.
47. Page C, Thompson C, Yacoub MH, Rose ML. Human endothelial stimulation of allogeneic T cells via a CTLA-4 independent pathway. Transplant Immunology 1994;2:342–7.
48. Pober JS, Orosz CG, Rose ML, Savage COS. Can graft endothelial cells initiate a host anti-graft response? Transplantation 1996;63 (*in Press*).
49. Linsley PS, Ledbetter JA. The role of the CD28 receptor during T cell responses to antigen. Ann Rev Immunol 1993;11:192–212.
50. Noelle RJ, Roy M, Shepherd DM, Stamenkovic I, Ledbetter JA, Aruffo A. A 39-kDa protein on activated helper T cells binds CD40 and transduces the signal for cognate activation of B cells. Proc Natl Acad Sci 1992;89:6550–4.
51. Buhlmann JE, Foy TM, Aruffo A, Crassi KM, Ledbetter JA, Green WR, Xu JC, Schultz LD, Roopesian D, Flavell RA. In the absence of CD40 signal, B cells are tolerogenic. Immunity 1995;2:645–53.
52. Muller DL, jenkins MK, Schwartz RH. Clonal expansion versus functional clonal inactivation: a costimulatory signaling pathway determines the outcome of T cell antigen receptor occupancy. Ann Rev Immunol 1989;7:445–80.
53. Pearson TC, Alexander DZ, Winn KJ, Linsley PS, Lowry RP, Larsen CP. Transplantation tolerance induced by CTLA4-Ig. Transplantation 1994;57:1701–6.
54. Larsen CP, Alexander DZ, Hollenbaugh D, Elwood ET, Ritchie SC, Aruffo A, Hendriz R, Pearson TC. CD40-gp39 interactions play a critical role during allograft rejection. Suppression of allograft rejection by blockade of the CD40-gp39 pathway. Transplantation 1996;61:4–9.
55. Larsen CP, Elwood ET, Alexander DZ, Ritchie SC, Hendriz R, Tucker P, Burden C, Cho HR, Aruffo A, Hollenbaugh D, Linsley PS, Winn KJ, Pearson TC. Long-term acceptance of skin and cardiac allografts after blocking CD40 and CDE28 pathways. Nature 1996;381:434–8.
56. Ruel RM, Fang JC, Denton MD, Geehan C, Long C, Mutchell RN, Ganz P, Briscoe DM. CD40 and CD40 liogand (CD154) are coexpressed on microvessels in vivo in human cardiac allograft rejection. Transplantation 1997;64:1765–74.

57. Mach M, Schonbeck U, Sukhova GK, Bourcier T, Bonnefoy JY, Pober JS, Libby P. Functional CD40 ligand is expressed on human vascular endothelial cells, smooth muscle cells and macrophages: implication for CD40-CD40 ligand signaling in atherosclerosis. Proc Natl Acad Sci 1997;94: 1931–6.
58. Houer LW, de los Santos RP, Hoyer JR. Antihaemophilic factor antigen: localization in endothelial cells by immunofluorescent microscopy. J Clin Investigation 1973;52:2737–44.
59. Labarrere CA, Pitts D, halbrook H, Faulk PW. Natural anticoagulant pathways in normal and transplanted human hearts. J Heart Lung Transplant 1992;11:342–7.
60. Schultz R, Panas DL, Catena R, Moncada S, Olley PM, Lopachuk GD. The role of nitric oxide in cardiac depression induced by interleukin-1 beta and tumor necrosis factor alpha. Br J Pharm 1995;114:27–34.
61. Arbustini E, Grasso M, Diegoli M, Bramerio M, Scott Foglienei A, Albertario M, Matinelli L, Gavazzi A, Goggi C, Camapna C, Vigano M. Expression of tumor necrosis factor in human acute cardiac rejection. An immunohistochemical and immunoblotting study. Am J Pathol 1991;139: 709–15.
62. Ruan XM, Qiao JH, Trento A, Czer LS, Blanche C, Fishbein MC. Cytokine expression and endothelial cell and lymphocyte activation in human cardiac allograft rejection: an immunocytohistochemical study of endomyocardial samples. J Heart Lung Transplant 1992;11:110–15.
63. Noronha IL, Eberlein Gonska M, Hartley B, Stephens S, Cameron JS, Waldherr R. in situ expression of tumor necrosis factor alpha, interferon gamma, and interleukin-2 receptors in renal allograft biopsies. Transplantation 1992;54:1017–24.
64. Cunningham DA, Dunn MJ, Yacoub MH, Rose ML. Local production of cytokines in the human cardiac allograft. Transplantation 1994;57:133–7.
65. Dallman MJ, Larsen CP, Morris PJ. Cytokine gene transcription in vascularized organ grafts: analysis using semiquantitative polymerase chain reaction. J Exper Med 1991;174:493–6.
66. Wu CJ, Lovett M, Wong-Lee J, Moeller F, Kitamura M, Goralski TJ, Billingham ME, Starnes VA, Clayberger C. Cytokine gene expression in rejecting cardaic allografts. Transplantation 1992;54: 326–32.
67. Azzawi M, Hasleton PS, Grant SCD, Stewart JP, Hutchinson IV. Interleukin-10 in human heart transplantation: an in situ hybridization study. J Heart Lung Transplant 1995;14:519–28.
68. Nickerson P, Steurer W, Stiger J, Zheng X, Steele AW, Strom TB. Cytokines and the Th1/Th2 paradigm in transplantation. Curr Opin Immunol 1994;6:757–64.
69. Seder RA, Gazzinelli R, Sher A, paul WE. Interleukin 12 acts directly on CDE4+ T cells to enhance priming for interferon gamma production and diminishes interleukin 4 inhibition of such priming. Proc Natl Acad Sci 1993;90:10188–92.
70. Giri JG, Ahdieh M, Eisenman J, Shanebeck K, Brabstein K, Kumaki S, Namen A, Park LS, Cosman D, Anderson D. Utilization of the beta and gamma chains of theIL-2 receptor by the novel cytokine IL-15. EMBO J 1994;13:2822–30.
71. Russell ME. Macrophage and transplant ateriosclerosis: known and novel molecules. J Heart Lung Transplant 1995;14:S111–15.
72. Pavlakis M, Strehlau J, Lipman M, Shapiro M, Maslinski W, Strom TB. Intragraft IL-15 transcripts are increased in human renal allograft rejection. Transplantation 1996;62:543–5.
73. van Gelder T, Baan CC, Balk AH, Knoop CJ, Holweg CT, van der Meer P, Mochtar B, Zondervan PE, Niesters HG, Weimar W. Blockade of interleukin (IL)-2/IL-2 receptor pathway with a monoclonal anti-IL-2 receptor antibody (BT 563) does not prevent the development of acute heart allograft rejection in humans. Transplantion 1998;65:405–10.
74. Yang X, Chowdhury N, Cai B, et al. Induction of myocardial nitric oxide synthase by cardiac allograft rejection. J Clin Invest 1994;94:714–21.
75. Worrall NK, Chang K, Suau GM, et al. Inhibition of inducible nitric oxide synthase prevents myocardial and systemic vascular barrier dysfunction during early cardiac allograft rejection. Circ Research 1996;78:769–79.
76. Worrall NK, Misko TP, Sullivan PM, Hui JJ, Rodi CP, Ferguson TB. Corticosteroids inhibit expression of inducible nitric oxide synthase during acute cardiac allograft rejection. Transplantation 1996;61:324–8.
77. Cai B, Roy DK, Sciacca R, Michler RE, Cannon PJ. Effects of immunosuppressive therapy on expression of inducible nitric oxide synthase (iNOS) during cardiac allograft rejection. Int J Cardiol 1995;50:243–51.
78. Cui S, Reichner JS, Mateo RB, Albina JE. Activated murine macrophages induce apoptosis in tumor cells through nitric oxide-dependent or—independent mechanisms. Cancer Res 1994;54:2462–7.
79. Szabolcs M, Michler RE, Yang X, et al. Apoptosis of cardiac myocytes during cardiac allograft rejection. Relation to induction of nitric oxide synthase. Circulation 1996;94:1665–73.
80. Szabolcs MJ, Ravalli S, Minanov O, Sciacca RR, Michler RE, Canjnon PJ. Apoptosis and increased

expression of inducible nitric oxide synthase in human allograft rejection. Transplantation 1998;65:804–12.
81. Patel R, Terasaki PI. Significance of the positive crossmatch test in kidney transplantation. N Eng J Med 1969;280:735–9.
82. Auchincloss H. Xenografting: a review. Transplantation Reviews 1990;4:14–27.
83. Brasile L, Zerbe T, Rabin B, et al. Identification of the antibody to vascular endothelial cells in patients undergoing cardiac transplantation. Transplantation 1985;40:672–5.
84. Trento A, Hardesty RL, Griffith BP, et al. Role of the antibody to vascular endothelial cells in hyperacute rejection in patients undergoing cardiac transplantation. J Thor and Cardiovasc Surg 1988;95:37–41.
85. Kemnitz J, Cremer J, Restropo-Specht I, et al. Hyperacute rejection in heart allografts. Path Res and Practice 1991;187:23–9.
86. Weill R, Clarke DR, Iwaki Y, et al. Hyperacute rejection of a transplanted human heart. Transplantation 1981;32:71–2.
87. Singh G, Thompson M, Griffith B, et al. Histocompatibility in cardiac transplantation with particular reference to immunopathology of positive serologic crossmatch. Clin Immunology and Immunopatholgy 1983;28:56–66.
88. Yacoub M, Ferstenstein H, Doyle P, et al. The influence of HLA matching in cardiac allograft recipients receiving cyclosporine and azathioprine. Transplant Proc 1987;19:2487–9.
89. McCloskey D, Ferstenstein H, Banner N, et al. The effect of HLA lymphocytotoxic antibody status and crossmatch on cardiac transplant survival. Transplan Proc 1989;21:804–6.
90. Smith JD, Danskine AJ, Laylor RM, et al. The effect of panel reactive antibodies and the donor specific crossmatch on graft survival after heart and lung transplantation. Transplant Immunology 1993;1:60–5.
91. Lavee J, Kormos RL, Duquesnoy RJ, et al. Influence of panel-reactive antibody and lymphocytotoxic crossmatch on survival after heart transplantation. J Heart Lung Transpl 1991;10:921–30.
92. Taylor CJ, Chapman JR, Ting A, et al. Characterization of lymphocytotoxic antibodies causing a positive crossmatch in renal transplantation. Transplantation 1989;48:953–8.
93. Cerilli J, Brasile L, Galouzis T, et al. The vascular endothelial cell antigen system. Transplantation 1985;39:286–9.
94. Billingham ME, Cary NRB, Hammond EH, et al. A working formulation for the standardization of nomenclature in the diagnosis of heart and lung rejection: heart rejection study group. J Heart Transp 1990;9:587–91.
95. Schuurman HJ, Jambroes G, Borleffs JCC, et al. Acute humoral rejection after heart transplantation. Transplantation 1988;46:603–5.
96. Schuurman HJ, Gmelig-Meyling FHJ, Wijngaard PLJ, et al. Endomyocardial biopsies after heart transplantation. Transplantation 1989;48:435–8.
97. Wijngaard PL, van der Meulen A, Schuurman HJ, et al. Cytoimmunologic monitoring for the diagnosis of acute rejection after heart transplantation. Transpl Proceedings 1989;21:2521–2.
98. Hammond EH, Yowell RL, Nunoda S, et al. Vascular (humoral) rejection in heart transplantation: pathologic observations and clinical implications. J Heart Transplant 1989;8:430–43.
99. Maisch B, Hufnagel G, Bauer E, et al. Value of immunohistological and immunoserological monitoring in cardiac transplantation. Eur Hear J 1987;8:29–34.
100. Harkiss GD, Cave P, Brown DL, et al. Anti-heart antibodies in cardiac allograft recipients. Int Arch Allergy and Applied Immunology 1984;73:18–22.
101. Lowry PJ, Thompson RA, Littler WA. Humoral immunity in cardiomyopathy. Br Heart J 1983; 50:390–4.
102. Cherry R, Nielson H, Reed E, Reemsta K, Suciu-Foca N, Marboe C. Vascular (humoral) rejection in human cardiac allograft biopsies: relation to circulating anti-HLA antibodies. J Heart Lung Transplantation 1992;11:24–30.
103. Labarrere CA, Pitts D, Halbrook H, Page Faulk W. Immunoglobulin M antibodies in transplanted human hearts. J Heart Lung Transplantation 1993;12:394–402.
104. Page Faulk W, Labarrere CA, Pitts D, Halbrook H. Vascular lesions in biopsy specimens devoid of cellular infiltrates: qualitative and quantitative immunocytochemical studies of human cardiac allografts. J Heart Lung Transplantation 1993;12:219–29.
105. Simmonds J, Price R, Corbett J, et al. Enhanced chemiluminescence detection of Western blotted proteins from two-dimensional SDS PAGE. In: Dunn MJ (ed):2-D PAGE '91: Proceedings of the International Meeting on Two-Dimensional Electrophoresis. London, NHLI, 1991, pp. 46–8.
106. Dunn MJ, Rose ML, Latif N, et al. Demonstration by Western blotting of antiheart antibodies before and after cardiac transplantation. Transplantation 1991;51:806–12.
107. Fenoglio J, Ho E, Reed E, et al. Anti-HLA antibodies and heart allograft survival. Transpl Proceedings 1989;21:807–9.

108. Smith JD, Danskine AJ, Rose ML, et al. Specificity of lymphocytotoxic antibodies formed after cardiac transplantation and correlation with rejection episodes. Transplantation 1992;53:1358–62.
109. Suciu-Foca N, Reed N, Marboe C, et al. The role of anti-HLA antibodies in heart transplantation. Transplantation 1991;51:716–24.
110. Opeltz G, Graver B, Mickey R, et al. Lymphocytotoxic antibody responses to transfusions in potential kidney transplant recipients. Transplantation 1981;32:177–83.
111. Scornick JC, Ireland JE, Howard J, et al. Assessment of the risk for broad sensitization by blood transfusions. Transplantation 1984;37:249–52.
112. Ross R. The pathogenesis of atherosclerosis-an update. N Eng J Med 1986;314:488–500.
113. Hornick P, Smith JS, Pomerance A, Mitchell A, Banner NJ, Rose ML, Yaoub MH. Influence of acute rejection episodes, HLA matching and donor/recipient phenotype on the development of early transplant-associated coronary artery disease. Circulation 1997;96: II-48-II-53.
114. Hornick P, Mason PD, Yacoub MH, Rose ML, Batchelor R, Lechler RL. Assessment of the contribution that direct allorecognition makes to the progression of chronic cardiac transplant rejection in humans. Circulation 1998;97:1257–63.
115. Dunn MJ, Crisp S, Rose ML, et al. Detection of anti-endothelial antibodies by Western blotting-positive correlation with coronary artery disease after cardiac transplantation. Lancet 1992;39: 1566–70.
116. Crisp SJ, Dunn MJ, Rose ML, Barbir M, Yacoub MH. Anti-endothelial antibodies after heart transplantation: the accelerating factor in transplant-associated coronary artery disease. J Heart Lung Transplant 1994;13:81–92.
117. Wheeler CH, Collins A, Dunn MJ, Crisp SJ, Yacoub MH, Rose ML. Characterization of endothelial antigens associated with transplant associated coronary artery disease. J Heart Lung Transplantation 1995;14:S188–97.

3. IMMUNOBIOLOGY OF CHRONIC CARDIAC ALLOGRAFT REJECTION

Petri Koskinen, Jussi Tikkanen, Roope Sihvola, Pekka Häyry, Karl Lemström
Transplantation Laboratory, Cardiopulmonary Research Group of Transplantation Laboratory, University of Helsinki, and Helsinki University Central Hospital, Helsinki, Finland

Cardiac transplantation is currently the only method available to return patients with end-stage heart disease to normal life. The success of intrathoracic organ transplantation has increased constantly over the past decade as a result of new surgical techniques, immunosuppressive protocols, and innovations in managing acute rejection and infection, particularly cytomegalovirus (CMV) infection. Despite the substantial improvement in early survival, the long-term survival rate has not increased during the past decade.

CLINICAL AND HISTOLOGICAL MANIFESTATIONS

Chronic rejection has emerged as a major obstacle affecting cardiac allograft survival in the long run.[1] In cardiac allografts, chronic rejection, i.e., cardiac allograft vasculopathy (CAV) manifests itself clinically as a diffuse decrease in ventricular performance with ultimate graft failure, acute myocardial infarction, or sudden death.[2] CAV is characterized histologically by persistent low-grade perivascular inflammation, smooth muscle cell (SMC) proliferation, and intimal thickening[3] (Figure 1, see color plates section, back of book) and usually affects the entire length of the vessel wall and, more importantly, also involves the small penetrating intramyocardial branches.[4] In endomyocardial biopsies activated T cells and macrophages are found in cellular infiltrates within the graft vasculature. Upregulation of MHC class II antigen expression on the vascular endothelial cells suggests the role of immunologically mediated mechanisms in the development of this disorder.[5]

Address correspondence to: Dr. Petri Koskinen, MD, Cardiopulmonary Research Group, of Transplantation Laboratory, University of Helsinki and Helsinki University Central Hospital, P.O. Box 21 (Haartmaninkatu 3), FIN-00014 Helsinki, Finland, Tel +358-9-1912 6590, Fax +358-9-2411 227, e-mail: Petri.Koskinen@Helsinki.Fi

IMMUNOLOGICAL AND NONIMMUNOLOGICAL RISK FACTORS FOR CHRONIC REJECTION

The pathophysiology and mechanisms of chronic rejection in intrathoracic organs are poorly known, but clinical studies have suggested several risk factors contributing to the development of chronic rejection. Histocompatibility is of prime importance.[6–8] Additional risk factors in cardiac allografts are the frequency and/or intensity of acute rejections,[9–13] and humoral immune response.[14]

Apart from immunological factors, risk factors of nonimmunological origin contribute to chronic rejection. Prolonged cold ischemia time,[15] hyperlipidemia,[16–19] recipient characteristics such as younger or older age, female gender, pretransplant ischemic heart disease, and donor characteristics such as older age and female gender have been reported to the development of CAV.[20] Cytomegalovirus infection may also be a contributing factor but its importance has been dispuuted by some investigators.[21–26]

IDENTIFIED RISK FACTORS IN EXPERIMENTAL TRANSPLANTATION

In rats, it has been clearly demonstrated that the stronger the histoincompatibility between strains, the more severe are the histological changes in the cardiac allografts attributable to CAV.[27] Acute rejection has been shown to be a clear risk factor for the development of CAV in rabbit cardiac allografts.[28] The role of hypercholesterolemia in the pathogenesis of CAV remains controversial in experimental studies. Alonso et al. demonstrated that hypercholesterolemia increases the severity of cardiac graft vasculopathy[29] whereas studies in the rat demonstrate that feeding the animals with cholesterol-rich diet did not enhance intimal thickening in aortic[30] or cardiac allografts.[31] However, combined hypercholesterolemia and hypertriglyceridemia significantly increased arteriosclerotic changes in rat aortic allografts.[32]

THE RELATIONSHIP OF CMV INFECTION AND CARDIAC ALLOGRAFT VASCULOPATHY

We became interested in the relationship between CMV infection and acute allograft rejection in mid-80's, when a very high frequency of late acute rejection was observed in CMV-infected renal transplant recipients.[33] Concomitant fine needle aspiration biopsies of the kidneys demonstrated high levels of class II expression in graft parenchymal cells in patients with prior CMV disease, and moderately elevated levels of serum creatinine. A plausible explanation for this finding was provided later by Rubin et al. (personal communication) who suggested that several disorders including sepsis and rejection, lead to release of tumor necrosis factor which, upon binding to its receptor, activates the Nuclear Factor-κB (NF-κB). Tumor necrosis factor (TNF)-α is also able to stimulate the activity of the CMV-IE enhancer/promoter region.[34] CMV infection of several cell lines leads to NF-kB activation.[35] NF-kB binding sites are present in regulatory regions of various cellular and viral genes including the IE enhancer region of CMV.[36] In a reciprocal situation, CMV infection, most likely via gamma-interferon, leads to upregulation of MHC antigens in the allograft and, thereby, increases its immunogenicity. Although other explanations may exist, for example sequence homology in CMV immediate early antigen and class II β-chain,[37] and the β2 microglobulin chain of class I serving as a receptor for CMV,[38] the NF-NF-1B pathway provides the most logical explanation for these findings.

Several groups later reported that CMV infection is related to accelerated cardiac allograft vasculopathy,[21–24] and a relationship between CMV infection and classical atherosclerosis was also suspected.[39,40] We confirmed these findings in the prospective Helsinki Protocol Biopsy Study,[41,42] and moreover, demonstrated in endomyocardial biopsy specimens that CMV infection leads to early morphological endothelial activation preceding the intimal proliferation and thickening.[43]

This observation lead to investigation of the mechanisms of this disorder in experimental animals, using aortic and cardiac allografts. The results can be summarized as follows: infection of the recipient rat with rat CMV virus resulted in an early inflammatory response in allograft vascular adventitia and in the intima (endothelialitis),[43] followed by an increase in intimal nuclear content and intimal thickness. These events temporally coincided with early activation of inflammatory leukocytes in the allograft adventitia (acute rejection), and increased expression of platelet derived growth factor (PDGF)-BB, transforming growth factor (TGF)-beta, and basic fibroblast growth factor (bFGF) mRNA by reverse transcriptase polymerase chain reaction.[44]

When the recipient rats were treated with gancyclovir (DHPG), the enhanced intimal response was entirely abolished.[45] Gancyclovir-treatment dramatically reduced the inflammatory response in the allograft[46] and thereby, growth factor synthesis in response to injury. However, gancyclovir did not prevent the expression of IE antigen of CMV.[47] Speir et al. demonstrated that SMC migrating to the intima in coronary restenosis express elevated levels of CMV IE antigen IE84 and tumor suppressor protein p53, suggesting that IE84 inactivates p53 and predisposes SMC to increased growth.[48]

Whether these observations are applicable to humans has recently been investigated by Valantine et al. Using coronary intravascular ultrasound as an endpoint, parenteral gancyclovir treatment for the first 28 days post transplantation, compared to placebo, reduced the incidence of transplant vaculopathy at 5 years from 60% to 40% in all patients and from 62% to 32% in patients not receiving concomitant calcium channel blockers (personal communication).

Taken together, CMV infection and (late) acute allograft rejection appear to be intimately linked, possibly with NF-kB as a common molecular mediator. CMV infection predisposes the recipient to chronic allograft rejection, and gancyclovir prophylaxis abolishes the enhanced response in experimental animals and decreases its likelihood in man.

CYTOKINES IN CARDIAC ALLOGRAFT VASCULOPATHY

In our laboratory, we have used a heterotopic rat cardiac allograft model from DA to WF rats under triple-drug immunosuppression (methylprednisolone

0.5 mg/kg/day, azathioprine 2 mg/kg/day, and three different doses of cyclosporine (CsA 5, 10, and 20 mg/kg/day)). Our results demonstrate that low level CsA (trough blood level 200 ug/l) is associated with severe intimal cell accumulation and intimal thickening in cardiac allograft arteries which nearly occludes the lumen of the vessels within 3 months after transplantation. Intermediate dose of CsA (blood trough level ranging from 400–900 ug/l) significantly inhibited intimal thickening, while the high dose of CsA (blood trough level ranging from >1200 ug/l) totally abolished the vascular changes of cardiac allograft.[49] These vasculopathic alterations were significantly associated with endothelial expression of P-selectin[50] and vascular cell adhesion molecule-1 (VCAM-1) as well as perivascular inflammation composed of ED3+ activated macrophages and CD4+ T cells.[49] In these allografts, the expression of TNF-α, a cytokine inducing both P-selectin and VCAM-1 expression, was upregulated in vascular media cells, intimal cells, and in interstitial mononuclear cells.[50] In nonimmunosuppressed rabbit cardiac allografts, a strong relationship exists between TNF-α expression and SMC proliferation in the coronary arteries of acutely rejecting hearts.[51] Furthermore, soluble TNF-α receptor reduced the incidence and intensity of intimal thickening in rabbit cardiac allografts.[52] Thus, TNF-α may provide an early marker of SMC activation and a novel therapeutic target for the prevention of CAV.

Messenger RNA (mRNA) transcript levels of additional cytokines such as IL1,[53] IFN-γ,[54] MCP-1,[55] iNOS,[56] AIF-1 and 2,[57] Gal/GalNac,[58] and ET-1[59] are also typically increased in cardiac allografts compared to syngeneic grafts and may contribute to the development of graft vasculopathy. These factors are expressed by a subset of the mononuclear cell population that infiltrate the perivascular space and interstitium.

PLATELET-DERIVED GROWTH FACTOR AND OTHER GROWTH FACTORS IN CARDIAC ALLOGRAFT VASCULOPATHY

Studies on PDGF ligand and receptor expression in ordinary atherosclerotic lesions have suggested a regulatory role for PDGF in vascular wall proliferative disease.[60] PDGF is a major mitogen for mesenchymally derived cells such as SMC and fibroblasts.[61] The PDGF ligand consists of a disulphide-linked dimer of two polypeptides, the PDGF-A and PDGF-B chains, and can be expressed in the form of homodimers (PDGF-AA or -BB) or a heterodimer (PDGF-AB).[61] Two separate PDGF receptors (PDGF-Rα and PDGF-Rβ) have been identified.[62] These receptors exist as monomers on the cell surface, but signal transduction by PDGF requires receptor dimerization.[63] PDGF-Rβ binds only the PDGF-B chain, whereas PDGF-Rα binds both the A and B chains.[63] Dimerization of receptor molecules, followed by autophosphorylation of the receptor protein-tyrosinase kinase, initiates the signalling cascades and leads to the biological responses of PDGF.[62,64]

Utilizing a panel of antibodies (Table 1), we have found that the expression of PDGF-AA, -Rα, and -Rβ- in intimal cells, and PDGF-BB in macrophages at the protein level correlates with the development of cardiac allograft vasculopathy.[65] Therefore, we hypothesized that PDGF may have a *rate-limiting* role in the devel-

Table 1. Correlation of Growth Factor and Cytokine Expression with Intimal Thickness in Chronically Rejecting Cardiac Allografts 3 Months after Transplantation

	Arteries and Arterioles							
Antigen	Perivascular infiltrate	Media	Neointima	Endothelium	Cardiomyocyte	Mononuclear Cells	Fibrotic Area	Capillary Endothel
PDGF-AA	0.497	0.853***	0.807***	0.428	0.173	0.534*	—	0.742**
PDGF-BB	0.118	0.524*	0.250	—	0.591*	0.570*	0.285	0.180
VEGF	0.271	0.385	0.669*	0.700**	0.848***	0.634*	0.183	—
TGF-pan	0.085	0.676**	0.667**	0.061	0.689**	0.135	0.380	0.441
TNF-α	0.071	0.549*	0.536*	0.441	0.271	0.596*	0.071	0.367

The ralatioship between intimal thickness and antigen expression was examined using a linear regression analysis, and the result given as correlation coefficients (*r*). *P < 0.05, **P < 0.01, ***P < 0.001.

opment of this disease. The hypothesis was tested in a rat model of heterotopic cardiac allografts. When recipient animals received CGP 53716, a PDGF-R protein-tyrosine kinase inhibitor, a significant reduction in the incidence and intensity of vasculopathic lesions was noted.[66] When smooth muscle cells (SMC) were stimulated *in vitro* with PDGF-AA or BB in the presence IL-1β or TNF-α, CGP 53716 significantly inhibited only A-ligand but not B-ligand induced replication. Concomitantly in quantitative RT-PCR, IL-1β or TNF-α stimulation specifically upregulated the expression of PDGF-Ra mRNA but not of other ligand or receptor genes in cultured SMC (Sihvola et al., submitted). Thus, it appears that a PDGF-A—Rα dependent cycle is induced in the generation of allograft vasculopathy which may be inhibited by blocking of signaling downstream of PDGF-R.

Additional growth factors that have been linked to the pathogenesis of CAV include TGF-β, bFGF, and VEGF (Lemström et al., unpublished observations) (Table 1). Of these, TGF-β, in addition to TNF-α, and IL-1, released by macrophages and T cells have been shown to induce autocrine stimulation of SMC by PDGF-AA. IL-1 and TNF-α also stimulate fibronectin production, which may serve to traffic and trap inflammatory cells (particularly in the subendothelium) into the wall and periphery of the vessels in the graft. In rat cardiac allografts with chronic rejection, bFGF was detected in mast cells and the intensity of intramyocardial mast cell infiltration was linked to the intensity of CAV (Koskinen et al., unpublished observations).

T CELL AND MACROPHAGE ACTIVATION PATHWAYS

The receptor-ligand pairs CD28-B7 and CD40-CD40L (gp39) are essential for the initiation and amplification of T cell dependent immune responses.[67,68] CD28-B7 interactions provide the second signals necessary for optimal T cell activation and IL-2 production,[69–71] whereas CD40-CD40L (gp39) signals costimulate B cell, macrophage, endothelial cell and T cell activation.[72–78] T cells that produce IL-2 and

IFN-γ, termed Th1 cells, are associated with T cell and macrophage activation. In contrast, T cells that produce IL-4 and IL-5, termed Th2 cells, augment humoral responses and inhibit Th1 responses. Activated macrophages secrete multipotent cytokines and growth factors[79] that may act synergistically or in concert in the inflammatory reactions of chronic rejection. Either blockade of CD28-B7 costimulatory pathway or blockade of the CD28 and CD40 pathways has been shown to inhibit the development CAV in rodents.[80,81]

KNOCK-OUT ANIMAL MODELS IN CHRONIC REJECTION

Studies in knock-out animals have confirmed alloantigen-related, alloantigen-unrelated and infectious origins of allograft vasculopathy. Murine heart allografts transplanted into severe combined immune deficient (SCID) mice generate no intimal response, but do so if the recipients are reconstituted with donor-directed cytotoxic antibody.[82] Depletion of T cells, humoral antibody response, CD4 cells and/or macrophages, all reduce allograft vasculopathy in murine knock-out models.[83] A recent study of heart transplants in IFN-γ, IL-4, and IL-10 knock-out mice revealed a reduced graft survival in IFN-γ and IL-10 knock-out recipients whereas IL-4 knock-out recipients had a graft survival time comparable to wild-type animals.[84] Decreased graft survival in IFN-γ knock-out recipients was related to higher levels of IL-2 transcripts and alterations with macrophage activation. In IL-10 knock-out recipients, increases in iNOS and IFN-γ-driven responses were observed. In grafts of IL-4 knock-out animals, higher levels of CD3 transcripts and TNF-α levels were recorded suggesting that IL-4 may regulate T cell infiltration through TNF-α mediated inflammatory cell recruitment.[84]

Working Hypothesis of Chronic Rejection

The end-point of CAV is a fibroproliferative lesion occluding the vascular lumen. The proliferative behaviour of smooth muscle cells is a key element in the disease processes. Smooth muscle cells exist in two different phenotypes, the so-called "contractile" phenotype which is prominent in adulthood, and the so called "synthetic" phenotype which is prominent during embryonal life. During the proliferative process, there is a phenotypic shift from the contractile to the synthetic type; only the latter type is able to replicate.[85] In vitro studies have demonstrated that a variety of molecules are expressed in the vascular wall during the development of obstructive arteriopathy that may potentially control the migration and proliferation of smooth muscle cell.[86] These molecules include peptide growth factors, cytokines, vasoactive hormones, and lipid mediators of inflammation.

Based upon experimental results, blockade of the T cell activation pathway by CsA attenuates cardiac allograft vasculopathy in a dose-dependent fashion, suggesting that T cell activation is a proximal event in the cascade that culminates in graft disease. We believe that the final immunological pathway in the development of sclerotic changes is mediated by a delayed-type hypersensitivity (DTH) like-reaction, whereby macrophages and CD4+ T cells have a major initiating role and the final effector molecules, cytokines and growth factors, are similar to those operating in other sclerotic arteriopathies (Figure 2).

Paul et al. have recently initiated a systematic study to investigate which additional genes may be expressed in the vascular wall during the development of vasculopathy. Using differential display (DD-) PCR of <10% of the RNA, preliminary results suggest that >300 genes are activated, in addition of these described above.

CURRENT PARADIGM FOR PREVENTION

Reduction of allograft vasculopathy by immunosuppressive treatment using high-dose cyclosporine,[49,87] rapamycin,[88] deoxyspergualin,[89] mycophenolate mofetil[90] or CTL4Ig,[91] all reflect an active immunological component to chronic rejection. Conversely, triple anti-hypertensive drug treatment,[92,93] essential fatty-acid deficient diet,[56] small molecular weight heparins[90] and treatment with anti-lipidemic 3-hydroxy-3-methyl-glutanyl-coenzyme A reductase inhibitors have been shown to inhibit allograft vasculopathy not only in rat models but also in humans,[95] speak for non-immunological contribution. A most powerful drug in the treatment of both experimental[46] and clinical chronic rejection in heart transplantation is the well-established anti-viral drug ganciclovir. This drug has two possible mechanisms of action: elimination of virus and the virus-induced inflammatory response which leads to stimulation of smooth mucle cells by cytokines, eikosanoids and growth factors[46] and/or inhibition of early viral protein IE84 -induced p53 inactivation in smooth muscle cells.[35]

As expected, a whole number of genes are differentially expressed at the induction and during the proliferation of allograft vasculopathy. They consist of adhesion ligands and their receptors in the graft endothelium and inflammatory leukocytes, including the Ig-superfamily genes (ICAM, VCAM, class II), selectins, integrins and lectins.[50] Considering the chemotactic events of leukocytes to abluminal direction and smooth muscle cells towards the lumen, it is not unexpected that a number of cytokines and chemokines are seen.[54] Also classical growth factors known to be related to smooth muscle cell replication or migration and/or to endothelial repair after injury are prominently expressed in both human and rat allografts undergoing chronic rejection.[96] Finally, and not unexpectedly, vasoactive hormones such as endothelin-1,[59] matrix metalloproteinases, tissue inhibitors of matrix metalloproteinases and inducible nitric oxide synthetase are frequently detected. Paul and Russell have identified still additional genes, either up- or down-regulated as a consequence of allograft vascular injury.[97,98] Thus, we may expect that between 100–300 differentially expressed genes may eventually be recorded when comparing chronically rejecting to stabile allografts. The question remains, which of these genes are rate-limiting, i.e., potential targets of therapy.

Although both clinical and experimental studies have clearly demonstrated that a large number of predisposing factors contribute to chronic rejection, most clinical investigators still believe that chronic rejection can be prevented by improving the quality of immunosuppressive therapy and by reducing the frequency of acute episodes of rejection.

Acute rejection is not a single entity. It may display itself with different intensi-

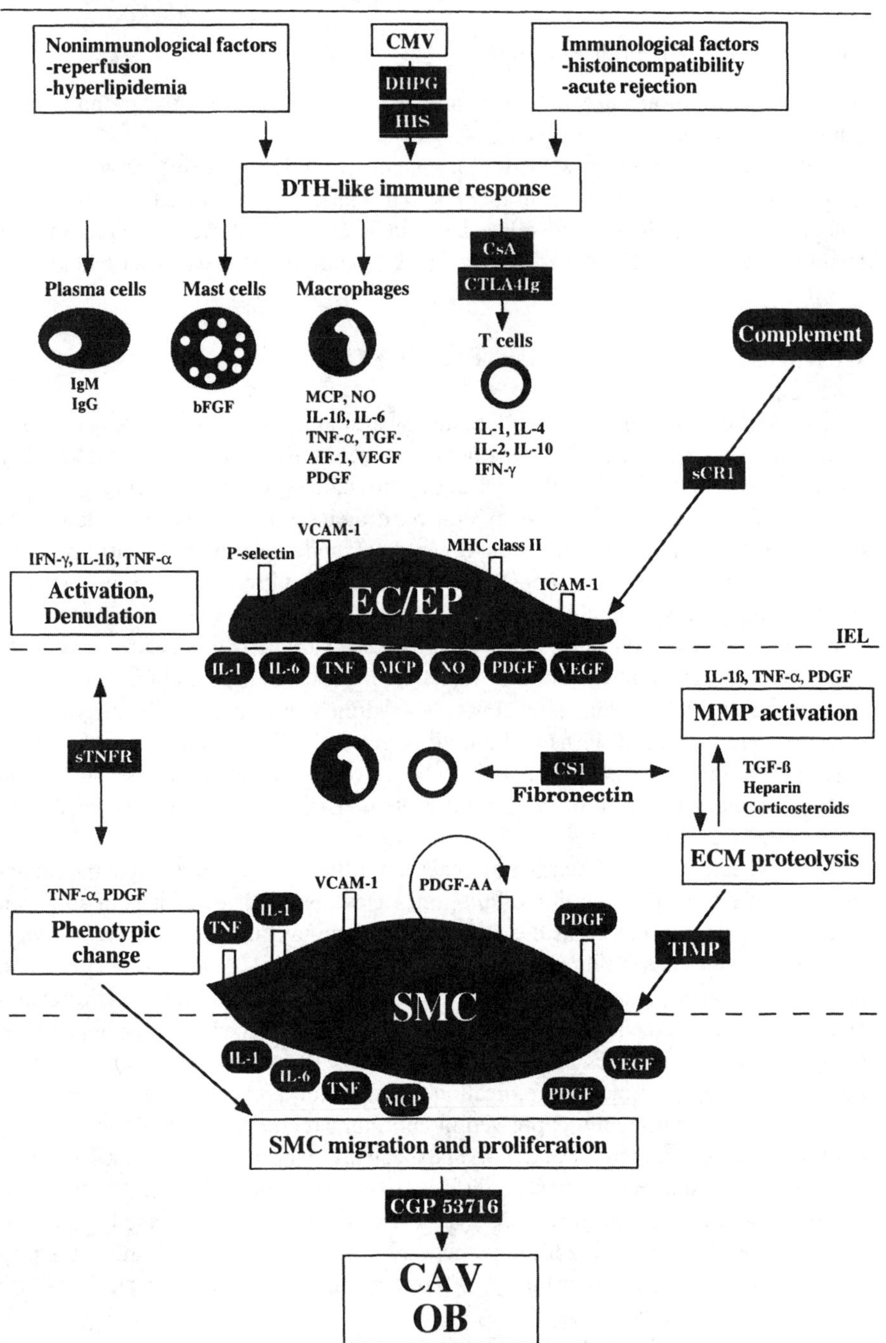

Figure 2. Summary of the major pathways of smooth muscle cell regulation in allograft vasculopthy (chronic rejection). The etiology of chronic rejection is most likely multifactorial. We hypothesize that nonimmune and immune-mediated inflammation induces persistent low-grade damage to vascular endothelium, which in turn secretes growth factors and cytokines in an attempt to repair the damage. This results in neighbouring smooth muscle cell replication in the allograft vascular wall, the influx of myocytes from the media into the intima, and generation of an arteriosclerotic lesion. Within the arterial wall, smooth muscle cells are embedded in and associated with a complex network of non-cellular structural elements, called extracellular matrix (ECM). The ECM is in a steady state of production and degradation. The degradation is mediated by a gene family of proteolytic enzymes called matrix metalloproteinases (MMP), which are secreted as inactive zymogens. They are activated by proteolytic cleavage reactions and their activity is also regulated by a family of specific protein inhibitors, i.e., tissue inhibitors of metalloproteinases (TIMP).

ties, length and histological pattern and at different time points after transplantation. Late acute rejections are considered more harmful than early acute rejections.[99] Of paramount importance is also the histological pattern. Van Saase et al.[100] and S. Olsen, H.E. Hansen and M. Madsen (unpublished) have conducted a study investigating the impact of the histological patten of rejection to long-term graft survival. Both groups demonstrated that a vascular pattern of acute rejection predicts a substantially inferior long-term graft survival and that late graft fucntion is highly dependent on the intensity of vasculitis in the acute biopsy histology. Consequently, as future trials aim to improve immunosuppression efficicay, the impact of experimental therapy on the histological pattern of acute rejection should be taken into account.

ADDITIONAL APPROACHES TO THERAPY

In order to define additional sites of intervention, we and others have initiated studies to interfere with the vascular response after preventive measures to eliminate risk factors and the effect of acute rejection have failed. In order to define the rate-limiting steps in the allograft vascular response, i.e., potential targets for therapy, investigators have focused on differentially-expressed genes and gene products within the allograft vascular wall. In classical organ models such as heart transplants, it is technically difficult to investigate individual hollow structures, such as grafted coronary arteries, for gene expression, as this process would require extensive dissection procedures. Therefore simple "tube models" have been developed where only the structures to be investigated are transplanted. This can be accomplished by aortic allografts or by using vascular wall endothelial trauma models (denudation of carotids or aorta) to induce an intimal response. Observations obtained in "tube models" can be analyzed in detail for smooth muscle cell migration and replication. In vitro results must subsequently be confirmed using more traditional organ models such as rodents and larger animals.

For targeted drug design, which specifically aims to agonize or antagonize a given receptor, ligand or enzyme, several modalities exist. Gene therapy is highly specific, but the delivery of genes to the target organ has been difficult regardless of whether live attenuated virus or conventional plasmid vectors are employed. The extreme selectivity and specificity of the immune system, has been exploited to develop monoclonal antibodies (chimeric or humanized) to target given (usually cell surface) proteins. Regardless of these modifications and their high specificity, monoclonal antibodies have inherent limitations: they require parenteral administration and are prone to generate antibodies which block their action in long-term use. This may be partially overcome by using peptides, particularly if based on D-aminoacid constructs, which are not degradable by naturally occurring peptidases. Although these drugs are also administrated parenterally, they do not usually evoke an immune response. Peptidomimetics have even better properties as they are organic compounds that lack the peptide bond; however, their development is particularly demanding. Nevertheless, some of these approaches have already been successfully employed (see below).

Somatostatin (SST) is the anti-hormone of somatotropin (growth hormone) and strongly inhibitory to insulin-like growth factor I (IGF-1) and other growth factors as demonstrated in vascular preparations by Delafontaine, Foegh and their associates.[101,102] Analogs of somatostatin have been shown to inhibit smooth muscle cell proliferation and intimal thickening in a variety of rodent and rabbit models of angioplasty injury.[103,104] In our own studies, significant inhibition in the expression of insulin-like growth factor 1 and particularly of platelet derived growth factor was observed in non-immunosuppressed aorta allografts; concomitantly, there was a decrease in the smooth muscle cell replication rate by 50–80% in both the media and the intima. The intensity of intimal thickening was reduced by 50%.[105] Studies in humans have, however, been met with less favorable results. One reason for this inconsistency may be that somatostatin employs five different receptors, which may be differently expressed in different tissues, and that the analogs studied may not have been targeted against the proper receptor.

Smooth muscle cells in their secretory (i.e., migratory and proliferative) state express a variety of receptors to a variety of ligands. Particularly interesting in this constellation are the IGF-1 receptor regulating the proliferation of smooth muscle cells, PDGF-Rα regulating the mitogenic response of smooth muscle cells, and -Rβ regulating both smooth muscle cell migration and replication. We have shown (Aavik et al., unpublished observations) that the mRNA expression levels of these receptors closely follow the migratory and proliferatory patterns of smooth muscle cells after denudation trauma to rat carotid.

In an attempt to interfere with the IGF-1 receptor we empoyed peptides resembling the D-domain of IGF-1, the key domain binding to the IGF-1 receptor. In order to prevent degradation by naturally occurring peptidases, we used D-amino acids in the construction of these peptides.[106] As reported in detail elsewhere,[111] some of these peptides strongly inhibited smooth muscle cell replication in vitro, whereas the "scrambled" peptides did not. They also inhibited both smooth muscle cell replication and intimal thickening after carotid denudation in vivo, although the maximal inhibitory effect was noted to be 70% and 30%, respectively.

Expression of matrix metalloproteinases is necessary for smooth muscle cell locomotion and their penetration through the extracellular matrix and the internal elastic lamina. It has been shown previously in several vascular trauma models[107,108] that inhibition of matrix metalloproteinases inhibits smooth muscle cell migration into the neointima. Potentially, interference with proteolysis of the extracellular matrix by elastase inhibitors[109] or by matrix metalloproteinase inhibitors, may offer another site for the inhibition of chronic rejection.

As already described, in our previous studies with chronically-rejecting rat cardiac allografts, we have demonstrated that the expression of PDGF-A in the media and intima and PDG-Rα and -Rβ in the intima and endothelium, are significantly correlated to intimal thickening. It was, therefore, of interest to investigate whether blocking of PDGF receptor signaling could inhibit chronic rejection. Highly specific protein tyrosine kinase inhibitors are now available for experimental use.[110] One such analogue inhibited PDGF A and B ligand-induced smooth muscle cell replication and migration in vitro and smooth muscle cell replication and migration after carotid denudation in vivo.[111] Most interestingly, both the number of affected vessels and the mean index of intimal obliteration in rat cardiac allografts. Were decreased (Sihvola et al., submitted). These observations remain to be confirmed in large animal models.

SUMMARY

The clinical condition of chronic rejection progresses histologically to proliferative allograft vasculopathy. This disorder reflects the cumulative trauma to the allograft, regardless of its origin. As a consequence of trauma, inflammation is generated within and around the allograft arteries leading to endothelial activation, smooth muscle cell replication and migration, and intimal thickening of the previously transplanted coronary arteries. Many changes in the graft parenchyma may be partially explained either on the basis of ischemic injury or on the basis of functional cross-reactivity of the graft parenchymal cells to growth factors regulating smooth muscle cells. According to the current paradigm, chronic rejection can be prevented in some animal models by more intensive and selective immunosuppression. Unfortunately, this is not true for human cardiac transplant recipients. On the other hand, retransplantation experiments in experimental animals suggest that elimination of histoincompatibility by retransplantation to donor strain, does not prevent the progression of the disorder after the initial stimulus has been sufficiently strong or long-lasting. In order to design additional sites of intervention after arterial injury and activation, attention has been focused on the regulation of the synthesis of growth factors stimulating smooth muscle cells, on the blocking and binding of the growth factors to their receptors, on the inhibition of signalling downstream of the receptor and on the inhibition of proteolytic enzymes necessary for the locomotion of the smooth muscle cells. Experimental studies demonstrate that by blocking these events it is possible to regulate the smooth muscle cell response in vitro and in vivo both in arterial injury model and particularly in the allograft. Unfortunately, despite encouraging experimental results, no current agent can completely inhibit the vasculopathic response. Future studies may demonstrate whether several approaches must be applied concomitantly, or whether the genes regulating several of these processes simultaneously can be identified and exploited.

REFERENCES

1. Hosenpud JD, Bennett LE, Keck BM, Fiol B, Novick RJ. The Registry of the International Societ for Heart and Lung Transplantation: fourteenth official report–1997. *J Heart Lung Transplan* 1997;16:691–712.
2. Billingham ME. Cardiac transplant atherosclerosis. *Transplant Proc* 1987;19:19–25.
3. Billingham ME. The pathologic changes in long-term heart and lung transplant survivors. *J Hea Lung Transplant* 1992;11:252–257.
4. Gao SZ, Alderman EL, Schroeder JS, Silverman JF, Hunt SA. Accelerated coronary vascular diseas in the heart transplant patient: coronary arteriographic findings. *J Am Coll Cardiol* 1988;1: 334–340.
5. Hruban RH, Beschorner WE, Baumgartner WA, Augustine SM, Ren H, Reitz BA, Hutchins GN Accelerated arteriosclerosis in heart transplant recipients is associated with a T-lymphocyt mediated endothelialitis. *Am J Pathol* 1990;137:871–882.
6. Olivari MT, Homans DC, Wilson RF, Kubo SH, Ring WS. Coronary artery disease in cardiac tran plant patients receiving triple-drug immunosuppressive therapy. *Circulation* 1989;80:111–115.
7. Stovin PG, Sharples L, Hutter JA, Wallwork J, English TA. Some prognostic factors for the deve opment of transplant-related coronary artery disease in human cardiac allografts. *J Heart Lu Transplant* 1991;10:38–44.
8. Costanzo-Nordin MR. Cardiac allograft vasculopathy: relationship with acute cellular rejection a histocompatibility. *J Heart Lung Transplant* 1992;11:90–103.
9. Uretsky BF, Murali S, Reddy PS, Rabin B, Lee A, Griffith BP, Hardesty RL, Trento A, Bahns

HT. Development of coronary artery disease in cardiac transplant patients receiving immunosuppressive therapy with cyclosporine and prednisone. *Circulation* 1987;76:827–834.
10. Narrod J, Kormos R, Armitage J, Hardesty R, Ladowski J, Griffith B. Acute rejection and coronary artery disease in long-term survivors of heart transplantation. *J Heart Lung Transplant* 1989; 8:418–421.
11. Radovancevic B, Poindexter S, Birovljev S, Velebit Vl, McAllister HA, Duncan JM, Vega D, Lonquist J, Burnett CM, Frazier OH. Risk factors for development of accelerated coronary artery disease in cardiac transplant recipients. *Eur J Cardio-Thorac Surg* 1990;4:309–313.
12. Young JB, Windsor NT, Kleiman NS, Lowry R, Cocanougher B, Lawrence EC. The relationship of soluble interleukin-2 receptor levels to allograft arteriopathy after heart transplantation. *J Heart Lung Transplant* 1992;11:79–82.
13. Deng MC, Bell S, Huie P, Pinto F, Hunt SA, Stinson EB, Sibley R, Hall BM, Valantine HA. Cardiac allograft vascular disease. Relationship to microvascular cell surface markers and inflammatory cell phenotypes on endomyocardial biopsy. *Circulation* 1995;91:1647–654.
14. Hammond EH, Yowell RL, Nunoda S, Menlove RL, Renlund DG, Bristow MR, Gay WA Jr, Jones KW, O'Connell JB. Vascular (humoral) rejection in heart transplantation: pathologic observations and clinical implications. *J Heart Lung Transplant* 1989;8:430–443.
15. Heroux AL, O'Sullivan EJ, Liao Y, Kao W, Johnson M, Mullen M, Pifarre R, Constanzo-Nordin MR. Early and late cardiac allogrfat arteriopathy: are they different entities? *J Am Coll Cardiol* 1992;19:174A.
16. Hess ML, Hastillo A, Mohanakumar T, Cowley MJ, Vetrovac G, Szentpetery S, Wolfgang TC, Lower RR. Accelerated atherosclerosis in cardiac transplantation: role of cytotoxic B-cell antibodies and hyperlipidemia. *Circulation* 1983;68:94–101.
17. Gao SZ, Schroeder JS, Hunt S, Stinson EB. Retransplantation for severe accelerated coronary artery disease in heart transplant recipients. *Am J Cardiol* 1988;62:876–881.
18. Winters GL, Kendall TJ, Radio SJ, Wilson JE, Costanzo-Nordin MR, Switzer BL, Remmenga JA, McManus BM. Posttransplant obesity and hyperlipidemia: major predictors of severity of coronary arteriopathy in failed human heart allografts. *J Heart Transp* 1990;9:364–371.
19. Eich D, Thompson JA, Ko DJ, Hastillo A, Lower R, Katz S, Katz M, Hess ML. Hypercholesterolemia in long-term survivors of heart transplantation: an early marker of accelerated coronary artery disease. *J Heart Lung Transplant* 1991;10:45–49.
20. Sharples LD, Caine N, Mullins P, Scott JP, Solis E, English TA, Large SR, Schofield PM, Wallwork J. Risk factor analysis for the major hazards following heart transplantation–rejection, infection, and coronary occlusive disease. *Transplantation* 1991;52:244–252.
21. Grattan MT, Moreno-Cabral CE, Starnes VA, Oyer PE, Stinson EB, Shumway NE. Cytomegalovirus infection is associated with cardiac allograft rejection and atherosclerosis. *JAMA* 1989;261: 3561–3566.
22. McDonald K, Rector TS, Braulin EA, Kubo SH, Olivari MT. Association of coronary artery disease in cardiac transplant recipients with cytomegalovirus infection *Am J Card* 1989;64:359–362.
23. Loebe M, Schuler S, Zais O, Warnecke H, Fleck E, Hetzer R. Role of cytomegalovirus infection in the development of coronary artery disease in the transplanted heart. *J Heart Transp* 1990;9:707–711.
24. Everett JP, Hershberger RE, Norman DJ, Chou S, Ratkovec RM, Cobanoglu A, Ott GY, Hosenpud JD. Prolonged cytomegalovirus infection with viremia is associated with development of cardiac allograft vasculopathy. *J Heart Lung Transplant* 1992;11:133–137.
25. Koskinen PK, Krogerus LA, Nieminen MS, Mattila SP, Häyry PJ, Lautenschlager IT. Quantitation of cytomegalovirus infection associated histoligal findings in endomyocardial biopsies of heart allografts. *J Heart Lung Transplant* 1993;12:343–354.
26. Rubin RH. Impact of cytomegalovirus infection on organ transplant recipients. *Rev Inf Dis* 1990;12:754–766.
27. Cramer DV, Qian SQ, Harnaha J, Chapman FA, Estes LW, Starzl TE, Makowka L. Cardiac transplantation in the rat. I. The effect of histocompatibility differences on graft arteriosclerosis *Transplantation* 1989;47:414–419.
28. Nakagawa T, Sukhova GK, Rabkin E, Winters GL, Schoen FJ, Libby P. Acute rejection accelerates graft coronary disease in transplanted rabbit hearts. *Circulation* 1995;92(4):987–993.
29. Alonso DR, Starek PK, Minick CR. Studies on the pathogenesis of atheroarteriosclerosis induced in rabbit cardiac allografts by the synergy of graft rejection and hypercholesterolemia. *Am J Patho* 1977;87:415–442.
30. Mennander A, Tikkanen MJ, Räisänen-Sokolowski A, Paavonen T, Ustinov J, Häyry P. Chronic rejection in rat aortic allografts. IV. Effect of hypercholesterolemia in allograft arteriosclerosis. *J Heart Lung Transplant* 1993;12:123–131.
31. Adams DH, Karnovsky MJ. Hypercholesterolemia does not exacerbate arterial intimal thickening in chronically rejecting rat cardiac allografts. *Transplant Proc* 1989;21:437–439.

32. Räisänen-Sokolowski A, Tilly-Kiesi M, Ustinov J, Mennander A, Paavonen T, Tikkanen MJ, Häyry P. Hyperlipidemia accelerates allograft arteriosclerosis (chronic rejection) in the rat. *Arteriosclerosis & Thrombosis* 1994;14:2032–2042.
33. von Willebrand E, Petterson E, Ahonen J, Häyry P. CMV infection, class II antigen expression, and human kidney allograft rejection. *Transplantation* 1986;42:364–367.
34. Fietze E, Prösch S, Reinke P, Stein J, Döcke W-D, Staffa G, Löning S, Devaux S, Emmrich F, von Baehr R, Krüger DH, Volk H-D. Cytomegalovirus infection in transplant recipients. The role of tumor necrosis factor. *Transplantation* 1994;58:675–680.
35. Speir E, Shibutani T, Yu ZX, Ferrans V, Epstein SE. Role of reactive oxygen intermediates in cytomegalovirus gene expression and in the response of human smooth muscle cells to viral infection. *Circ Research* 1996;79(6):1143–1152.
36. Cherrington JM, Mocarski ES. Human cytomegalovirus ie 1 transactivates the alpha promoter-enhancer via an 18-base-pair repeat element. *J Virol* 1989;63:1435–1440.
37. Fujinami RS, Nelson JA, Walker L, Oldstone MBA. Sequence homology and immunologic cross-reactivity of human cytomegalovirus with HLA-DR beta chain: a means for graft rejection and immunosuppression. *J Virol* 1988;62:100–105.
38. Beck S, Barrell BG. Human cytomegalovirus encodes a glycoprotein homologous to MHC class-I antigens. *Nature* 1988;331(6153):269–272.
39. Hendrix MGR, Dormans PHJ, Kitslaar P, Bosman F, Bruggeman CA. The presence of cytomegalovirus nucleic acids in arterial walls of atherosclerotic and nonatherosclerotic patients. *Am J Pathol* 1989;134:1151–1157.
40. Melnick JL, Adam E, Debakey ME. Possible role of cytomegalovirus in atherogenesis. *JAMA* 1990;263:2204–2207.
41. Koskinen PK, Krogerus LA, Nieminen MS, Mattila SP, Häyry PJ, Lautenschlager IT. Cytomegalovirus infection and accelerated cardiac allograft vasculopathy in human cardiac allografts. *J Heart Lung Transplant* 1993;12:343–354.
42. Koskinen PK, Nieminen MS, Krogerus LA, Lemström KB, Mattila SP, Häyry PJ, Lautenschlager IT. Cytomegalovirus infection accelerates cardiac allograft vasculopathy: correlation between angiographic and endomyocardial biopsy findings in heart transplant patients. *Transplant Int* 1993;6:341–347.
43. Koskinen P, Lemström K, Bruggeman C, Lautenschlager I, Häyry P. Acute cytomegalovirus infection induces a subendothelial inflammation (endothelialitis) in the allograft vascular wall. A possible linkage with enhanced allograft arteriosclerosis. *Am J Pathol* 1994;144(1):41–50.
44. Lemström KB, Aho PT, Bruggeman CA, Häyry PJ. Cytomegalovirus infection enhances mRNA expression of platelet-derived growth factor-BB and transforming growth factor-beta 1 in rat aortic allografts. Possible mechanism for cytomegalovirus-enhanced graft arteriosclerosis. *Arterioscler Thromb* 1994;14:2043–2052.
45. Lemström KB, Bruning JH, Bruggeman CA, Lautenschlager IT, Häyry PJ. Triple drug immunosuppression significantly reduces immune activation and allograft arteriosclerosis in cytomegalovirus-infected rat aortic allografts and induces early latency of viral infection. *Am J Pathol* 1994;144:1334–1347.
46. Lemström KB, Bruning JH, Bruggeman CA, Koskinen PK, Aho PT, Yilmaz S, Lautenschlager IT, Häyry PJ. Cytomegalovirus infection-enhanced allograft arteriosclerosis is prevented by DHPG prophylaxis in the rat. *Circulation* 1994;90(4):1969–1978.
47. Neyts J, Snoeck R, Schols D, Balzarini J, De Clercq. Selective inhibition of human cytomegalovirus DNA synthesis by (S)-1-(3-hydroxy-2-phosphonylmethoxypropyl)cytosine [(S)-HPMPC] and 9-(1,3-dihydroxy-2-propoxymethyl)guanine (DHPG). *Virology* 1990;179(1):41–50.
48. Speir E, Modali R, Huang ES, Leon MB, Shawl F, Finkel T, Epstein SE. Potential role of human cytomegalovirus and p53 interaction in coronary restenosis. *Science* 1994;265(5170):391–394.
49. Koskinen PK, Lemström KB, Häyry PJ. How cyclosporine modifies histological and molecular events in the vascular wall during chronic rejection of rat cardiac allografts. *Am J Pathol* 1995;146:972–980.
50. Koskinen PK, Lemström KB. Adhesion molecule P-selectin and vascular cell adhesion molecule-1 in enhanced heart allograft arteriosclerosis in the rat. *Circulation* 1997;95:191–196.
51. Tanaka H, Swanson SJ, Sukhova G, Schoen FJ, Libby P. Smooth muscle cells of the coronary arterial tunica media express tumor necrosis factor-alpha and proliferate during acute rejection of rabbit cardiac allografts. *Am J Pathol* 1995;147(3):617–626.
52. Clausell N, Molossi S, Sett S, Rabinovitch M. In vivo blockade of tumor necrosis factor-alpha in cholesterol-fed rabbits after cardiac transplant inhibits acute coronary artery neointimal formation. *Circulation* 1994;89(6):2768–2779.
53. Clausell N, Molossi S, Rabinovitch M. Increased interleukin-1β and fibronectin expression are early features of the development of the postcardiac transplant coronary arteriopathy in piglets. *Am J Pathol* 1993;142:1772–1786.

54. Russell ME, Wallace AF, Hancock WW, Sayegh MH, Adams DH, Sibinga NE, Wyner LR, Karnovsky MJ. Upregulation of cytokines associated with macrophage activation in the Lewis-to-F344 rat transplantation model of chronic cardiac rejection. *Transplantation* 1995;59(4):572–578.
55. Russell ME, Adams DH, Wyner LR, Yamashita Y, Halnon NJ, Karnovsky MJ. Early and persistent induction of monocyte chemoattractant protein 1 in rat cardiac allografts. *Proc Natl Acad Sci USA* 1992;90:6086–6090.
56. Russell ME, Wallace AF, Wyner LR, Newell JB, Karnovsky MJ. Upregulation and modulation of inducible nitric oxide synthase in rat cardiac allografts with chronic rejection and transplant arteriosclerosis. *Circulation* 1995;92(3):457–464.
57. Utans U, Quist WC, McManus BM, Wilson JE, Arceci RJ, Wallace AF, Russell ME. Allograft inflammatory factor-1. A cytokine-responsive macrophage molecule expressed in transplanted human hearts. *Transplantation* 1996;61(9):1387–1392.
58. Russell ME, Utans U, Wallace AF, Liang P, Arceci RJ, Karnovsky MJ, Wyner LR, Yamashita Y, Tarn C. Identification and upregulation of galactose/N-acetylgalactosamine macrophage lectin in rat cardiac allografts with arteriosclerosis. *J Clin Invest* 1994;94(2):722–730.
59. Watschinger B, Sayegh MH, Hancock WW, Russell ME. Upregulation of endothelin-1 mRNA and peptide expression in rat cardiac allografts with rejection and arteriosclerosis. *Am J Pathol* 1995;146(5):1065–1072.
60. Ross R. The pathogenesis of atherosclerosis: a perspective for the 1990s. *Nature* 1993;362:801–809.
61. Ross R, Raines EW, Bowen-Pope DF. The biology of platelet-derived growth factor. *Cell* 1986;46: 155–169.
62. Heldin CH, Westermark B. Platelet-derived growth factor: three isoforms and two receptor types. *Trends Genet* 1989;5:108–111.
63. Seifert RA, Hart CE, Phillips PE, Forstrom JW, Ross R, Murray MJ, Bowen-Pope DF. Two different subunits associate to create isoform-specific platelet-derived growth factor receptors. *J Biol Chem* 1989;264:8771–8778.
64. Williams LT. Signal transduction by the platelet-derived growth factor receptor. *Science* 1989;243: 1564–1570.
65. Lemström KB, Koskinen PK. Expression and localization of platelet-derived growth factor ligand and receptor protein during acute and chronic rejection of rat cardiac allografts. *Circulation* 1997;96:1240–1249.
66. Buchdunger E Zimmermann J, Mett H, Meyer T, Müller M, Regenass U. Selective inhibition of the platelet-derived growth factor signal transduction pathway by a protein-tyrosine kinase inhibitor of the 2-phenylaminopyrimidine class. *Proc Natl Acad Sci USA* 1995;92:2558–2562.
67. Bluestone JA. New perspectives of CD28-B7-mediated T cell costimulation. *Immunity* 1995; 2:555–559.
68. Banchereau J, Bazan F, Blanchard D, Briere F, Galizzi JP, van Kooten C, Liu YJ, Rousset F, Saeland S. The CD40 antigen and its ligand. *Ann Rev Immunol* 1994;12:881–922.
69. Jenkins MK, Taylor PS, Norton SD, Urdahl KB. CD28 delivers a costimulatory signal involved in antigen-specific IL-2 production by human T cells. *J Immunol* 1991;147:2461–2466.
70. Schwartz RH. Costimulation of T lymphocytes: the role of CD28, CTLA-4, and B7/BB1 in interleukin-2 production and immunotherapy. *Cell* 1992;71(7):1065–1068.
71. Boussiotis V, Freeman GJ, Gray G, Gribben J, Nadler LM. B7 but not intercellular adhesion molecule-1 costimulation prevents the induction of human alloantigen-specific tolerance. *J Exp Med* 1993;178:1753–1763.
72. Grewal IS, Xu J, Flavell RA. Impairment of antigen-specific T-cell priming in mice lacking CD40 ligand. *Nature* 1995;378:617–620.
73. van Essen H, Ikutani H, Gray D. CD40 ligand-transduced co-stimulation of T cells in the development of helper function. *Nature* 1995;378:620–623.
74. Hollenbaugh D, Mischel-Petty N, Edwards CP, Simon JC, Denfeld RW, Kiener PA, Aruffo A. Expression of functional CD40 by vascular endothelial cells. *J Exp Med* 1995;182:33–40.
75. Armitage RJ, Fanslow WC, Strockbine L, Sato TA, Clifford KN, Macduff BM, Anderson DM Gimpel SD, Davis-Smith T, Maliszewski CR, et al. Molecular and biological characterization of a murine ligand for CD40. *Nature* 1992;357:80–82.
76. Cayabyab M, Phillips JH, Lanier LL. CD40 preferentially costimulates activation of CD4+ T lymphocytes. *J Immunol* 1994;152:1523–1531.
77. Noelle RJ, Roy M, Shepherd DM, Stamenkovic I, Ledbetter JA, Aruffo A. A 39-kDa protein on activated helper T cells binds CD40 and transduces the signal for cognate activation of B cells. *Proc Nat Acad Sci USA* 1992;89:6550–6554.
78. Alderson MR, Armitage RJ, Tough TW, Strockbine L, Fanslow WC, Spriggs MK. CD40 expression by human monocytes: regulation by cytokines and activation of monocytes by the ligand for CD40. *J Exp Med* 1993;178:669–674.

79. Johnston RB Jr. Current concepts: immunology. Monocytes and macrophages. *N Engl J Med* 1988;318(12):747–752.
80. Russell ME, Hancock WW, Akalin E, Wallace AF, Glysing-Jensen T, Willett TA, Sayegh MH. Chronic cardiac rejection in the LEW to F344 rat model. Blockade of CD28-B7 costimulation by CTLA4Ig modulates T cell and macrophage activation and attenuates arteriosclerosis. *J Clin Invest* 1996;97(3):833–838.
81. Larsen CP, Elwood ET, Alexander DZ, Ritchie SC, Hendrix R, Tucker-Burden C, Cho HR, Aruffo A, Hollenbaugh D, Linsley PS, Winn KJ, Pearson TC. Long-term acceptance of skin and cardiac allografts after blocking CD40 and CD28 pathways. *Nature* 1996;381:434–438.
82. Russell PS, Chase CM, Winn HJ, Colvin RB. Coronary atherosclerosis in transplanted mouse hearts. II. Importance of humoral immunity. *J Immunol* 1994;152(10):5135–5141.
83. Shi C, Lee WS, He Q, et al. Immunologic basis of transplant-associated arteriosclerosis. *Proc Natl Acad Sci USA* 1996;93(9):4051–4056.
84. Räisänen-Sokolowski A, Mottram PL, Flysing-Jensen T, Satoskar A, Russell ME. Heart transplants in interferon-gamma, interleukin 4, and interleukin 10 knockout mice. Recipient environment alters graft rejection. *J Clin Invest* 1997;100(10):2449–2456.
85. Thyberg J, Hedin U, Sjölund M, Palmberg L, and Bottger BA. Regulation of differentiated properties and proliferation of arterial smooth muscle cells. *Arteriosclerosis* 1990;10:966–990.
86. Ross R. The pathogenesis of atherosclerosis: a perspective for the 1990s. *Nature* 1993;362:801–809.
87. MacDonald AS, Sabr K, MacAuley MA, McAlister VC, Bitter SH, Lee T. Effects of leflunomide and cyclosporine on aortic allograft chronic rejection in the rat. *Transplant Proc* 1994; 26(6):3244–3245.
88. Gregory CR, Huang X, Pratt RE, et al. Treatment with rapamycin and mycophenolic acid reduces arterial intimal thickening produced by mechanical injury and allows endothelial replacement. *Transplantation* 1995;59(5):655–661.
89. Räisänen SA, Yilmaz S, Tufveson G, Häyry P. Partial inhibition of allograft arteriosclerosis (chronic rejection) by 15-deoxyspergualin. *Transplantation* 1994;57(12):1772–1777.
90. Räisänen SA, Vuoristo P, Myllärniemi M, Yilmaz S, Kallio E, Häyry P. Mycophenolate mofetil (MMF, RS-61443) inhibits inflammation and smooth muscle cell proliferation in rat aortic allografts. *Transpl Immunol* 1995;3(4):342–3451.
91. Russell ME, Hancock WW, Akalin E, et al. Chronic cardiac rejection in the LEW to F344 rat model. Blockade of CD28-B7 costimulation by CTLA4Ig modulates T cell and macrophage activation and attenuates arteriosclerosis. *J Clin Invest* 1996;97(3):833–838.
92. Kingma I, Chea R, Davidoff A, Benediktsson H, Paul LC. Glomerular capillary pressures in long-surviving rat renal allografts. *Transplantation* 1993;56(1):53–60.
93. Benediktsson H, Chea R, Davidoff A, Paul LC. Antihypertensive drug treatment in chronic renal allograft rejection in the rat. Effect on structure and function. *Transplantation* 1996;62(11):1634–1642.
94. Akyurek LM, Funa K, Wanders A, Larsson E, Fellstrom BC. Inhibition of transplant arteriosclerosis in rat aortic grafts by low molecular weight heparin derivatives. *Transplantation* 1995;59(11):1517–1524.
95. Kobashigawa JA, Katznelson S, Laks H, et al. Effect of pravastatin on outcomes after cardiac transplantation. *N Engl J Med* 1995;333(10):621–627.
96. Häyry P, Isoniemi H, Yilmaz S, Mennander A, Lemström K, Räisänen-Sokolowski A, Koskinen P, Ustinov J, Lautenschlager I, Taskinen E, Krogerus L, Aho P, Paavonen T. Chronic allograft rejection. *Immunol Rev* 1993;134:33–81.
97. Utans U, Liang P, Wyner LR, Karnovsky MJ, Russell ME. Chronic cardiac rejection: identification of five upregulated genes in transplanted hearts by differential mRNA display. *Proc Natl Acad Sci USA* 1994;91(14):6463–6467.
98. Chen J, Myllärniemi M, Akyurek LM, Häyry P, Marsden PA, Paul LC. Identification of differentially expressed genes in rat aortic allograft vasculopathy. *Am J Pathol* 1996;149(2):597–611.
99. Basadonna GP, Matas AJ, Gillingham KJ, et al. Early versus late acute renal allograft rejection impact on chronic rejection. *Transplantation* 1993;55(5):993–995.
100. van Saase JL, van der Woude FJ, Thorogood J, et al. The relation between acute vascular and interstitial renal allograft rejection and subsequent chronic rejection. *Transplantation* 199 59(9):1280–1285.
101. Delafontaine P, Lou H, Alexander RW. Regulation of insulin-like growth factor I messenger RN levels in vascular smooth muscle cells. *Hypertension* 1991;18(6):742–747.
102. Foegh ML, Ramwell PW. Angiopeptin: experimental and clinical studies of inhibition of myointimal proliferation. *Kidney Int Suppl* 1995:S18–22.
103. Lundergan C, Foegh ML, Vargas R, et al. Inhibition of myointimal proliferation of the rat carot artery by the peptides, angiopeptin and BIM 23034. *Atherosclerosis* 1989;80(1):49–55.

104. Foegh ML, Asotra S, Conte JV, et al. Early inhibition of myointimal proliferation by angiopeptin after balloon catheter injury in the rabbit. *J Vasc Surg* 1994;19(6):1084–1091.
105. Häyry P, Räisänen A, Ustinov J, Mennander A, Paavonen T. Somatostatin analog lanreotide inhibits myocyte replication and several growth factors in allograft arteriosclerosis. *Faseb J* 1993;7(11): 1055–1060.
106. Häyry P, Myllärniemi M, Aavik E, et al. Stabile D-peptide analog of insulin-like growth factor-1 inhibits smooth muscle cell proliferation after carotid ballooning injury in the rat. *Faseb J* 1995;9(13):1336–1344.
107. Zempo N, Koyama N, Kenagy RD, Lea HJ, Clowes AW. Regulation of vascular smooth muscle cell migration and proliferation in vitro and in injured rat arteries by a synthetic matrix metalloproteinase inhibitor. *Arterioscler Thromb Vasc Biol* 1996;16(1):28–33.
108. Bendeck MP, Irvin C, Reidy MA. Inhibition of matrix metalloproteinase activity inhibits smooth muscle cell migration but not neointimal thickening after arterial injury. *Circ Res* 1996;78(1):38–43.
109. Cowan B, Baron O, Crack J, Coulber C, Wilson GJ, Rabinovitch M. Elafin, a serine elastase inhibitor, attenuates post-cardiac transplant coronary arteriopathy and reduces myocardial necrosis in rabbits afer heterotopic cardiac transplantation. *J Clin Invest* 1996;97(11):2452–2468.
110. Levitzki A. Targeting signal transduction for disease therapy. *Curr Opin Cell Biol* 1996;8(2): 239–244.
111. Myllärniemi M, Calderon L, Lemström K, Buchdunger E, Häyry P. Inhibition of platelet-derived growth factor receptor tyrosine kinase inhibits vascular smooth muscle cell migration and proliferation. *Faseb J* 1997;11(13):1119–1126.

4. INFLAMMATORY CELL INFILTRATION, CYTOKINES, AND MECHANISMS OF MYOCYTE NECROSIS IN CARDIAC TRANSPLANT REJECTION

Jay Bruce Sundstrom,
Kimberley Cecile Jollow, and Aftab Ahmed Ansari
Emory University School of Medicine, Department of Pathology and Laboratory Medicine, Atlanta GA

INTRODUCTION

Successful engraftment or rejection of the cardiac allograft depends on the function and viability of each of the lineages of cells that comprise cardiac tissue, the major lineage being highly specialized, terminally differentiated parenchymal cardiac myocytes. The traditional approach to optimizing survival of the allograft has been to target what have been considered as immune-mediated mechanisms of rejection. However, it is now becoming increasingly clear that the rejection pathways that evolve are determined not only by the nature of the allogeneic antigenic signals which initiate the allo-response, but also by the inflammatory environment in which these responses develop. Therefore, effective clinical strategies to prevent graft rejection must address antigen-independent as well as antigen-dependent processes involved in both direct and indirect mechanisms of cardiac myocyte cell death or "drop out". In this review we will describe how both the complex interaction of the immune response to alloantigen displayed by distinct lineages of cells that comprise donor tissues possessing different intrinsic antigen presentation capabilities and the inflammatory "response to injury" lead to the direct and/or indirect destruction of cardiac myocytes and the remodeling and reinforcement of damaged tissues within the cardiac allograft.

THE NATURE OF CARDIAC ALLOGRAFT REJECTION

The earliest and rarest form of immune response, seen within minutes to hours of transplantation, is hyperacute rejection. It is characterized by polymorphonuclear infiltration within the vasculature, fibrin thrombi formation, interstitial edema, and diffuse hemorrhages throughout the myocardium. Hyperacute rejection is initiated by the presence of preformed antibodies to MHC II or blood group antigens, generally from previous transfusions, allografts or pregnancies. Due to the use of pre-transplantation cross-match tests, the incidence of hyperacute rejection is now less than 1%. Within the first year post-transplantation, the major immunological threat to the patient is acute cellular rejection. This form of rejection is usually reversible with the use of increased doses of immunosuppressive drugs. The nature of the lymphocytic infiltrate and its relation to myocyte necrosis is discussed in detail below. The major cause of late post-transplant mortality in cardiac transplant recipients, however, is chronic rejection, also known as graft vascular disease. It is characterized by proliferation of smooth muscle cells and fibroblasts, endothelial cell hypertrophy, collagen deposition, and lymphocytic infiltration within both the arterial and venous blood vessels. The result of this proliferation and deposition is concentric intimal thickening of the vessels and eventual obstruction of the graft vasculature.

TRIGGERING EVENTS LEADING TO IMMUNE-MEDIATED ALLOGRAFT REJECTION

The first step in immune mediated rejection occurs when resting T cells of the host immune system become sensitized to allogeneic MHC molecules expressed on donor tissues within the allograft. However, for such sensitization to occur, allogeneic MHC molecules must be properly presented to the T cell. Full activation of resting T cells requires an antigen-specific signal but also an antigen-independent signal termed a co-stimulatory signal delivered optimally and efficiently by the same antigen presenting cell (APC). The ability to deliver the full set of T cell activation signals is assigned to a select group of "professional" APCs. Once activated, the T cells become less dependent on antigen-independent co-stimulation and are able to unleash their effector or potentiating functions after encountering appropriately presented cognate antigen presented by APCs which do not express detectable levels of co-stimulatory molecules and are referred to as "non-professional" APCs. How alloantigen specific signals are translated into T cell responses depends on the APC and the cytokine environment in which T cell allo-activation takes place.

The Nature of Allogeneic MHC Molecules

T cells are unable to detect whole proteins or conformational epitopes. Instead, they recognize discrete oligomeric peptide fragments of protein antigens displayed by MHC antigens on antigen presenting cells.[1] Anchor residues within the peptide-binding groove on the MHC molecule fix the orientation of the antigenic peptide. For T cell activation to occur such specific peptide residues complexed with MHC molecules must be recognized by clonally rearranged cognate T cell receptors (TCR).[1] The peptide-MHC complex thus forms the antigenic epitope that is specifically recognized by cognate TCRs expressed on the surface of T cells. These T cell epitopes are derived from two major antigen processing pathways within the antigen presenting cell.[2,3] The Class I pathway processes antigenic peptides from endogenous proteins for presentation by MHC Class I for $CD8^+$ restricted T cell recognition. The Class II pathway processes exogenous proteins into antigenic peptides for presentation by MHC Class II molecules for $CD4^+$ restricted T cell recognition (Figure 1). In the absence of foreign antigen, the peptides displayed by MHC antigens are derived exclusively from self proteins. Tolerance to these self antigens is maintained by deleting cognate T cells from the repertoire during thymic education. However, when the same processed self-peptide is presented by allo-MHC it will be recognized and perceived as foreign to self-restricted T cells. This is because a) the peptide anchoring residues which determine the orientation of the bound processed peptides vary among the different allelic forms of MHC molecules and b) allelic differences in the constant or framework regions of the allo-MHC molecules themselves may also contribute to the "foreign" features of the allotope. Thus, in the context of the transplanted allograft, where APCs of either donor or host origin are able to present antigen to host T cells, allo-immune responses may be triggered by the recognition of 1) allo-antigens (e.g. processed peptides from allo-MHC molecules) presented by allo-MHC (allo-restricted), 2) self-antigens presented by allo-MHC (allo-restricted), 3) allo-antigens presented by self-MHC (self-restricted).[4]

In any given individual, the frequency of T cell clones able to recognize alloantigen is 50 to 100 times greater than the T cell precursor frequency for nominal antigens such as tetanus toxoid.[4] This is because the typical APC is able to display a significantly greater variety of allo-antigenic determinants and can therefore recruit a proportionately greater number of T cells in the response to allo-antigen (Figure 2, see color plates section, back of book). On the other hand, a single processed nominal antigen may yield only a limited number of antigenic peptides for self-restricted MHC presentation by the APC, and accordingly the precursor frequency of T cells able to respond to foreign antigen is proportionately smaller. APCs use the same MHC class II antigen processing pathway for self-restricted presentation of exogenous allo-antigen (indirect pathway) or nominal antigen. Therefore, it is expected that immune responses to indirectly presented alloantigen share the same relative strength and kinetics as responses to exogenous nominal antigen. Thus, cellular immune responses leading to acute rejection are most likely triggered by direct recognition of allo-antigen, whereas indirect allo-recognition has a more dominant role in the immuno-pathogenesis of chronic rejection.

Tissue Matching and Opportunities for Therapeutic Intervention

The effects of histocompatibility matching, especially at MHC class I (HLA-A and HLA-B) and MHC class II (HLA-DR) loci on cardiac allo-graft survival have been evaluated in several multi-center studies.[5] Although, donor-recipient matching at the MHC loci are not routinely performed for cardiac transplants out of concern for organ preservation time, results of these studies show that HLA compatibility, particularly at the HLA-DR loci, strongly correlates with increased graft survival.[6]

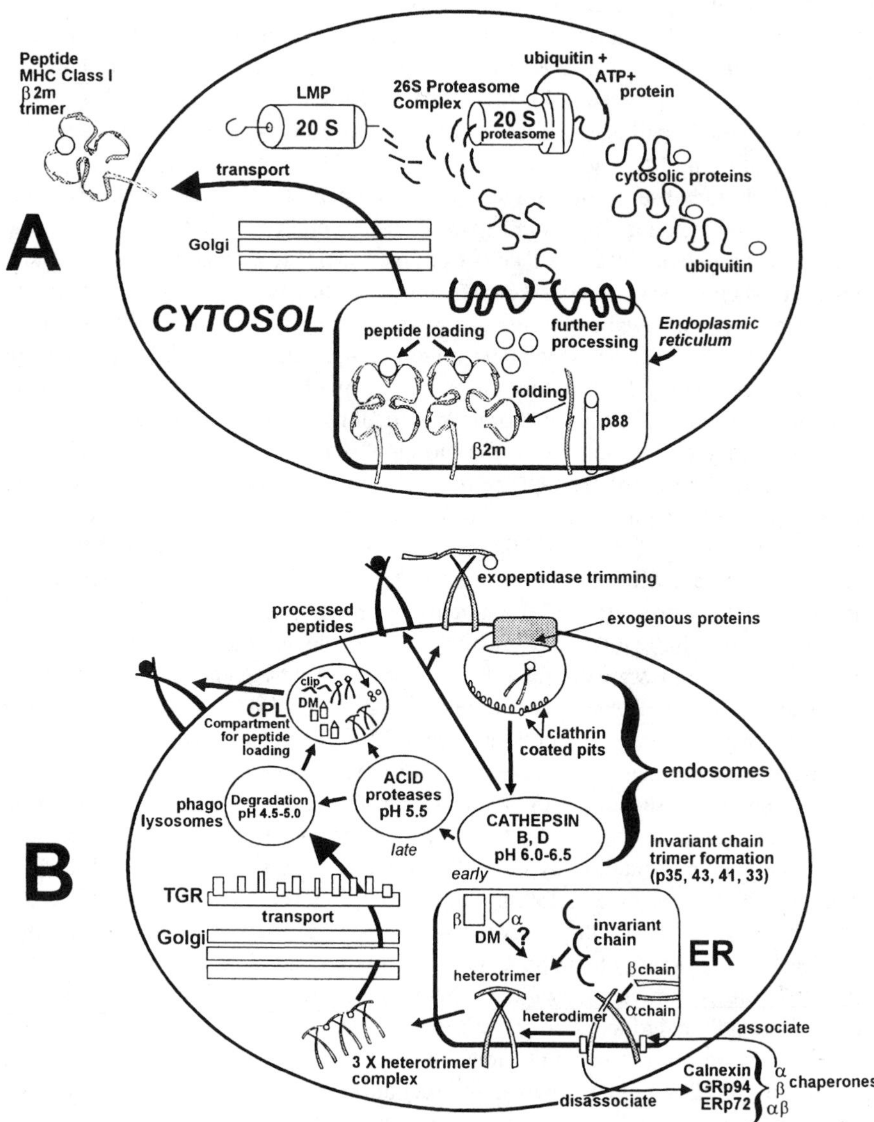

"Professional vs. Semi-Professional" Antigen Presentation

Full activation of resting T lymphocytes requires at least two signals delivered simultaneously by an APC.[7] One signal is antigen specific and is mediated through cognate interactions between the TCR and MHC Class I/II antigens bearing an appropriate oligomeric peptide derived through processing of the parent protein antigen by one of the two major pathways mediated by antigen degradation by APCs (Figure 1). The other (co-stimulatory) signal is not antigen specific and is delivered

Figure 1. A. MHC class I processing. Processing of endogenous antigens for presentation by MHC class I begins in the cytosol with the proteolytic degradation of ubiquitin-tagged proteins by the multicatalytic proteasome (LMP). The Transporter of Antigenic Peptides (TAP) delivers size-selected processed oligomeric peptides from the cytosol into the ER where they may undergo further processing. Inside the ER nascent MHC class I molecule associate with chaperone proteins (e.g. p. 88) to facilitate proper folding of the molecule into its α1, α2, and α3 domains. Then as properly processed peptides (8–11 residues in length) bind to the peptide loading groove (defined by the α1 and α2 domains) a heavy chain/peptide/β2-microglobulin complex forms and the chaperone disassociates. The stable MHC I/peptide trimer is then transported through the golgi and expressed on the cell surface. **B. MHC class II processing.** Processing of extracellular antigens occurs as exogenous proteins are internalized via phagocytosis, pinocytosis, or receptor mediated endocytosis in clathrin coated pits and shuttled into an endocytic route from early to late endosomes and eventually to phagolysosomes with concomitant proteolytic degradation by acid proteases (e.g. cathepsins). MHC class II assembly occurs independently of endocytic antigen processing. Nascent MHC class II, synthesized in the ER, associates with chaperone proteins which facilitate proper folding of the MHC Class II α and β heavy chains and retards egress of MHC II from the ER until they are properly configured and associated in a trimeric complex with the invariant chain (Ii). The peptide antigen binding groove formed by the MHC II heterodimer binds to a conserved region of the invariant chain referred to as the class II invariant peptide (CLIP). The MHCαβ-Ii heterotrimer (nonameric complex) dissociates from the calnexin chaperone and is transported through the golgi and transgolgi reticulum (TGR) to a late endosomal compartment for peptide loading (CPL) where the heterodimeric molecule DM facilitates the replacement of CLIP with processed antigenic peptide. Once loaded with peptide the MHC class II-peptide complex is transported to and expressed on the cell surface.

Table 1. Role of co-stimualtory molecules (CSMs) and cellular adhesion molecules (CAMs) in triggering alloactivation. List of two classes of CSMs and CAMs that co-stimulate synergistically with or independent of T cell receptor induced signalling events

	Costimulatory Molecule/Cellular Adhesion Molecule		
APC ligand	T cell CSM/CAM	TCR dependent co-signal	TCR independent co-signal
ICAM-1,2,3	LFA-1/MAC-1	+	
LFA-1	ICAM-1	+	
LFA-3	CD2	+	
VCAM-1	VLA-4	+	
MHC class I	CD8	+	
MHC class II	CD4	+	
MHC class I/II	TCR	+	
B7-1,2,3	CD28/CTLA-4		+
HSA	HSA		+
Ii-CS	CD44		+
4-1BB-L	4-1BB		+
CD40	CD40-L (CD154)		+

through the engagement of co-stimulatory molecules on the T cell and their specific counter-ligands on the APC. Second signals mediated by CSMs associated with professional APCs (e.g. B7-1, CD40, HSA, 4-1BB-L) are transduced through biochemical pathways that are distinct from the cyclosporine-sensitive circuits used for signaling mediated through the TCR.[8–13] Other more broadly distributed CSMs (e.g. ICAM-1, LFA-1, LFA-3) help stabilize interactions between T cells and APCs while providing co-stimulation through TCR signal transduction pathways (Table 1). The net effect of CSMs is to work synergistically with the antigen-specific signals to enhance gene expression for lymphokines and their receptors.

Professional APCs, such as dendritic cells and macrophages, contain a density and array of MHC Class I/II and co-stimulatory molecules that is sufficient for full activation of resting T cells. Professional APCs of donor origin may be present as "passenger" cells within the allograft. Larsen et al.[14] have shown that donor passenger dendritic cells emigrate from the heart and migrate to the spleen within 40 hours after transplantation.

However, in addition to these passenger APCs, parenchymal cells of other tissue lineages within the allograft, which normally are unable to allo-activate resting T cells, may be conscripted for duty as facultative APCs through the actions of pro-inflammatory cytokines (e.g. IFN-γ, TNF-α, and IL-1β) which up-regulate their surface expression of MHC I/II and co-stimulatory molecules. For example it has been shown that HLA-A, B, C, and HLA-DR as well as the co-stimulatory molecule CD40 expression on cultured endothelial cells can be enhanced by treatment with IFN-γ.[15] These CD40 expressing endothelial cells can then interact with $CD4^+$ T cells to alter their activated phenotype.[16] In our own laboratory we have shown that pretreatment of human cardiac microvascular endothelial cells with IFN-γ leads to enhanced surface expression of CD40 and HLA-DR. Subsequent co-culture of these CD40 expressing cells with a transfected HeLa cell line expressing CD40 ligand (CD40L) induces the expression of B7-1 on the activated cardiac microvascular EC and enables them to allo-activate resting T cells (16a). This data is in agreement with previous reports from other laboratories[17,18] for a prominent role for CD40 in cardiac allograft rejection.

Resting previously primed memory T cells can receive the requisite antigen-specific and antigen-nonspecific activation signals from either professional or facultative APCs. However, naive T cells that receive antigen-specific signals in the absence of appropriate second (antigen non-specific) signals are rendered refractory or anergic.[19,20] Thus, the nature of such requisite co-stimulatory signals for "naive" T cell activation has been the focus of strategies aimed at prolonging allo-graft survival by blocking the initiation of T cell responses which may lead to rejection. This is exemplified by the finding from other laboratories that have demonstrated that antibodies which block co-stimulatory signaling through CD4, ICAM-1, CD40, B7-1, or VCAM-1 can result in improvement in allo-graft survival in experimental cardiac allograft rejection.[18,21–23]

Not all cell lineages within the cardiac allograft can be induced to present allo-antigen. Our laboratory has shown that IFN-γ pretreated human fetal cardiac myocytes expressing MHC class I and II, ICAM-1, and LFA-3 are unable to induce proliferative responses in allogeneic peripheral blood lymphocytes from normal donors.[24] It is, however, important to remember that once activated, T cells may engage in cognate interactions with allo-antigen and discharge their effector functions (e.g. cytolysis, or potentiation) without a requirement for co-stimulation by the target cell.

How Cytokines Influence the Allo-Immune Response

Evidence suggests that humoral and cellular immune responses develop along unique pathways which are associated with and most likely governed by separate sets of non-overlapping cytokines.[25] TH1 responses, which govern cell-mediated immune responses, are associated with IL-2, IFN-γ, and IL-12, whereas TH2 responses, which influence humoral immune responses, are associated with IL-3, IL-4, IL-5, IL-6, IL-10, and IL-13.

The direction in which the allo-immune response develops is primarily determined by events surrounding the initial allo-activation of the naive T cell. Such activation initially induces synthesis of IL-2 with little or no synthesis of IL-4 or IFN-γ by the naive T cell. These newly activated T cells soon develop a TH0 phenotype, expressing an intermediate set of cytokines (e.g. IFN-γ, IL-2, IL-4, and IL-5). These TH0 T cells will then make a developmental commitment to either a TH1 or TH2 phenotype depending on external cytokine signals.[25] TH0 T cells developing under the influence of IFN-γ become TH1, whereas TH0 T cells developing under the influence of IL-4 become TH2. APCs are also capable of influencing which developmental pathway is chosen by the TH0 T cell.

Measuring and interpreting cytokine levels in episodes of cardiac allograft rejection is a complex task. It was originally believed that since cellular immune responses were responsible for acute rejection, that TH1 cytokine responses were responsible for driving the immune rejection. Studies in which serum levels of TH1 vs. TH2 cytokines levels were measured by ELISA following transplantation have shown no correlation with TH1 or TH2 cytokine patterns and acute rejection.[26] However, in another study,[27] cytokines patterns of donor-specific graft-infiltrating lymphocytes (GILs) isolated from serial endomyocardial biopsies (EMB) revealed a strong correlation of TH1 (IL-2/IFN-γ) cytokines but not TH2 (IL-4) cytokines in GILs isolated from EMBs with a histological evidence of acute rejection. These observations are consistent with the concept that $CD8^+$ GILs are able to inhibit the development of TH2 responses thus allowing the TH1 responses to develop. However, other studies reveal that although mice depleted of $CD8^+$ CTLs do indeed show altered cytokine responses skewed toward TH2 profiles, they still are able to acutely reject heterotropic cardiac allografts.[28] In this case it is possible that allograft rejection is mediated by infiltrating eosinophils which respond to TH2 cytokines, e.g. IL-4 and IL-5.[29] Eosinophilia in cardiac transplant recipients is uncommon an may be due to the influence of certain sets of cytokines that selectively induce infiltration by eosinophils.[29]

Lymphocyte Trafficking and Transendothelial Migration

Chemotactic signals and cellular adhesion molecules (CAMs) on activated ECs function together as a physiological beacon to hail responding lymphocytes to sites of inflammation within the allograft. These trafficking signals act in an allo-antigen independent fashion favoring the recruitment of neutrophils, monocytes and activated or memory lymphocytes to sites of focal inflammation within the allograft. A three-step model for leukocyte recruitment and migration through the activated endothelium has been proposed (Figure 3, see color plates section, back of book).[30] Initially, leukocyte attachment and rolling along the inflamed endothelium is initiated through tethering by selectins and their ligands. Chemokines and other soluble inflammatory products (e.g. PAF, LTB4, C5a, FMLP) that are either produced by the activated endothelium or captured from the extracellular environment, become concentrated on the activated endothelium where they are posted on proteoglycans of the EC glycocalyx. Engagement of these chemokines with their receptors displayed on microvilli of the rolling leukocyte leads to the second step: triggering of a cholera toxin sensitive (G-protein mediated) activation pathway that results in the enhanced affinity of leukocyte β2-integrins for EC (Ig supergene family) ligands. These actions lead to the third step: strong adhesion and transendothelial migration. *In vitro* studies under flow conditions have shown that the entire process of attachment, rolling, arrest, and diapedesis of leukocytes through (cytokine) activated endothelium occurs rapidly, within minutes.[31]

Leukocyte migration occurs across chemotactic gradients by a multi-step process. Activated leukocytes bristling with a variety of chemokine receptors must successfully navigate across a field of multiple chemokine concentration gradients. In the complex inflammatory environment of the injured or rejecting allograft, only those leukocytes possessing the requisite sets of receptors will be capable of correctly interpreting and responding to the cacophony of chemotactic signals directing them to sites of focal inflammation.[31,32]

Thus the initiation and implementation of immune responses toward the allograft involves proper recognition of allo-activation signals from different cells and allo-antigens within the graft interpreted within a context of inflammation that develops in response to tissue injury. The business of sorting out these complex activation and chemotactic signals determines which immune cells (and their products) are recruited to participate in the immune response which also determines the type of immune response that develops. For instance, the inflammatory response to injury may "sound the alarm" recruiting all granulocytes, macrophages, activated lymphocytes to the scene. However, there may be only a small percentage of allo-activated lymphocytes among the responding graft-infiltrating leukocytes. A general scheme for the sequence of events for the initiation, development, and implementation of the antigen-specific immune response that partitions these events into an "Afferent Phase, Central Phase, and Efferent Phase" is outlined in Figure 4 (see color plates section, back of book).

PHENOTYPIC AND FUNCTIONAL CHARACTERIZATION OF CELLULAR INFILTRATES

The Quilty Effect

The Quilty Effect was not observed until the introduction of cyclosporine therapy, even though its occurrence is not directly linked to cyclosporine dosage.[33] The Quilty Effect has been divided into two subclasses by the International Society for Heart and Lung Transplantation (ISHLT). The first, Quilty Type A, is noninvasive and is characterized by cellular infiltration into the subendocardial region without myocyte necrosis or loss of function. In Quilty Type B, the subendocardial infiltration extends into the myocardium and may be associated with myocyte injury. Despite the occurrence of myocyte damage in Quilty Type B, neither form is associated with acute rejection or requires increased immunosuppression.[33,34]

No link has been found between the phenomenon and the incidence of infections with viruses such as cytomegalovirus or Epstein-Barr virus or the development of lymphoproliferative disorders.[35] Overall, approximately 50% of patients post transplant develop Quilty lesions. However, there is no difference in mortality between the patients who develop Quilty lesions after cardiac allograft transplantation and those who do not.

Within these lesions, the majority of the infiltrate consists of T lymphocytes, along with smaller foci of B cells. Occasional macrophages and plasma cells can also be seen, although fewer macrophages are seen compared to acute rejection. The T cells exhibit a CD4 to CD8 ratio of approximately 3 : 1[34] and morphologically appear small, with round nuclei, no nucleoli, and no observable mitotic activity.

Nature and Function of Cellular Infiltrates

Approximately 50% of cardiac allograft recipients will experience episodes of acute cellular rejection, most of which occur during the first six months post transplantation.[4] Such events are characterized by an infiltration of lymphocytes into the myocardium, with or without myocyte damage. The grade of the rejection is determined according to the size of the infiltrate and the presence of damage to the myocytes, with higher grades treated with increased immunosuppression[36] (see Chapters 9 and 10)

The composition of the EMB visualized lymphocytic infiltrate has changed with more recent alterations in immunosuppressive treatments. Using regimens of azathioprine and corticosteroids, the infiltrate was primarily composed of $CD8^+$ T lymphocytes.[37] Upon the introduction of cyclosporine therapy, however, the cellular infiltrate consisted primarily of $CD4^+$ T lymphocytes, with macrophages and $CD8^+$ T cells also present albeit in lower numbers.[38,39] The composition of the cellular infiltrate also appears to be distinctly correlated with the level of rejection. With moderate rejection in cyclosporine-treated patients, eosinophils may be seen within the myocardium, and in severe rejection both eosinophils and neutrophils may be present.[36] Additionally, macrophages are seen in increasing numbers with higher levels of rejection.[40]

One method of studying the phenomenon of acute rejection that has been used by several laboratories, including ours, has been the culture of lymphoid cells from EMBs. The working hypothesis has been that such cultured cells represent enriched populations of host mononuclear cells that are specifically involved in graft rejection and/or maintenance. These *in vitro* culture-propagated cells have been studied for their phenotypes,[41] donor specificity,[42,43] cytokine expression,[44] and even for the measurement of the efficacy of new immunosuppressive drug therapies.[45] However, we found that more than 85% of the mononuclear cells in EMB specimens that scored as grade 3A rejection appeared to have undergone apoptosis, at least as defined by the TUNEL technique.[46] Thus, it may be far more important to study cellular infiltrates from tissues and biopsies prior to a rejection event, an approach which is extremely labor-intensive and requires continuous sequential monitoring studies.[47]

Although the phenotype of the cellular infiltrate has been determined, the precise cell lineage responsible for myocyte death, and the mechanism by which this is mediated, is unknown. As stated above, when phenotypically characterized $CD8^+$

cytotoxic T lymphocytes (CTLs) were found to be present in endomyocardial biopsies, early interest focused strategies on the elimination of this cell lineage.[48] However, studies soon thereafter proved that $CD8^+$ T cells do not by themselves play a major role in rejection. In an important study utilizing the murine model of cardiac allo-transplantation, Bishop et al. depleted $CD8^+$ T cells and saw no cytotoxic T lymphocytes (CTLs) within the infiltrate, but rejection still occurred.[49] Supporting this view was the findings of Wagoner et al. who obtained enriched populations of $CD8^+$ CTLs from rejecting murine allografts and found that they had only limited ability to lyse donor myocytes.[50] Finally, Krieger et al., who using CD8 knockout mice, still saw rejection of major histocompatibility complex mismatched skin and heart allografts.[51]

One possible explanation for the diminished role of $CD8^+$ T cells in cardiac rejection may lie in the recently published findings of Mingari et al.[52] They found that IL-15, and to a lesser extent IL-2, could induce the expression of the natural killer (NK) cell receptor CD94/NKG2A on mature $CD8^+$ T cells. In NK cells, this receptor interacts with MHC I expressed by the target cell and inhibits NK-mediated cytolysis. In $CD8^+$ T cells, a similar result was found, as CD94/NKG2A-expressing CTLs failed to lyse MHC I positive allogeneic cells except in the presence of anti CD94 blocking antibody. The importance of such MHC class I recognizing killer cell inhibitory receptors (KIRs) in the field of transplantation has been highlighted by the finding that expression of the appropriate KIR in transgenic mice can prevent rejection of a bone marrow graft expressing the corresponding MHC class I allele.[53] Since cardiac myocytes are known to express MHC class I especially post transplantation either directly (due to trauma/ischemia, reperfusion injury, etc.) or indirectly by cytokines released by inflammatory cells, these MHC class I molecules could serve as a mechanism for inhibition of infiltrating $CD8^+$ CTL-mediated cytolysis and, in addition, inhibit NK cell mediated function.

Attention next focused on the role of the $CD4^+$ T cell. Reinforcing this trend were the findings of studies in CD4 knockout mice, which revealed long-term acceptance of allogeneic skin and heart allografts, a process that was reversed with the transfusion of recipient strain wild type syngeneic $CD4^+$ T cells which reconstituted CD4 mediated rejection.[51] As described above, activation of these $CD4^+$ T cells could occur either directly, by interaction with allogeneic donor MHC II expressing cells, or indirectly, through presentation of shed donor antigens by host antigen presenting cells (APCs). Whichever pathway is used, activation of naive $CD4^+$ T cells requires the interaction between potent co-stimulatory molecules and their natural ligands, such as B7 and CD28.[54–56] Further support for the importance of $CD4^+$ T cells comes from studies that show that blocking this pathway causes long-term allograft acceptance.[57–59]

Although these studies indicate that CD4 cells play a central role in acute rejection, they do not indicate the mechanism of myocyte death. One possibility is direct cytolysis of cardiac myocytes by $CD4^+$ T cells. The major mechanism for cytolysis by $CD4^+$ T cells is through the fas/fas ligand pathway. In this pathway, fas ligand (CD95L) bearing $CD4^+$ T cells interact with fas (CD95) expressing target cells, and induce the target cells to undergo apoptosis. However, despite the discovery of constitutive fas expression in murine cardiac allografts,[60] Larsen et al. showed that non fas expressing donor cardiac allografts were still rejected providing evidence that this pathway is not required for acute rejection.[61]

Another major mechanism of T cell induced cytolysis is through the release of lytic granules containing molecules such as perforin and granzyme. Although cytotoxicity mediated by these molecules is primarily associated with $CD8^+$ T cells, $CD4^+$ T cells can also employ them to induce target cell death.[62,63] Together these molecules act to form pores in the target cell membrane, and induce apoptosis. Nevertheless, these molecules may not play a major and/or exclusive role in myocyte death, as it has been reported that rejection occurs even in perforin knockout mice.[64] In the end, a role for $CD4^+$ T cells in allograft rejection must be sought beyond the model of direct cytolysis. Bolstering this view is the work of VanBuskirk et al., who have found that $CD4^+$ cytolytic activity is not needed for acute cardiac allograft rejection but instead is mediated by non-cytolytic $CD4^+$ T cells.[65]

Currently, the most likely role for $CD4^+$ T cells in allograft rejection may be through the delayed type hypersensitivity (DTH) response. In DTH responses, primed $CD4^+$ T cells of the TH1 phenotype respond to a second presentation of the same antigen by elaborating cytokines and chemokines, and by activating macrophages. These DTH activated macrophages are capable of achieving target cell death both by inducing apoptosis and by directly causing necrosis.

In regard to DTH in the transplant model, it has been shown that allogeneic DTH reactions correlate with acute rejection while tolerance is accompanied by a lack of an allogeneic DTH.[66] Additionally, mRNA transcripts for inducible nitric oxide synthase (iNOS) and tumor necrosis factor alpha (TNF-α), two cytokines important in DTH responses, were found to be increased in murine cardiac allograft rejection compared to normal or syngeneic transplants.[60] Opinions remain divided as to the actual role of DTH activated macrophages in myocyte death. While one study in a rat cardiac allograft model found direct lysis of myocytes by macrophages,[67] another study utilizing the same model observed no direct lysis but rather an inhibition of myocyte contractions.[68,69]

The possible contribution of other components of the cellular infiltrate cannot be overlooked. Neutrophils, while most prominently seen in the humoral-associated hyperacute rejection, are also found in a high frequency of biopsies classified as representing acute rejection.[36] These polymorphonuclear cells (PMNs) are capable of inducing target cell death by the release of proteolytic enzyme- and toxin-filled granules and by the production of oxygen radicals with membrane-bound NADPH oxidase. Accordingly, these neutrophil-generated reactive oxygen intermediates (ROI) have been shown to cause severe cardiac dysfunction in a canine model.[70]

In this canine model, the mechanism of cardiac injury appears to begin with adhesion between the CD11/CD18 integrins on the canine neutrophil and ICAM-1 on the myocyte. ICAM-1 is not normally expressed on canine myocytes, but can be induced by cytokines such as TNF-α, IL-1, and IL-6.[71] The interaction results in intracellular oxidative injury to the myocyte and subsequent contracture and death.[72] Interestingly, human cardiac myocytes have been found to express ICAM-1 during acute rejection.[73] Furthermore, administration of anti-ICAM-1 antibodies has prolonged allograft survival in a mouse model, inhibiting myocyte necrosis but not lymphocytic infiltration.[74]

Natural killer (NK) cells are best known for host defense against viral infection and tumors, but may also participate in allogeneic immune responses. Since there is no current evidence for the influence of cyclosporine on NK cell mediated function[75] and this lineage of hematopoietic cells do not require prior priming for activation, it is most likely that NK cells are among the first cell lineage of the immune system to respond to the allograft. Supporting this view is that finding that, in rat cardiac allografts, NK cells along with macrophages predominate during the first three days following non-immunosuppressed transplantation.[76,77] Phenotypically marked NK cells have also been reported to constitute part of the lymphocytic infiltrate within the human myocardium and in increased numbers in the coronary sinus in biopsies reflecting acute rejection.[78,79] Although NK cells, like CTLs, can induce target cell death through the granzyme and perforin pathways as well as by apoptosis, their mode of target recognition is completely different. While CTLs require cognate interaction between CD8/MHC I interaction for killing, NK cells induce target cell death specifically in response to a lack of MHC class I expression on the target cell. Petersson et al. examined this in Wistar Furth to Brown Norway rat cardiac allografts and found NK cell activation and specific alloreactive cell killing.[80] Other studies have reported that the kinetics and magnitude of NK cell activity was similar in both cyclosporine treated and untreated cardiac allograft recipient rats.[81] These authors concluded therefore that this lineage of effector cells do not play a major role in rejection.[81]

Nevertheless, NK cells may have an effect on allograft rejection beyond direct myocyte lysis. As producers of IFN-γ and IL-2, NK cells have the potential to promote a TH1 environment and may thus help determine the quality and magnitude of the host response.[76] NK cells may also influence alloactivation through their effect on microvascular endothelial cells. One study showed that NK cells, through cytokine production, induced MHC class II expression on human microvascular endothelial cells.[82] These MHC class II positive MECs have been shown to induce allo-proliferative responses and thus could participate in initiation and maintenance of allograft rejection

Eosinophils are best known for defense against parasites but are also seen in the lymphocytic infiltrate of acute rejection in both lung and heart transplantation.[83,84] While they are capable of direct killing through the release of toxin-containing granules, this is not considered to be a likely method of myocyte death. Instead, it is possible that eosinophils, which are responsive to the TH2 cytokines IL-4 and IL-5, may play an effector role by the TH2 effector cell pathway. Support for a role for eosinophils is provided by results of one study of a mouse cardiac allograft model that found when CTLs were depleted and a TH2 environment created, acute allograft rejection still occurred. However, in this case instead of T lymphocytes, the infiltrate consisted primarily of eosinophils.[85]

RESPONSE TO INJURY

We have described how allo-activation triggers a cascade of humoral and cellular events that evoke targeted immunopathogenesis that is amplified by an ensuing inflammatory response to injury. The model we have used to describe these events proposes that recognition of allo-antigen leads to activation of T lymphocytes, which then commit to a certain type of immune response (e.g. cellular vs. humoral), resulting in destruction of graft myocardial tissue, causing inflammation to occur, which drives and amplifies the immune response. However, it is more likely, especially with the clinical application of modern anti-immunosuppressive drug therapies, that myocardial injury precedes the initiation of an anti-graft immune response and defines the inflammatory environment in which allo-responses are engendered and develop. For instance, the nature of the cardiac injury will determine which sets of inflammatory signals are induced and thus will influence 1) which cell lineages are recruited to the site of injury, 2) how allo-antigen will be presented (by which APC), and 3) how allo-antigenic signals will be interpreted (nature of allo-antigen and cytokine environment). We will now consider non-immune mechanisms of myocardial injury which may play a role in allograft rejection.

Non-Immune Mechanisms of Cardiac Myocyte Injury

Mature terminally differentiated cardiac myocytes do not undergo mitotic division. Consequently, myocardial injuries that cause death of the myocyte result in a permanent impairment of heart function. Nevertheless, cardiac myocytes have been shown to be very resilient to mechanical and chemical stress or trauma. Thus, depending on the severity, injury to cardiac myocytes can be classified as reversible or irreversible. Reversible injury (e.g. as seen in some ischemia/reperfusion injuries) is characterized by reduction in myocyte contractilility and reduced left ventricular function both of which are restored after the insult is removed. Despite transient metabolic changes that may occur under anoxic conditions, there are no lasting ultrastructural changes in the myocardium. On the other hand, irreversible injury leads to cell death either by apoptosis, by necrosis, or a combination of both[86,87] (see Chapter 5). In the transplant setting both reversible and irreversible damage to myocyte may occur by non-immune mechanisms, e.g. oxidative stress (ischemia/reperfusion), mechanical injury, cytotoxicity of anti-rejection drugs, or viral infections. Depending on the type and severity of the trauma to the myocardium, different sets of inflammatory signals are generated from each insult that helps to promote and define ensuing allo-immune responses.

Oxidative Stress, Ischemia/Reperfusion

Ischemia and reperfusion injuries leading to rejection of the transplanted heart may arise at any time during the life of the allograft. For instance, the initial surgical harvesting of the donor heart involves subjecting the organ to periods of cold ischemia lasting from one to three hours followed by reperfusion of the implanted cardiac allograft with recipient blood. Also, post-transplantation both acute and chronic vascular rejection may cause occluding epicardial and microvascular damage that results in ischemia. Pathologies that arise from these types of oxidative stress occur in two phases: ischemic injury followed by reperfusion injury.[88,89]

The progression from reversible to irreversible ischemic injury is subtle and depends on the relative oxygen demand. However, advanced stages of ischemia (e.g. >60 min. in contracting myocardium) is associated with disruption of the sarcolemma and mitochondrial swelling, characteristic of necrotic death. If the supply of oxygenated blood is re-established during the reversible phase, the ischemic myocyte can recover from the wasting effects of anaerobic metabolism. However, reperfusion ironically triggers a new set of events that also can cause irreversible myocyte injury.[88] The pathology of reperfusion injuries involves ROI, e.g. molecular oxygen, hydrogen peroxide, superoxide anion, or the hydroxyl radical. These are formed during ischemia and reperfusion in a variety of tissues, including the parenchyma, vascular endothelial cells, and the infiltrating white blood cells and through a variety of chemical pathways. Cellular injury is caused either by the direct oxidation or biochemical modification of DNA, membrane lipids, and proteins or indirectly by mediating the recruitment and activation of granulocytes which inflict immune-mediated injury as well as the generation of more ROIs. Further damage may result from the cellular disruption of ischemic myocardial tissues that become swollen due to intracellular osmotic load and which are then suddenly exposed to increased hemodynamic pressures during reperfusion.

Ischemic events also induce the activation of complement components, e.g. C5a, the generation of arachidonic acid and its metabolic products via the lipoxygenase pathway, e.g. LTB4, and the release of peptide mediators, e.g. PAF, that are chemotactic for granulocytes and that activate neutrophils.[90] Reperfusion promotes the diffusion of these inflammatory mediators throughout the microvasculature where they also activate endothelial cells and up regulate expression of CAMs e.g. CD62P, thereby strengthening neutrophil-endothelial adhesion. These inflammatory events can lead to the accumulation of neutrophils in the involved microvasculature of the ischemic heart resulting in a blockage that is another manifestation of reperfusion injury also referred as the no-reflow phenomena. In such a setting, the abundance of infiltrating activated neutrophils concentrated in focal areas within the myocardium favors the expansion of vascular and myocardial necrosis.

Mechanical Injury

Myocyte dropout (due to any of the mechanisms of injury discussed above) imposes an increased physiological burden on the surviving myocytes, which are responsible for maintaining proper heart function. This leaves the heart muscle weakened and often, especially during ischemia, forced to operate under increased hemodynamic loads. Since the myocardium cannot compensate for such irreversible injury by myocyte replacement or hyperplasia, ventricular myocytes undergo a condition of volume overload hypertrophy leading to wall thinning and left ventricular dilation. This leads to overstretching of enlarged contracting myocytes that may trigger apoptosis and further loss of myocyte tissue. These events trigger tissue repair and replacement activities that lead to collagen deposition with fibroblast proliferation.

Cytotoxicity from Anti-Rejection Drugs

To limit the effects of cellular immune-mediated rejection, immunosuppressive drugs that target T cell activation and inhibit such activation are routinely administered. Although combination therapy is effective in muting the anti-graft immune response, each drug can cause both reversible and irreversible myocyte damage. For example, CsA causes lipid peroxidation, especially in the presence of its carrier, cremophor (which is toxic by itself). This can lead to the generation of H_2O_2 and other ROIs which injure myocardial tissues by mechanisms described above.[91] CsA cytoxicity also results from its blocking of the Ca^{++}/calmodulin mediated reactions involving Ca^{++} ATPase and NOS, which affects the downstream activities of Ca^{++} ATPase and NOS.[92]

Viral Infections

The direct injury of the human myocytes due to viral infection and active replication of the virus within this cell lineage remains uncertain. Murine models of viral myocarditis have shown that murine cardiac myocytes infected with coxsackie B3 virus are destroyed by virus specific $CD8^+$ CTL *in vitro*.[93,94] Our lab has shown that the human fetal cardiac myocyte cell line, W-1, is able to process and present flu matrix protein and serve as targets for human MHC class I restricted CTLs specific for the 58–66 flu matrix peptide (manuscript in preparation). However, in the absence of reagents and methodologies that can be utilized to assess cardiac myocyte-directed specific immune responses, information on the direct cytopathic effects of viral infection on human cardiac myocytes becomes limited. This issue gains importance in the case of cardiac transplant recipients whose biopsies prior to transplant show evidence of myocarditis highly suspected to be due to a viral infection.

TISSUE REPAIR AND REMODELING

Tissue repair and remodeling is a physiological response to injury. Such injuries may occur during the immuno-pathogenesis of allo-graft rejection. In these situations repair and remodeling programs that are initiated to resolve the tissue damage, can ironically contribute to the process of chronic rejection. Repair and remodeling is also engendered following non-immune mediated injuries such as surgical trauma or ischemic injury.

Although these terms are often used together, repair and remodeling are not synonymous. Tissue repair is an acute phenomena that involves the expression of genes and cellular proteins that are necessary for immediate structural reinforcement as well as for the recruitment of specialized cells, e.g. granulocytes and monocytes, which manage the clean up and removal of damaged proteins and tissue. Remodeling may proceed chronically and involves a transition to different phenotypes by the vascular and parenchymal cells. In the heart such phenotypic modulation is controlled by the induction of reserve genetic programs (once active during fetal development) that include homeo-box genes, immediate early proto-oncogenes, genes coding for structural elements, as well as genes coding for new sets of specific growth receptors.[95–97] Growth factors elaborated in the remodeling environment bind either in an endocrine, paracrine, or juxtacrine fashion to their receptors on target cells, which undergo phenotypic transition in the remodeling process. Transduction of these receptor-mediated signals initiates the transcription of different sets of genes causing for instance the expression of fetal isoforms of structural proteins, the proteins that direct the recruitment and proliferation of other cells, and enzymes involved in the resorption and deposition of extracellular matrix proteins which contribute to the remodeling process.[98–100]

Structural Changes in the Myocardium

The heart is comprised of a collection of different cellular components including contractile myocytes, endothelial cells, fibroblasts, vascular muscle cells, endocardial cells, macrophages, mast cells and non-cellular components, e.g. type I and type III fibrillar collagen. Although myocytes numerically represent approximately 30% of the cells, they occupy 70 to 75% of the volume in the healthy heart. Weber[101] has proposed a model of heart disease in which these cells are arranged into two compartments: a myocyte and non-myocyte compartment. In the healthy heart these two compartments are organized in an efficient working relationship to maintain proper cardiac function. However, disease or injury causes a disruption in the structural balance of the two compartments either directly (e.g. by myocyte drop out) or indirectly (by tissue repair and remodeling).

The cellular phenotype and structural architecture of the heart is maintained in a dynamic equilibrium regulated by chemical and mechanical signals with opposing functions. For example, hypertension causes the release of NO by endothelial cells which induces vasodilation and a drop in blood pressure. Vascular injury causes thrombin activation which induces PDGF from platelets which activates endothelial cells and macrophages which produce inflammatory chemokines and cytokines, including TGF-β, which then attenuate the production of PDGF. Nevertheless, cells undergoing phenotypic alterations during remodeling may change their sensitivity to growth factors, mitogens or growth inhibitors, or mechanical stress forces, thus affecting their underlying spatial relationships and structural design. In pathologies involving the heart muscle, e.g. ischemia and mechanical overload, these changes cause hypertrophy and hyperplasia of cardiac myocytes, replacement and interstitial fibrosis, and left ventricular dilation. In vascular trauma the pathological effects of remodeling cause the phenotypic modulation of VSMCs from a non-proliferating contractile form to the proliferating synthetic form as is seen in transplantation associated vasculopathy, and in restenosis. Many of the growth hormone, cytokines, chemokines, and bioactive peptides that control and perpetuate the remodeling process show pleiotropic effects that overlap with the allo-immune response (Table 2). Thus, in the transplantation setting, the interactions between the inflammatory and the immune responses may disrupt the dynamics of the repair and remodeling programs leading to either accelerated or chronic rejection.[102]

Table 2. Chemokines, growth factors, and bio-active molecules involved in injury, repair, and remodeling of cardiac tissues

FACTOR	SOURCE	Target	Effect
C-X-C Chemokines			
PF4	α-granules of platelets	Fibroblasts, platelets, MC	Release of mediators (e.g. histamine, LTB4) by MC; chemotaxis by fibroblasts; inhibition of EC proliferation
IL-8	Multiple lineages including EC, T Cells, monocyte/macrophages	Neutrophils, T cells	Neutrophil chemotaxis
IP-10	EC, monocytes, fibroblasts	Monocytes, EC, NK, activated CD4 + T cells	Chemotaxis of monocytes, NK cells, and T cells; inhibits EC proliferation
C-C Chemokines			
MIP-1α	Fibroblasts, monocytes, eosinophils, neutrophils, lymphocytes, VSMC, platelets, MC	T cells, basophils, NK cells, monocytes, neutrophils, MC, DC	Chemotaxis and Ca^{++} mobilization in T cells, monocytes, NK cells, neutrophils, and DC; chemotaxis and degranulation of Eosinophils; histamine release by MC.
MIP-1β	T and B cells, Neutrophils, VSMC, MC, monocytes, fibroblasts	Monocytes, T cells, basophils	Chemotaxis and Ca^{++} mobilization of T cells; chemotaxis and enzyme release by monocytes; histamine release by basophils
MCP-1	Multiple lineages including EC, fibroblasts, monocytes/	Monocytes, T cells, basophils, eosinophils,	Activation and chemotaxis of monocytes, T cells, basophils, and eosinophils; chemotaxis of MC, and DC; CD54 induction on
CM	macrophages, VSMC, cardiac myocytes,	mast cells, NK cells, DC, cardiac myocytes	
RANTES	T cells, monocytes, fibroblasts, NK cells, platelets	T cells, monocytes, MC, DC, NK cells, eosinophils, basophils	Chemotaxis, activation, and release of enzymes by monocytes; chemotaxis and activation of T cells, chemotaxis and Ca^{++} mobilization of DC, chemotaxis, degranulation, and activation of basophils, and eosinophils; chemotaxis of NK cells and MC.
Polypeptide growth factors			
PDGF	Platelets, EC, Macrophages, VSMC	VSMC, fibroblasts, monocytes	Chemotactic for cardiac fibroblasts and VSMC
aFGF	Multiple sources including vascular EC and cardiac myocytes	Myocytes, VSMC, fibroblasts, EC	Mitogen
bFGF	Multiple sources including vascular EC and cardiac myocytes	Myocytes, VSMC, fibroblasts, EC	Mitogen

Table 2. (continued)

FACTOR	SOURCE	Target	Effect
VEGF	VSMC, macrophage	Monocyte/macrophage, EC	Chemotactic for monocyte/macrophage; causes EC proliferation and increased paracellular permeability.
IGF-1	EC, VSMC, Platelets	VSMC, Myocyte	Stimulates collagen release and matrix formation; mitogenic for cardiac myocytes
HB-EGF	Macrophages, EC, VSMC,	VSMC	Mitogenic for VSMC
Proinflammatory Cytokines/Interleukins			
TGF-β	Platelets, EC, T lymphocytes, monocytes/macrophages	VSMC, cardiac fibroblasts/myocytes, EC, monocytes/ macrophages, neutrophils, B and T cells	Inhibits proliferation of T/B cells and NK cells; inhibits CTL activity; nhibits (at low concentrations) and promotes (at high concentrations) proliferation of VSCM; promotes collagen release and matrix formation by fibroblasts
IL-1β	Macrophages, fibroblasts, EC, neutrophils, NK cells, T/B cells, VSMC	VSCM, T cells, EC, fibroblasts	T cell, NK cell, and fibroblast activation and proliferation; neutrophil chemotaxis; EC activation of macrophages
IFN-γ	(Allo) activated T cells and NK cells	Macrophages, T cells, EC, parenchymal cells	Induces MHC gene expression on somatic cells; activates macrophages; drives TH1 immune responses.
TNF-α	Macrophage/monocytes, neutrophils, NK cells, T cells	Pleiotropic activities: cytotoxicity,	Pleiotropic activities: cytotoxic for certain tissues; mitogenic for neutrophils; activates EC, induces chemokine/cytokine production in fibroblasts & EC, induces collagen release and matrix formation.
Bioactive molecules and hormones			
Endothelin	EC	VSMC, fibroblasts	Vasoconstriction; proliferation of VSCM and fibroblasts
Nitric Oxide	ECs, Macrophages	EC, macrophage/ monocytes	Vasodilation of EC and toxicity of cardiac myocytes
Angiotensin-2	Fibroblasts, myocytes, kidney-derived renin	Myocytes, fibroblasts, VSMC	Increases vasoconstriction; causes cardiac fibroblast proliferation, collagen release, and matrix formation; induces growth factors and autocrine mitogenesis in VSMC

Abbreviations: MC = mast cell, DC = dendritic cell, NK = natural killer, VSMC—vascular smooth muscle cell, EC = endothelial cell.

There are several possible examples of how such immunopathologies might occur. In one scenario local tissue damage from an ischemic event, infection, or vascular lesion causes platelet activation and the granular release of 1) platelet factor 4 (PF4) and β-thromboglobin, which in turn attract and activate fibroblasts, 2) LTB4, which attracts neutrophils, 3) PDGF, which attracts and activates fibroblasts and VSCMs and induces expression of the small inducible gene family encoding chemotractants, e.g. MCP-1. Monocytes migrating to the site of injury secrete 1) TGF-β, which causes fibroblasts to release matrix proteins (collagen and fibronectin) mediating replacement fibrosis, and 2) TNF-α and IL-1 which activate endothelial cells causing the up- regulation of CAMs and chemokines e.g. RANTES, MIP-1α, and MIP-1β, which recruit activated and memory $CD8^+$ and $CD4^+$ lymphocytes. Infiltrating T cells responding to these chemotactic signals encounter allo-antigen presented indirectly by macrophages and release IFN-γ. Macrophages respond to IFN-γ by producing ROI which causes further tissue damage while donor tissues respond to IFN-γ by up-regulating processing of (endogenous and exogenous) peptides and the presentation of MHC antigens. The allo-response is thus perpetuated and perhaps enhanced by the presentation of antigenic peptides derived from unique fetal isoforms of structural proteins induced during myocardial remodeling.[99,102] This model represents only one of many possible complex series of events that can be regulated by a variety of other inflammatory factors.[103,104] Thus, it is the consequence of interactions between the host's immune system and the inflammatory processes of response to injury which will ultimately direct the clinical outcome towards tissue repair or rejection.

REFERENCES

1. Davis, MD, Boniface, JJ, Reich, Z, Lyons, D, Hampl, J, Arden, B, and Chien, Y. Ligand recognition by alpha/beta T cell receptors. *Annual Reviews of Immunology* 16:523–544, 1998.
2. Cresswell, P. Assembly, transport, and function of MHC class II molecules. *Annual. Reviews of Immunology* 12:259–293, 1994.
3. Lehner, PJ and Cresswell, P. Processing and delivery of peptides presented by MHC class I molecules. [Review] *Current Opinion in Immunology* 8(1):59–67, 1996.
4. VanBuskirk, AM, Pidwell, DJ, Adams, PW, and Orosz, CG. Transplantation Immunology. [Review] *JAMA* 278(22):1993–1999, 1997.
5. Opelz, G and Wujciak, T. The influence of HLA compatibility on graft survival after heart transplantation. The Collaborative Transplant Study. *New England Journal of Medicine* 330(12):816–819, 1994.
6. Costanzo-Nordin, MR, Fisher, SG, O'Sullivan, EJ, Johnson, M, Heroux, A, Kao, W, Mullen, GM, Radvany, R, and Robinson, J. HLA-DR incompatibility predicts heart transplant rejection independent of immunosuppressive prophylaxis. *Journal of Heart & Lung Transplantation* 12(5):779–789, 1993.
7. Bretscher, P. The two-signal model of lymphocyte activation twenty-one years later. *Immunology Today* 13(2):74–76, 1992.
8. June, CH, Bluestone, JA, Nadler, LM, and Thompson, CB. The B7 and CD28 receptor families. *Immunology Today* 15(7):321–331, 1994.
9. Hubbe, M and Altevogt, P. Heat-stable antigen/CD24 on mouse T lymphocytes: evidence for a co-stimulatory function. *European Journal of Immunology* 24(3):731–737, 1994.
10. Naujokas, MF, Morin, M, Anderson, MS, Peterson, M, and Miller, J. The chondroitin sulfate form of invariant chain can enhance stimulation of T cell responses through interaction with CD44. *Cell* 74(2):257–268, 1993.
11. Liu, Y, Wenger, RH, Zhao, M, and Nielsen, PJ. Distinct costimulatory molecules are required for

the induction of effector and memory cytotoxic T lymphocytes. *Journal of Experimental Medicine* 185(2):251–262, 1997.

12. Shuford, WW, Klussman, K, Tritchler, DD, Loo, DT, Chalupny, J, Siadak, AW, Brown, TJ, Emswiler, J, Raecho, H, Larsen, CP, Pearson, TC, Ledbetter, JA, Aruffo, A, and Mittler, RS. 4-1BB costimulatory signals preferentially induce CD8+ T cell proliferation and lead to the amplification in vivo of cytotoxic T cell responses. *Journal of Experimental Medicine* 186(1):47–55, 1997.
13. Robey, E and Allison, JP. T-cell activation: Integration of signal from the antigen receptor and costimulatory molecules. *Immunology Today* Vol 16(7):(pp 306–310), 1995.
14. Larsen, CP, Morris, PJ, and Austyn, JM. Donor dendritic leukocytes migrate from cardiac allografts into recipients' spleens. *Transplantation Proceedings* 22(4):1943–1944, 1990.
15. Mach, F, Schonbeck, U, Sukhova, GK, Bourcier, T, Bonnefoy, JY, Pober, JS, and Libby, P. Functional CD40 ligand is expressed on human vascular endothelial cells, smooth muscle cells, and macrophages: implications for CD40-CD40 ligand signaling in atherosclerosis. *Proceedings of the National Academy of Sciences of the United States of America* 94(5):1931–1936, 1997.
16. Karmann, K, Hughes, CC, Fanslow, WC, and Pober, JS. Endothelial cells augment the expression of CD40 ligand on newly activated human CD4+ T cells through a CD2/LFA-3 signaling pathway. *European Journal of Immunology* 26(3):610–617, 1996.

16a. Jallow, KC, Zimring, JC, Sundstrom, JB, Ansari, AA. CD40 ligation induced phenotypic and functional expression of CD80 by human cardiac microvascular endothelial cells. Transplantation 68:430–439, 1999.

17. Hancock, WW, Sayegh, MH, Zheng, XG, Peach, R, Linsley, PS, and Turka, LA. Costimulatory function and expression of CD40 ligand, CD80, and CD86 in vascularized murine cardiac allograft rejection. *Proceedings of the National Academy of Sciences of the United States of America* 93(24):13967–13972, 1996.
18. Larsen, CP and Pearson, TC. The CD40 pathway in allograft rejection, acceptance, and tolerance. [Review]. *Current Opinion in Immunology* 9(5):641–647, 1997.
19. Lasalle, JM and Hafler, DA. T cell anergy. *FASEB Journal* 8(9):601–608, 1994.
20. Gimmi, CD, Freeman, GJ, Gribben, JG, Gray, G, and Nadler, LM. Human T-cell clonal anergy is induced by antigen presentation in the absence of B7 costimulation. *Proceedings of the National Academy of Sciences of the United States of America* 90(14):6586–6590, 1993.
21. Orosz, CG, Huang, EH, Bergese, SD, Sedmak, DD, Birmingham, DJ, Ohye, RG, and VanBuskirk, AM. Prevention of acute murine cardiac allograft rejection: anti-CD4 or anti-vascular cell adhesion molecule one monoclonal antibodies block acute rejection but permit persistent graft-reactive alloimmunity and chronic tissue remodelling. *Journal of Heart & Lung Transplantation* 16(9): 889–904, 1997.
22. Rehman, A, Tu, Y, Arima, T, Linsley, PS, and Flye, MW. Long-term survival of rat to mouse cardiac xenografts with prolonged blockade of CD28-B7 interaction combined with peritransplant T-cell depletion. *Surgery* 120(2):205–212, 1996.
23. Larsen, CP, Elwood, ET, Alexander, DZ, Ritchie, SC, Hendrix, R, Tucker-Burden, C, Cho, HR, Aruffo, A, Hollenbaugh, D, Linsley, PS, Winn, KJ, and Pearson, TC. Long-term acceptance of skin and cardiac allografts after blocking CD40 and CD28 pathways. *Nature* 381(6581):434–438, 1996.
24. Sundstrom, JB, Mayne, A, Kanter, K, Herskowitz, A, and Ansari, AA. Mechanisms of human cardiac allograft rejection: absence of co-stimulatory molecules and cell adhesion molecules on major histocompatibility complex class I/II+ human cardiac myocytes does not induce anergy. *Transplantation Proceedings* 27:1310–1313, 1997.
25. Paul, WE and Seder, RA. Lymphocyte responses and cytokines. *Cell* 76(2):241–251, 1994.
26. Grant, SC, Lamb, WR, Brooks, NH, Brenchley, PE, and Hutchinson, IV. Serum cytokines in human heart transplant recipients. Is there a relationship to rejection? *Transplantation* 62:480–491, 1996.
27. Van, BNM, Daane, CR, Vaessen, LM, Balk, AH, Claas, FH, Zondervan, PE, Jutte, NH, and Weimar, W. Different patterns in donor-specific production of T-helper 1 and 2 cytokines by cells infiltrating the rejecting cardiac allograft. *Journal of Heart & Lung Transplantation* 14:816–823. 1995.
28. Chan, SY, Debruyne, LA, Goodman, RE, Eichwald, EJ, and Bishop, DK. In vivo depletion of CD8+ T cells results in Th2 cytokine production and alternate mechanisms of allograft rejection. *Transplantation* 59:1155–1161, 1995.
29. Gravanis, MB and Ansari, AA. Myocarditis and dilated cardiomyopathy. *Emory University Journal of Medicine* 4(3):205–209, 1990.
30. Springer, TA. Traffic signals on endothelium for lymphocyte recirculation and leukocyte emigration. *Annual Review of Physiology* 57:827–872, 1995.
31. Campbell, JJ, Hedrick, J, Zlotnik, A, Siani, MA, Thompson, DA, and Butcher, EC. Chemokines and the arrest of lymphocytes rolling under flow conditions. *Science* 279(5349):381–384, 1998.

32. Butcher, EC and Picker, LJ. Lymphocyte homing and homeostasis. *Science* 272(5258):60–66, 1996.
33. Forbes, CR, Rowan, RA, and Billingham, ME. Endocardial infiltrates in human heart transplants: a serial biopsy analysis comparing four immunosuppression protocols. *Human Pathology* 21:850–855, 1990.
34. Kottke-Marchant, K and Ratliff, NB. Endomyocardial lymphocytic infiltrates in cardiac transplant recipients: incidence and characterization. *Archives of Pathology and Laboratory Medicine* 113: 690–698, 1989.
35. Joshi, A, Masek, M, Brown, B, Weiss, L, and Billingham, ME. "Quilty" revisited: a 10 year perspective. *Human Pathology* 26:547–557, 1995.
36. Billingham, ME. The diagnosis of acute cardiac rejection by endomyocardial biopsy. Biblthca cardiol. Karger No 43, 83–102, 1988.
37. Rose, ML, Gracie, JA, Fraser, A, Chisholm, P, and Yacoub, MH. Use of monoclonal antibodies to quantitate T lymphocyte subpopulations in human cardiac allografts. *Transplantation* 38:230–234, 1984.
38. Ouwehand, AJ, Baan, CC, Vaessen, LM, Jutte, NH, Balk, AH, Bos, E, Claas, FH, and Weimar, W. Characteristics of graft-infiltrating lymphocytes after human heart transplantation. HLA mismatches and the cellular immune response within the transplanted heart. *Human Immunology* 39:233–242, 1994.
39. Carlquist, JF, Greenwood, JH, Hammond, EH, and Anderson, JL. Phenotype and serine esterase production of human cardiac allograft-infiltrating lymphocytes. *Journal of Heart & Lung Transplantation* 12:748–755, 1993.
40. Weintraub, D, Masek, M, and Billingham, ME. The lymphocyte subpopulations in cyclosporine-treated human heart rejection. *Heart Transplantation* 4:213–216, 1985.
41. Vaessen, L, Ouwehand, A, Baan, C, Jutte, N, Balk, A, Claas, F, and Weimar, W. Phenotypic and functional analysis of T cell receptor gamma delta-bearing cells isolated from human heart allografts. *Journal of Immunology* 147:846–852, 1991.
42. Vaessen, L, Baan, C, Ouwehand, A, Jutte, N, Balk, A, Mochtar, B, Claas, F, and Weimar, W. Acute rejection in heart transplant patients is associated with the presence of committed donor-specific cytotoxic lymphocytes in the graft but not in the blood. *Clin Exp Immunol* 88:213–219, 1992.
43. Ouwehand, A, Baan, C, Roelen, D, Vaessen, L, Balk, A, Jutte, N, Bos, E, Claas, F, and Weimar, W. The detection of cytotoxic T cells with high-affinity receptors for donor antigens in the transplanted heart as a prognostic factor for graft rejection. *Transplantation* 56:1223–1229, 1993.
44. Van Besouw, N, Daane, C, Vaessen, L, Balk, A, Claas, F, Zondervan, P, Jutte, N, and Weimar, W. Different patterns in donor-specific production of T-helper 1 and 2 cytokines by cells infiltrating the rejecting cardiac allograft. *Journal of Heart and Lung Transplantation* 14:816–823, 1995.
45. Ouwehand, A, Baan, C, Groeneveld, K, Balk, A, Jutte, N, Bos, E, Claas, F, and Weimar, W. Altered specificity of alloreactive cardiac graft-infiltrating cells by prophylactic treatment with OKT3 or horse anti-lymphocyte globulin. *Transplantation* 55:154–158, 1993.
46. Jollow, K, Sundstrom, JB, Gravanis, M, Kanter, K, Herskowitz, A, and Ansari, A. Apoptosis of mononuclear cell infiltrates in cardiac allograft biopsy specimens questions studies of biopsy-cultured cells. *Transplantation* 63:1482–1489, 1997.
47. Ansari, A, Mayne, A, Sundstrom, JB, Gravanis, M, Kanter, K, Sell, K, Villanger, F, Siu, C, and Herskowitz, A. Frequency of hypoxanthine guanine phosphoribosyltransferase (HPRT-) T cells in the peripheral blood of cardiac transplant recipients. *Circulation* 92:862–874, 1995.
48. Sell, KW, Kanter, K, Rodey, GE, Wang, YC, and Ansari, AA. Characterization of human heart-infiltrating cells after transplantation, V: suppression of donor-specific allogeneic responses by cloned T-cell lines isolated from heart biopsy specimens of patients after transplantation. *Journal of Heart and Lung Transplantation.* 11:500–510, 1992.
49. Bishop, DK, Chan, S, Li, W, Ensley, RD, XU, S, and Eichwald, EJ. CD4-positive helper T lymphocytes mediate mouse cardiac allograft rejection independent of donor alloantigen specific cytotoxic T lymphocytes. *Transplantation* 56:892–897, 1993.
50. Wagoner, LE, Zhao, L, Bishop, KD, Chan, S, Xu, S, and Barry, WH. Lysis of adult ventricular myocytes by cells infiltrating rejecting murine cardiac allografts. *Circulation* 93:111–119, 1995.
51. Krieger, NR, Deng-Ping, Y, and Fathman, CG. CD4+ but not CD8+ cells are essential for allorejection. *Journal of Experimental Medicine* 184:2013–2018, 1996.
52. Mingari, MC, Ponte, M, Bertone, S, Schiavetti, F, Vitale, C, Bellomo, R, Moretta, A, and Moretta, L. HLA class I-specific inhibitory receptors in human T lymphocytes: Interleukin 15-induced expression of CD94/NKG2A in superantigen- or alloantigen-activated CD8+ T cells. *Proceedings of the National Academy of Sciences* 95:1172–1177, 1998.
53. Cambiaggi, A, Verthuy, C, Naquet, P, Romagne, F, Ferrier, P, Biassoni, R, Moretta, A, Moretta, L, and Vivier, E. Natural killer cell acceptance of H-2 mismatch bone marrow grafts in transgenic mice

expressing HLA-Cw3 specific killer cell inhibitory receptor. *Proceedings of the National Academy of Sciences* 94:8088–8092, 1997.

54. Lai, D, Tsai, SP, and Hardy, RJ. Impact of HIV/AIDS on life expectancy in the United States. *AIDS* 11:203–207, 1997.
55. Cetta, F and Michels, VV. The natural history and spectrum of idiopathic dilated cardiomyopathy, including HIV and peripartum cardiomyopathy. *Current Opinion in Cardiology* 10:332–338, 1995.
56. Lenschow, DJ, Walunas, TL, and Bluestone, JA, CD28/B7 system of T cell co-stimulation. *Annual Review of Immunology* Vol 14:233–258, 1996.
57. Lakkis, FG, Konieczny, BT, Saleem, S, Baddoura, FK, Linsley, PS, Alexander, DZ, Lowry, RP, Pearson, TC, and Larsen, CP. Blocking the CD28-B7 T cell co-stimulation pathway induces long term cardiac allograft acceptance in the absence of IL-4. *Journal of Immunology* 158:2443–2448, 1997.
58. Pearson, TC, Alexander, DZ, Corbascio, M, Hendrix, R, Ritchie, SC, Linsley, PS, Faherty, D, and Larsen, CP. Analysis of the B7 costimulatory pathway in allograft rejection. *Transplantation* 63:1463–1469, 1997.
59. Larsen, CP, Elwood, ET, Alexander, DZ, Ritchie, SC, Hendrix, R, Tucker-Burden, C, Cho, HR, Aruffo, A, Hollenbaugh, D, Linsley, PS, Winn, KJ, and Pearson, TC. Long-term acceptance of skin and cardiac allografts after blocking CD40 and CD28 pathways. *Nature 381*:434–438, 1996.
60. Alexander, DZ, Pearson, TC, Hendrix, R, Ritchie, SC, and Larsen, CP. Analysis of effector mechanisms in murine cardiac allograft rejection. *Transplant Immunology* 4:46–48, 1996.
61. Larsen, CP, Alexander, DZ, Hendrix, R, Ritchie, SC, and Pearson, TC. Fas-mediated cytotoxicity. An immuno-effector or immuno-regulatory pathway in T cell-mediated immune responses? *Transplantation* 60:221–224, 1995.
62. Vergelli, M, Hemmer, B, Muraro, PA, Tranquill, L, Biddison, WE, Sarin, A, McFarland, HF, and Martin, R. Human autoreactive CD4+ T cell clones use perforin- or Fas/Fas ligand-mediated pathways for target cell lysis. *Journal of Immunology* 158:2756–2761, 1997.
63. Blazar, BR, Taylor, PA, and Vallera, DA. CD4+ and CD8+ T cells each can utilize a perforin-dependent pathway to mediate lethal graft-versus-host disease in major histocompatibility complex-disparate recipients. *Transplantation* 64:571–576, 1997.
64. Schulz, M, Schuurmann, HJ, and Joegensen, J, Steiner, C, Meerloo, T, Kagi, D, Hengartner, H, Zinkernagel, RM, Schrier, MH, and Burki, K. Acute rejection of vascular heart allografts by perforin-deficient mice. *European Journal of Immunology* 25:474–480, 1995.
65. VanBuskirk, AM, Wakely, ME, and Orosz, CG. Acute rejection of cardiac allografts by noncytolytic CD4+ T cell populations. *Transplantation* 62; 300–302, 1996.
66. Sirak, J, Orosz, CG, Wakely, E, and Van Buskirk, AM. Allocreative delayed-type hypersensitivity in graft recipients. Complexity of responses and divergence from acute rejection. *Transplantation* 63:1300–1307, 1997.
67. Pinsky, DJ, Cai, B, Yang, X, Rodriguez, C, Sciacca, RR, and Cannon, PJ. Nitric oxide dependent killing of myocytes by adjacent macrophages. *Circulation* 90(suppl I):1–192, 1994.
68. Christmas, SE and MacPherson, GG. The role of mononuclear phagocytes in cardiac allograft rejection in the rat, II: characterization of mononuclear phagocytes extracted from rat cardiac allografts. *Cellular Immunology* 69:271–280, 1982.
69. Christmas, SE and MacPherson, GG. The role of mononuclear phagocytes in cardiac allograft rejection in the rat, III: the effect of cells extracted from rat cardiac allografts upon beating heart cell cultures. *Cellular Immunology* 69:281–290, 1982.
70. Rowe, GT, Eaton, LR, and Hess, ML. Neutrophil-derived, oxygen free radical-mediated cardiovascular dysfunction. *Journal of Molecular and Cellular Cardiology*. 16(11):1075–1079, 1984.
71. Entman, ML, Youker, K, Shappel, SB, Siegel, C, Rothlein, R, Dreyer, WJ, Schmalsteig, FC, and Smith, CW. Neutrophil adherence to isolated adult canine myocytes. *Journal of Clinical Investigation* 85:1497–1506, 1990.
72. Entman, ML, Youker, K, Shoji, T, Kukielka, G, Shappell, SB, Taylor, AA, and Smith, CW. Neutrophil induced oxidative injury of cardiac myocytes. *Journal of Clinical Investigation* 90:1335–1345, 1992.
73. Herskowitz, A, Mayne, AE, Willoughby, SB, Kanter, K, and Ansari, AA. Patterns of myocardial cell adhesion molecule expression in human endomyocardial biopsies after cardiac transplantation. Induced ICAM-1 and VCAM-1 related to implantation and rejection. *American Journal of Pathology* 145:1082–1094, 1994.
74. Isobe, M, Yagita, H, Okamura, K, and Ihara, A. Specific acceptance of cardiac allograft after treatment with antibodies to ICAM-1 and LFA-1. *Science* 255:1125–1127, 1992.
75. Petersson, E, Qi, Z, Ekberg, H, Ostraat, O, Dohlsten, M, and Hedlund, G. Activation of alloreactive natural killer cells is resistant to cyclosporine. *Transplantation* 63:1138–1144, 1997.

76. Dresske, B, Zhu, X, Herwartz, C, Brotzmann, K, and Fandrich, F. The time pattern of organ infiltration and distribution of natural killer cells and macrophages in the course of acute graft rejection after allogeneic heart transplantation in the rat. *Transplantation Proceedings* 29:1715–1716, 1997.
77. Hayashi, T, Nozawa, M, Otsu, H, Deguchi, H, Kitaura, Y, and Kawamura, K. Cell-mediated cytotoxicity in acute rat cardiac allograft rejection: an immunological and ultrastructural study. Virchows Archiv—A, *Pathological Anatomy and Histopathology*. 418:41–50, 1991.
78. Marboe, CC, Knowles, DM, Chess, L, Reemtsma, K, and Fenoglio, JJ. The immunologic and ultrastructural characterization of the cellular infiltrate in acute cardiac allograft rejection: prevalence of cells with the natural killer (NK) phenotype. *Clinical Immunology and Immunopathology* 27:141–151, 1983.
79. Holzinger, C, Zuckermann, A, Laczkovics, A, Seitelberger, R, Laufer, G, Andert, S, Kink, F, Hovart, R, and Wolner, E. Monitoring of mononuclear cell subsets isolated from the coronary sinus and the right atrium in patients after allograft heart transplantation. *Journal of Thoracic and Cardiovascular Surgery* 102:215–222, 1991.
80. Petersson, E, Ostraat, O, Ekberg, H, Hansson, J, Simanaitis, M, Brodin, T, Dohlsten, M, and Hedlund, G. Allogeneic heart transplantation activates alloreactive NK cells. *Cellular Immunology* 175:25–32, 1997.
81. Uhteg, LC, Kupiec-Weglinski, JW, Rocher, LL, Salomon, DR, Tilney, NL, and Carpenter, CB. Systemic natural killer activity following cardiac engraftment in the rat: lack of correlation with graft survival. *Cellular Immunology* 100:274–279, 1986.
82. McDoall, RM, Batten, P, McCormack, A, Yacoub, MH, and Rose, ML. MHC class II expression on human heart microvascular endothelial cells: exquisite sensitivity to interferon-gamma and natural killer cells. *Transplantation* 64:1175–1180, 1997.
83. Gollub, SB, Huntrakoon, M, Dunn, MI. The significance of eosinophils in mild and moderate acute rejection. *American Journal of Cardiovascular Pathology* 3:21–26, 1990.
84. Riise, GC, Schersten, H, Nilsson, F, Ryd, W, and Andersson, BA. Activation of eosinophils and fibroblasts assessed by eosinophilic cationic protein and hyaluronan in BAL. Association with acute rejection in lung transplant recipients. *Chest* 110:89–96, 1996.
85. Chan, SY, DeBruyne, LA, Goodman, RE, Eichwald, EJ, and Bishop, DK. In vivo depletion of CD8+ T cells results in Th2 cytokine production and alternate mechanisms of allograft rejection. *Transplantation* 59:1155–1161, 1995.
86. Anversa, P, Olivetti, G, Leri, A, Liu, Y, and Kajstura, J. Myocyte cell death and ventricular remodeling. *Current Opinion in Nephrology & Hypertension* 6(2):169–176, 1997.
87. Kroemer, G, Dallaporta, B, and Resche-Rigon, M. The mitochondrial death/life regulator in apoptosis and necrosis. *Annual Review of Physiology* 60:619–642, 1998.
88. Granger, DN and Korthuis, RJ. Physiologic mechanisms of postischemic tissue injury. *Annual Review of Physiology* 57:311–332, 1995.
89. Jennings, RB and Reimer, KA. The cell biology of acute myocardial ischemia. *Annual Review of Medicine* 42:225–246, 1991.
90. Lucchesi, BR. Modulation of leukocyte-mediated myocardial reperfusion injury. *Annual Review of Physiology* 52:561–576, 1990.
91. Tatou, E, Mossiat, C, Maupoil, V, Gabrielle, F, David, M, and Rochette, L. Effects of cyclosporin and cremophor on working rat heart and incidence of myocardial lipid peroxidation. *Pharmacology* 52(1):1–7, 1996.
92. Hutcheson, AE, Rao, MR, Olinde, KD, and Markov, AK. Myocardial toxicity of cyclosporin A: inhibition of calcium ATPase and nitric oxide synthase activities and attenuation by fructose-1,6-diphosphate in vitro. *Research Communications in Molecular Pathology & Pharmacology* 89(1):17–26, 1995.
93. Van Houten, N and Huber, SA. Role of cytotoxic T cells in experimental myocarditis. *Springer Seminars. in Immunopathology* 11(1):61–68, 1989.
94. Guthrie, M, Lodge, PA, and Huber, SA. Cardiac injury in myocarditis induced by Coxsackievirus group B, type 3 in Balb/c mice is mediated by Lyt 2+ cytolytic lymphocytes. *Cellular. Immunology* 88(2):558–567, 1984.
95. Lyons, GE. Vertebrate heart development. *Current Opinion in Genetics & Development* 6(4): 454–460, 1996.
96. Lyons, GE. In situ analysis of the cardiac muscle gene program during embryogenesis. *Trends in Cardiovascular Medicine* 4(2):70–77, 1994.
97. Gorski, DH, Patel, CV, and Walsh, K. Homeobox transcription factor regulation in the cardiovascular system. *Trends in Cardiovascular Medicine* 3(5):184–190, 1993.
98. Struijker-Boudier, HA, Smits, JF, and De May, JG. Pharmacology of cardiac and vascular remodeling. *Annual Review of Pharmacology & Toxicology* 35:509–539, 1995.

99. Parker, TG and Schneider, MD. Growth factors, proto-oncogenes, and plasticity of the cardiac phenotype. *Annual Review of Physiology* 53:179–200, 1991.
100. Deuel, TF, Kawahara, RS, Mustoe, TA, and Pierce, AF. Growth factors and wound healing: Platelet-derived growth factor as a model cytokine. *Annual Review of Medicine* 42:567–584, 1991.
101. Weber, KT and Brilla, CG. Pathological hypertrophy and cardiac interstitium. Fibrosis and renin-angiotensin-aldosterone system. *Circulation* 83(6):1849–1865, 1991.
102. Orosz, CG and Pelletier, RP. Chronic remodeling pathology in grafts. *Current Opinion in Immunology* 9(5):676–680, 1997.
103. Waltenberger, J, Wanders, A, Fellstrom, B, Miyazono, K, Heldin, C, and Funa, K. Induction of transforming growth factor-beta during cardiac allograft rejection. *Journal of Immunology* 151:1147–1153, 1993.
104. Orosz, CG and Sedmak, DD. Concerns regarding the current paradigm for chronic allograft rejection. *Transplant Immunology* 5(3):169–172, 1997.

5. APOPTOSIS IN CARDIAC TRANSPLANT REJECTION

Mireia Puig[†], Navneet Narula*, Jagat Narula[†]
[†]Center for Heart Failure, Transplantation Research, Hahnemann University Hospital, Philadelphia, Pennsylvania
*Department of Radiology, Hahnemann University Hospital Philadelphia, Pennsylvania

Apoptosis is a genetically programmed process of cell death which is distinct from necrosis and occurs normally in dividing tissues. Such a process is mandatory for tissue development and growth in order to maintain the balance between new and old cells. Contrary to necrosis, apoptosis is an active energy-requiring process and is genetically programmed (Kerr 1972). Ultrastructural characterization of the process of apoptosis reveals that it involves individual cells which separates from the surrounding cells, the nucleus and cytoplasm undergo condensation, nuclear chromatin aggregates in dense masses under the nuclear envelope and intact organelles become closely packed in cytoplasmic protuberances. These protuberances are rounded by membrane and released as apoptotic bodies which are readily removed by professional scavenger or the neighboring cells. The apoptotic bodies are not accompanied by inflammatory cell infiltration because the intracellular contents are not released. The apoptotic bodies in hematoxylin-eosin stained slides are observed as small spherical or ovoid cytoplasmic bodies with pyknotic nuclear remnants (Kerr 1972). Unlike a programmed apoptotic process, necrosis involves clusters of cells; their cellular contents are exteriorized, and an intense inflammatory reaction ensues.

In contrast to random DNA fragmentation in necrosis, the DNA damage during apoptosis occurs in most orderly pattern wherein DNA is fragmented to the olignucleosomal or polyoligonucleosomal sizes. The DNA fragmentation can be identified by either gel electrophoresis or by in situ end labeling (TUNEL) in the histologic sections of the tissues. The electrophoresis resolves low molecular weight DNA fragments of oligonucleosomal size (180 bp) or its multiples displayed in the form of equidistant ladder rungs. The in situ labeling identifies individual nuclei in the tissue that contain fragmented DNA.

Apoptosis usually occurs as a physiological process in dividing tissues and has been well-described in normal embryogenesis (Glüksmann 1951, Saunders 1966, Farbman 1968), during renewal of healthy tissues such as endometrium and intestinal epithelium (Kerr 1965, Kerr 1971) and upon physiologic involution of various organs such as that of thymus and senescent prostate. On the other hand, it has been tacitly believed that apoptosis does not occur in tissues that do not divide, such as

Table 1. Differences between necrotic and apoptotic cell death

	Necrosis	Apoptosis
Infiltration	Inflammatory infiltrate	No inflammatory infiltrates
Distribution	Contiguous cells involved	Scattered cells
Cell Volume	Increased	Decreased
Appearance	Cell Rupture	Cell fragmentation
Membrane	Altered permeability	Preserved permeability
Subcellular Organelles	Destroyed	Preserved
Mitochondria	Intramitochondrial densities	Structurally preserved, leaky envelope, altered membrane potential, loss of cytochrome C
DNA fragmentation	Random	Nucleosomic 180 bp or multiples
Chromatin	Small aggregates	Large aggregates
Energy Requirement	Not required	Required

neuronal or myocardial cells. A non-physiologic presence of excessive apoptosis in such terminally-differentiated tissues may lead to disorders, such as congestive heart failure, and Alzheimer's disease.

MOLECULAR AND CELLULAR BASIS OF APOPTOSIS

Our understanding of apoptosis is derived from studies of development in a nematode *C.elegans*. The characterization of the death genes ced-3 and ced-4 which are involved in apoptosis in the nematodes has facilitated the identification of their mammalian homologues. These proteases which have been referred to as *caspases* (cysteine aspartic acid-specific proteases) are proteolytically cleaved from their precursors and in turn fragment various cytoplasmic, mitochondrial and nuclear proteins. Of the family of mammalian caspases, caspase 1, 4, 5 and 8 are involved in cytokine processing; 2, 8, 9, and 10 in signal transduction and 3, 6 and 7 in enzymatic digestion of intracellular proteins (Yeh 1998).

Multiple pathways trigger apoptosis (Figure 1). TNF receptor superfamily which is activated following interaction with Fas ligand and cytokines such as TNF leads to assembly of death domains such as TRADD (TNF-receptor associated death domain); TRAF2 (TNF receptor associated factor 2) and FADD (Fas-associated death domain) and contribute to apoptosis by activating caspase 1 or ICE (interleukin-1-beta converting enzyme) (Nagata 1997). Other varieties of stress including DNA damaging and non-DNA damaging stimuli may lead to apoptosis by release of cytochrome C from mitochondria (Liu et al. 1996). The mitochondrial respiratory chain protein-cytochrome c, which is localized between the outer and inner mitochondrial membranes, is released into the cytoplasm before the execution of apoptosis and has also been shown to induce apoptotic changes in nuclei in a cell free system in vitro. The mechanism of cytochrome C release is not well understood. One mechanism has recently been proposed wherein caspase-8 mediates cleavage of Bid and the carboxy-terminal fragment of Bid mediates the cytochrome c release (Luo et al. 1998). It has also been hypothesized that JNK or stress activated protein kinase may translocate to mitochondria and overwhelm Bcl-2 protection of cytochrome c release (Narula 1998a). The cytochrome c release facilitates formation of a complex of Apaf-1 and recently cloned mammalian homologue of ced-4

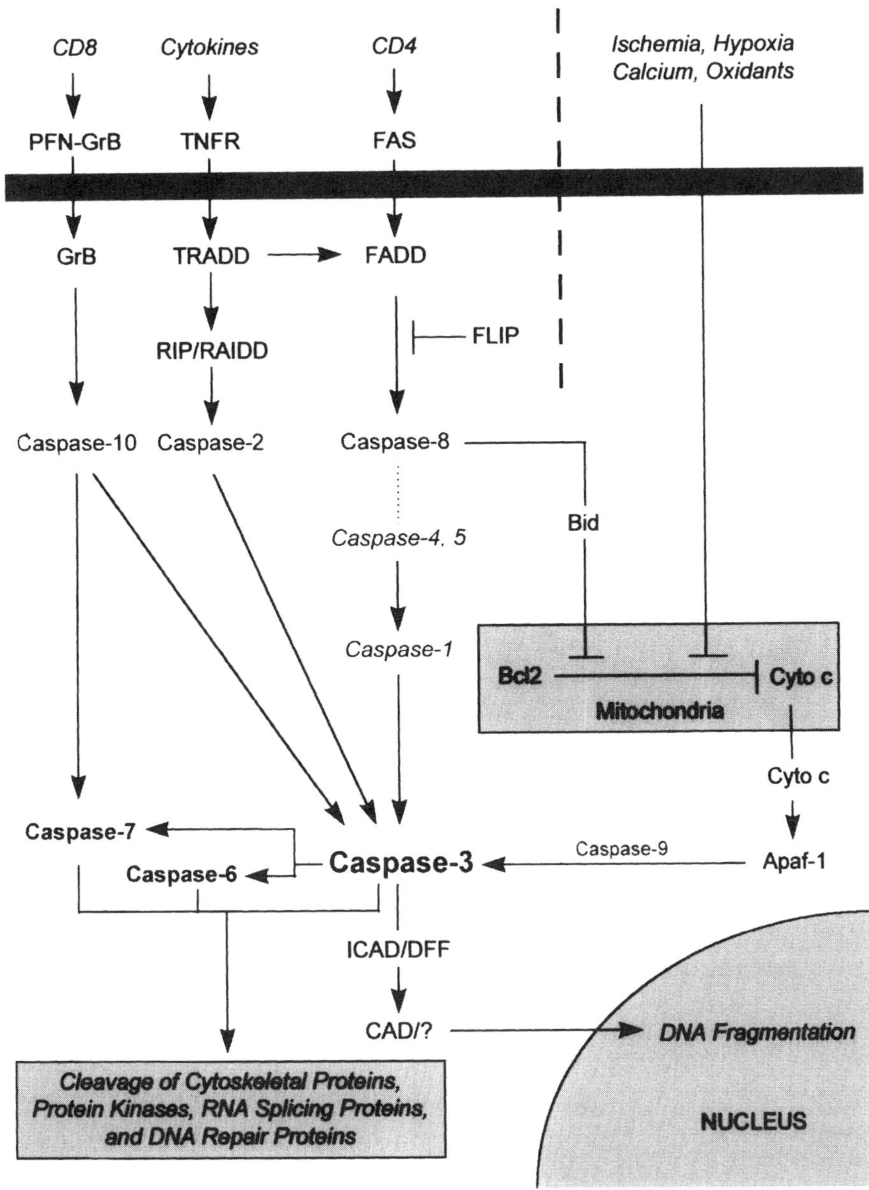

Figure 1. *Molecular and cellular basis of apoptosis, abbreviations*–PFN-GrB : Perforin-granzyme B; GrB: granzyme B; TNFR: Tumor Necrosis Factor Receptor; TRADD: TNF Receptor Associated Death Domain; RIP/RAIDD: Receptor Interacting Protein/RIP-Associated Ich-1/CED Homologue Protein with Death Domain; FADD: Fas Associated Death Domain; FLIP: Flice-Inhibitory Protein; Cytoc: Cytochrome C; Apaf-1: Apoptosis Activation Factor 1; ICAD/DFF: Inhibitor of Caspase Activated Deoxyribonuclease/DNA Fragmentation Factor.

which eventually activates caspase-3 (Li et al. 1997). In addition, it has recently been demonstrated that granzyme B in association with perforin may lead to apoptosis by activation of caspase-10 or direct involvement in proteolysis (Froelich 1998).

APOPTOSIS IN HEART TRANSPLANT REJECTION

Apoptosis has been described in the context of organ transplantation in humans. In liver transplantation apoptosis contributes to death of hepatocytes (Afford 1995) and biliary duct cells (Nawaz 1994, Afford 1995, Gapany 1997). In renal transplantation, apoptosis has been detected in both acute (Ito 1995, Olsen 1989, Matsuno 1994, Matsuno 1997) and chronic rejection states (Laine 1997). The process of programmed cell death has been observed in human intestinal transplantation (Lee 1996a, Lee 1996b), as also in pancreatic transplantation (Knoop 1991; Boonstra 1997). In cardiac transplantation, the role of apoptosis of various myocardial cells is being defined in animals and humans.

Evidence of Apoptosis in Animal Models of Transplant Rejection

Numerous recent experimental studies have demonstrated relevance of apoptosis in heart transplant rejection. Szábolcs and associates (1996) performed heterotopic abdominal transplants of hearts from Lewis to Wistar Furth rats; Lewis to Lewis grafts served as controls. Apoptosis was observed in allogeneic but not in syngeneic animals. The prevalence of apoptotic cardiac myocytes increased from day 3 (0.30/sq. mm ventricular myocardial tissue) to day 5 (1.30/sq. mm). Maximum apoptosis was seen on the fifth day after transplantation which coincided with severe rejection. Apoptosis was seen adjacent to macrophage-rich inflammatory infiltrates. Severity of apoptosis correlated with the degree of inducible nitric oxide synthase expression (iNOS), and iNOS mRNA. In addition to myocytes, a large number of interstitial and endothelial cells also demonstrated apoptosis.

Kageyama et al. (1998) confirmed the findings of apoptosis in allograft rejection of disparate Lewis (RT^1 to RT^a) rats. Only a few cardiac myocytes (apoptotic index, 0.011 ± 0.021; cellular rejection) and lymphocytes demonstrated apoptosis on the first day that concurred with mild transplant rejection (ISHLT grade 1A). Apoptosis of myocytes progressively increased by the third post operative day (apoptotic index, 0.065 ± 0.007; cellular rejection, ISHLT grade 2) and the fifth day (apoptotic index, 0.094 ± 0.017; cellular rejection, ISHLT grade 3A-3B). Apoptosis in the cardiomyocytes was accompanied by increased expression of Fas ligand transcripts, granzyme B and perforin mRNA upregulation. Apoptosis of only infiltrating cells was observed in isografts. The experiment suggested that Fas/Fas-ligand and granule-mediated mechanisms constitute the basis of apoptosis of myocardial cells during allograft rejection.

Apoptosis in Human Cardiac Allograft Rejection

Laguens et al. (1996) studied 63 endomyocardial biopsy specimens from 6 patients, obtained 1 week to 5 months after transplantation. Apoptosis was observed in all specimens with ISHLT grade 3A or higher rejection, approximately half the specimens with grade 2 rejection and only occasionally in grade 1B rejection. Apoptosis did not occur in biopsy samples with grade 1A or 0 rejection. Apoptosis was subjacent to the areas of infiltration. However, no correlation was detected between the intensity of apoptosis and the degree of rejection. In addition, apoptosis of interstitial cells and endothelial cells was seen in all degrees of rejection; it was more prevalent in severe forms. In contrast to the observations of Laguens and associates, Jollow et al., observed more significant apoptosis of inflammatory cells compared to that of myocytes in their study of 22 endomyocardial biopsie specimens from cardiac allograft recipients (1997). All biopsies showed moderately severe rejection, classified as ISHLT grade 3A at different time points after transplantation, only one biopsy specimen with no inflammatory infiltrates and no myocyte damage (ISHLT grade 0) was included as control. Apoptosis of myocytes and inflammatory cells was seen in all biopsy specimens.

In a subsequent study, Szabolcs et al. replicated their observations in endomyocardial biopsies obtained from 30 allograft recipients. Of these, 18 biopsy specimens demonstrated inflammatory cell infiltration associated with myocyte damage (ISHLT grade 3A-B). The cellular infiltrate was rich in CD68+ macrophages and CD4+ lymphocytes in the regions with myocyte necrosis but the infiltrates were composed predominantly of CD8+ T cells in myocardial areas with less myocyte damage. No inflammatory infiltrates or myocyte damage was present in the remaining 12 biopsy specimens. Apoptosis was abundantly seen in the biopsies with allograft rejection and was seen near foci of myocyte damage, associated predominantly with macrophage-rich mixed inflammatory infiltrates. Cardiac myocyte apoptosis, however, was also observed occasionally in areas without inflammation in the severely rejecting (ISHLT grade 3B) allografts. Minimal apoptosis of cardiac myocytes was observed in biopsies from the group with no allograft rejection (ISHLT grade 0). There was a 30-fold increase in the total number of apoptotic cells in rejecting (2.49 apoptotic nuclei per mm^2 of myocardium) compared with the control (0.08 apoptotic neclei) biopsy specimens.

Puig et al. studied apoptosis in 40 endomyocardial biopsies at different time intervals after transplantation (1998). The myocardial uptake of radiolabeled antimyosin antibody was used to detect the severity of allograft rejection (Ballester et al. 1990, 1992, 1997, 1998, Hosenpud 1992). Apoptosis was observed in cardiomyocytes, and also in vascular endothelial cells, interstitial cells and lymphocytes. Apoptotic myocytes were predominantly observed in the vicinity of mononuclear cell infiltration; apoptosis was most prevalent in the specimens that contained significant macrophage infiltration (>5 cells per high power field). Prevalence of apoptosis increased progressively in parallel to the severity of rejection.

Recently, radiolabeled annexin V imaging has been reported in cardiac allograft recipients for the noninvasive detection of apoptosis (Narula 2000). Annexin V binds to phosphatidyl serine that gets exteriorized from the inner to outer leaflet of sarcolemmal lipid bilayer during apoptosis. Of the 13 allograft recipients, 8 had no uptake of annexin V in cardiac region; all patients had unremarkable endomyocardial biopsy and no evidence of apoptosis. Of the 5 remaining patients, 3 had focal and 2 had diffuse annexin uptake. Three patients with focal scans demonstrated ISHLT grade 2/4 rejection in EMB specimens; the presence of apoptosis was supported by caspase 3 upregulation in scattered cardiomyocytes. Of the two patients with diffuse annexin V uptake, one had an evidence of ISHLT grade 3A/4 rejection in EMB specimen and upregulation of caspase 3 in candiomyocytes, in terstitial and endothelial cells. The remaining patient with diffuse annexin scan demonstrated aggressive vascular rejection with intense caspase upregulation in vascular endothelial cells and occasional cardiomyocytes.

Role of Cytokines and Nitric Oxide in Apoptosis Associated with Transplant Rejection

Constitutive NOS is expressed in the endothelial cells and produces small amounts of NO, whereas cytokine-mediated inducible nitric oxide synthetase (iNOS) in macrophages produces larger amounts of NO for prolonged periods (Szabolcs et al.). iNOS expression during allograft rejection is likely to be associated with cytokines such as IL-1β and interferon-γ (Wu et al. 1992). In addition, activated T helper cells can induce iNOS by contact-dependent signaling involving CD40 ligand-CD40 interactions with macrophages (Tian et al. 1995). In fact, monoclonal antibodies directed against CD40 have been used to abrogate acute cellular rejection as well as the chronic vasculopathy (Larsen et al. 1996).

Using a rat model of heterotopic abdominal cardiac transplantation, Szabolcs et al. and Yang et al., demonstrated progressive increase in expression of iNOS mRNA and iNOS protein, which paralleled the time course of apoptosis in cardiac myocytes (Szabolcs 1996). iNOS expression was observed most intensely in myocytes adjacent to macrophage-rich inflammatory infiltrates and the iNOS expression was proportional to the distribution of nitrotyrosine. These results were further substantiated by Worrall et al. who reported that treatment with a relatively selective iNOS inhibitor prolonged survival, improved performance, and reduced the pathological changes in the cardiac allografts. Szabolcs et al. (1998) confirmed the role of nitric oxide mediated mechanisms in endomyocardial biopsies obtained from cardiac allograft recipients. Their immunohistochemical studies for iNOS showed strong cytoplasmic reactivity in macrophages and cardiac myocytes in rejecting grafts. Cardiac myocytes adjacent to macrophage-rich inflammatory infiltrates contained high levels of nitrated amino acids as determined by their strong immunoreactivity for nitrotyrosine.

Alexander et al. (1996) underscored that the nitric oxide-mediated mechanisms were operative in transplant rejection even in the absence of Fas, CD8 and B cells. Rejection in these animals was associated with upregulation of macrophage effector transcripts such as iNOS and TNFα.

Granule-Mediated Mechanisms Associated with Apoptosis in Transplant Rejection

Granule-mediated apoptosis is known to participate in both innate (natural killer cells) and adaptive defense (cytotoxic T cells) mechanisms against intracellular pathogens, tumors and non-self cells, and this process is entirely independent of perforin-mediated cellular necrosis (Froelich et al. 1998). Apoptosis is induced through combined action of the pore-forming protein perforin and a family of granule-associated serine proteases referred to as granzymes (Tschopp and Nabholz 1990). Gene deletion studies in mice have demonstrated that granzyme type B is important for apoptosis (Heusel et al. 1994). During granule-mediated apoptosis induced by CD8 lymphocytes, granzyme B possibly enters target cells by receptor-dependent endocytosis with plasma membrane containing sublytic perforin pores. The granzyme B escapes to the cytosol due to disruption of leaky endocytic vesicle or when vesicle fuses with an endosome (Froelich et al. 1998, to activate caspase-10 and eventually caspase-3 (Figure 1). While various inducers of apoptosis follow a linear cascade, granzyme B involves multiple pathways including less important substrates and direct processing of cytosolic, mitochondrial and intranuclear proteins.

Kageyama et al. demonstrated progressive upregulation of granzyme B and perforin mRNA with apoptosis in the rejecting hearts in murine model of heart transplantation (1998). Although Alexander et al. also observed upregulation of granzyme B 5–12 days after transplantation, they demonstrated that CD8 cytotoxic lymphocytic activity was not necessary for rejection. CD8-deficient mice reject allografts normally and the contribution of granzyme B to apoptosis in transplant rejection will need to be critically studied.

Fas-Related Mechanisms in Apoptosis in Allograft Rejection

Interaction of Fas/Fas-ligand invokes death receptors and death domains to activate caspase 8 and 1 and eventually caspase 3 enroute to apoptosis. In a murine model of heart transplantation, gradually progressive expression of Fas-ligand has been reported after transplantation; Fas-ligand remained essentially undetected in syngeneic grafts (Kageyama et al. 1998). On the other hand, Fas transcripts were expressed in both syngeneic and allogeneic grafts and their magnitude was not altered during the course after transplantation. While this study implicated direct role of Fas/Fas-ligand interaction in induction of cardiomyocyte death, another study has questioned its role in immunoeffector function (Larsen et al. 1995). Although the latter study has found the upregulation of Fas transcripts in both allografts and isografts as well as Fas-ligand upregulation only in allografts, the absence of an intact Fas/Fas-ligand system did not alter the process of graft rejection even in CD4-dependent model. This elegant study by Larsen et al. (1995) utilized various graft combinations to prove their point. Fas-deficient *lpr/lpr* donor hearts implanted in Fas-ligand deficient mutant *gld/gld* homozygote mice were rejected normally suggesting that the Fas system is not functionally involved in rejection. The rejection of Fas-deficient donor hearts occurred normally even in (therefore, CD4-dependent) recipient mice. The study suggested that Fas pathway may not be involved in immunoeffector function and could be principally responsible for regulation of clonal expansion and subsequent contraction of alloreactive T cell population towards development of immunological tolerance to graft.

Peripheral immunological tolerance is developed by the ability of lymphocytes to kill themselves using Fas/Fas-ligand interactions (Abbas 1996). In fact both *lpr/lpr* and *gld/gld* homozygous mouse models of systemic autoimmunity have demonstrated defective expresion of Fas or a mutation of Fas ligand (Nagata and Suda, 1995). Defective expression of Fas also leads to systemic autoimmune disorders in humans (Rieux-Laucaut et al., 1995; Fisher et al., 1995). Helper T lymphocytes challenged repeatedly by antigen, express high levels of Fas and Fas-ligand. Upregulation of Fas and Fas-ligand on the same cells facilitates self-destruction or these cells may kill each other leading to contraction of alloreactive or self-active lymphocyte clones. However, Fas-mediated systems do not participate in thymic selection of developing T cells and are only involved in peripheral deletion of mature T cells in lymphoid tissues (Singer and Abbas, 1994).

Although the role of Fas/Fas-ligand mediated myocardial damage has been questioned, it is likely that TNFα may be utilizing a death domain assembly in myocardial damage. TNF is widely expressed in allografts even in the absence of cellular and clinical evidence of rejection (Torre-Amione et al. 1998) and TNFα levels are known to be elevated in selective coronary sinus samples in allograft recipients (Fyfe et al. 1993). Although, no direct evidence of TNF mediated apoptosis is available in human heart transplantation, it is possible that chronic TNFα upregulation may be involved in ongoing apoptotic cell death.

Apoptosis in Allograft Vasculopathy

It has been proposed that apoptosis may play an important role in slowing the process of chronic rejection and allograft vasculopathy. White et al. (1997) observed greater intimal thickening, apoptosis and Fas-Ligand mRNA expression in allograft vessels than isograft vessels in rats. On the other hand, Dong et al. (1996) studied apoptosis in coronary arteries from 2 cardiac allograft recipients and compared them with severe native atherosclerotic coronary artery disease and normal coronary vessels. Almost all endothelial cells and one-third of the T cells were Fas-positive in allograft vessels (Table 2). Of the T cells and macrophages that expressed Fas, only one-fifth demonstrated evidence of DNA fragmentation in the mild and moderate vasculopathy as compared to the majority of inflammatory cells in severe transplant vasculopathy. On the other hand, most endothelial cells were apoptotic in mild-to-moderate vasculopathy as compared with minimal endothelial damage in the severe vasculopathy group. In contrast to transplant vasculopathy, apoptosis was observed mainly in macrophages of the lipid-rich cores of atherosclerotic disease; these cells were Fas-negative. In most normal arteries, occasional Fas and TUNEL positive endothelial and T cells were seen. In transplanted hearts, MHC class I and

Table 2. Percent prevalence of apoptosis in endothelial cells and macrophages in allograft vasculopathy

	Allograft Vasculopathy		
		DNA Fragmentation in Fas	
	Fas Overexpression	Early Vasculopathy	Late Vasculopathy
Endothelial Cells	100	75	10
Macrophages/T cells	30	20	80

II antigens are expressed on vascular endothelial cells which may lead to induction of humoral and cellular immune response and accumulation of T lymphocytes and antibodies in the subendothelial space (Hruban et al. 1990). The injury to the endothelial cells results in secretion of various growth factors and cytokines such as PDGF, TGF-β, IL-1 and IL-6, that mediate vascular remodeling (Gibbons and Dzau 1994). Data from Dong et al. (1997) reveals that during early vasculopathy, only a few lymphocytes demonstrate evidence of apoptosis. It could be assumed that in early vasculopathy the alloreactive lymphocytes which are freshly stimulated by alloantigen may be resistant to cell death (Miyawaki et al. 1992) but inflict severe endothelial cell damage (Dong et al. 1997).

CONCLUSIONS

Apoptosis of myocytes occurs in human cardiac allograft rejection. Myocyte apoptosis may occur with all degrees of rejection, and even in its absence. The prevalence and severity of apoptosis is predominantly determined by the intensity of macrophage infiltration and is likely mediated by nitric oxide-related mechanisms. Apoptosis of interstitial, endothelial and inflammatory cells also occurs in the allograft and suggests an immunoregulatory role. Studies of the role of nitric oxide in myocyte damage and Fas and Fas ligand in peripheral tolerance have raised the exciting possibility that these pathways can be exploited in a beneficial way.

REFERENCES

1. Abbas AK. Die and let live: eliminating dangerous lymphocytes. Cell 1996;84:655–657.
2. Afford SC, Hubscher S, Strain AJ, Adams DH, Neuberger JM. Apoptosis in the human liver during allograft rejection and end-stage liver disease. J Pathol 1995;176:373–380.
3. Alexander DZ, Pearson TC, Hendrix R, Ritchie SC, Larsen CP. Analysis of effector mechanisms in murine cardiac allograft rejection. Transplant Immunol 1996;4:46–48.
4. Ashkenazi A and Dixit VM. Death receptors: signaling and modulation. Science 1998;281:1305–1308.
5. Ballester M, Bordes R, Tazelaar T, Carrió I, Marrugat J, Narula J, Billingham ME. An evaluation of biopsy classification for rejection: relation to the detection of myocardial damage by ^{111}In-monoclonal antimyosin antibody imaging. J Am Coll Cardiol 1998;31:1357–61.
6. Ballester M, Carrió I. Noninvasive detection of acute cardiac rejection: the quest for the perfect test. J Nucl Cardiol 1997;4:249–55.
7. Ballester M, Obrador D, Carrió I, Moya C, Augè JM, Bordes R, Martí V, Bosch I, Bernà L, Estorch M, Pons G, Cámara ML, Padró JM, Arís A, Caralps JM. Early postoperative reduction of monoclonal antimyosin antibody uptake is associated with absent rejection-related complications after heart transplantation. Circulation 1992;85:61–68.
8. Beckman JS, Koppenol WH. Nitric oxide, superoxide, and peroxynitrite: the good, the bad and the ugly. Am J Physiol 1996;271(Cell Physiol 40): C1424.
9. Beranek JT. Apoptosis is the main mechanism of cardiomyocyte death in hyperacute rejection of heart xeno and allografts. Transplantation 1997;64:1632–1633.
10. Beranek JT. Eosinophilic droplets similar to red cells are present in the hyperacute rejection of heart xenograft. J Intern Med 1997a;241:89.
11. Beranek JT. Myocardial pseudovascular tubes are present in the delayed rejection of heart xenografts. Transplantation 1997b;63:3486.
12. Bergese SD, Klenotic SM, Wakely ME, Sedmak DD, Orosz CG. Apoptosis in murine cardíac grafts. Transplantation 1997;63(2):320–325.
13. Boonstra SG, Wever PC, Lateveer SC: Apoptosis of acinar cells in panreas allograft rejection. Translantation 1997;64:1211–1213.

14. Cui S, Reichner JS, Mateo RB, Albina JE. Activated murine macrophages induce apoptosis in tumor cells through nitric oxide-dependent or independent mechanisms. Cancer Res 1994;54:2462.
15. Dec GW, Hajjar RJ, Narula J. Apoptosis in heart failure. Cardiol Clinics 1998;16:691–710.
16. Dong C, Wilson JE, Winters GL, McManus BM. Human transplant coronary artery disease. Pathological evidence of Fas-mediated apoptotic cytotoxicity in allograft arteriopathy. Lab Invest 1996;74: 921–937.
17. Dong C, Winters GL, Wilson JE, McManus BM. Enhanced lymphocyte longevity and absence of proliferation and lymphocyte apoptosis in Quilty effects of human heart allografts. Am J Pathol 1997;151:121–130.
18. Farbman AI. Electron microscope study of palate fusion in mouse embryos. Devl Biol 1968;18:93.
19. Finkel MS, Oddis CV, Jacob TD, Watkins SC, Hattler BG, Simmons RL. Negative inotropic effects of cytokines on the heart mediated by nitric oxide. Science 1992;257:387–389.
20. Fisher GH, Rosenberg FJ, Strauss SE, Dale JK, Middelton LA, Lin AY, Strober W, Leonardo MJ, Puck JM. Dominant interfering Fas gene mutations impair apoptosis in a human autoimmune lymphoproliferative syndrome. Cell 1995;81:935–946.
21. Froelich CJ, Dixit VM, Yang X. Lymphocyte granule-mediated apoptosis: matters of viral mimicry and deadly proteases. Immunol Today 1998;19:30–36.
22. Fuks Z, Persaud RS, Alfieri A et al. Basic fibroblast growth factor protects endothelial cells against radiation-induced programmed cell death in vitro and in vivo. Cancer Res 54:2582–2890.
23. Fyfe A, Daly P, Galligan L, Pirc L, Feindel C, Cardella C. Coronary sinus sampling of cytokines after heart transplantation: evidence for macrophage activation and interleukin-4 production within the graft. J Am Coll Cardiol 1993;21:171.
24. Gapany C, Zhao M, Zimmermann A. The apoptosis protector, bcl-2 protein, is downregulated in bile duct epithelial cells of human liver allografts. J Hepatol 1997;26:535–542.
25. Gibbons GH, Dzau VJ. The emerging concept of vascular remodeling. N Engl J Med 1994;330: 1431–1438.
26. Glüksmann A. Cell death in normal vertebrate ontogeny. Biol Rev 1951;26:59.
27. Heusel JW, Wesselschmidt RL, Shresta S, Russell JH, Ley TJ. Cytotoxic lymphocytes require granzime B for the rapid induction of DNA fragmentation and apoptosis in allogenic target cells. Cell 1994;76:977–987.
28. Hori S, Havaux X, Rubay R, Latinne D, Bazin H, Gianello P. Effects of graft preservation and IgM depletion on guinea pig to rat cardiac xenograft survival. Transplantation 1997;63:1554.
29. Hosenpud JD. Noninvasive diagnosis of cardiac allograft rejection. Another of many searches for the grail. Circulation 1992;85:368–371.
30. Hruban RH, Beschorner WE, Baumgartner WA, Augustine SM, Ren H, Reitz BA, Hutchins GM. Accelerated arteriosclerosis in heart transplant recipients is associated with a T-lymphocyte-mediated endothelialitis. Am J Pathol 1990;137:871–881.
31. Ito H, Kasagi N, Shomori K, Osaki M, Adachi H. Apoptosis in the human allografted kidney. Analysis by terminal deoxynucleotidyl transferase-mediated dUTP-botin nick end labeling. Transplantation 1995;60(8):794–798.
32. James TN. Complete heart block and fatal right ventricular failure in an infant. Circulation 1996; 1588–1600.
33. Jollow KC, Sundstorm JB, Gravanis MB, Ka-ter K, Herskowitz A, Ansari AA. Apoptosis of mononuclear cell infiltrates in cardiac allograft biopsy specimens questions studies of biopsy cultured cells. Transplantation 1997;63:1487–1489.
34. Kageyama Y, Li XK, Suzuki S, Suzuki H, Suzuki K, Kazui T, Harada Y. Apoptosis is involved in acute cardiac allograft rejection in rats. Ann Thorac Surg 1998;65:1604–1609.
35. Kerr JFR, Wyllie AH, Currie AR. Apoptosis: a basic biological phenomenon with wide ranging implications in tissue kinetics. Br J Cancer 1972;26:239–257.
36. Kerr JFR. A histochemical study of hypertrophy and ischaemic injury of rat liver with special reference to changes in lysosomes. J Path Bact 1965;90:419.
37. Kerr JFR. Shrinkage necrosis: a distinct mode of cellular death. J Pathol 1971;105:13.
38. Knoop M, McMahon RFT, Jones CJP, Hutchinson IV. Apoptosis in pancreatic allograft rejection-ultrastuctural observations. Exp Pathol 1991;41:219–224.
39. Kondo S, Yin D, Aoki T, Takahashi J, Morimura T, Takeuchi J. Bcl-2 gene prevents apoptosis of basic fibroblast growth factor-deprived murine aortic endothelial cells. Exp Cell Res 1994;213: 428–432.
40. Kubota T, McTiernan CF, Frye CS, Slawson SE, Lemster BH, Koretsky AP, Demetris AJ, Feldman AM. Dilated cardiomyopathy in transgenic mice with cardiac-specific overexpression of tumor necrosis factor-alpha. Circ Res 1997;81:627.
41. Laguens RP, Cabeza Meckert PM, San Martino J, Perrone S, Favaloro S. Identification of programmed cell death (apoptosis) in situ by means of specific labeling of nuclear DNA fragments in heart biopsy samples during acute rejection episodes. J Heart Lung Transplant 1996;15:911–918.

42. Laine J, Etelämäki P, Holmberg C, Dunkel L. Apoptotic cell death in human chronic renal allograft rejection. Transplantation 1997;63(1):101–105.
43. Larsen C, Elwwod D, Alexander D et al. Long-term acceptance of skin and cardiac allografts after blocking CD40 and CD28 pathways. Nature 1996;381:434.
44. Larsen CP, Alexander DZ, Hendrix R, Ritchie SC, Pearson TC. Fas-mediated cytotoxicity: an immunoeffector or immunoregulators pathway in T cell mediated immune responses. Transplantation 1995;60:221–224.
45. Lee RG, Nakamura K, Tsamandas AC et al. Pathology of human intestinal transplantation. Gastrenterology 1996a;110:1820–1834.
46. Lee RG, Tsamanda AC, Abu-Elmagd K et al. Histologic spectrum of acute cellular rejection in human intestinal allografts. Transplant Proc 1996b;28(5):2767.
47. Li P, Nijhawan D, Budihardjo I, Srinivasulo SM, Ahmed M, Alnemri ES, Wang X. Cytochrome C and dATP dependent formation of Apaf-1/Caspase 9 complex initiates an apoptotic protease cascade. Cell 1997;91:479–489.
48. Liu X, Kim CN, Yang J, Jemmerson R, Wang X. Induction of apoptotic program in cell-free extracts requirements for dATP and Cytochrome C. Cell 1996;86:147–157.
49. Luo X, Budihardjol I, Zon H, Slaughter C, Wang X. Bid, a Bcl-2 interacting protein, mediates Cytochrome C release from mitochondria in response to activation of cell surface death receptors. Cell 1998;94:481–490.
50. Mallat Z, Tedgui A, Fontaliran F et al. Evidence of apoptosis in arrhythmogenic right ventricular dysplasia. N Engl J Med 1996;335:1190–1197.
51. Marsh CB, Anderson CL. Lowe MP, Wewers MD. Monocyte IL-8 release is induced by two independent Fc gamma-R-mediated pathways. J Immunol 1996;157:2632–2637.
52. Marsh CB, Gadek JE, Kindt GC, Moore SA, Wewers MD. Monocyte Fc gamma receptor cross-linking induces IL-8 production. J Immunol 1995;155:3161.
53. Marsh CB, Love MP, Rovin BH, Parker JM, Liao Z, Knoell DL, Wewers MD. Lymphocytes produce IL-1 beta in response to Fc gamma receptor cross-linking effects on parenchymal cell IL-8 release. J Immunol 1998;160:3942–3948.
54. Marsh CB, Wewers MD, Tan LC, Robin BH. Fc gamma receptor cross-linking induces peripheral blood mononuclear cell MCP-1 expression. J Immunol 1997a;158:1078–1084.
55. Matsuno T, Nakagawa K, Sasaki H et al. Apoptosis in acute tubular necrosis and acute renal allograft rejection. Transplant Proc 1994;26(4):2170–2173.
56. Matsuno T, Sasaki H, Nakagawa K et al. Fas antigen expression and apoptosis in kidney allografts. Trasplant Proc 1997;29:177–178.
57. McConkey DJ, Orrenius S. The role of calcium in the regulation of apoptosis. J Leukoc Biol 1996;59:775.
58. Miyakawi T, Uehara T, Nibu R, Tsuji I, Yachie A, Yonehara S, Taniguchi N. Differential expression of apoptosis-related Fas antigen on lymphocyte subpopulations in human peripheral blood. J Immunol 1992;149:3753–3758.
59. Nagata S, Suda T. Fas and Fas-Ligand: lpr and gld mutations. Immunol Today 1995;16:39–43.
60. Nagata S. Apoptosis by death factor. Cell 1997;88:355–365.
61. Narula J, Chandrashekhar Y, Dec GW. Apoptosis in heart failure: a saga of heightened expectations, unfulfilled promises and broken hearts ... Apoptosis, 1999;3:309–315.
62. Narula J, Haider N, Virmani R et al. Apoptosis in myocytes in end-stage heart failure. N Engl J Med 1996;335:1182–1189.
63. Narula J, Kharbanda S, Khaw BA. Apoptosis in heart disease. Chest 1997;112:1358–1362.
64. Kharbanda S, Pandey P, Saxena S, Haider N, Iskandrian AE, Narula J. Translocation of SAPK to mitochondria and release of cytochrome C during apoptosis. Circulation 1998;98:683.
65. Nathan C. Natural resistance and nitric oxide. Cell 1995;82:873.
66. Nawaz S, Fennell RH. Apoptosis of bile duct epithelial cells in hepatic allograft rejection. Histopathology 1994;25:137–142.
67. Olsen S, Burdick JF, Keown PA, Wallace AC, Racusen LC, Solez K. Primary acute renal failure ("Acute tubular necrosis") in the transplanted kidney: Morphology and pathogenesis. Medicine 1989; 68(3):173–187.
68. Pinsky DJ, Cai B, Yang X, Rodriguez C, Sciacca RR, Marsh CB. The letal effects of cytokine induced nitric oxide on cardiac myocytes are blocked by nitric oxide synthase antagonism or transforming growth factor beta. J Clin Invest 1995;95:677–685.
69. Puig M, Ballester M, Matias-Guiu X, Bordes R, Carrió I, Aymat MR, Marrugat J, Padró JM, Caralps JM, Narula J. Apoptosis of myocytes in cardiac allograft rejection: An additional mechanism of myocardial damage away from Foci of Myocyte Necrosis (submitted for publication, 1998).
70. Reiter Y, Ciobotariu A, Jones J, Morgan BP, Fishelson Z. Complement membrane attack complex, perforin, and bacterial exotoxins induce in K562 cells calcium-dependent cross-protection from lysis. J Immunol 1995;155:2203.

71. Rieux-Laucaut F, Le Deist F, Hivroz C, Rogerts IAG, Debatin KM, Fischer A, Villartay JP. Mutations in Fas associated with human lymphoproliferative syndrome and auto immunity. Science 1995;268:1347–1349.
72. Rose AG, Cooper DK. A histopathologic grading system of hyperacute (humoral, antibody-mediated) cardiac xenograft and allograft rejection. J Heart Lung Transplant 1996:15:804.
73. Sashida H, Uchida K, Abiko Y. Changes in cardiac ultrastructure and myofibrillar proteins during ischemia in dogs, with special reference to changes in Z lines. J Moll Cell Cardiol 1984;16:1161.
74. Saunders JW. Death in embryonic systems. Science 1966;154:604.
75. Singer GG, Abbas AK. The Fas antigen is involved in peripheral but not thymic deletion of T lymphocytes in T cell receptor transgenic mice. Immunity 1994;1:365–371.
76. Steel GG. Cell loss as a factor in the growth rate of human tumors. Eur J Cancer 1967;3:381.
77. Szabolcs M, Michler RE, Yang X et al. Apoptosis of cardiac myocytes during cardiac allograft rejection. Relation to induction of nitric oxide synthase. Circulation 1996;94(7):1665–1673.
78. Szabolcs MJ, Rawalli S, Minanov O, Sciacca R, Michler RE, cannon PJ. Apoptosis and increased expression of inducible nitric oxide synthetase in human allograft rejection. Transplantation 1998;65:804–812.
79. Torre-Amione G, MacLellan W, Kapadia S, Weilbacher D, Farmer J, Young J, Mann D. Tumor necrosis factor-alpha is persistently expressed in cardiac allografts in the absence of histological or clinical evidence of rejection. Transplant Proc 1998;30:875–877.
80. Tschopp J, Nabholz M. Perforin-mediated target cell lysis by cytolytic T lymphocytes. Annu Rev Immunol 1990;8:279–302.
81. Wewers MD, Marsh CB. Role of the antibody in the pathogenesis of transplant vascular sclerosis: a hypothesis. Transplant Immunol 1997;5:283–288.
82. White WL, Zhang YL, Shelby J et al. Myocardial apoptosis in a heterotopic murine heart transplantation model of chronic rejection and graft vasculopathy. J Heart Lung Transplant 1997;16:250–255.
83. Wu C, Lovett M, Wong-hee J et al. Cytokine gene expression in rejecting cardiac allografts. Transplantation 1992;54:236.
84. Yeh ETH. Life and death of cell. Hospital Practice. August 15, 1998;85–92.
85. Yokoyama T, Vaca L, Rossen RD, Durante W, Hazarika P, Mann DL. Cellular basis for the negative inotropic effects of tumor necrosis factor-alpha in the adult mammalian heart. J Clin Invest 1993;92:2303–2312.
86. Yoshida K, Inui M, Harda K et al. Reperfusion of rat heart after brief ischemia induces proteolysis of calspectin (non-erythroid spectrin) during apoptosis. J Biol Chem 1995;270:6425.

6. PATHOLOGY OF CARDIAC ALLOGRAFT VASCULAR (MICROVASCULAR) REJECTION: IMPACT ON PATIENT OUTCOMES

Elizabeth H. Hammond, M.D.,
Robert L. Yowell, M.D., Ph.D, Dale G. Renlund, M.D
Cardiac Transplant Program Utah Transplantation Affiliated Hospitals (Utah) Salt Lake City, Utah

INTRODUCTION

Pathologic descriptions of allograft rejection of solid organs have long recognized several forms of vascular involvement as part of the rejection process. Renal allografts commonly display vasculitis involving the arteries and arterioles of the cortex with or without cellular infiltrates invading tubules in the severest forms of acute rejection.[1–3] This vascular inflammatory process, often termed acute vascular rejection, is identified in 50% of acutely rejecting kidneys and is frequently associated with allograft injury or loss in spite of increased immunosuppressive therapy.[2–4] By contrast, arteritis is rarely identified in cardiac allografts on endomyocardial biopsy although it has been associated with poor allograft survival.[5,6]

Studies of allograft rejection in animals have shown that the microvasculature is the earliest structure to be destroyed.[7,8] Destruction of the microvasculature of human skin allografts has also been shown to be the central event in first set rejection; in fact, the destruction of the capillary bed is likely more damaging to the allograft than piecemeal destruction of the allograft parenchyma.[9]

Since infiltrating cells arrive in all solid organ allografts via the blood, adherence and penetration of the capillaries, arterioles and venules by lymphoid cells is often considered as part of the rejection process (Table 1)[10–16]. In the liver, the endothelialitis involving venules is necessary to exclude other causes of inflammation of portal regions.[15] Capillaritis is considered an important component of acute allograft rejection in the lung.[14] Interstitial edema, a consequence of microvascular alteration, is seen as an important part of the rejection process in renal and lung allo-

Address: Department of Pathology, Lds Hospital, 8th Ave and C Street, Salt Lake City, Utah 84143, Phone: 801 321-1029, Fax: 801 321-5020

Table 1. Acute Cellular Rejection Features

	Primary Target	Endothelial Target	Differential Diagnosis
KIDNEY	tubular epithelial cells	microvasculature, arterioles 50% of acute rejection involves arterioles	infection, ischemia, cyclosporine toxicity, acute tubular damage, interstitial nephritis
HEART	myocytes	none specified as part of process; arteriolitis rare	ischemia, biopsy site artifact, Quilty lesion, infection
LIVER	bile duct epithelium	venulitis of portal and central veins; endothelialitis secures diagnosis of rejection	hepatitis, drug toxicity, bile duct obstruction, sepsis, ischemia, hyperalimentation toxicity
LUNG	bronchioles, alveolar lining cells	arteriolitis/venulitis necessary for diagnosis of moderate rejection	infection, BALT tissue, biopsy site, ischemia
BONE MARROW (GVHD)	keratinocytes, intestinal lining cells, bile duct epithelium, salivary glands	none known	chemotherapy, radiation effects

BALT: bronchoalveolar lavage.

grafts.[11] In the cardiac allograft, perivascular and intravascular inflammation are considered elements of early mild cellular rejection.[17] Acute microvascular changes, such as endothelialitis (adherence of leukocytes to enlarged endothelial cells) and interstitial edema have largely been ignored in cardiac allograft pathology.[17] Experimental studies have documented that microvascular alterations do occur in cardiac rejection and are associated with increased allograft water content and increased extracellular hyaluronan.[18,19]

Rejection responses of the various solid organ allografts are reflective of differences in the underlying structure of these organs. Unlike the liver, kidney and lung, the heart is supplied with nutrients by a single vascular supply; changes in the single capillary bed directly effect myocardial oxygenation. Other features also affect the organ response to rejection. In the liver, there is a large population of resident antigen presenting cells.[20] These cells can effectively deal with virtually any humoral immune response, making such effects less serious in the liver allograft. In the kidney, direct cyclosporine effects on the vasculature compromise the tubular reserve in rejection responses.[21] Finally, in pulmonary allografts, pulmonary lymphoid tissues constitute an important additional source of donor immune competent cells which can alter allograft responses.[22]

In this chapter, pathologic features of acute and chronic rejection involving the microvasculature (capillaries and venules) are described as they have been studied and reported from the Utah Transplantation Associated Hospitals (UTAH) Cardiac Transplant program (682 patients receiving cardiac allografts between 1985–1998).[23–29] Most of these patients were treated with immunoprophylactic protocols, including anti-thymocyte globulin (ALG) or murine monoclonal antibody against the CD 3 receptor (OKT3).[26–28] The morphologic observations in this chapter detail the types of microvascular changes that can be encountered in endomyocardial biopsies, explanted hearts, and autopsies from these patients.[23–25,28,29]

In all histologic investigations, it is important to remember that histopathologic observations are static and that the rejection processes are dynamic. Thus, the real importance of types of the infiltrating cells in a biopsy or the presence of immune complexes, *if not demonstrated consistently over time*, may not be relevant to the mechanism by which rejection occurs. To be clinically relevant, any pathologic observation must be related to long term allograft and patient survival in clinical correlative studies. Assessment of mechanisms responsible for pathologic findings must also account for the impact of immunosuppression, and its effectiveness in treatment of rejection.

IMMUNOCYTOCHEMICAL DETERMINANTS OF MICROVASCULAR REJECTION AND THE ROLE OF IMMUNOFLUORESCENCE MICROSCOPY IN PATIENT MANAGEMENT

Initial criteria for the diagnosis of microvascular rejection of cardiac allografts were the demonstration of immunoglobulin and complement components co-localized to the microvasculature of frozen sections of endomyocardial biopsy samples. Routine immunofluroescence microscopy, analogous to methods used on renal biopsies, was employed in these studies. Just as has been found in renal biopsies, immunocytochemical examination of fixed, paraffin embedded samples cannot be used for this evaluation because of the large amounts of non specific binding encountered.[30,31]

Significant controversy exists about the role of immunofluorescence microscopy in the followup of cardiac transplant patients.[31,32,33] In the UTAH program, all patients are routinely followed for 6 weeks with immunofluorescence microscopy so that a predominant pattern of rejection can be assigned. Patients who show co-localization of immunoglobulin and complement ***on at least 3 biopsies*** continue to be followed with this method. One or two biopsies may be positive for immunoglobulin and complement in patients with other forms of rejection as a predominant pattern. We recently reviewed our experience with immunofluorescence staining (Table 2). We analyzed the first occurrence of positive immunofluorescence in our rejection pattern (cellular, vascular or mixed) groups. (Patients are categorized as to rejection pattern groups after reviewing biopsy pathology from the first 3 months following transplant.) Sixty percent of patients categorized as displaying a vascular rejection pattern and 45% of patients categorized as displaying a mixed rejection pattern had positive biopsies within the first 2 weeks post transplant. If immunofluorescence was performed for 6 weeks, 88% of vascular and 83% of mixed rejection pattern patients will have exhibited these findings, allowing clinicians to continue surveillance by immunofluorescence. By contrast, only 4% of patients who were ultimately classified as displaying a cellular rejection pattern had positive biopsies during this early period. Overall, positive immunofluorescent findings were much more common in the early post tranplant period: 373 of 682 heart transplant recipients (55%) had at least one positive biopsy. *It is the repetitive occurrence of positivity that allows for the recognition of the predominant rejection pattern.* This difference in methodology accounts for much of the confusion in the literature on

Table 2. Categories of Microvascular Rejection and their Corresponding Ishlt Grades

	No evidence of microvascular rejection	Equivocal for microvascular rejection	Definite microvascular rejection	Severe microvascular rejection
ISHLT grade	0	0	0	4
Histology of venules and capillaries	normal	+/– endothelial cell changes	+/– endothelial cell changes +/– capillaritis* +/– venulitis* +/– leukocytoclasis*	endothelial injury vasculitis and leukocytoclasis
interstitial edema	0	yes/no	yes	abundant
myocyte contraction band or coagulative necrosis	0	0	yes/no	yes/no
Immune complexes by IF	no	no; may see Ig or C	yes	yes/ no
Fibrin by IF	no	no	yes/no intravascular and interstitial; if yes*	++intravascular and interstitial
MHC II expression on venules and capillaries	no	yes/no	yes	yes usually; no when severe vascular damage
ATT expression on vessels	yes	yes	yes/no	no, usually
tPA expression on arterioles	yes	yes	yes/no	no
PAI-1 complexes	no	no	yes/no	yes/no

* indicates evidence that microvascular rejection process is more significant on spectrum of mild to severe.
ISHLT is International Society of Heart and Lung Transplantation.
IF is immunofluorescence method to demonstrate immune reactants.
ATT: anti-thrombin III.
tPA: tissue plasminogen activator.
PAI-1: plasminogen activator inhibitor-1.

this point. Series by Lones and Bonnard both report similar frequencies of early immunofluorescence positivity (52% and 60%, respectively); they do not report how many of their patients had at least 3 biopsies which are immunofluorescent positive.[34]

From a patient management perspective, immunofluorescence can only be useful if uniformly applied to all endomyocardial biopsies for at least 6 weeks post transplant so that the pattern assignment can be made. In questionable cases, further immunofluorescence testing can be performed to establish the correct pattern assignment.

Since the original publication of the first prospective series of patients with microvascular rejection, other investigators have confirmed and extended these observations to include other immunocytochemical markers of microvascular alteration.[34–37] Faulk and Labarrere have documented the relevance of immunocytochemical studies of anticoagulant and fibrinolytic pathway markers in assessing microvascular damage. They have noted that antithrombin III (ATT), a marker of the natural anticoagulant pathway, is normally expressed by the arterioles and venules and is lost in instances of microvascular damage.[32] Furthermore, tissue plasminogen activator (tPA), normally present in smooth muscle cells of myocardial arterioles, is similarly lost in allograft microvascular injury. Associated with this loss of tPA is the accumulation of microvascular complexes of tPA with plasminogen activator inhibitor-1 (PAI-1). Fibrin and plasmin are found in the interstitium of such biopsies. Alteration of the expression of these molecules clearly precedes permanent microvascular injury of cardiac allografts and has been correlated with cardiac allograft loss.[33]

Lones and colleagues have also noted that biopsies with microvascular rejection have a large number of intravascular macrophages accumulating in the microvessels which are often confused with activated endothelial cells.[34] These cells can be shown to be macrophages immunocytochemically, using antibodies directed against macrophage antigens, KP-1 and CD 68. The prominence of intravascular macrophages has been documented by ultrastructural examination of endomyocardial biopsies reported by Ratliff et al.[35,36] Antibody directed against Factor VIII-related antigen (FVIII ra) or CD 34 can be used to highlight endothelial cells.[37–38] The association of prominent intravascular macrophages and dysregulation of fibrinolysis and anticoagulation is potentially important to understanding this process: macrophages are able to directly and indirectly alter fibrinolytic processes, at least in atherosclerotic lesions. Tipping et al. have reported that macrophages from these lesions are able to make PAI-1 and also stimulate production of PAI-1 by endothelial cells (but do not stimulate tPA production), probably through augmented secretion of interleukin 1(IL-1) and tumor necrosis factor alpha (TNF).[39]

MHC Class I backbone determinants can be evaluated with immunocytochemical methods, but probably provide no useful information, since they are so pervasively expressed on endothelial and myocardial cell surfaces.[40] Similarly, we do not recommend that endomyocardial biopsies be routinely evaluated for immunophenotyping of lymphocytes, since studies of this type have not yet yielded clinically useful information.[41–43]

Other immunocytochemical studies may prove useful in the future in defining the role of endothelial cells and macrophages in the microvascular rejection process. Different populations of macrophages can be characterized, as well as evidence of markers of macrophage (CD14) or lymphocyte (CD25) activation.[44,45] Markers of macrophage effector function can also be sought, including mRNA for inducible nitric oxide synthetase (iNOS), protein expression or enzyme activity.[46] Macrophage, endothelial and myocyte apoptosis can also be evaluated immunocytochemically, using ISEL, ISNT or TUNEL techniques which have been successfully applied to cardiac allografts.[46,47] However, human allografts have not been extensively studied using these techniques.

Vascular adhesion marker expression may also be evaluated in cardiac allografts. A longitudinal study of 20 allograft recipients suggested that increased expression of the vascular cell adhesion molecule-1 (VCAM-1) and the intercellular adhesion molecule-1 (ICAM-1) on the microvasculature was found to be temporally related to cellular rejection.[48] VCAM expression was restricted to venules surrounded by infiltrating CD3 positive lymphocytes which may provide a necessary co-factor for its expression. The temporal relationship of ICAM-1 to rejection events is consistent with the proposed role of this adhesion molecule as a mediator of high affinity binding and transmigration events, as well as its co-stimulator function in antigen dependent activation of T lymphocytes.[49] Since ICAM can also be induced by ischemic injury, its presence may be non-specific. In vitro studies have shown that anti-HLA antibodies can also stimulate ICAM expression by cultured endothelial cells. By contrast, endothelial leukocyte adhesion molecule-1 (ELAM-1 or E-selectin) precedes cellular rejection and is only expressed transiently. Its expression is highly correlated with subsequent rejection.[50] In animal models of allograft rejection, ICAM-1 and VCAM-1 expression have been demonstrated during rejection using PCR to detect mRNA.; antibodies directed against VCAM-1 were efficacious in abrogating the rejection.[51–54] This finding is confirmatory of the relationship of lymphocyte adhesion and infiltration but is not diagnostically useful. If upregulation of these adhesion molecules can be consistently demonstrated before infiltration of lymphocytes or if they can be correlated with the need for treatment, they may prove important monitoring criteria (see Chapter 18). To date, no studies have established their monitoring utility.

Another important marker of endothlial function is endothelin-1 (ET-1), a potent vasoconstricting peptide. Endothelial injury or activation may stimulate release of ET-1 from endothelial cells of the microvasculature, as has been shown to occur in the vascular remodeling of chronic rejection.[55] Elevated serum levels of ET-1 have been found in the serum of liver and kidney transplant patients with acute rejection as well.[56,57] The role of ET-1 in acute cardiac rejection is yet undefined.

Studies in human and animal allografts have attempted to characterize cytokine expression using PCR to detect mRNA or using immunocytochemistry or in situ hybridization. MRNA of IL-1, IL-6, TNF, lymphotoxin (LT), and (transforming growth factor-beta)TGFb can be found in isografts, but mRNA of IL-2, IL-4, and gamma interferon were only found in allografts.[58–61] Platelet derived growth factors (PDGF-A and PDGF-B) have also recently been evaluated in allograft biopsies by immunocytochemistry and in situ hybridization. PDGF-A can be considered a marker of injured or activated endothelial cells and is expressed largely by endothelial and smooth muscle cells; PDGF-B is principally localized to infiltrating macrophages.[61]

CLASSIFICATION OF MICROVASCULAR REJECTION

Categories are defined on the basis of histologic and immunocytochemical findings (Chapter 9).[25,30] Similar features have also been described in treated animal xenografts in which acute vascular rejection has been prolonged to several days or weeks.[62–64] Microvascular rejection in individual biopsies can be separated into distinct categories including negative, equivocal, definite and severe, based on a combination of immunofluorescence and histologic criteria (Table 2).

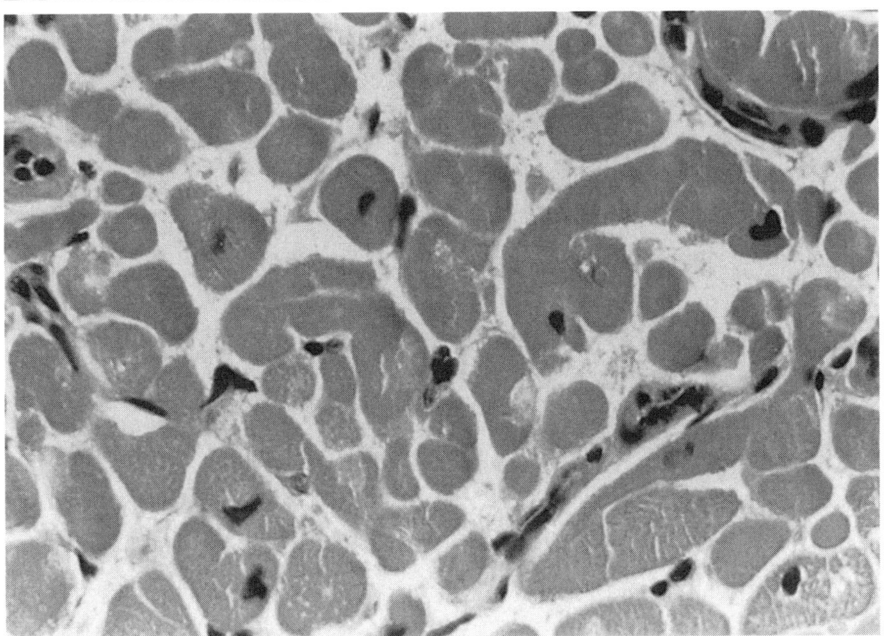

Figure 1. Endomyocardial biopsy with slight interstitial edema (increased interstitial spaces) and endothelial cell prominent in included capillaries. This biopsy is equivocal for vascular rejection. If the immunofluorescence microscopy of the same fragment showed immune complexes, this histologic appearance would be consistent with definite vascular rejection. See Table 2. Magnification 200X, hematoxylin and eosin stain.

No Evidence of Microvascular Rejection

In this category, are included all biopsies which show no light or immunofluorescent evidence of vascular rejection. By light microscopy, the biopsy has normal capillaries, venules and arterioles. Interstitial edema and hemorrhage are not present. By immunofluorescence, negative biopsies show no significant immune reactants. Vessels express strong uniform ATT expression of arterioles and venules without expression by capillaries.[33] Tissue plasminogen activator (tPA) is expressed exclusively by smooth muscle cells of the arterioles within the heart.[33]

Equivocal Evidence of Microvascular Rejection

By light microscopy, equivocal biopsies show histologic endothelial cell activation or damage with/without associated edema or hemorrhage, interstitial inflammation or thrombosis (Figure 1). Histologically, the biopsies are designated as ISHLT grade 0. Equivocal histologic changes are ubiquitous in the first weeks post transplant in patients undergoing induction immunosuppression with monoclonal anti CD3 (OKT3) which has been shown to produce transient lymphocytic activation and release of cytokines such as tumor necrosis factor (TNF) and Interleukin-1.[65,66] Since these factors lead to vascular permeability and endothelial

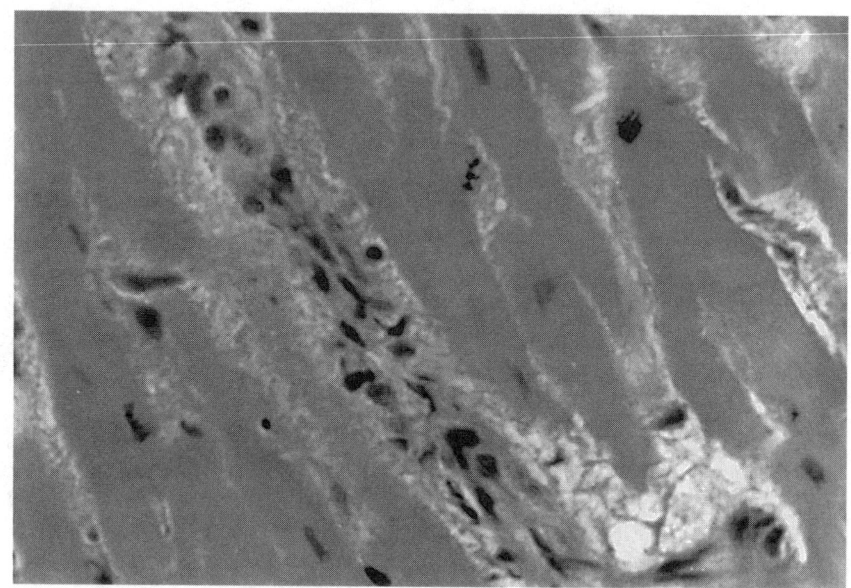

Figure 2. In this biopsy, marked perivascular edema is seen along with endothelial cell prominence and luminal adherence of macrophages in the illustrated capillary. Immunofluorescence microscopy demonstrated immune complexes; the biopsy was diagnostic for acute vascular rejection. Magnification 200X, hematoxylin and eosin stain. Photograph used with permission (Figure 4, Cardiovascular Pathology 2:1993, p. 25).

activation, it is not surprising that patients frequently display these features during OKT3 therapy.[67,68] Equivocal biopsy findings can alsobe seen in patients with systemic viral illnesses especially those caused by cytomegalovirus.[12,25,69]

Another equivocal histologic feature is the presence of focal myocyte necrosis or healing necrosis with granulation tissue. Focal ischemic injury is commonplace in the first weeks post transplant and complicates the diagnosis of both acute cellular and microvascular rejection.[70] By contrast, the finding of myocyte necrosis of either coagulation or contraction band type in the interval of months to years post transplant, is a feature strongly suggestive of either allograft coronary vasculopathy or global ischemic damage.[24,25]

By immunofluorescence, equivocal biopsies may show microvascular accumulation of immunoglobulin or complement components but not both. MHC Class II antigen expression may be upregulated on the microvasculature.[23,25] Expression of ATT may be lost from venules but not arterioles. Tissue plasminogen activator may show focal loss from arteriolar smooth muscle.[31,32]

Acute Microvascular Rejection

Acute microvascular rejection may have a deceptively negative histologic appearance, resembling equivocal biopsies. Interstitial edema is always present, recognized as the expansion of interstitial or perivascular spaces (Figure 2). Venules

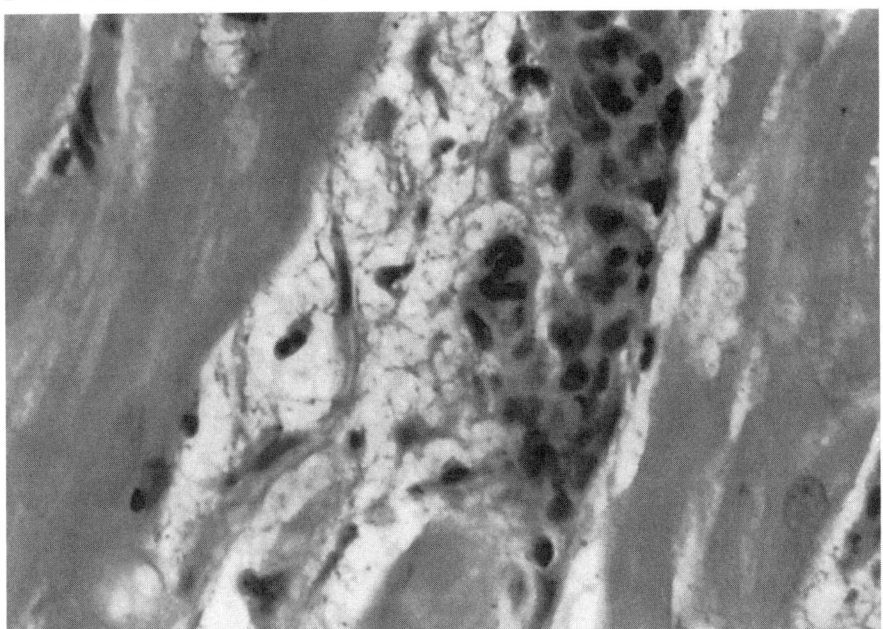

Figure 3. This hematoxylin and eosin-stained section of endomyocardial biopsy shows a vessel with adherent leukocytes and prominent perivascular edema. Immunofluorescence microscopy demonstrated immune complexes. Diagnosis is acute vascular rejection. Magnification 400X. Photograph used with permission (Figure 8, Journal of Heart Lung Transplant 8:1989, p. 438).

and capillaries may show evidence of injury or endothelial cell activation or they may show adherence of macrophages and /or other inflammatory cells (capillaritis) or leukocytoclastic vasculitis (Figure 3). In the absence of cellular rejection, demonstration of vasculitis qualifies the biopsy for a diagnosis of acute vascular rejection. In diagnostic vasculitis, the vessels may show prominent accumulation of nuclear dust. Invading inflammatory cells may be neutrophils as well as lymphocytes and macrophages; this histologic appearance can lead to confusion with healing ischemic myocardial damage. Unlike healing damage, microvascular rejection is a diffuse process with generalized vascular alterations and generalized interstitial edema. If the histologic appearance is not diagnostic, immunofluorescence is particularly useful in establishing the diagnosis of acute vascular rejection.

By immunofluorescence, the biopsies will show co-localization of immunoglobulin and complement components in capillaries and venules with the possible intravascular localization of small amounts of fibrin (Figure 4). In some cases, particularly in longstanding vascular rejection, only intravascular and interstitial fibrin may be detected.[24,25] In significant and long standing acute vascular rejection, ATT and tPA expression are usually completely lost and tPA-PAI-1 complexes are often present. This pattern of expression is often clinically associated with hemodynamic compromise.[23,28] Upregulation of MHC class II antigen is also uniformly seen[25,71] (Figure 5). Rarely, vasculitis can be caused by cellular immune

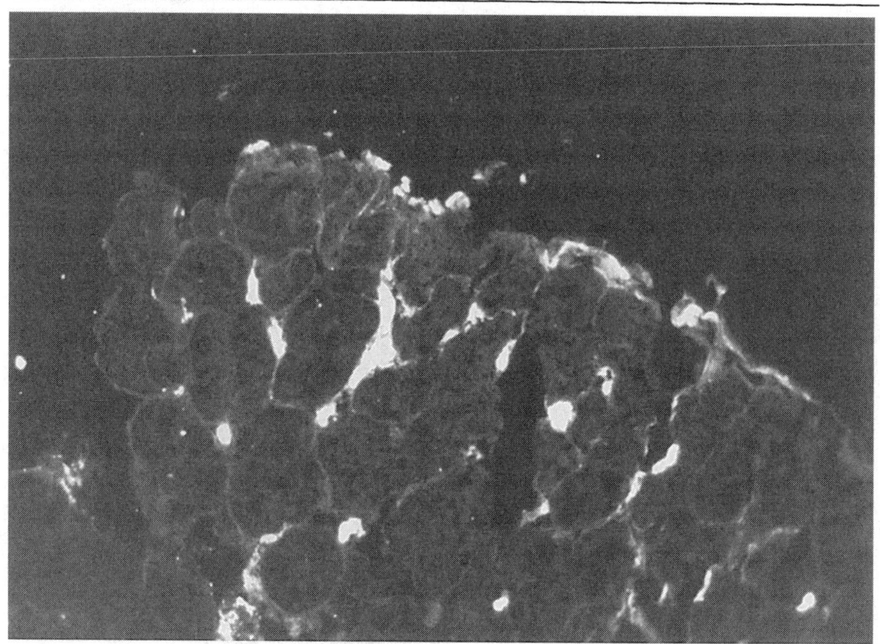

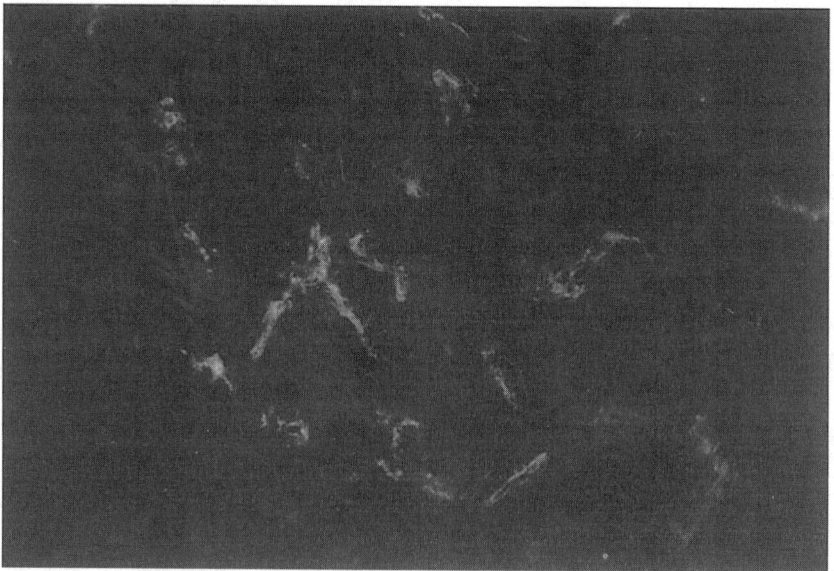

Figure 5. Photomicrograph of prominent HLA-DR accumulation in the microvasculature of a patient with acute vascular rejection. Magnification 250X. Photograph used with permission (Figure 16, Cardiovascular Pathology 2:1933, p. 28).

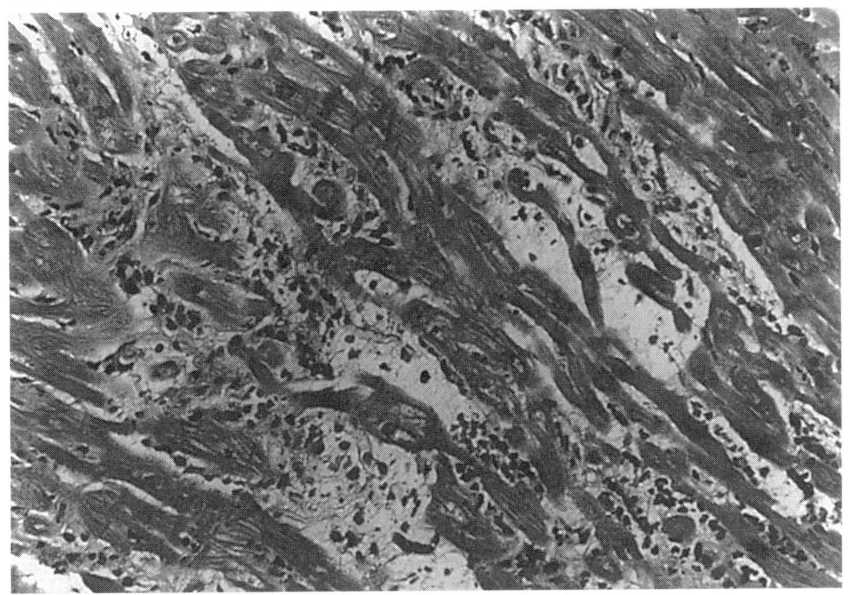

Figure 6. In this photomicrograph, marked interstitial edema, vasculitis and myocyte damage are all easily appreciated. The biopsy has the typical appearance of severe cellular and vascular rejection, ISHLT 4. Magnification 100X, hematoxylin and eosin stain. Photograph used with permission (Figure 16, Chapter 28: Pathology of Microvascular Rejection in the Transplantation and Replacement of Thoracic Organs DKC Cooper, LW Miller and GA Patterson, editors 1996, p. 246. Kluwer Academic Publishers, Dordecht/Boston/London).

mechanisms and in such cases, immune complexes are not demonstrated in vessel walls. We have seen this pattern in only 3 of 75 patients with vascular rejection, but it has been more frequent in the experience of others.[72,73]

Severe Microvascular Rejection

Severe microvascular rejection is morphologically indistinguishable from severe cellular rejection (ISHLT grade 4). It is the end result of any severe rejection process. The endomyocardial biopsy shows a diffuse, mixed leukocytic infiltration which include neutrophils and eosinophils. Vasculitis is often obvious. Myocyte necrosis and interstitial edema and hemorrhage may be prominent. Myocyte necrosis, when associated with interstitial mixed inflammation, can be confused with healing ischemic myocyte necrosis (Figure 6).[70,74–76]

Immunocytochemically, biopsies with severe cellular/vascular rejection will often have vascular deposits of immunoglobulin and complement as well as interstitial and vascular accumulation of fibrin. Complement components may also be distributed within the interstitium. Examination of biopsies for ATT and tPA will show loss of these reactants. tPA-PAI-1 complexes may be present.[32,33] The microvasculature may paradoxically show a lack of MHC Class II expression resulting from the relentless vascular injury. This can be highlighted by immunoperoxidase staining of vessels with Factor VIIIra. In severe rejection, the endothelium is ragged or frayed or may show areas where endothelial cells are missing.[12,25]

Severe Hyperacute (Microvascular) Rejection

Hyperacute rejection of cardiac allografts is very rare and catastrophic. Acute cardiac dysfunction results from deposition of preformed antibody (immunoglobulin IgG or IgM) and complement components in the microvasculature of the allograft. This process has been reported to occur even in the presence of a negative lymphocytotoxic cross match. Allograft dysfunction results from endothelial damage, vascular permeability, interstitial edema and hemorrhage which cause myocardial ischemia. If the process persists for several hours, an infiltrate of neutrophils within and around vessels can be seen.[77,78]

In the absence of immunomodulatory treatment, hyperacute rejection is routinely seen in xenotransplantation (see Chapter 7).[62–64,79] The pathologic process is characterized by prominent interstitial edema followed by interstitial hemorrhage and swelling of the capillary and venular endothelium. Inflammatory infiltrates are not a feature because of the rapid time course of the process which leads to xenograft loss within minutes or hours. Hyperacute rejection is mediated by the deposition of xenospecific antibodies in the donor heart. If the process is abrogated by depletion or inhibition of natural antibodies or inhibition of complement activation, the histologic findings often include inflammation and venular thrombosis. Ischemic myocyte injury with myocytolysis and eventual coagulative necrosis is seen in xenografts surviving several weeks. A pattern of rejection identical to severe mixed acute cellular and vascular rejection (ISHLT grade 4) is observed in xeonografts in whom complement function returns.[64]

RELATIONSHIP OF MICROVASCULAR REJECTION TO ISHLT GRADING SCHEMA

The current ISHLT grading scheme for acute cardiac allograft rejection does not include the categorization of microvascular changes.[16] The relationship between microvascular rejection categories and the ISHLT grading schema are shown in Table 2, based on the authors' experience examining over 20,000 endomyocardial biopsies. Because the features of the microvasculature (endothelial alterations, endothelialitis, interstitial edema) are ignored in the current grading schema, the presence of microvascular changes cause difficulty in interpretation and lead to interpretive disagreements, even among experienced pathologists.[80] Although outcome studies have demonstrated the utility of recognizing acute vascular rejection, alterations of patient immunosuppressive therapy are not usually undertaken unless allograft dysfunction is present.[81] Such allograft dysfunction is manifest by hemodynamic derangements and echocardiographic evidence of systolic and/or diastolic dysfunction.[82]

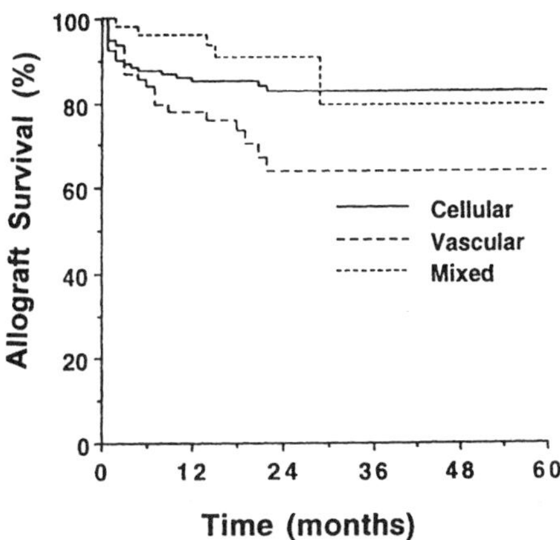

Figure 7. Kaplan-Meier analysis of percent of allograft survival at 5 years, stratified by rejection pattern. The curve demonstrates a higher mortality in patients with the vascular rejection pattern. Tarone Ware test was significant among the groups ($P < 0.027$). Proportional hazard regression model showed that the vascular rejection pattern patients were significantly different ($P = 0.012$) from the combined groups of cellular and mixed rejection pattern patients. (Used with permission, Journal of Heart Lung Transplant 11:1992, p. S117.)

CLASSIFICATION OF MIXED (CELLULAR AND VASCULAR) REJECTION

Mixed cellular and microvascular rejection may be manifest simultaneously in an endomyocardial biopsy.[12,25] Independent grades for each process can be assigned. The ISHLT cellular rejection grading criteria have been extensively reported.[12,17] Vascular rejection grades are assigned according to the criteria described earlier in this chapter (Table 2). Mixed rejection, as defined in this chapter, is not recognized in the ISHLT schema; such biopsies are designated only by their cellular grade. As mentioned previously, vasculitis is often ignored in the ISHLT schema except in the case of severe rejection (grade 4) where it is almost always manifest. Vasculitis discovered histologically in a biopsy with cellular rejection would qualify biopsy as showing mixed rejection.

DESIGNATION OF THE DOMINANT PATHOLOGIC REJECTION PATTERN

Four separate reports have shown that the designation of patients by their predominant rejection type is prognostically useful.[23,24,28,29] In prospectively conducted studies, patients who demonstrate a recurring pattern of microvascular rejection during the first 3 months after transplantation have a significantly worse survival (Figure 7). Assignment to a pattern group is based on the results of biopsies obtained during the first 3 months post transplant. If the patient has three biopsies which are positive for microvascular rejection during that period, he/she is categorized as a

Table 3. Relationship of Patient Mortality to Rejection Pattern Utah Cardiac Transplant Program 1985–1996

	Number of patients (% of total patients)	Number of deaths	Percent deaths by pattern
Cellular pattern	352 (60%)	107	30
Vascular pattern	110 (18%)	70	64
Mixed pattern	135 (22%)	52	39

vascular rejector, especially if those episodes occurred prior to cellular rejection episodes. To be considered a mixed rejector, a patient must have multiple episodes of mixed rejection prior to any cellular rejection episodes. Usually, patients with one predominant histologic pattern of rejection subsequently display that pattern of rejection.

Recently, we reviewed survival in cardiac transplant patients, transplanted in Utah between March 1985 and September 1996. In a population of 587 transplant recipients, survival rates varied nearly two fold when patients were stratified by rejection pattern. Nineteen percent were classifiable as vascular rejectors, when prospectively assigned. Twenty-two percent of patients were mixed rejectors. Cellular rejectors, 60% of patients, comprise the remainder of the population (Table 3). Mortality was only 30% in patients classified as cellular rejector compared to a mortality rate of 64% in those classified as vascular rejectors ($p = <0.001$). When causes of mortality were reviewed, vascular rejectors were found to be much more likely to die of cardiovascular causes, (death due to allograft coronary artery disease, myocardial infarction, and heart failure) compared to cellular rejectors. (49% versus 27%, $p = <0.001$) (Figure 8). Similarly, mixed rejection pattern patients were much more likely to die of cardiovascular causes (44% versus 27%, $p = <0.008$) when compared to those demonstrating only a cellular rejection pattern. Mortality due to other causes was not significantly different when patients were stratified by rejection pattern. Other causes tabulated included infection, malignancy and "other", which includes death due to multi organ failure and miscellaneous causes.

Interestingly, although mixed rejectors have an overall mortality rate similar to cellular rejectors, we have previously reported that they have a four-fold higher risk of developing allograft coronary artery disease; vascular rejection pattern patients have an eight to nine fold greater risk of allograft coronary artery disease (Figure 9). These risks are irrespective of the time post transplantation.[24] The relationship of rejection patterns to the occurrence of allograft coronary artery disease is very impressive, especially when reviewed in the light of other published associations of allograft coronary artery disease risk.[83]

CLINICAL RESPONSE TO DIAGNOSIS OF ACUTE VASCULAR REJECTION

Given the grave prognostic implications for a patient who demonstrates a repetitive pattern of microvascular cardiac allograft rejection, heightened vigilance is

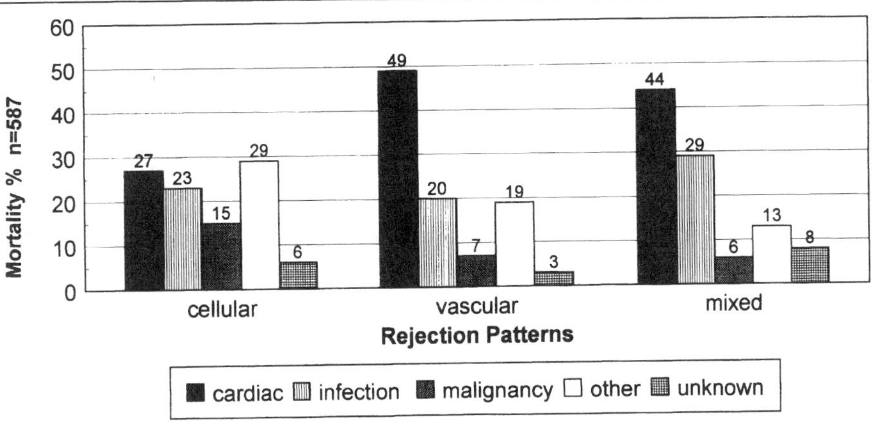

Figure 8. Bar graph illustrating causes of death in UTAH cardiac transplant patients stratified by pattern of rejection. Vascular and mixed rejecter pattern patients were much more likely to die of cardiovascular causes that cellular rejecter pattern patients. (Vascular versus cellular pattern patients $P < 0.001$; Mixed versus cellular pattern patients $P < 0.008$) EHH and RLY, unpublished observations.

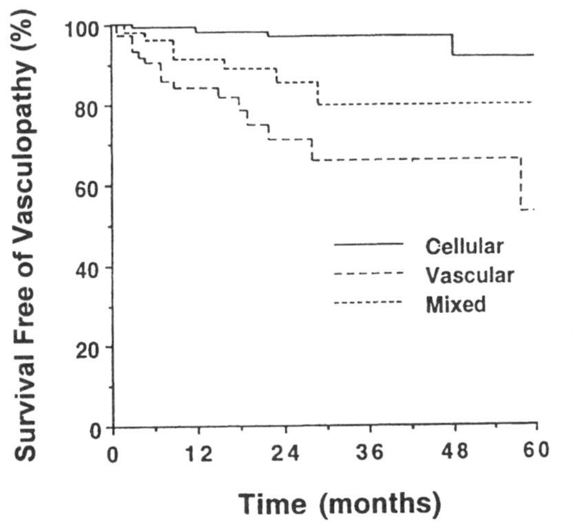

Figure 9. Kaplan-Meier analysis of percent of patients surviving without allograft coronary vasculopathy, stratified by rejection pattern types. Tarone Ware test was significant among the groups ($P < 0.001$). The stepwise proportional hazard model showed that the risk of developing allograft coronary vasculopathy within 5 years was higher for vascular rejection pattern patients ($P = 0.001$; odds ratio = 8.63 ± 1 SE = (4.86–15.35)) and for the mixed rejection pattern group ($P < 0.014$; odds ratio = 4.72 ± 1 SE = (2.52–8.85)) when compared with the cellular rejection pattern group. (Used with permission, Journal of Heart Lung Transplant 11:1992, pp. S115–S116.)

mandated. Immunosuppressive medications are tapered more slowly and surveillance echocardiography is performed more frequently. Worsening of parameters of systolic and/or diastolic function are promptly investigated by an endomyocardial biopsy. Although surveillance endomyocardial biopsies are not necessarily performed more frequently, immunofluorescence staining of the biopsies is continued until microvascular rejection is consistently absent. At times, changing from azathioprine to cyclophosphamide or mycophenolate mofetil has appeared helpful.

In general, in the absence of echocardiographic or clinical signs of allograft dysfunction, the diagnosis of mild microvascular rejection on a single endomyocardial biopsy does not prompt augmentation in immunosuppression. However, even in the absence of evidence of allograft dysfunction, moderate microvascular rejection diagnosed on a single endomyocardial biopsy is cause for concern. At the very least, an earlier subsequent echocardiogram and endomyocardial biopsy are performed and maintenance immunosuppression is optimized.

In the presence of echocardiographic findings and clinical signs of allograft dysfunction, the diagnosis of moderate or even mild microvascular cardiac allograft rejection on the endomyocardial biopsy is most helpful, since augmentation of immunosuppression can be life-and-allograft-saving. Plasmapheresis, heparin anticoagulation, and high-dose corticosteroid with or without antilymphocyte antibody treatment have reversed severe cardiac allograft dysfunction due to microvascular rejection. In these dire situations, the use of a short course of high-dose cyclophosphamide may be beneficial. Severely compromised patients require inotropic support until cardiac allograft function is stabilized and improved.

RELATIONSHIP OF ACUTE MICROVASCULAR REJECTION TO CHRONIC ALLOGRAFT VASCULOPATHY

There is significant clinical and pathologic interest in the pathology and pathogenesis of chronic allograft vasculopathy, a form of chronic rejection that afflicts all solid allografts. The form usually recognized and studied in heart is manifested pathologically by diffuse concentric subintimal fibrosis of epicardial coronary arteries, with or without inflammation and/or with involvement of penetrating branches of epicardial vessels.[84] We have recognized and described another manifestation of chronic rejection, common particularly in patients with vascular rejection pattern. This form of chronic rejection, studied in detail in explant and autopsy hearts from our transplant patient population, involves the smallest penetrating arteries and arterioles within the myocardium as well as the epicardial coronaries. The history and pathologic features are usually quite specific. The patient develops evidence of heart failure manifest by a decreasing ejection fraction with its usual signs and symptoms, despite the absence of angiographic evidence of significant epicardial coronary artery disease, other than vessel pruning. On endomyocardial biopsy, a distinctive group of morphologic features are demonstrated. Focal areas of myocyte dropout are evident, in which myocytes are replaced by loose connective tissue and eventually by dense collagen. Surrounding myocytes are often hypertrophied and vacuolated. Inflammatory cells, such as lymphocytes and macrophages, may be seen, but they are limited to the areas of myocyte dropout or scarring. Capillaries are scarce and endothelial activation is absent.[12,24,25,70,75,76] The patchy nature of this process and its predilection for the subendocardial region suggests that the myocyte loss is due to generalized microvascular damage which includes small arteries and arterioles outside of the field of examination on endomyocardial biopsy. The process may be termed, "global myocardial ischemia".[12,25] The histologic changes are also seen in patients with coronary allograft vasculopathy. If these changes are encountered on repeated endomyocardial biopsies in patients with slowly worsening cardiac function, the prognosis is poor. Such patchy myocyte loss is distinctive from that loss usually associated with myocardial infarction in which large zones of myocyte necrosis are ultimately replaced by dense scarring.

By immunocytochemistry, patients with global myocardial ischemia or allograft coronary vasculopathy usually show generalized increased MHC Class II (HLA-DR) staining of microvasculature of the endomyocardial biopsy in the absence of other pathologic evidence of acute rejection.[85-87] The immunocytochemical findings of microvascular immunoglobulin and complement components may be decreased from previous biopsies or may be totally absent. ATT is often absent in the microvasculature and tPA in undetectable in smooth muscle. This pattern of ATT and tPA expression was detected in 7 of 11 hearts examined at autopsy in whom global ischemic changes were the predominant cause of heart failure (EH, unpublished observations). We have seen biopsies from several patients who lack microvascular damage but have coronary vasculopathy; ATT and tPA staining were not diminished. The amount of fibrin staining is often decreased over previous biopsies. We believe that these altered morphologic expressions in the microvasculature may be the results of attempted repair of chronic damage of the microvasculature.[87]

Ultrastructural observations of biopsies from patients with histological evidence of chronic damage of large and small blood vessels have shown changes analogous to those found in ischemic hearts of experimental animals; these hearts show a prominent loss of actin rather than myosin in intact myofilament bundles, giving a coarse appearance to the myofilaments.[85] In addition, large numbers of myocyte cytoplasmic organelles are often scattered about the interstitium and associated with a patchy, haphazard collection of collagen fibrils. The vessels usually have irregular profiles and may show irregular endothelial cell swelling. Reduplication of basal lamina is common and generalized.[85]

DRUG-INDUCED VASCULAR PROCESSES SIMULATING VASCULAR REJECTION

In patients treated with antibodies raised in various animal species such as horse, rabbit, sheep or mice, an immune complex-mediated response to these foreign proteins may develop.[88-90] The immunosuppressive function of the monoclonal antibody is abrogated by the production of antibodies against the immunosuppressive agent and early rejection may develop due to the lack of immunosuppression.[91] Alternatively, patients may show a serum sickness-like process within the allograft microvasculature related to the deposition of immune complexes of the monoclonal antibody and the host anti-idiotypic antibody directed against it.[92] In our institutions, where many patients have been treated with OKT3, all patients are routinely evaluated by immunocytochemistry for the accumulation of murine immunoglobulin (the antigen) in cardiac vessels.[93] Typically, the efficacy of OKT3 therapy is monitored by following total daily T-lymphocyte counts or in the case of OKT3, CD3 lymphocyte counts. This method is an insensitive way to detect early anti-idiotypic antibody accumulation; a better method is the flow cytometric assay described which detects declines in steady state plasma levels of the OKT3 (due to complexing of antigen with anti-idiotypic antibody) one to three days earlier than the rise of CD3 positive cells in the serum.[94] We have demonstrated that continuing OKT3 treatment despite the presence of anti-idiotypic antibodies universally results in humorally mediated microvascular alterations.[93] When therapy is promptly aborted at the first suggestion of OKT3 sensitization, (a fall in steady state OKT3 levels), improvement in allograft survival is seen.[95] Furthermore, patients without OKT3 sensitization during early rejection prophylaxis also did not develop sensitization if retreatment was necessary. Routine immunocytochemical monitoring may be very helpful in understanding the nature of the immunologic response. Morphologically, endomyocardial biopsies have features of microvascular alteration identical to those found in vascular rejection patients. The only different feature is the presence of mouse immunoglobulin in a distribution identical to the human immunoglobulin and complement components.

PATHOGENESIS OF MICROVASCULAR REJECTION

The changes described in this chapter suggest that endothelial cell activation and injury associated with leukocyte homing, vascular permeability and subsequent inflammation with myocyte degeneration are prominent features in patients displaying light microscopic, and immunocytochemical alterations associated with microvascular rejection. Investigations of endothelial cell biology have shown that endothelial cells are capable of many important functions which can be altered in the allograft.[68,96–100] Endothelial cells provide a natural anticoagulated surface through their binding of antithrombin three and thrombomodulin, although the evidence in cardiac transplants suggests that the former pathway is more important than the latter.[86] Endothelial cells produce diverse cytokines which can modulate the biologic behavior of cells in the myocardial tissue. These cytokines are produced in inflammation, ischemia, and many other circumstances commonly operative in allotransplantation, such as infection and lymphocyte activation.[96–101] Endothelial activation can also be the result of immunosuppression or immunoprophylaxis utilizing monoclonal anti-T cell antibodies. The therapy can generate T cell activation, as a result of interaction of the antibody and the CD-3 or T-cell receptor antigen on the lymphocyte surface.[102] A predominant cytokine released is tumor necrosis factor alpha; antibody directed against this cytokine is effective in abrogating the first dose response commonly seen in these patients.[103,104] Other reports suggest that such lymphocyte activation leads to increased release of IL2 and gamma interferon which promotes further endothelial cell activation.

We have observed that patients with the persistent morphologic pattern of microvascular rejection (vascular rejectors) include patients sensitized to OKT3 while undergoing immunoprophylaxis. It is also the most common rejection pattern in patients who have a positive, donor-specific cross-match at the time of transplantation (Figure 10). OKT3 induced microvascular rejection is related to humoral immune responses with probable altered B-lymphocyte immune regulation or polyclonal B-lymphocytic activation.[65,66] The morphologic changes are very similar to those described in patients with serum sickness, and experimental animals with

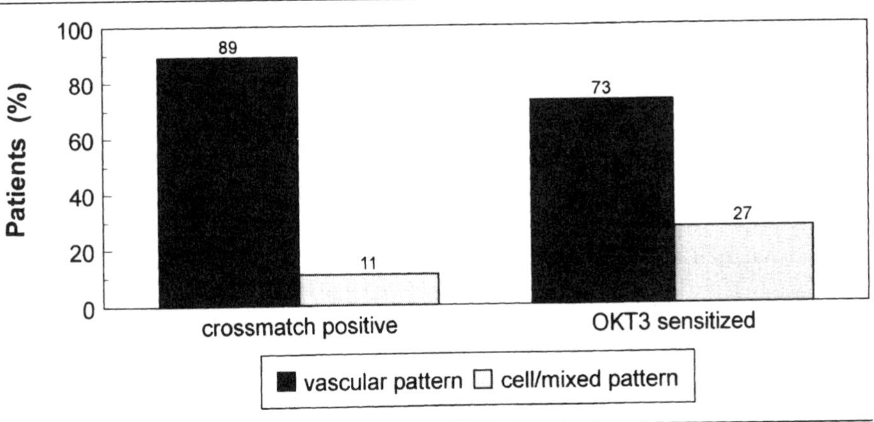

Figure 10. Bar graph displaying the proportion of vascular rejection pattern patients with either a positive cross match or clinically detected sensitization to immunoprophylaxis with OKT3. The overall percentage of patients with vascular rejection pattern in the UTAH Cardiac Transplant Program was 22%. Rejection pattern category was determined independently from knowledge of either of these clinical features.

leukocytoclastic vasculitis, the Arthus phenomenon and animals rejecting xenografts in whom antibody levels or complement activity have been decreased.[62–64,88–90] The pathogenic mechanisms responsible for these vascular inflammatory processes (where an antigen-antibody complex process is definitely implicated) involve complement activation, cytokine release and chemotaxis and activation of neutrophils and macrophages with concomitant activation of their potent inflammatory repertoire.[100]

Recent work has shed light on the pathogenesis of microvascular rejection in our transplant population.[29] We examined the incidence of the vascular rejection pattern in our patients related to the duration of OKT3 early rejection prophylaxis (Figure 11). We found a statistically significant association of the vascular rejection pattern and duration of OKT3 treatment greater than 7 days. The association of the vascular rejection pattern and OKT3 duration in early rejection prophylaxis, in multivariate analysis was independent of previously recognized predictors of vascular rejector pattern: patient sex, patient age, positive crossmatch and positive panel reactive antibody status. Patients with OKT3 sensitization were also excluded from the analysis. The association of the vascular rejection pattern with duration of OKT3 greater than 7 days suggests that anti-idiotypic antibody production, which occurs to some degree in all patients after 7 days of induction, synergizes with the humoral rejection response so that it becomes the predominant pattern in susceptible patients.[29]

An alternative hypothesis is that the OKT3 early rejection prophylaxis for greater than 7 days alters cytokine production, such as TNF production. It is well recognized that TNF is the cytokine responsible for the first dose OKT3 reaction.[104] Recent studies have shown that TNF may play a significant role in allograft rejection.[52,53] TNF recruits cells to the site of antigenic challenge, activates

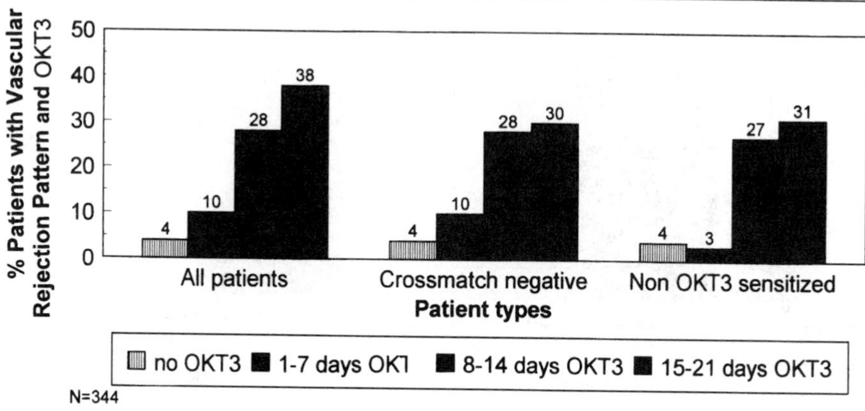

Figure 11. Bar graph illustrating the relationship of duration of OKT3 early rejection prophylaxis to vascular pattern of rejection. With increasing duration of OKT3 administration, the proportion of patients developing the vascular rejection pattern increases. ($P < 0.0001$). The association persists even after excluding patients with a positive crossmatch ($P = 0.001$) or patients sensitized to OKT3 ($P = 0.0001$).

immunocompetent cells, augments the expression of MHC class I and class II antigens, and induces the production of other cytokines. Lymphocytes, macrophages and endothelial cells are all able to produce TNF alpha and are activated by its actions. Elevation of mRNA for TNF alpha is detected in rat cardiac allografts in advance of clinical rejection.[105] Antibody against TNF alpha has also been shown to be effective, in combination with cyclosporine A, in prolonging rat cardiac allograft survival. Elevation of circulating levels of TNF have been detected in cardiac and renal transplant recipients.[106,107] Thus, it is likely that TNF is produced concomitantly with each dose of OKT3 that is given so that the amount of TNF produced in patients treated for 14 or 21 days is significantly greater than in patients receiving the drug for only 7 days. Furthermore, activation of macrophages and endothelial cells, which promote further TNF production, are accelerated by binding of these cells to immune complexes, like complexes of OKT3 and its anti-idiotypic antibody. Thus, circumstances are favorable for the increased production of TNF in patients receiving prolonged OKT3 administration. TNF enhances immunologic responsiveness and would be expected to accelerate rejection responses in patients as it has been shown to do in experimental animals. If this hypothesis is correct, antibody directed against TNF alpha may be an effective strategy to prevent microvascular rejection in this patient population.

The likelihood that microvascular rejection is mediated by TNF or other cytokines in addition to humoral immune mechanisms cannot be differentiated by the present or previous studies. We have consistently seen up-regulation of HLA-DR on the large and small vessels of the cardiac allograft which, at least in experimental situations, is produced exclusively by interaction of endothelial cells with interferon gamma.[96] This finding, as well as the prominent fibrin deposition and endothelial activation, suggests that cytokine mediated (delayed-type) hypersensitivity may also be implicated in this process.[108]

SUMMARY

The consequence of either a humoral or cellular immune response directed against the vascular endothelium would ultimately be compromised myocardial oxygenation. Important inflammatory participants in this process include neutrophils and macrophages which can be activated by immune complexes, cytokines, complement components, endotoxin, and platelet activating factor. Such activation can result in the production of various leukotrienes, arachidonic acid metabolites, and a variety of cytokines which lead to vascular permeability, leukocyte adherence via various specifically induced adhesion molecules, and the activation of proteolytic enzymes such as protein kinase C. The ability of endothelial cells to express adhesion molecules (ELAM-1, ICAM-1, VCAM-1) in response to inflammatory stimuli or cytokine release such as IL1 can create the morphologic expression of vascular rejection including endothelial activation and capillaritis. Studies of chronic rejection of cardiac and renal allografts have demonstrated a remarkably similar panoply of inflammatory effects which also stimulate proliferation of arterial smooth muscle cells.[100] These effects lead to chronic rejection and are likely operative to some extent in all allografts, regardless of rejection type. Microvascular rejection of cardiac allografts represents a subset of rejection responses in which inflammatory and proliferative effects are multiplied by the role of antibody. Studies reported in this chapter illustrate the importance of clinical recognition of these humoral responses; patients who are vascular rejectors are more likely to have hemodynamic compromise associated with acute rejection episodes, are more likely to develop chronic rejection or allograft vasculopathy, and have higher mortality rates from cardiovascular causes. The challenge that remains is designing immunosuppressive therapies that diminish or remove these consequences.

REFERENCES

1. Jeannet M, Pinn V, Flax M, Winn HJ, Russell PS. Humoral Antibodies in renal allotransplantation in man. N Engl J Med 1970;282:111–117.
2. Farnsworth A, Hall BM, Ng ABP, et al. Renal biopsy morphology in renal transplantation. Am J Surg Pathol 1984;8:243–252.
3. Salmela KT, von Willebrand EO, Kyllonen LEJ, Acute vascular rejection in renal transplantation-diagnosis and outcome. Transplantation 1992;54:858–862.
4. Colvin, Robert B. Kidney Transplantation. In: Diagnostic Immunopathology. RB Colvin, AT Bhan and RT McCluskey (editors). NY: Raven Press 1995;329–366.
5. Herskowitz A, Soule LM, Ueda K, Tamura F, Baumgartner WA, Borton AM, Reitz BA, Achuff SC, Traill TA, Baughman KL. Arteriolar vasculitis on endomyocardial biopsy: a histologic predictor of poor outcome and cyclosporine-treated heart transplant recipients. J Heart Transplant 1987; 6:127–136.
6. Smith SH, Kirklin JK, Geer JC, Caulfield JB, McGiffin DC. Arteritis and cardiac rejection after transplantation. Am J Cardiology 1987; 59:1171–1173.
7. Forbes RDC, Guttman RD, Gomersall M, Hibberd J. A controlled serial ultrastructural tracer study of first set cardiac allograft rejection in the rat. Am J Pathol 1983;111:184–196.
8. Leszcynski D, Laszcyska M, Halttunen J, Hayry P. Renal target structures in acute allograft rejection: a histochemical study. Kidney Int 1987;31:1311–1316.
9. Dvorak HF, Mihm MC, Dvorak AM, et al. Rejection of first set skin allografts in man: the microvasculature is the critical target of the immune response. J Exp Med 1979;150:322–337.
10. Butcher EC. The regulation of lymphocyte traffic. Curr Top Microbiol Immunol. 1986;128: 85–122.

11. Berg EL, Goldstein LA, Jutila MA, et al. Homing receptors and vascular addressins: cell adhesion molecules that direct lymphocyte migration. Immunol Rev 1989;108:5–18.
12. Hammond EH. Cardiac transplantation. In: Diagnostic Immunopathology RB Colvin, A Bhan and R McCluskey, editors NY: Raven Press 1995, p. 367.
13. Demetris AJ, Lasky S, Van Thiel DH, et al. Pathology of hepatic transplantation: A review of 62 adult allograft recipients immunosuppressed with a cyclosporine/steroid regimen. Am J Pathol 1985;118:151–161.
14. Stewart S. Pathology of lung transplantation. Seminars in Diagnostic Pathology 1992;9:210–217.
15. Snover DC, Freese DK, Sharp HL, et al. Liver allograft rejection: an analysis of the use of biopsy in determining outcome of rejection. Am J Surg Pathol 1987;11:1–10.
16. Hammond EH. Transplant Pathology. In: Principles and Practice of Surgical Pathology and Cytopathology, Third Edition. SG Silverberg, RA DeLellis, WJ Frable, editors. NY: Churchill Livingstone 1997, p. 253.
17. Billingham ME, Cary NRB, Hammond ME, et al. A working formulation for the standardization of nomenclature in the diagnosis of heart and lung rejection: heart rejection study group. J Heart Transplant 1990;9:587–592.
18. Waldenstrom A, Martinussen HJ, Gerdin B, Hallgren R. Accumulation of hyaluronan and tissue edema in experimental myocardial infarction. J Clin Invest 1991;88(5):1622–1628.
19. Hallgren R, Gerdin B, Tengblad A, Tufveson G. Accumulation of hyaluronan (hyaluronic acid) in myocardial interstitial tissue parallels development of transplantation edema in heart allografts in rats. J Clin Invest 1990;85(3):668–673.
20. Demetris AJ, Murase N, Ye Q, Galvao FH, Richert C, Saad R, Pham S, Duquesnoy RJ, Zeevi A, Fung JJ, Starzl TE. Analysis of chronic rejection and obliterative arteriopathy. Possible contributions of donor antigen-presenting cells and lymphatic disruption. Am J Pathol 1997;150(2): 563–578.
21. Watschinger B, Sayegh MH. Endothelin in organ transplantation. Am J Kidney Dis 1996;27(1): 151–161.
22. Prop J, Kuijpers K, Petersen AH, Bartels HL, Nieuwenhuis P, Wildevuur CR. Why are lung allografts more vigorously rejected than hearts? J Heart Transplant 1985;4(4):433–436.
23. Hammond EH, Yowell RL, Nunoda S, et al. Vascular (humoral) rejection in heart transplantation: pathologic observations and clinical implications. J Heart Transplant 1989;8:430–443.
24. Hammond EH, Yowell RL, Price GD, et al. Vascular rejection and its relationship to allograft coronary artery disease. J Heart Transplant 1992;11:111–119.
25. Hammond EH, Hansen J, Spencer LS, et al. Vascular rejection in cardiac transplantation: Histologic, immunopathologic, and ultrastructural features. Cardiovasc Pathol 1993;2:21–34.
26. Woodley SL, Renlund DG, O'Connell JB, Bristow MR. Immunosuppression following cardiac transplantation. J Heart Transplant, Cardiology Clinics 1990;8:83–87.
27. Renlund DG, O'Connell JB, Gilbert EM. A prospective comparison of murine monoclonal CD-3 (OKT3) antibody-based and equine antithymocyte globulin-based rejection prophylaxis in cardiac transplantation. Transplantation 1989;47:599–605.
28. Ensley RD, Hammond EH, Renlund DG, et al. Clinical manifestations of vascular rejection in cardiac transplantation. Transplant Proc 1991;23:1130–1132.
29. Ma H, Hammond EH, Taylor DO, Yowell RL, Bristow MR, O'Connell JB, Renlund DG. The repetitive histologic pattern of vascular cardiac allograft rejection. Increased incidence associated with longer exposure to prophylactic murine monoclonal anti-CD3 antibody (OKT3). Transplantation 1996;62(2):205–210.
30. Hammond EH, Hansen LK, Spencer LS, et al. Immunofluorescence of endomyocardial biopsy specimens: methods and interpretation. J Heart Lung Transplant 1993;12:S113–S124.
31. Loy TS, Bulatao IS, Darkow GV, Demmy TL, Reddy HK, Curtis J, Bickel JT. Immunostaining of cardiac biopsy specimens in the diagnosis of acute vascular (humoral) rejection: a control study. J Heart Lung Transplant 1993 Sep; 12(5):736–740.
32. Labarrere CA, Pitts D, Nelson DR, Faulk WP. Vascular tissue plasminogen activator and the development of coronary artery disease in heart-transplant recipients. N Engl J Med 1995;333(17): 1111–1116.
33. Labarrere CA, Pitts D, Halbrook H, Faulk WP. Tissue plasminogen activator, plasminogen activator inhibitor-1, and fibrin as indexes of clinical course in cardiac allograft recipients: An immunocytochemical study. Circulation 1994;89:1599–1608.
34. Lones MA, Czer LS, Trento A, Harasty D, Miller JM, Fishbein MC. Clinical-pathologic features of humoral rejection in cardiac allografts: a study in 81 consecutive patients. J Heart Lung Transplant 1995;14(1 Pt 1):151–162.
35. Hook S, Caple JF, McMahon JT, Myles JL, Ratliff NB. Comparison of myocardial cell injury in acute cellular rejection versus acute vascular rejection in cyclosporine-treated heart transplants. J Heart Lung Transplant 1995;14(2):351–358.

36. Ratliff NB, McMahon JT. Activation of intravascular macrophages within myocardial small vessels is a feature of acute vascular rejection in human heart transplants. J Heart Lung Transplant 1995; 14(2):338–345.
37. Rand JH, Wu XX, Potter BJ, et al. Co-localization of von Willebrand factor and type VI collagen in human vascular subendothelium. Am J Pathol 1993;142:843–850.
38. Suster S, Wong TY. On the discriminatory value of anti-HPCA-1 (CD-34) in the differential diagnosis of benign and malignant cutaneous vascular proliferations. Am J Dermatopathol 1994; 16:355–363.
39. Tipping PG, Davenport P, Gallicchio M, et al. Atheromatous plaque macrophages produce plasminogen activator inhibitor type-1 and stimulate its production by endothelial cells and vascular smooth muscle cells. Am J Pathol 1993;143:875–885.
40. Sell KW, Talaat T, Wang YC, et al. Studies of major histocompatibility complex class I/II expression on sequential human heart biopsy specimens after transplantion. J Heart Transplant 1988; 7:407–418.
41. Marboe CC, Schierman SW, Rose E, et al. Characterization of mononuclear cell infiltrates in human cardiac allografts. Transplant Proc 1984;16:1598–1599.
42. Colvin RB. Diagnostic use in transplantation, clinical applications of monoclonal antibodies in renal allograft biopsies. Am J Kidney Dis 1988;11:2,126–130.
43. Hengstenberg C, Rose ML, Page C, Taylor PM, Yacoub MH. Immunocytochemical changes suggestive of damage to endothelial cells during rejection of human cardiac allografts. Transplantation 1990;49(5):895–899.
44. Gassel AM, Hansmann ML, Radzun HJ, Weyland M. Human cardiac allograft rejection. Correlation of grading with expression of different monocyte/macrophage markers. Am J Clin Pathol 1990; 94:274–279.
45. Paul LC, Grothman GT, Benediktsson H, Davidoff A, Rozing J. Macrophage subpopulations in normal and transplanted heart and kidney tissues in the rat. Transplantation 1992;53(1):157–162.
46. Szabolcs M, Michler RE, Yang X, Aji W, Roy D, Athan E, Sciacca RR, Minanov OP, Cannon PJ. Apoptosis of cardiac myocytes during cardiac allograft rejection. Relation to induction of nitric oxide synthase. Circulation 1996;94(7):1665–1673.
47. Jollow KC, Sundstrom JB, Gravanis MB, Kanter K, Herskowitz A, Ansari AA. Apoptosis of mononuclear cell infiltrates in cardiac allograft biopsy specimens questions studies of biopsy-cultured cells. Transplantation 1997;63(10):1482–1489.
48. Briscoe DM, Yeung AC, Schoen EL, Allred EN, Stavrakis G, Ganz P, Cotran RS, Pober JS. Predictive value of inducible endothelial cell adhesion molecule expression for acute rejection of human cardiac allografts. Transplantation 1995;59:204–211.
49. Lemstrom K, Koskinen P, Hayry P. Induction of adhesion molecules on the endothelia of rejecting cardiac allografts. J Heart Lung Transplant 1995;14:205–213.
50. Hosenpud JD, Shipley GD, Morris TE, et al. The modulation of human aortic endothelial cell ICAM-1 expression by serum containing high titers of anti-HLA antibodies. Transplantation 1993; 55:405–411.
51. Deng MC, Bell S, Huie P. Cardiac allograft vascular disease: relationship to microvascular cell surface markers and inflammatory cell phenotype on endomyocardial biopsy. Circulation 1995; 91:1647–1654.
52. Bolling SF, Kunkel SL, Lin H. Prolongation of cardiac allograft survival in rats by anti-TNF and cyclosporine combination therapy. Transplantation 1992;53:283–286.
53. Imagawa DK, Millis JM, Seu P, Olthoff KM, Hart J, Wasef E, Dempsey RA, Stephens S, Busuttil RW. The role of tumor necrosis factor in allograft rejection. III. Evidence that anti-TNF antibody therapy prolongs allograft survival in rats with acute rejection. Transplantation 1991 Jan; 51(1):57–62.
54. Sadahiro M, McDonald TO, Allen MD. Reduction in cellular and vascular rejection by blocking leukocyte adhesion molecule receptors. Am J Pathol 1993;142:675–683.
55. Forbes RD, Cernacek P, Zheng S, Gomersall M, Guttmann RD. Increased endothelin expression in a rat cardiac allograft model of chronic vascular rejection. Transplantation 1996;61(5):791–797.
56. Yokoi Y, Nakamura S, Serizawa A, Nishiyama R, Nishiwaki Y, Baba S. The role of endothelin in the pathophysiology of renal impairment during acute liver rejection. Transplantation 1994; 58(2):144–149.
57. Watschinger B, Sayegh MH. Endothelin in organ transplantation. Am J Kidney Dis 1996; 27(1):151–161.
58. Jordan SC, Czer L, Toyoda M. Serum cytolkine levels in heart allograft recipients: correlation with findings on endomyocardial biopsy. J Heart Lung Tranplant 1993;12:333–337.
59. Morgan CJ, Pelletier RP, Hernadez CJ, et al. Alloantigen dependent endothelial phenotype and lymphokine mRNA expression in rejectiong murine cardiac allografts. Transplantation 1993; 55:919–924.

60. Russell ME, Wallace AF, Hancock WW, Sayegh MH, Adams DH, Sibinga NE, Wyner LR, Karnovsky MJ. Upregulation of cytokines associated with macrophage activation in the Lewis-to-F344 rat transplantation model of chronic cardiac rejection. Transplantation 1995;59(4):572–578.
61. Alpers CE, Davis CL, Barr D, Marsh CL, Hudkins KL. Identification of platelet-derived growth factor A and B chains in human renal vascular rejection. Am J Pathol 1996;148(2):439–451.
62. Leventhal JR, Sakiyalak P, Witson J, Simone P, Matas AJ, Bolman RM, Dalmasso AP. The synergistic effect of combined antibody and complement depletion on discordant cardiac xenograft survival in nonhuman primates. Transplantation 1993;57:974–977.
63. Kobayashi T, Taniguchi S, Ye Y, Niekrasz M, Kosanke S, Neethling FA, Wright LJ, Rose AG, White DJ, Cooper DK. Delayed xenograft rejection in C3-depleted discordant (pig-to-baboon) cardiac xenografts treated with cobra venom factor. Transplant Proc 1996;28(2):560–560.
64. Leventhal JR, Matas AJ, Sun LH, Reif S, Bolman RM III, Dalmasso AP, Platt JL. The immunopathology of cardiac xenograft rejection in the guinea pig-to-rat model. Transplantation 1993;56:1–8.
65. Breisblatt WM, Schulman DS, Stein K, et al. Hemodynamic response to OKT3 in 6 orthotopic heart transplant recipients: Evidence of reversible myocardial dysfunction. J Heart Lung Transplant 1991; 10:359–365.
66. Abramowicz D, Schandene L, Goldman M, et al. Release of tumor necrosis factor, interleukin-2, and gamma-interferon in serum after injection of OKT3 monoclonal antibody in kidney transplant recipients. Transplantation 1989;47:606–608.
67. Pober JS, Doukas J, Hughes CC, Savage CO, Munro JM, Cotran RS. The potential roles of vascular endothelium in immune reactions. Hum Immunol 1990;28(2):258–262.
68. Cotran RS, Pober JS, Gimbrone MA, Springer TA, Wiebke EA, Gaspari AA, Rosenberg SA, Lotze MT. Endothelial activation during interleukin 2 immunotherapy: a possible mechanism for the vascular leak syndrome. J Immunol 1987;139:1883–1888.
69. Toyoda M, Galfayan K, Galera OA, Petrosian A, Czer LS, Jordan SC. Cytomegalovirus infection induces anti-endothelial cell antibodies in cardiac and renal allograft recipients. Transpl Immunol 1997;5(2):104–111.
70. Gaudin PB, Rayburn BK, Hutchins GM. Peritransplant injury to the myocardium associated with the development of accelerated arteriosclerosis in heart transplant recipients. Am J Surg Pathol 1994; 18:338–346.
71. Carlquist JF, Hammond EH, Yowell RL, et al. Correlation between class II antigen (DR) expression and interleukin 2 induced lymphocyte proliferation during acute cardiac allograft rejection. Tranplantation 1990;50:582–588.
72. Miller LW, Wesp A, Jennison SH, et al. Vascular rejection in heart transplant recipients. J Heart Lung Transplant 1993;12:S147–152.
73. Costanzo-Nordin MR, Heroux AL, Radvany R, Koch D, Robinson JA. Role of humoral immunity in acute cardiac allograft dysfunction. J Heart Lung Transplant 1993 Mar; 12(2): S143–S146.
74. Hammond EH, Yowell RL. Pathologic evaluation of early cardiac allograft dysfunction. Pathology Case Reviews 1998;3:1–7.
75. Neish AS, Loh E, Schoen FJ. Myocardial changes in cardiac transplant-associated coronary arteriosclerosis: Potential for Timely Diagnosis. J Am Coll Cardiol 1992;19:586–592.
76. Winters GL, Schoen FJ. Graft arteriosclerosis-induced myocardial pathology in heart transplant recipients: predictive value of endomyocardial biopsy. J Heart Lung Transplant 1997 Oct; 16(10):985–993.
77. Zehr KJ, Herskowitz A, Lee PC, et al. Neutrophil adhesion inhibition prolongs survival of cardiac allografts with hyperacute rejection. J Heart Lung Tranplant 1993;12:837–844.
78. Trento A, Hardesty RL, Griffith BP, et al. Role of the antibody to vascular endothelial cells in hyperacute rejection in patients undergoing cardiac transplantation. J Thorac Cardiovasc Surg 1988; 95:37–41.
79. Rose AG, Cooper DK. A histopathologic grading system of hyperacute (humoral, antibody-mediated) cardiac xenograft and allograft rejection. J Heart Lung Transplant 1996; 15(8):804–817.
80. Loy TS, Demmy T. Interobserver variability in the diagnosis of cardiac rejection. Modern Pathol 1995;8:29A.
81. Olsen SL, Wagoner LE, Hammond EH, Taylor DO, Yowell RL, Ensley RD, Bristow MR, O'Connell JB, Renlund DG. Vascular rejection in heart transplantation: clinical correlation, treatment options, and future considerations. J Heart Lung Transplant1993;12:S135–S142.
82. Gill EA, Borrego C, Bray BE, Renlund DG, Hammond EH, Gilbert EM. Left ventricular mass increases during cardiac allograft vascular rejection. J Am Coll Cardiol 1995;25:922–6.
83. Marboe CC. Cardiac Transplant Vasculopathy. in *Solid Organ Transplantation Pathology*, EH Hammond, editor, WB Saunders Co, Philadelphia, 1994,p.111.
84. Billingham ME. Pathology and etiology of chronic rejection of the heart. Clin Transplant 1994; 8(3 Pt 2):289–292.

85. Hammond EH, Yowell RL. Ultrastructural findings in cardiac transplant recipients. Ultrastructural Pathol 1994;18:213–220.
86. Labarrere CA, Nelson DR, Faulk WP. Endothelial activation and development of coronary artery disease in transplanted human hearts. JAMA 1997;278(14):1169–1175.
87. Hammond EH. Microvascular cardiac rejection. In: Transplantation and Replacement of Thoracic Organs. DKC Cooper, LW Miller, GA Patterson, editors. Boston. Kluwer Academic Publishers, 1996, p. 239–252.
88. Bielory L, Gascon P, Lawley TJ, Young NS, Frank MM. Human serum sickness: a prospective analysis of 35 patients treated with equine anti-thymocyte globulin for bone marrow failure. Medicine (Baltimore). 1988;67(1):40–57,89.
89. Lawley TJ, Bielory L, Gascon P. A prospective clinical and immunologic analysis of patients with serum sickness. N Engl J Med 1984;311:1407–1413.
90. Prin Mathieu C, Renoult E, Kennel De, March A, Bene MC, Kessler M, Faure GC. Serum anti-rabbit and anti-horse IgG, IgA, and IgM in kidney transplant recipients. Nephrol Dial Transplant. 1997;12(10):2133–2139.
91. Suthanthiran M, Fotino M, Riggio RR, et al. OKT3 Associated Adverse Reactions: Mechanistic basis and therapeutic options. Am J Kidney Dis 1989;14:39–44.
92. Jaffers GJ, Fuller TC, Cosimi B, et al. Monoclonal antibody therapy: anti-idiotypic and non anti-idiotypic to OKT3 arising despite intense immunosuppression. Transplantation 1986;41:572–578.
93. Hammond EH, Wittwer CT, Greenwood J, et al. Relationship of OKT3 sensitization and vascular rejection in cardiac transplant patients receiving OKT3 rejection prophylaxis. Transplantation 1990; 50:776–782.
94. Wittwer CT, Knape WA, Bristow MR, Gilbert EM, Renlund DG, O'Connell JB, DeWitt CW. Quantitative flow cytometric plasma OKT3 assay: potential application in cardiac transplantation. Transplantation 1989;48:533–535.
95. Hammond E, Yowell R, Greenwood J, et al. Monitoring of patients for OKT3 sensitization prevents adverse outcome. Transplantation 1993;55:1061–1063.
96. Pober JS, Cotran RS. The role of endothelial cells in inflammation. Transplantation 1990; 50:537–544.
97. Cines DB. Disorders associated with antibodies to endothelial cells. Rev Infect Dis 1989; 11 Suppl 4:S705–S711.
98. Pober JS, Orosz CG, Rose ML, Savage CO. Can graft endothelial cells initiate a host anti-graft immune response? Transplantation 1996;61(3):343–349.
99. Shaddy RE, Prescott SM, McIntyre TM, Zimmerman GA. Role of Endothelial Cells in Tranplant Rejection. in *Solid Organ Transplantation Pathology*, EH Hammond, editor, WB Saunders Co, Philadelphia, 1994, p. 35.
100. Lemstrom K, Koskinen P, Hayry P. Molecular mechanisms of chronic renal allograft rejection. Kidney Int Suppl 1995;52:S2–S10.
101. Miltenburg AM, et al. Induction of antibody-dependent cellular cytotoxicity against endothelial cells by renal transplantation. Transplantation 1989;48:681–684.
102. Caillat-Zucman S, Blumenfeld N, Legendre C, et al. The OKT3 immunosuppressive effect: in situ modulation of human graft infiltrating T cells. Transplantation 1990;49:156–160.
103. Chatenoud L, Ferran C, Reuter A, et al. Systemic reaction to the monoclonal antibody OKT3 in relation to serum levels of tumor necrosis factor and interferon gamma. N Engl J Med 1989; 320:1420–1422.
104. Ferran C, Dautry F, Merite S, Sheehan K, Schreiber R, Grau G, Bach JF. Chatenoud L Anti-tumor necrosis factor modulates anti-CD3-triggered T cell cytokine gene expression in vivo. J Clin Invest 1994;93(5):2189–2196.
105. Pizarro TT, Malinowska K, Kovacs EJ, et al. Induction of TNFa and TNFb gene expression in rat cardiac transplants during allograft rejection. Transplantation 1993;6:399–404.
106. Maury CPJ, Teppo AM. Raised serum levels of cachetin tumor necrosis factor a in renal allograft rejection. J Exp Med 1987;166:1132–1137.
107. Chollet-Martin S, Depoix JP, Hvass U, et al. Raised plasma levels of tumor necrosis factor in heart allograft rejection. Transplant Proc 1990;22:283–286.
108. Dvorak HF, Galli SJ, Dvorak AM. Cellular and vascular manifestations of cell-mediated immunity. Hum Pathol 1986;17:122–137.

7. STRATEGIES FOR THE INDUCTION OF ALLOGRAFT TOLERANCE

Thomas Wekerle*, Josef Kurtz and Megan Sykes
Bone Marrow Transplantation Section, Transplantation Biology Research Center, Massachusetts General Hospital/Harvard Medical School, MGH-East, Bldg. 149-5102, 13th Street, Boston, MA 02129, USA

INTRODUCTION

The principal causes of graft loss, acute rejection, chronic rejection, malignancy and infections, could potentially be avoided by a drug-free state of immunological tolerance. Though factors other than alloreactivity can contribute to chronic rejection,[1] it is becoming increasingly clear that alloreactivity is essential for the full picture of chronic rejection to be seen[2,3] and that the experimental induction of tolerance prevents chronic rejection.[4,5] The induction of donor-specific tolerance to xenografts would obviate the need for excessive immunosuppression,[6] and would be an advance that could help to make xenotransplantation clinically applicable.

Thus, the appeal of tolerance induction lies in its potential to revolutionize the clinical practice of transplantation medicine. The reliable induction of a robust state of tolerance would transform the course of allotransplant recipients from a life-long dependency on an admixture of partially effective and toxic drugs, to a drug-free state of stable graft function, ideally limited only by the life-expectancy of the recipient, not the graft. This chapter covers an overview of the different mechanisms of T cell tolerance and their use in experimental models for tolerance induction, discusses tolerance which develops spontaneously in organ transplant recipients, and views strategies to actively induce tolerance in the clinical setting.

MECHANISMS OF T CELL TOLERANCE

T cell-dependent immune reactions are the centerpiece of alloreactivity. Consequently, T cell tolerance is regarded as the key to achieving transplantation tolerance.[7,8] Three broad mechanisms for T cell tolerance are generally recognized:

* Current address: Dept. of Surgery! Vienna General Hospital, Waehringer Guertel A1090, Vienna, Austria

clonal deletion, *anergy* and *suppression*. *Clonal deletion* leads to the elimination of T cells with a certain antigen specificity; *anergy* is characterized by the presence of T cells that are functionally inactivated and do not become fully reactive upon encounter with antigen; and *suppression* involves a population of cells that actively inhibits responding T cells. Tolerance mechanisms are further classified as either *central* if they occur during development of T cells in the thymus (the central organ of T cell development) or as *peripheral* if they take place extrathymically and hence involve mature peripheral T cells.

Clonal Deletion

Clonal deletion describes the elimination of T cells with a certain antigen specificity. T cells undergo two selection processes during their maturation in the thymus.[9,10] During *positive selection*, T cells with a T cell receptor (TCR) capable of recognizing self-MHC plus peptides are rescued from "death by neglect" (occurring when the TCR does not recognize any peptides) and are allowed to differentiate further.[11,12] T cells expressing TCRs specific for self-antigens, in contrast, are *negatively selected* and are eliminated by an apoptotic mechanism.[13,14] Antigens presented on a variety of cell populations can mediate negative selection, including thymic stroma[15] and bone marrow derived cells,[16,17] with dendritic cells probably being the most efficient mediators. Clonal deletion is a major mechanism by which a self-tolerant T cell repertoire is generated.

In addition to negative selection in the thymus, extrathymic clonal deletion has been described in several experimental models,[18–20] demonstrating that under certain circumstances clonal deletion can eliminate mature peripheral T cells. Apoptosis by activation-induced cell death may be an important mechanism in this peripheral deletion process.[21]

Clonal deletion has been evaluated experimentally in two ways: 1) by determining the rate of occurrence of certain V beta ($V\beta$) products on T cells; and 2) by using transgenic mice with a TCR specific for a transplantation antigen. Certain superantigens bind to MHC (major histocompatibility) class II (I-E in mice) at unique sites, and are specifically recognized by T cells expressing certain V regions of the β-chain of their TCR, regardless of the specificity of the TCR.[13,22–25] Mice have endogenous retroviruses in their genome that encode such superantigens. This information has been used to demonstrate the deletion of self-reactive maturing thymocytes,[13] and provides a tool for assessment of deletional tolerance in transplantation models. By using recipient strains that encode the superantigen but lack the MHC (i.e. I-E) molecule required to present it, in combination with donor strains that provide the required MHC for expression of the superantigen, the deletion of donor-reactive T cells can be determined. Since superantigens might behave differently from allo-antigens, however, a more direct way to look at alloreactive T cells is to use recipients with transgenic TCR specific for a transplantation antigen (e.g. either H-Y or L^d).[26,27]

Since clonal deletion can lead to the complete absence of donor-reactive cells, it is the most robust form of tolerance and the most desirable mechanism for clinical tolerance induction. Models creating mixed hematopoietic chimerism depend on central deletion for inducing and maintaining tolerance, and will be discussed below. Models using intrathymic injection of donor antigen may also rely in part on deletional processes,[28,29] but peripheral mechanisms also play a significant role.[29–31] The utility of intrathymic injection has not been demonstrated in large animal models[32] or in the clinical setting.

Anergy

In addition to the TCR recognizing a specific antigen in the context of MHC antigens, T cells require additional signals in order to become fully activated.[33,34] In the absence of these additional "costimulatory" signals, T cells become functionally unresponsive to subsequent stimulation with antigen, and are termed anergic. A variety of costimulatory signals have been identified, including soluble factors,[35–37] and cell to cell surface interactions.[34,38–40] Among the signals of central importance for T cell-dependent immune responses is the costimulation mediated by interactions of CD28 and CD40 ligand (CD40L, gp39, CD154) on T cells with B7 (CD80 and CD86)[41,42] and CD40,[43,44] respectively, on an antigen presenting cell (APC). Additional signals required for T cell activation come from adhesion molecules, including LFA-1 and ICAM-1.[38] Classical anergy is associated with a lack of interleukin-2 (IL-2) production and can be overcome by the provision of exogenous IL-2.[34] In some systems of anergy, however, IL-2 cannot reverse the anergic state.[45] In some cases, anergy is accompanied by down-modulation of the TCR.[46–48] The induction of anergy is an active process requiring some degree of intracellular signaling, as has been shown by the prevention of anergy induction by blocking signaling through CTLA-4.[49,50] In addition to activation without adequate costimulation, anergy can be induced by stimulation with low affinity peptide ligands.[11,45] Tolerance relying on anergy is often not very stable and may be overcome by infections[51,52] or removal of antigen from the environment.[53,54]

Several experimental models for inducing transplantation tolerance rely mainly on anergy. One way in which anergy can be induced is by presenting antigen on donor APCs that do not provide adequate costimulatory signals. This can be achieved by depleting the graft of APCs,[55] by impairing APC function by UV-irradiation,[56] or by injecting splenocytes which contain a large fraction of non-professional APCs (i.e. cell types that do not have all the phenotypic and functional characteristics needed for effective antigen presentation; e.g. resting B cells). Donor-specific transfusions probably improve graft survival by a similar mechanism,[57] but deletion may be another mechanism contributing to their effectiveness.[58] The administration of antibodies against adhesion molecules can cause anergy and indefinite graft survival in a rodent cardiac allograft model.[59,60] Anergy may also play a role in inducing tolerance by treatment with anti-T cell monoclonal antibodies (mAb),[61–64] but immune deviation and suppression have also been implicated in these models.[65,66] Recently, long-term renal allograft survival was achieved in rhesus monkeys after profound T cell depletion with a new anti-CD3 mAb.[32] CTL activity declined in these animals, while anti-donor MLR (mixed lymphocyte reaction) reactivity and antibody production were preserved.[67] The mechanisms responsible for this state of so-called "split tolerance" are unknown.

Recently, blocking costimulatory pathways has attracted considerable interest for the induction of tolerance in transplantation.[68–70] Simultaneous interference with the CD28 and CD40 pathways may be a promising approach to induce graft acceptance. CTLA4Ig has been widely used to block the interaction between CD28, CTLA-4 and B7, and antibodies specific for CD40L have been used to block the CD40-CD40L interaction.

The administration of CTLA4Ig or anti-CD40L can lead to indefinite survival of vascularized grafts or islet grafts in rodents,[71–73] with optimal results obtained when both pathways are blocked simultaneously.[74,75] Though prolongation of skin graft survival has been shown,[69,71,74] primary skin graft tolerance is not achieved by costimulatory blockade on its own.[71,76] Mechanisms other than anergy have been described to explain T cell hyporesponsiveness after costimulatory blockade and may contribute to the tolerance-inducing effect.

CTLA4Ig plus anti-CD40L as the sole treatment was also recently evaluated in a primate kidney transplantation model.[75] This regimen was highly effective in preventing acute rejection episodes and prolonging graft survival. However, *in vitro* reactivity against donor antigen persisted, indicating that tolerance was not established. Costimulatory blocking reagents, like other approaches for inducing tolerance, appear less effective when tested in primate rather than rodent models.

Suppression

Active suppression has been implicated in various transplantation models as a mechanism for establishing or maintaining tolerance.[66,79–83] Despite the wealth of functional data supporting the existence of suppressive mechanisms, it has been difficult to clone suppressor cells or to identify specific markers for suppressor cell populations, and their existence has therefore remained controversial. So-called natural suppressor (NS) cells act in an antigen-non-specific, non-MHC-restricted manner,[84–86] and have been found in the bone marrow of many species, including humans.[87–89] Although NS cells in some studies do not express surface markers for T cells, B cells or macrophages ("null" phenotype),[84,86,87] T cells and NK cells with NS-like activity have been described.[85,90–92] They are found at sites of active hematopoiesis[86,87] and have been shown to play a role in suppressing graft-versus-host-disease (GVHD) in some models.[86,87,93] The effector mechanism(s) by which these cells cause suppression probably includes the secretion of soluble molecules, including cytokines, such as transforming growth factor β (TGF-β).[94] Nitric oxide[95] and prostaglandins[96] have also been implicated. In fact, NS cells are a likely factor in the observed state of non-specific immunosuppression leading to an increased incidence of severe viral infections that has been observed in organ transplant patients receiving bone marrow (BM) augmentation.[97]

Specific suppression has been implicated in numerous experimental transplantation models.[98–100] One effector mechanism may involve the dichotomy of T helper cell function. Th1 and Th2 subsets of T helper cells are characterized by distinct patterns of cytokine production. Th2 cells produce large quantities of IL-4 and IL-10 and have been implicated in promoting graft acceptance.[42,80,81] Th1 cells are characterized by high levels of interferon-γ (IFN-γ) and IL-2 production and have been associated with graft rejection. However, recently it has become increasingly clear that the concept of distinct, non-overlapping roles for Th1 versus Th2 subpopulations is an oversimplification, and that Th2 cells can also mediate graft rejection.[101–104]

Antigen-specific suppression has also been implicated as a major mechanism in models in which tolerance is induced by oral antigen feeding.[105] Oral administration of purified proteins or of cells carrying the desired epitopes, causes systemic unresponsiveness in various autoimmune[106,107] and transplantation models.[108,109] Depending on the dose of antigen, deletion, anergy or suppression contribute to tolerance induction. A unique cell population, termed Th3, has been shown to play an important role in these models.[110] Th3 cells secrete primarily TGF-β, use IL-4 as a growth and differentiation factor, and are able to downregulate Th1 and Th2 responses. It has recently been recognized that both CD4+ and CD8+ Th3 cells are generated after oral antigen administration.[111]

Of great interest is the recent demonstration of T regulatory cells (designated Tr1) that produce IL-10, IL-5 and TGF-β, but not IL-2 or IL-4, and thus are neither classical Th1 nor Th2 cells.[112] These suppressor cells have been shown to prevent T cell responses *in vitro* and autoimmune colitis *in vivo* in an antigen-specific manner, and a potential role for such a cell population in "spontaneously" occurring graft acceptance could be envisioned.

The induction of anergy and suppression can be linked phenomena, as has been demonstrated by anergic T cells acting as specific suppressor cells.[113] In this situation the APC serves as the link through which anergic or suppressor cells can influence other populations recognizing the same or associated antigens on the APC.[114] This seems also to occur in the case of "infectious tolerance".

Veto cells inactivate or delete CTL recognizing antigens expressed on the veto cell,[115] and are another type of specific suppressor cells. Several different cell phenotypes with veto activity have been described.[116–118] Veto activity has been proposed to contribute to graft-versus-host tolerance,[119] marrow engraftment[120] and the transfusion effect.[121] It also has been shown to be important in a rhesus monkey model of renal transplantation combined with bone marrow infusion,[82,122] and has been proposed as a mechanism by which microchimerism could potentially prolong graft survival.[123] Recent data indicating that CTL undergo apoptosis when signals through surface MHC class I and TCR are triggered at the same time suggest a possible effector mechanism of veto activity mediated by $CD8^+$ cells, which can signal via class I molecules on CTL.[124]

Relationship between Central and Peripheral Tolerance Mechanisms

Peripheral and central mechanisms may contribute to tolerance induction in the same model, and may depend on each other. Recently, it has been shown in a swine model that the induction of peripheral tolerance is dependent on the presence of the host thymus at the time of transplantation.[125,126] Possible links between peripheral and central mechanisms include the recirculation of T cells after activation in the periphery through the thymus where they may be then eliminated or inactivated,[127]

Table 1. Mechanisms of T cell tolerance

A. Clonal deletion:
* *intrathymic*: negative selection
* *extrathymic*: activation-induced cell death, veto cells
B. Anergy:
* inadequate costimulatory signals, CTLA4 signaling
C. Suppression:
* natural suppresser cells, Th1/2 immune deviation, Th3 cells, Tr1 cells, veto cells

and the migration of donor antigen to the thymus leading to the production of dominant suppressive cell populations.[128,129]

DEVELOPMENT OF TOLERANCE IN ALLOGRAFT RECIPIENTS

Hyporesponsiveness or Tolerance under Conventional Immunosuppressive Therapy

Before discussing specific therapeutic regimens designed to induce tolerance, the occurrence of "spontaneous" tolerance in organ recipients needs to be discussed. It has been proposed that conventional immunosuppressive therapies can lead to a state of hyporesponsiveness, or even tolerance, that allows allograft recipients to safely stop their drug therapy at some point after transplantation. Indeed, several reports exist of liver transplant recipients who stopped all immunosuppressive therapy because of non-compliance or for medical reasons, and who nevertheless accepted their grafts for long periods of time thereafter.[130] The intentional withdrawal of immunosuppression has recently been evaluated. Long-term liver transplant recipients with a history of stable graft function were selected for the gradual discontinuation of their maintenance immunosuppression under close monitoring.[131,132] However, only a minority of patients could be successfully weaned from all immunosuppressive therapy. A substantial number of patients developed biopsy-proven rejection, after a mean interval of more than a year, and as late as 42 months after drug discontinuation. Even when a drug-free state can be achieved, spontaneous unresponsiveness is a precarious state and rejection can occur as a consequence of undefined stimuli.

Although stable graft function after cessation of all immunosuppression has also been described in renal transplant recipients, almost half of the patients were reported to subsequently lose graft function.[133] An attempt to withdraw immunosuppression prospectively has recently been undertaken in long-term acceptors of living related renal transplants.[134] Several patients were successfully withdrawn in this preliminary study. Of note, however, some patients demonstrating donor-specific unresponsiveness *in vitro* by MLR at the initial evaluation developed significant reactivity against the donor after weaning despite continuous normal graft function, implying that complete tolerance was not present. Cardiac transplant recipients have not been subjected to trials of complete withdrawal of immunosuppression because of the obvious risks involved. There have been attempts, however, to discontinue steroids in heart allograft recipients receiving triple drug therapy.[135–138] In a recent study, steroids were withdrawn by six months after heart transplantation in patients receiving triple-drug therapy.[138] When compared to patients continuing on standard immunosuppression, the withdrawal group demonstrated an approximately fourfold increase in the incidence of acute rejection episodes. Thus, neither tolerance nor reliable hyporesponsiveness occur routinely, and even the withdrawal of one element from standard immunosuppressive therapy can significantly increase the risk of rejection.

The clinical relevance of "spontaneously" occurring tolerance is further diminished by the lack of laboratory tests to reliably predict whether a specific patient could be successfully weaned from immunosuppression. Evaluation of the immunological state of transplant recipients by *in vitro* tests for donor hyporesponsiveness, such as MLR and cell-mediated-lympholysis (CML), has generally been of little value.[97,134,139,140]

Microchimerism as a Potential Cause of Allograft Acceptance

Microchimerism has been invoked as a putative cause for hyporesponsiveness and hypothetical tolerance occurring under conventional immunosuppression after allotransplantation.[130,142–144] Microchimerism describes a state where donor cells (or donor nucleic acids) are detectable in tissues of the recipient other than the grafted organ. Due to their small number, donor cells can in most cases only be detected with exquisitely sensitive methods, usually by PCR-based techniques. Some degree of microchimerism can be detected in many allograft recipients at some point after transplantation.[146] The long-term presence of donor cells could reflect either constant shedding of cells from the graft, or may reflect engraftment of donor hematopoietic stem cells that provide a constant supply of donor cells of various lineages. The disappearance of microchimerism after graftectomy, as reported in one patient, supports shedding from the graft as the major source of donor cells or nucleic acids.[146] In other cases, however, microchimerism persisted after retransplantation,[147] and donor progenitor cells have been found in organ recipients also receiving donor bone marrow,[97] arguing in favor of hematopoietic cell engraftment. In theory, several mechanisms could be envisioned by which microchimerism might have a tolerance-inducing effect. Non-professional APCs, if among the donor cells contributing to microchimerism, could anergize recipient T cells in the periphery. Otherwise, donor hematopoietic cells, which can be found in substantial numbers especially in liver grafts,[148,149] could migrate to the recipient thymus after transplantation and tolerize newly developing T cells. A third possible mechanism would be veto activity, by which donor T cells or NK cells eliminate host anti-donor CTL.[123]

It remains unclear at present whether microchimerism is the cause for graft acceptance, the consequence of effective immunosuppression or hyporesponsiveness, or is completely unrelated to the issue of graft acceptance. Available evidence supports the notion that microchimerism *per se* does not play a causative role in the occurrence of tolerance in immunosuppressed transplant recipients. Hematopoietic chimerism has been detected in numerous patients undergoing graft rejection.[146,147] In addition to microchimeric patients undergoing rejection, patients accepting grafts without demonstrable chimerism have been reported.[150,151] Furthermore, the occurrence of microchimerism does not predict either rejection or allograft acceptance.[147,152–156] Current clinical and experimental evidence do not provide strong support for the concept that microchimerism plays a central role in the induction of tolerance or hyporesponsiveness in allograft recipients treated with conventional immunosuppressive regimens.

Infusion of Bone Marrow to Augment Microchimerism

Clinical and experimental studies have been performed to evaluate the potential of BM infusions to organ transplant recipients to augment microchimerism and promote tolerance induction.[97,140,157,158] In the largest series to date, liver transplant recipients received unmodified donor BM according to several different treatment schedules, without specific preconditioning.[158] The infusion of two or more doses of BM led to improved graft and patient survival at short term follow-up in this preliminary study (92.5% versus 72% in the control group). However, no significant decrease in the incidence of rejection episodes occurred in the groups showing improved survival. Moreover, a trend toward a higher incidence of multiple rejection episodes was observed in groups receiving BM on the day of transplantation, underscoring the substantial risk of sensitization when BM is administered into non-T-cell-depleted recipients. The risk for severe GVHD also was increased after the administration of large quantities of BM. Reports on renal transplant patients receiving BM have yielded various results, overall with no clear improvement of long-term outcome.[97,140,141,157]

A potential explanation for how graft survival could be improved by treatment with donor BM is provided by the demonstration of a regulatory role for donor bone marrow cells on proliferative and cytotoxic T cell reactions *in vitro*.[159] This non-specific immunosuppressive effect could also account for the increased risk of severe viral infections in renal transplant recipients treated with BM.[97] In primate studies, in which treatment with anti-thymocyte globulin (ATG) and BM prolongs renal graft survival, a veto effect was proposed to explain the decrease in donor-specific cytotoxic T cell function.[82,122,160] The tolerance-inducing effect of ATG plus BM occurs only in a fraction of monkeys, however, and tolerance induction required sharing of one DR-allele between donor and recipient.[161]

STRATEGIES FOR THE INDUCTION OF TOLERANCE IN CLINICAL ORGAN TRANSPLANTATION

A clinical regimen for the induction of tolerance in organ transplant recipients should meet several criteria: *Reliability:* A strategy is needed that works not only in a small fraction, but in the vast majority of patients. This degree of reliability is especially important in view of the excellent short-term graft survival rates achieved with modern immunosuppressive therapies. *Acceptable toxicity:* The toxicity of a tolerance-inducing regimen has to be acceptable for routine clinical use, in view of the transplant-related morbidity currently seen in allograft recipients. Although a non-toxic strategy has to be the eventual goal, any short-term risk of a tolerance-inducing regimen has to be weighed against the morbidity and mortality associated with chronic immunosuppressive therapy used for conventional transplants. *Specificity:* Tolerance by definition is a state of non-reactivity against specific antigens, which in the case of transplantation tolerance are those of donor origin. A tolerance-inducing conditioning regimen has to leave the recipient otherwise immunocompetent in order to avoid the risks of non-specific hyporeactivity or immunosuppression. *Robustness:* To realize the full potential of tolerance induction, the state of tolerance has to be permanent, ideally lasting for the remaining life of the recipient. It also should be robust enough not to be perturbed by intercurrent diseases, or other events that may occur during the life of the patient. *Feasibility:* The selected strategy has to be feasible under most, if not all, clinical situations. Though regimes useful for living-donor transplants would be an important step forward, the eventual goal requires an approach workable for recipients of cadaveric organs.

The Case for Mixed Hematopoietic Chimerism

There is no shortage of experimental strategies for the induction of tolerance. Numerous regimens leading to the indefinite acceptance of vascularized grafts have been developed in rodent models over the last decades. However, most of these regimens fail to achieve similar results in large animal models. When developing a regimen in rodents, it is therefore of crucial importance to use the most stringent tests for tolerance induction, and to have a concept whose workability has been confirmed in primate studies and, ideally, in humans. Models using hematopoietic mixed chimerism are the only ones successful in reliably meeting the strongest experimental test for tolerance, permanent primary skin graft acceptance across a full MHC mismatch. Mixed chimerism induces central deletional tolerance. Non-human primate studies of mixed chimerism have achieved long-term acceptance of renal allografts without chronic immunosuppression.[162,163] Finally, the clinical potential of hematopoietic chimerism is illustrated by reports of patients who have undergone allogeneic bone marrow transplantation (BMT) for hematological indications, who subsequently received a kidney transplant from the same donor.[164–166] These patients accepted the renal graft without immunosuppression, even across major MHC barriers.[166] This evidence suggests that hematopoietic chimerism is a promising experimental approach to be developed for clinical use.[167,168]

The history of tolerance induction using hematopoietic cells began more than forty years ago, when Owen observed that in cattle twins sharing a common placental circulation "a mixture of two distinct types of erythrocytes" can be found long after birth.[169] Shortly thereafter, Medawar showed that these chimeric twins were tolerant to skin grafts from their twin sibling.[170,171] The group of Medawar also was first to actively induce tolerance experimentally by injecting a tissue suspension containing hematopoietic cells into embryos or neonatal mice.[172] These studies provided the basis for using BMT to induce donor-specific tolerance. First, full allogeneic BM chimeras were created by administering BM into myeloablated recipients.[173] This approach was further refined by the introduction of mixed hematopoietic chimerism,[174] which describes a state wherein hematopoietic populations of both the

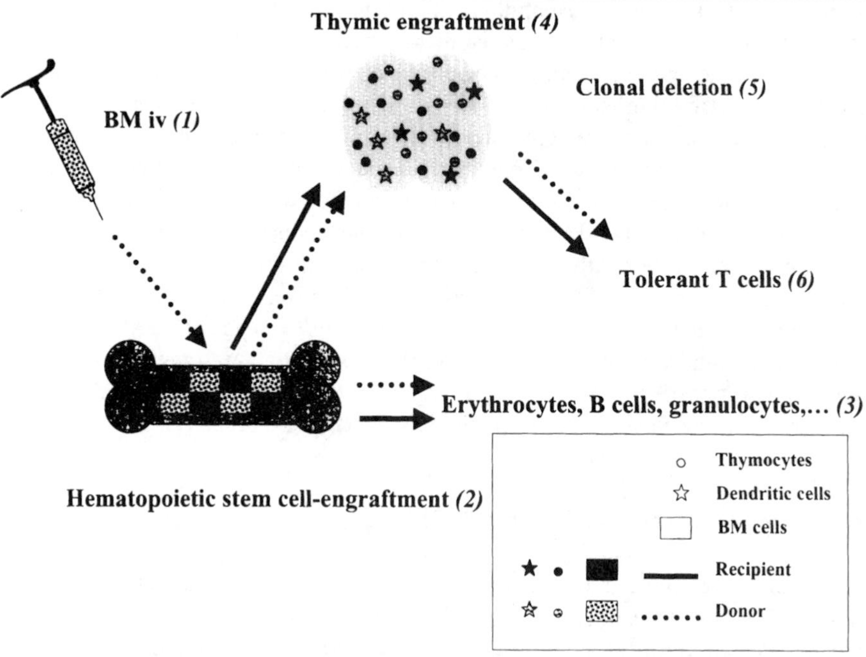

Figure 1. Schematic illustration of the concept of tolerance induction through mixed chimerism. Donor hematopoietic stem cells contained in the BM inoculum (1) engraft in the recipient's BM compartment, where they permanently co-exist with hematopoietic cells from the host (2). Both host and donor stem cells give rise to cells of all hematopoietic lineages (3), including progenitor cells that engraft in the thymus (4), where they give rise to dendritic cells mediating clonal deletion (5) and to thymocytes. These newly maturing thymocytes (of both host and donor origin) emigrating from the thymus are tolerant towards both host antigens and donor antigens, which are now treated as self antigens (6).

recipient and the donor co-exist in the recipient. Mixed chimerism offers several advantages over full chimerism, by overcoming the problem of immunoincompetence associated with fully MHC-mismatched allogeneic chimerism,[175] by eliminating the risk of death due to engraftment failure of the donor BM, and by reducing the susceptibility to GVHD.[86,176] Numerous experimental conditioning regimens for the induction of mixed chimerism have since been reported.[177–180] The main obstacle precluding the introduction of this approach into the clinical setting has been the toxicity associated with the host conditioning necessary to achieve engraftment of allogeneic BM.

The Concept of Tolerance Induction through Mixed Chimerism

Before describing specific strategies for the creation of mixed chimerism in detail, the principal features of this approach will be discussed briefly (Figure 1). The fundamental goal of tolerance through mixed hematopoietic chimerism is to "trick" the recipient's immune system into treating donor antigens as self antigens.

Several steps are necessary to achieve this goal. Hematopoietic stem cells contained in the donor BM inoculum need to "home" to the BM compartment of the recipient. For sufficient levels of engraftment to occur, some form of irradiation is usually necessary. Once stem cells have engrafted, they co-exist with recipient stem cells and give rise to cells of all hematopoietic lineages. In addition, hematopoietic progenitor cells seed the thymus, giving rise to both T cells and dendritic cells.[181] Antigens expressed on cells of hematopoietic origin within the thymus are the most effective mediators of negative selection. In the case of mixed chimeras, hematopoietic cells from both the recipient and the donor locate to the thymus and hence mediate the elimination of both self-reactive and donor-reactive T cells by negative selection.[10,182] Consequently, the newly-developing T cell repertoire in mixed chimeras is tolerant towards the donor and remains so as long as chimerism persists. Since in an adult recipient mature T cells with anti-donor reactivity already exist in the periphery, all peripheral T cells usually have to be destroyed by the host conditioning, to provide a "clean slate" for the newly developing T cell repertoire. This elimination of mature T cells is usually also necessary to prevent the rejection of the infused donor BM. When all of these steps are successfully accomplished, the most robust state of central, deletional tolerance is achieved.

Experimental Induction of Mixed Chimerism with a Non-Myeloablative Conditioning Regimen

Stable multi-lineage hematopoietic chimerism can be induced in mice conditioned with depleting doses of anti-CD4 and anti-CD8 mAbs, a non-myeloablative dose of whole body irradiation (WBI) and additional selective irradiation to the thymic area (TI), followed by the infusion of a conventional dose of unseparated fully MHC-mismatched allogeneic BM. (Figure 2).[177] Chimeras prepared with this regimen demonstrate donor-specific tolerance, as they permanently accept donor skin grafted any time after BMT. At the same time they demonstrate full immunocompetence, as shown by the rejection of third-party grafts in the usual time frame, and by other parameters.[183,184] This normal immunocompetence distinguishes them from full allogeneic chimeras, which suffer some degree of immunoincompetence.[175]

Central deletion of donor-reactive T cells is the main mechanism responsible for tolerance in this[185] and other models involving mixed chimerism.[186] Host and donor thymocytes bearing Vβ that recognize superantigens presented by donor MHC are specifically and permanently deleted in the thymus, and are consequently absent from the spleen and lymph nodes soon after the induction of mixed chimerism. More recently, the central deletion of alloreactive T cells was directly demonstrated in a mixed chimerism model using TCR transgenic recipients. In hosts with a transgenic TCR (2C) specific for a donor class I antigen, H-2L^d, central deletion of donor-reactive (anti-H-2L^d) CD8 cells could be shown by the disappearance of CD8 single positive thymocytes expressing the transgenic TCR.[187] In these mixed chimeras, donor cells with histological morphology resembling dendritic cells, which are potent mediators of negative selection, can be found in the thymus throughout follow-up, beginning as early as a few days after BMT.[185] The role of central deletion as the only significant mechanism by which tolerance is maintained in this

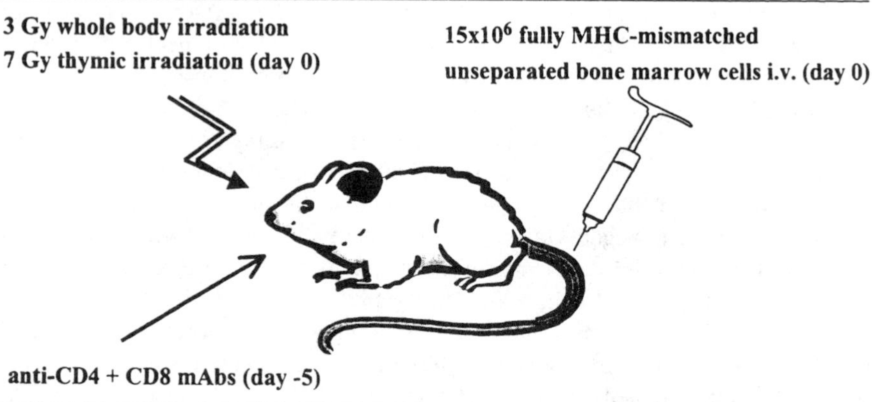

Figure 2. Non-myeloablative conditioning regimen for the induction of mixed chimerism and tolerance in mice.

non-myeloablative model is also supported by the lack of evidence for anergy or suppression.[188] Active suppression does not play a major role either, as chimerism and tolerance are easily broken in established chimeras by the infusion of naive host-type spleen cells or by the removal of antigen when the host thymus is left intact so that non-tolerant T cells are subsequently generated.[188]

GVHD is one of the biggest concerns in clinical allogeneic BMT. GVHD, however, is not seen in rodent models of mixed chimerism, nor in a related primate model,[162,189] despite the use of unseparated bone marrow cells (BMC). This is most readily explained by the continued presence of the T cell depleting antibodies in the host at the time of BMT,[185,190] but may also reflect the inherently decreased susceptibility of mixed chimeras to GVHD.[86,176]

Thymic irradiation can be replaced in the above non-myeloablative model for the induction of chimerism (Figure 2) by the repeated administration of anti-CD4 and anti-CD8 mAbs,[190,191] further reducing the potential toxicity of the conditioning regimen. Even though a single injection of T cell depleting mAbs leads to near-complete depletion of the peripheral T cell pool, donor-reactive thymocytes persist in the thymus and cause "intrathymic rejection", which ultimately leads to failure to tolerize the initially-recovering T cell repertoire (B. Nikolic and M. Sykes, in press). Chimerism is not stable, but starts to decline soon after BMT, even if relatively high levels of chimerism are initially achieved.[190] The repeated administration of anti-T cell mAbs would be of concern in the clinical setting, however, as it prolongs the period of exhaustive T cell depletion and thus increases the risk of potentially life-threatening infections. A considerably less toxic way to overcome the need for thymic irradiation is accomplished by the use of T cell costimulatory blocking reagents. The use of either CTLA4Ig or an anti-CD40L mAb in combination with a single dose of T cell-depleting mAbs leads to stable, lasting chimerism and donor-specific tolerance without thymic irradiation or prolonged T cell depletion, and thus promises to be of potential use in clinical chimerism protocols.[190b]

Although the exact long-term risk to a patient receiving a non-myeoloablative dose of whole body irradiation is presently unknown, it may be associated with substantial morbidity. It would be highly desirable to eliminate WBI from a clinical tolerance protocol. In an unconditioned host, even syngeneic pluripotent hematopoietic stem cells do not readily engraft. At least 1.5 to 3.0 Gy WBI is required for the induction of long-lasting stable chimerism in an essentially syngeneic mouse model.[192] This requirement for conditioning, however, can be overcome by injecting extremely large quantities of syngeneic BMC.[193,194] By extending these findings to the allogeneic mixed chimerism model, it has been possible to replace the WBI with the injection of a mega-dose of BM.[195] Mice are conditioned with T cell depleting mAbs, TI and a total of 200×10^6 unseparated BMC (approximately thirteen-fold higher than the conventional dose). Substantial chimerism and donor-specific tolerance are established in approximately 80% of mice. Intrathymic deletion has been confirmed as the major mechanism for tolerance induction in this modified protocol, and GVHD did not occur in any recipients. Recent advances in stem cell mobilization[196] and in *in vitro* hematopoietic stem cell expansion could make this approach clinically feasible.[197,198] This model represents the first minimally myelosuppressive conditioning regimen for the induction of allogeneic mixed chimerism. Thymic irradiation, however, is a key component of this regimen and a completely irradiation-free strategy for the induction of mixed chimerism remains a major goal.

Other conditioning regimens for the induction of mixed chimerism have been reported.[178–180,199] Of special note, a synthetic peptide mimicking the CDR3-D1 domain of the CD4 molecule was demonstrated to enhance chimerism and tolerance induction in haploidentical and isolated MHC class II mismatched strain combinations.[200] A new population of BM derived facilitating cells ($CD3^+$, $TCR\alpha\beta^-$, $TCR\gamma\delta^-$, $CD8^+$) has recently been reported,[201] but other studies have shown that facilitating cells are $CD8^+TCR^+$.[202] The $CD8^+TCR^+$ phenotype indicates that these are T cells, which have long been known to have the capacity to promote alloengraftment, even in the absence of their ability to recognize host antigens as allogeneic.[203–207]

Mixed Chimerism without T Cell Depletion or Myeloablation

In these protocols, recipient T cells have been eliminated in a non-specific way involving exhaustive depletion or myeloablation in order to permit the induction of stable mixed chimerism. Recently, it has been shown that it is possible to achieve allogeneic chimerism without T cell depletion by using T cell costimulatory blocking reagents. Mice receiving a non-myeloablative dose of WBI, a conventional dose of fully MHC-mismatched BM and costimulatory blockade with single injections of CTLA4Ig and anti-CD40L (Figure 3), demonstrated high levels of stable multilineage chimerism, and permanently accepted donor-type skin.[208] It is also of note that the conditioning in this model starts on the day of transplantation, which thus makes it theoretically applicable to cadaveric transplants.

Mixed Chimerism in a Non-Human Primate Model

Tolerance induction through mixed chimerism has been extended to a non-human primate model. Cynomolgus monkeys were conditioned with ATG for three

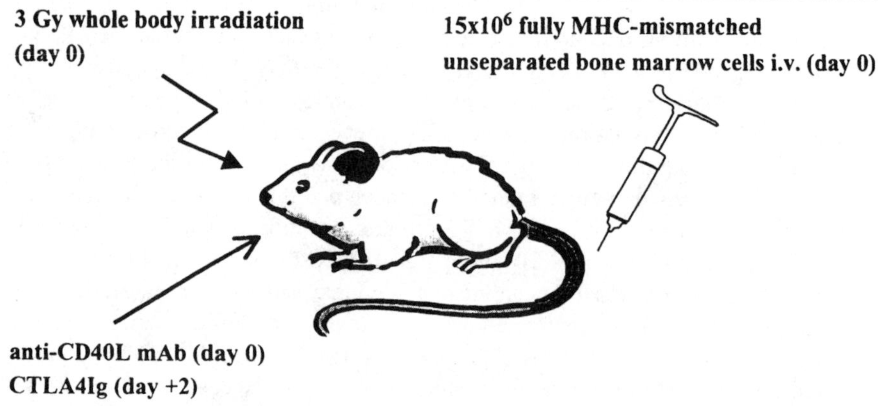

Figure 3. Protocol for the induction of mixed chimerism and tolerance without T cell depletion or myeloablation. The use of costimulatory blockade in the conditioning allows the induction of mixed chimerism in the presence of a mature T cell repertoire, avoiding host T cell depletion and thymic irradiation.

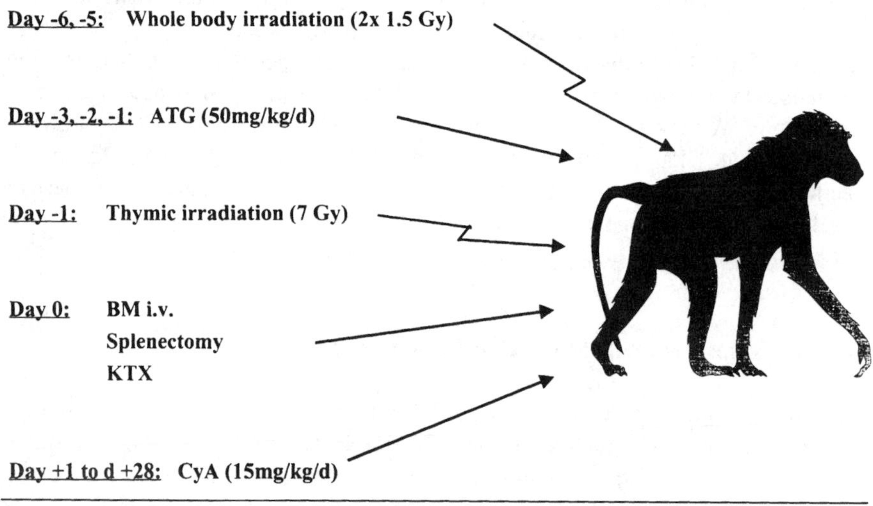

Figure 4. Protocol for the induction of mixed chimerism and tolerance in Cynomolgus monkeys.

days before bone marrow transplantation and kidney transplantation from the same donor, fractionated WBI (3 Gy), and local TI, splenectomy and cyclosporine (CyA) for four weeks after BMT,[162,163] with no further immunosuppression (Figure 4). The short course of CyA is presumably necessary to suppress residual donor-reactive host T cells not depleted by ATG. Multi-lineage chimerism was detectable in peripheral blood lymphocytes for up to 68 days after BMT and long-term stable graft function (for over 2.5 years) was achieved. The transient nature of chimerism in this primate model may be explained in part by the incompleteness of the depletion of mature T cells afforded by ATG. Control animals receiving the conditioning without BM infusion consistently rejected their grafts,[163] indicating that BMT is necessary for tolerance to occur in this model. However, tolerance persisted long after chimerism has declined, implying that the kidney graft itself probably participated in the long-term maintenance of tolerance. Therefore, other mechanisms in addition to central deletion may play a role in tolerance in this model, and the induction of stable chimerism remains to be achieved in primates.

Tolerance Induction in Xenogeneic Transplant Models

The mixed chimerism approach has been successfully extended to xenotransplantation models, including concordant rodent combinations[174,209,210] and a concordant primate model.[189] In a rat to mouse model using a non-myeloablative regimen for the induction of mixed chimerism, skin graft acceptance was achieved, even though chimerism was not stable.[210] Non-immune factors have been found responsible for this decline in chimerism[211] and are an additional obstacle to the achievement of stable mixed chimerism in xenogeneic systems.[212] Due to the existence of pre-formed natural antibodies, B cell tolerance is of even greater importance in the xenogeneic situation than in allotransplantation. Mixed chimerism can achieve both T cell tolerance and B cell tolerance, even in the presence of preformed, natural antibodies.[213] The potential to induce B cell tolerance for the most important antigens recognized by human natural antibodies on porcine donors has been clearly demonstrated after the induction of mixed chimerism in αgal-knock-out hosts receiving αgal-expressing BM.[214] It remains to be determined which mechanism of B cell tolerance is induced by mixed chimerism.[215]

Because of the even greater difficulty in achieving chimerism in discordant species combinations, thymic transplantation has been developed as an approach to inducing tolerance.[216,217] By transplanting fetal swine thymus into T cell and NK cell-depleted, thymectomized mice, permanent skin graft tolerance was achieved across a discordant xenogeneic barrier.[217] Mouse T cells develop in the pig thymus quite normally, and excellent immunocompetence is achieved in these mice.[218,219]

CONCLUSION

Despite many advances in the field of transplantation, clinical tolerance induction is still a much-needed goal. Inducing central deletional tolerance through mixed chimerism presently offers the most promising experimental approach to meet this challenge. A better understanding of the different mechanisms of T cell tolerance, and recent progress in developing a non-toxic conditioning regimen to induce chimerism justify optimism that this strategy can be introduced into clinical practice in the foreseeable future.

ACKNOWLEDGMENTS

We would like to thank Drs. Pierre Theodore and Yong Zhao for critical review of the manuscript and Diane Plemenos for expert secretarial assistance. T.W. is a recipient of fellowships from the Max Kade Foundation and the Austrian Science Fund (FWF). Some of the work described herein was supported by a sponsored research agreement between Massachusetts General Hospital and BioTransplant, Inc., and by NIH Grants RO1 HL49915-04 and PO1 AI 39755.

REFERENCES

1. Tullius, SG and NL Tilney. 1995. Both alloantigen-dependent and -independent factors influence chronic allograft rejection. *Transplantation* 59:313.
2. Russell, PS, CM Chase, HJ Winn, and RB Colvin. 1994. Coronary atherosclerosis in transplanted mouse hearts. I. Time course and immunogenetic and immunopathological considerations. *Am. J. Path.* 144:260.
3. Russell, PS, CM Chase, HJ Winn, and RB Colvin. 1994. Coronary atherosclerosis in transplanted mouse hearts. II. Importance of humoral immunity. *J. Immunol.* 152:5135.
4. Madsen, JC, K Yamada, JS Allan, JK Choo, AE Erhorn, MR Pins, L Vesga, JK Slisz, and DH Sachs. 1998. Transplantation tolerance prevents cardiac allograft vasculopathy in major histocompatibility complex class I-disparate miniature swine. *Transplantation* 65:304.
5. Colson, YL, K Zadach, M Nalesnik, and ST Ildstad. 1995. Mixed allogeneic chimerism in the rat. Donor-specific transplantation tolerance without chronic rejection for primarily vascularized cardiac allografts. *Transplantation* 60:971.
6. Sykes, M. 1996. Hematopoietic cell transplantation for the induction of allo- and xenotolerance. *Clin. Transplantation* 10:367.
7. Charlton, B, H Auchincloss Jr, and CG Fathman. 1994. Mechanisms of transplantation tolerance. *Annu. Rev. Immunol.* 12:707.
8. Sykes, M, DH Sachs, and S Strober. 1994. Mechanisms of tolerance. In: Bone Marrow Transplantation. SJ Forman, ED Thomas, and KG Blume, editors. Blackwell Scientific Publications, Inc., Cambridge. 204.
9. Robey, E and BJ Fowlkes. 1994. Selective events in T cell development. *Ann. Rev. Immunol.* 12:675.
10. Nikolic, B and M Sykes. 1996. Clonal deletion as a mechanism of transplantation tolerance. *J. Heart and Lung Transplant.* 15:1171.
11. Allen, PM. 1994. Peptides in positive and negative selection: a delicate balance. *Cell* 76:593.
12. Alam, SM, PJ Travers, JL Wung, W Nasholds, S Redpath, SC Jameson, and NRJ Gascoigne. 1996. T-cell-receptor affinity and thymocyte positive selection. *Nature* 381:616.
13. Kappler, JW, N Roehm, and P Marrack. 1987. T cell tolerance by clonal elimination in the thymus. *Cell* 49:273.
14. Pullen, AM, JW Kappler, and P Marrack. 1989. Tolerance to self antigens shapes the T-cell repertoire. *Immunol. Rev.* 107:125.
15. Oukka, M, E Colucci-Guyon, PL Tran, M Cohen-Tannoudji, and K Kosmatopoulos. 1996. CD4 T cell tolerance to nuclear proteins induced by medullary thymic epithelium. *Immunity* 4:545.
16. Brocker, T, M Riedinger, and K Karjalainen. 1997. Targeted expression of major histocompatibility complex (MHC) demonstrates that dendritic cells can induce negative but not positive selection in vivo. *J. Exp. Med.* 185:541.
17. Schonrich, G, G Strauss, K-P Muller, L Dustin, DY Loh, N Auphan, A-M Schmitt-Verhulst, B Arnold, and GJ Hammerling. 1993. Distinct requirements of positive and negative selection for selecting cell type and CD8 interaction. *J. Immunol.* 151:4098.
18. Rocha, B and H Von Boehmer. 1991. Peripheral selection of the T cell repertoire. *Science* 251:1225.
19. Webb, SR, C Morris, and J Sprent. 1990. Extrathymic tolerance of mature T cells: clonal elimination as a consequence of immunity. *Cell* 63:1249.
20. Moskophidis, D, F Lechner, H Pircher, and RM Zinkernagel. 1993. Virus persistence in acutely infected immunocompetent mice by exhaustion of antiviral cytotoxic effector T cells. *Nature* 362:758.
21. Van Parijs, L, A Ibraghimov, and AK Abbas. 1996. The roles of costimulation and Fas in T cell apoptosis and peripheral tolerance. *Immunity* 4:321.
22. Acha-Orbea, H and E Palmer. 1991. Mls- a retrovirus exploits the immune system. *Immunol. Today* 12:356.
23. Tomonari, K and S Fairchild. 1991. The genetic basis of negative selection of Tcrb-Vβ11$^+$ T cells. *Immunogenetics* 33:157.

24. Dyson, PJ, AM Knight, S Fairchild, E Simpson, and K Tomonari. 1991. Genes encoding ligands for deletion of Vβ11 T cells cosegregate with mammary tumour virus genomes. *Nature* 349:531.
25. Bill, J, O Kanagawa, D Woodland, and E Palmer. 1989. The MHC molecule I-E is necessary but not sufficient for the clonal deletion of Vβ11 bearing T cells. *J. Exp. Med.* 169:1405.
26. Sha, WC, CA Nelson, RD Newberry, DM Kranz, JH Russell, and DY Loh. 1988. Positive and negative selection of an antigen receptor on T cells in transgenic mice. *Nature* 336:73.
27. Von Boehmer, H and P Kisielow. 1990. Self-nonself discrimination by T cells. *Science* 248: 1369.
28. Jones, ND, NC Fluck, DL Roelen, AL Mellor, PJ Morris, and KJ Wood. 1998. Deletion of alloantigen-reactive thymocytes as a mechanism of adult tolerance induction following intrathymic antigen administration. *Eur. J. Immunol.* 27:1591.
29. Chen, W, MH Sayegh, and SJ Khoury. 1998. Mechanism of acquired thymic tolerance in vivo: intrathymic injection of antigen induces apoptosis of thymocytes and peripheral T cell anergy. *J. Immunol.* 160:1504.
30. Sayegh, MH, N Perico, L Gallon, O Imberti, WW Hancock, G Remuzzi, and CB Carpenter. 1994. Mechanisms of acquired thymic unresponsiveness to renal allografts. Thymic recognition of immunodominant allo-MHC peptides induces peripheral T cell anergy. *Transplantation* 58:125.
31. Odorico, JS, T O'Connor, L Campos, CF Barker, AM Posselt, and A Naji. 1993. Examination of the mechanisms responsible for tolerance induction after intrathymic inoculation of allogeneic bone marrow. *Ann. Surg.* 218:525.
32. Knechtle, SJ, D Vargo, J Fechner, Y Zhai, J Wang, MJ Hanaway, J Scharff, H Huaizhong, L Knapp, D Watkins, and DM Jr Neville. 1997. FN18-CRM9 immunotoxin promotes tolerance in primate renal allografts. *Transplantation* 63:1.
33. Lafferty, KJ and J Woolnough. 1977. The origin and mechanism of the allograft rejection. *Immunol. Rev.* 35:231.
34. Schwartz, RH. 1992. Costimulation of T lymphocytes: the role of CD28, CTLA-4, and B7/BB1 in interleukin-2 production and immunotherapy. *Cell* 71:1065.
35. Jenkins, MK, DM Pardoll, J Mizuguchi, TM Chused, and RH Schwartz. 1987. Molecular events in the induction of a nonresponsive state in interleukin 2-producing helper T-lymphocyte clones. *Proc. Natl. Acad. Sci. USA* 84:5409.
36. Murphy, EE, G Terres, SE Macatonia, C-S Hsieh, J Mattson, L Lanier, M Mysocka, G Trinchieri, K Murphy, and A O'Garra. 1994. B7 and interleukin 12 cooperate for proliferation and interferon gamma production by mouse T helper clones that are unresponsive to B7 costimulation. *J. Exp. Med.* 180:223.
37. Yanagida, T, T Kato, O Igarashi, T Inoue, and H Nariuchi. 1994. Second signal activity of IL-12 on the proliferation and IL-2R expression of T helper cell-1 clone. *J. Immunol.* 152:4919.
38. Van Seventer, GA, Y Shimizu, KJ Horgan, and S Shaw. 1990. The LFA-1 igand ICAM-1 provides an important costimulatory signal for T cell receptor-mediated activation of resting T cells. *J Immunol.* 144:4579.
39. Bachmann, MF, K Mckall-Faienza, R Schmits, D Bouchard, J Beach, DE Speiser, TW Mak, and PS Ohashi. 1997. Distinct roles for LFA-1 and CD28 during activation of naive T cells: Adhesion versus costimulation. *Immunity* 7:549.
40. DeBenedette, MA, A Shahinian, TW Mak, and TH Watts. 1997. Costimulation of CD28-T lymphocytes by 4-1BBL. *J. Immunol.* 158:551.
41. Linsley, PS and JA Ledbetter. 1993. The role of the CD28 receptor during T cell responses to antigen. *Ann. Rev. Immunol.* 11:191.
42. Sayegh, MH, E Akalin, WW Hancock, ME Russell, CB Carpenter, PS Linsley, and LA Turka. 1995. CD28-B7 blockade after alloantigenic challenge in vivo inhibits Th1 cytokines but spares Th2. *J. Exp. Med.* 181:1869.
43. Foy, TM, A Aruffo, J Bajorath, JE Buhlmann, and RJ Noelle. 1996. Immune regulation by CD40 and its ligand gp39. *Annu. Rev. Immunol.* 14:591.
44. Hancock, WW, MH Sayegh, R Peach, PS Linsley, and LA Turka. 1996. Costimulatory function of CD40L, CD80 and CD86 in vascularized murine cardiac allograft rejection. *Proc. Natl. Acad. Sci. U.S.A.* 93:13967.
45. Ryan, KR and BD Evavold. 1998. Persistence of peptide-induced $CD4^+$ T cell anergy in vitro. *J. Exp. Med.* 187:89.
46. Schonrich, G, U Kalinke, F Momburg, M Malissen, A-M Schmitt-Verhulst, B Malissen, GJ Hammerling, and B Arnold. 1991. Down-regulation of T cell receptors on self-reactive T cells as a novel mechanism for extrathymic tolerance induction. *Cell* 65:293.
47. Akkaraju, S, WY Ho, D Leong, K Canaan, MM Davis, and CC Goodnow. 1997. A range of CD4 T cell tolerance: Partial inactivation to organ-specific antigen allows nondestructive thyoriditis or insulitis. *Immunity* 7:255.

48. Ferber, I, G Schonrich, J Schenkel, AL Mellor, GJ Hammerling, and B Arnold. 1994. Levels of peripheral T cell tolerance induced by different doses of tolerogen. *Science* 263:674.
49. Perez, VL, L Van Parijs, A Biuckians, XX Zheng, TB Strom, and AK Abbas. 1997. Induction of peripheral T cell tolerance in vivo requires CTLA-4 engagement. *Immunity* 6:411.
50. Ramsdell, F and BJ Fowlkes. 1990. Clonal deletion versus clonal anergy: the role of the thymus in inducing self tolerance. *Science* 248:1342.
51. Rocken, M, JF Urban, and EM Shevach. 1992. Infection breaks T cell tolerance. *Nature* 359:79.
52. Ehl, S, J Hombach, P Aichele, T Ruelicke, B Odermatt, H Hengartner, R Zinkernagel, and H Pircher. 1998. Viral and bacterial infections interfere with peripheral tolerance induction and activate $CD8^+$ T cells to cause immunopathology. *J. Exp. Med.* 187:763.
53. Rocha, B, C Tanchot, and H Von Boehmer. 1993. Clonal anergy blocks in vivo growth of mature T cells and can be reversed in the absence of antigen. *J. Exp. Med.* 177:1517.
54. Ramsdell, F and BJ Fowlkes. 1992. Maintenance of in vivo tolerance by persistence of antigen. *Science* 257:1130.
55. Lechler, RI and JR Batchelor. 1982. Restoration of immunogenecity to passenger cell-depleted kidney allografts by the addition of donor strain dendritic cells. *J. Exp. Med.* 155:31.
56. Kobata, T, Y Ohnishi, N Urushibara, TA Takahashi, and S Sekiguchi. 1993. UV irradiation can induce in vitro clonal anergy in alloreactive cytotoxic T lymphocytes. *Blood* 82:176.
57. Bushell, A, PJ Morris, and KJ Wood. 1994. Induction of operational tolerance by random blood transfusion combined with anti-CD4 antibody therapy. A protocol with significant clinical potential. *Transplantation* 58:133.
58. Yang, L, B DuTemple, Q Khan, and L Zhang. 1998. Mechanism of long-term donor-specific allograft survival induced by pretransplant infusion of lymphocytes. *Blood* 91:324.
59. Isobe, M, H Yagita, K Okumura, and A Ihara. 1992. Specific acceptance of cardiac allograft after treatment with antibodies to ICAM-1 and LFA-1. *Science* 255:1125.
60. Isobe, M, J Suzuki, H Yagita, K Okumura, S Yamazaki, R Nagai, Y Yazaki, and M Sekiguchi. 1994. Immunosuppression to cardiac allografts and soluble antigens by anti-vascular cellular adhesion molecule-1 and anti-very late antigen-4 monoclonal antibodies. *J. Immunol.* 153:5810.
61. Alters, SE, JA Shizuru, J Ackerman, D Grossman, KB Seydel, and CG Fathman. 1991. Anti-CD4 mediates clonal anergy during transplantation tolerance induction. *J. Exp. Med.* 173:491.
62. Darby, CR, PJ Morris, and KJ Wood. 1992. Evidence that long-term cardiac allograft survival induced by anti-CD4 monoclonal antibody does not require depletion of $CD4^+$ cells. *Transplantation* 54:483.
63. Pearson, TC, JC Madsen, CP Larsen, PJ Morris, and KJ Wood. 1992. Induction of transplantation tolerance in adults using donor antigen and anti-CD4 monoclonal antibody. *Transplantation* 54:475.
64. Shizuru, JA, KB Seydel, TF Flavin, AP Wu, CC Kong, EG Hoyt, N Fujimoto, ME Billingham, VA Starnes, and CG Fathman. 1990. Induction of donor-specific unresponsiveness to cardiac allografts in rats by pretransplant anti-CD4 monoclonal antibody therapy. *Transplantation* 50:366.
65. Mottram, PL, W-R Han, LJ Purcell, IFC. McKenzie, and WW Hancock. 1995. Increased expression of IL-4 and IL-10 and decreased expression of IL-2 and interferon-gamma in long-surviving mouse heart allografts after brief CD4-monoclonal antibody therapy. *Transplantation* 59:559.
66. Yin, D and CG Fathman. 1995. CD4-positive suppressor cells block allotransplant rejection. *J. Immunol.* 154:6339.
67. Fechner, JH Jr, DJ Vargo, EK Geissler, C Graeb, J Wang, MJ Hanaway, DI Watkins, M Piekarczyk, DM Jr. Neville, and SJ Knechtle. 1997. Split tolerance induced by immunotoxin in a rhesus kidney allograft model. *Transplantation* 63:1339.
68. Sayegh, MH and LA Turka. 1998. The role of T cell costimulatory activation pathways in transplant rejection. *N. Engl. J. Med.* 338:1813.
69. Pearson, TC, DZ Alexander, KJ Winn, PS Linsley, RP Lowry, and CP Larsen. 1994. Transplantation tolerance induced by CTLA4Ig. *Transplantation* 57:1701.
70. Larsen, CP and TC Pearson. 1997. The CD40 pathway in allograft rejection, acceptance, and tolerance. *Curr. Opin. Immunol.* 9:641.
71. Markees, TG, NE Phillips, RJ Noelle, LD Shultz, JP Mordes, DL Greiner, and AA Rossini. 1997. Prolonged survival of mouse skin allografts in recipients treated with donor splenocytes and antibody to CD40 ligand. *Transplantation* 64:329.
72. Linsley, PS, PM Wallace, J Johnson, MG Gibson, JL Greene, JA Ledbetter, C Singh, and MA Tepper. 1992. Immunosuppression in vivo by a soluble form of the CTLA-4 T cell activation molecule. *Science* 257:792.
73. Parker, DC, DL Greiner, NE Phillips, MC Appel, AW Steele, FH Durie, RJ Noelle, JP Mordes, and AA Rossini. 1995. Survival of mouse pancreatic islet allografts in recipients treated with allogeneic small lymphocytes and antibody to CD40 ligand. *Proc. Natl. Acad. Sci. U.S.A.* 92: 9560.

74. Larsen, CP, ET Elwood, DZ Alexander, SC Ritchie, R Hendrix, C Tucker-Burden, H Rae Cho, A Aruffo, D Hollenbaugh, PS Linsley, KJ Winn, and TC Pearson. 1996. Long-term acceptance of skin and cardiac allografts after blocking CD40 and CD28 pathways. *Nature* 381:434.
75. Kirk, AD, DM Harlan, NN Armstrong, TA Davis, Y Dong, GS Gray, X Hong, D Thomas, JH Fechner Jr, and SJ Knechtle. 1997. CTLA4-Ig and anti-CD40 ligand prevent renal allograft rejection in primates. *Proc. Natl. Acad. Sci. U.S.A.* 94:8789.
76. Konieczny, BT, Z Dai, ET Elwood, S Saleem, PS Linsley, FK Baddoura, CP Larsen, TC Pearson, and FG Lakkis. 1998. IFN-γ is critical for long-term allograft survival induced by blocking the CD28 and CD40 ligand T cell costimulation pathways. *J. Immunol.* 160:2059.
77. Henn, V, JR Slupsky, M Graefe, I Anagnostopoulos, R Foerster, G Mueller-Berghaus, and RA Kroczek. 1998. CD40 ligand on activated platelets triggers an inflammatory reaction of endothelial cells. *Nature* 391:591.
78. Kuchroo, VK, MP Das, JA brown, AM Ranger, SS Zamvil, RA Sobel, HL Weiner, N Nabavi, and LH Glimcher. 1995. B7-1 and B7-2 costimulatory molecules activate differentially the Th1/Th2 developmental pathways: application to autoimmune disease therapy. *Cell* 80:707.
79. Qin, S, SP Cobbold, H Pope, J Elliott, D Kioussis, J Davies, and H Waldmann. 1993. "Infectious" transplantation tolerance. *Science* 259:974.
80. Hancock, WW, MH Sayegh, CA Kwok, HL Weiner, and CB Carpenter. 1993. Oral, but not intravenous, alloantigen prevents accelerated allograft rejection by selective intragraft Th2 activation. *Transplantation* 55:1112.
81. Onodera, K, WW Hancock, E Graser, M Lehmann, MH Sayegh, TB Strom, HD Volk, and JW Kupiec-Weglinski. 1997. Type 2 helper T cell-type cytokines and development of "infectious" tolerance in rat cardiac allograft recipients. *J. Immunol.* 158:1572.
82. Thomas, JM, FM Carver, J Kasten-Jolly, CE Haisch, LM Rebellato, U Gross, SJ Vore, and FT Thomas. 1994. Further studies of veto activity in rhesus monkey bone marrow in relation to allograft tolerance and chimerism. *Transplantation* 57:101.
83. Field, EH, Q Gao, N Chen, and TM Rouse. 1997. Balancing the immune system for tolerance. *Transplantation* 64:1.
84. Oseroff, A, S Okada, and S Strober. 1984. Natural suppressor (NS) cells found in the spleen of neonatal mice and adult mice given total lymphoid irradiation (TLI) express the null surface phenotype. *J. Immunol.* 132:101.
85. Hertel-Wulff, B, S Okada, A Oseroff, and S Strober. 1984. In vitro propagation and cloning of murine natural suppressor (NS) cells. *J. Immunol.* 133:2791.
86. Sykes, M, A Eisenthal, and DH Sachs. 1988. Mechanism of protection from graft-vs-host disease in murine mixed allogeneic chimeras. I. Development of a null cell population suppressive of cell-mediated lympholysis responses and derived from the syngeneic bone marrow component. *J. Immunol.* 140:2903.
87. Sykes, M, Y Sharabi, and DH Sachs. 1990. Natural suppressor cells in spleens of irradiated, bone marrow reconstituted mice and normal bone marrow: lack of Sca-1 expression and enrichment by depletion of Mac1-positive cells. *Cell. Immuol.* 127:260.
88. Sugiura, K, S Ikehara, N Gengozian, M Inaba, EE Sardina, H Ogata, SM Seong, and RA Good. 1990. Enrichment of natural suppressor activity in a wheat germ agglutinin positive hematopoietic progenitor-enriched fraction of monkey bone marrow. *Blood* 75:1125.
89. Mortari, F, MA Bains, and SK Singhal. 1986. Immunoregulatory activity of human bone marrow. Identification of suppressor cells posessing OKM1, SSEA-1, and HNK-1 antigens. *J. Immunol.* 137:1133.
90. Strober, S, S Dejbachsh-Jones, P Van Vlassalaer, G Duwe, S Salimi, and JP Allison. 1989. Cloned natural suppressor cell lines express the CD3+CD4–CD8– surface phenotype and the A, B heterodimer of the T cell antigen receptor. *J. Immunol.* 143:1118.
91. Sykes, M, KA Hoyles, ML Romick, and DH Sachs. 1990. In vitro and in vivo analysis of bone marrow derived $CD3^+$, $CD4^-$, $CD8^-$, $NK1.1^+$ cell lines. *Cell. Immunol.* 129:478.
92. Hertel-Wulff, B, T Lindsten, R Schwadron, DM Gilbert, MM Davis, and S Strober. 1987. Rearrangement and expression of T cell receptor genes in cloned murine natural suppressor cell lines. *J. Exp. Med.* 166:1168.
93. Strober, S, V Palathumpat, R Schwadron, and B Hertel-Wulff. 1987. Cloned natural suppressor cells prevent lethal graft-vs-host disease. *J. Immunol.* 138:699.
94. Yamamoto, H, M Hirayama, C Genyea, and J Kaplan. 1994. TGF-β mediates natural suppressor activity of IL-2-activated lymphocytes. *J. Immunol.* 152:3842.
95. Langrehr, JM, RA Hoffman, JR Lancaster Jr, and RL Simmons. 1993. Nitric oxide—a new endogenous immunomodulator. *Transplantation* 55:1205.
96. Snijdewint, FGM, P Kalinski, EA Wierenga, JD Bos, and ML Kapsenberg. 1993. Prostaglandin E2 differentially modulates cytokine secretion profiles of human T helper lymphocytes. *J. Immunol.* 150:5321.

97. Garcia-Morales, R, M Carreno, JM Mathew, K Zucker, R Cirocco, G Ciancio, G Burke, D Roth, D Temple, L Fuller, V Esquenazi, T Karatzas, C Ricordi, A Tzakis, and J Miller. 1997. The effects of chimeric cells following donor bone marrow infusions as detected by PCR-flow assays in kidney transplant recipients. *J. Clin. Invest.* 99:1118.
98. Tomita, Y, H Mayumi, M Eto, and K Nomoto. 1990. Importance of suppressor T cells in cyclophosphamide-induced tolerance to the non-H-2-encoded alloantigens. Is mixed chimerism really required in maintaining a skin allograft tolerance. *J. Immunol.* 144:463.
99. Lancaster, F, YL Chui, and JR Batchelor. 1985. Anti-idiotypic T cells suppress rejection of renal allografts in rats. *Nature* 315(6017):336.
100. Maki, T, R Gottshalk, ML Wood, and AP Monaco. 1981. Specific unresponsiveness to skin allografts in anti-lymphocyte serum-treated, marrow-injected mice: participation of donor marrow-derived suppressor T cells. *J. Immunol.* 127:1433.
101. VanBuskirk, AM, ME Wakely, and CG Orosz. 1996. Transfusion of polarized Th2-like cell populations into SCID mouse cardiac allograft recipients results in acute allograft rejection. *Transplantation* 62:229.
102. Picotti, JR, SY Chan, RE Goodman, J Magram, EJ Eichwald, and DK Bishop. 1998. IL-12 antagonism induces T helper 2 responses yet exacerbates cardiac allograft rejection. Evidence against a dominant protective role for T helper 2 cytokines in alloimmunity. *J. Immunol.* 157:1951.
103. Chan, SY, LA DeBruyne, RE Goodman, EJ Eichwald, and DK Bishop. 1995. In vivo depletion of CD8+ T cells results in Th2 cytokine production and alternate mechanisms of allograft rejection. *Transplantation* 59:1155.
104. Piccotti, JR, SY Chan, AM VanBuskirk, EJ Eichwald, and DK Bishop. 1997. Are Th2 helper T lymphocytes beneficial, deleterious, or irrelevant in promoting allograft survival? *Transplantation* 63:619.
105. Weiner, HL. 1997. Oral tolerance: immune mechanisms and treatment of autoimmune diseases. *Immunol. Today* 18:335.
106. Lider, O, LMB. Santos, CSY. Lee, PJ Higgins, and HL Weiner. 1989. Suppression of experimental autoimmune encephalomyelitis by oral administration of myelin basic protein. *J. Immunol.* 142:748.
107. Nussenblatt, RB, RR Caspi, R Mahdi, C-C Chan, F Roberge, O Lider, and HL Weiner. 1990. Inhibition of S-antigen induced experimental autoimmune uveoretinitis by oral induction of tolerance with S-antigen. *J. Immunol.* 144:1689.
108. Sayegh, MH, ZJ Zhang, WH Hancock, CA Kwok, CB Carpenter, and HL Weiner. 1992. Down-regulation of the immune response to histocompatibility antigens and prevention of sensitization by skin allografts by orally administered alloantigen. *Transplantation* 53:163.
109. Sayegh, MH, SJ Khoury, WW Hancock, HL Weiner, and CB Carpenter. 1992. Induction of immunity and oral tolerance with polymorphic class II major histocompatibility complex allopeptides in the rat. *Proc. Natl. Acad. Sci. U.S.A.* 89:7762.
110. Miller, A, O Lider, AB Roberts, MB Sporn, and HL Weiner. 1992. Suppressor T cells generated by oral tolerization to myelin basic protein suppress both in vitro and in vivo immune responses by the release of transforming growth factor β after antigen-specific triggering. *Proc. Natl. Acad. Sci. U.S.A.* 89:421.
111. Chen, Y, J Inobe, and HL Weiner. 1995. Induction of oral tolerance to myelin basic protein in CD8-depleted mice: Both CD4+ and CD8+ cells mediate active suppression. *J. Immunol.* 155:910.
112. Groux, H, A O'Garra, M Bigler, M Rouleau, S Antonenko, JE de Vries, and MG Roncarolo. 1997. A $CD4^+$ T-cell subset inhibits antigen-specific T-cell responses and prevents colitis. *Nature* 389:737.
113. Lombardi, G, S Sidhu, R Batchelor, and R Lechler. 1994. Anergic T cells as suppressor cells in vitro. *Science* 264:1587.
114. Frasca, L, P Carmichael, R Lechler, and G Lombardi. 1997. Anergic T cells effect linked suppression. *Eur. J. Immunol.* 27:3191.
115. Thomas, JM, KM Verbanac, FM Carver, J Kasten-Jolly, CE Haisch, U Gross, and JP Smith. 1994. Veto cells in transplantation tolerance. *Clin. Transplant.* 8:195.
116. Muraoka, S and RG Miller. 1980. Cells in bone marrow and in T cell colonies grown from bone marrow can suppress generation of cytotoxic T lymphocytes directed against their self antigens. *J. Exp. Med.* 152:54.
117. Claesson, MH and RG Miller. 1984. Functional heterogeneity in allospecific cytotoxic T lymphocyte clones I. CTL clones express strong anti-self suppressive activity. *J. Exp. Med.* 160:1702.
118. Azuma, E and J Kaplan. 1988. Role of lymphokine-activated killer cells as mediators of veto and natural suppression. *J. Immunol.* 141:2601.
119. Azuma, E, H Yamamoto, and J Kaplan. 1989. Use of lymphokine-activated killer cells to prevent bone marrow graft rejection and lethal graft-vs-host disease. *J. Immunol.* 143:1524.

120. Nakamura, H and RE Gress. 1990. Interleukin 2 enhancement of veto suppressor cell function in T-cell-depleted bone marrow in vitro and in vivo. *Transplantation* 49:931.
121. Heeg, K and H Wagner. 1990. Induction of peripheral tolerance to class I major histocompatibility complex (MHC) alloantigens in adult mice: transfused class I MHC-incompatible splenocytes veto clonal response of antigen-reactive Lyt-2+ T cells. *J. Exp. Med.* 172:719.
122. Thomas, JM, FM Carver, PRG. Cunningham, LC Olson, and FT Thomas. 1991. Kidney allograft tolerance in primates without chronic immunosuppression—the role of veto cells. *Transplantation* 51:198.
123. Burlingham, WJ, AP Grailer, JH Fechner Jr, S Kusaka, M Trucco, M Kocova, FO Belzer, and HW Sollinger. 1995. Microchimerism linked to cytotoxic T lymphocyte functional unresponsiveness (clonal anergy) in a tolerant renal transplant recipient. *Transplantation* 59:1147.
124. Sambhara, SR and RG Miller. 1991. Programmed cell death of T cells signaled by the T cell receptor and the alpha-3 domain of class I MHC. *Science* 252:1424.
125. Yamada, K, PR Gianello, FL Ierino, T Lorf, A Shimizu, S Meehan, RB Colvin, and DH Sachs. 1997. Role of thymus in transplantation tolerance in miniature swine. I. Requirement of the thymus for rapid and stable induction of tolerance in class I-mismatched renal allografts. *J. Exp. Med.* 186:497.
126. Fishbein, JM, BR Rosengard, P Gianello, V Nickeleit, PC Guzzetta, CV Smith, K Nakajima, D Vitiello, GM Hill, and DH Sachs. 1994. Development of tolerance to class II-mismatched renal transplants after a short course of cyclosporine therapy in miniature swine. *Transplantation* 57:1303.
127. Agus, DB, CD Surh, and J Sprent. 1991. Reentry of T cells to the adult thymus is restricted to activated T cells. *J. Exp. Med.* 173:1039.
128. Blancho, G, P Gianello, S Germana, M Baetscher, DH Sachs, and C LeGuern. 1995. Molecular identification of porcine interleukin 10: regulation of expression in a kidney allograft model. *Proc. Natl. Acad. Sci. U.S.A.* 92:2800.
129. Pearce, NW, A Spinelli, KE Gurley, and BM Hall. 1993. Specific unresponsiveness in rats with prolonged cardiac allograft survival after treatment with cyclosporine. V. Dependence of CD4+ suppressor cells on the presence of alloantigen and cytokines, including interleukin-2. *Transplantation* 55:374.
130. Starzl, TE, AJ Demetris, and M Trucco. 1993. Cell migration and chimerism after whole organ transplantation: the basis of graft acceptance. *Hepatology* 17:1127.
131. Ramos, HC, J Reyes, K Abu-Elmagd, A Zeevi, N Reinsmoen, A Tzakis, AJ Demetris, JJ Fung, B Flynn, J McMichael, F Ebert, and TE Starzl. 1995. Weaning of immunosuppression in long-term liver transplant recipients. *Transplantation* 59:212.
132. Mazariegos, GV, J Reyes, IR Marino, AJ Demetris, B Flynn, W Irish, J McMichael, JJ Fung, and TE Starzl. 1997. Weaning of immunosuppression in liver transplant recipients. *Transplantation* 63:243.
133. Zoller, KM, SI Cho, JJ Cohen, and JT Harrington. 1980. Cessation of immunosuppressive therapy after successful transplantation: A national survey. *Kidney International* 18:110.
134. Mazariegos, GV, H Ramos, R Shapiro, A Zeevi, JJ Fung, and TE Starzl. 1995. Weaning of immunosuppression in long-term recipients of living related renal transplants: a preliminary study. *Transplant. Proc.* 27:207.
135. Kobashigawa, JA, LW Stevenson, ED Brownfield, JD Moriguchi, N Kawata, R Fandrich, DC Drinkwater, and H Laks. 1992. Initial success of steroid weaning late after heart transplantation. *J. Heart Lung Transplant.* 11:428.
136. Miller, LW, T Wolford, LR McBride, P Peigh, and DG Pennington. 1992. Successful withdrawal of corticosteroids in heart transplantation. *J. Heart Lung Transplant.* 11:431.
137. Canter, CE, S Moorhead, JE Saffitz, CB Huddleston, and TL Spray. 1994. Steroid withdrawal in the pediatric heart transplant recipient initially treated with triple immunosuppression. *J. Heart Lung Transplant.* 13:74.
138. Olivari, MT, ME Jessen, BJ Baldwin, VP Horn, CW Yancy, WS Ring, and RL Rosenblatt. 1995. Triple-drug immunosuppression with steroid discontinuation by six months after heart transplantation. *J. Heart Lung Transplant.* 14:127.
139. Reinsmoen, NL, A Jackson, C McSherry, D Ninova, RH Wiesner, M Kondo, RA Krom, MI Hertz, RM Bolman, and AJ Matas. 1995. Organ-specific patterns of donor antigen-specific hyporeactivity and peripheral blood allogeneic microchimerism in lung, kidney, and liver transplant recipients. *Transplantation* 60:1546.
140. Shapiro, R, AS Rao, P Fontes, A Zeevi, M Jordan, VP Scantlebury, C Vivas, HA Gritsch, RJ Corry, F Egidi, MT Rugeles, H Rilo, A Aitouche, AJ Demetris, G Rosner, M Trucco, W Rybka, W Irish, JJ Fung, and TE Starzl. 1995. Combined simultaneous kidney/bone marrow transplantation. *Transplantation* 60:1421.

141. Starzl, TE, AJ Demetris, M Trucco, A Zeevi, H Ramos, P Terasaki, WA Rudert, M Kocova, C Ricordi, S Ildstad, and N Murase. 1993. Chimerism and donor-specific nonreactivity 27 to 29 years after kidney allotransplantation. *Transplantation* 55:1272.

142. Starzl, TE, AJ Demetris, N Murase, ST Ildstad, C Ricordi, and M Trucco. 1992. Cell migration, chimerism, and graft acceptance. *Lancet* 339:1579.

143. Starzl, TE, M Trucco, A Zeevi, M Kocova, S Ildstad, AJ Demetris, H Ramos, WA Rudert, C Ricordi, and N Murase. 1992. Systemic chimerism in human female recipients of male livers. *Lancet* 340:876.

144. Suberbielle, C, S Calliat-Zucman, and C Legendre. 1997. Peripheral microchimerism in long-term cadaveric-kidney allograft recipients. *Lancet* 343:1468.

145. Starzl, TE, AJ Demetris, N Murase, M Trucco, AW Thomson, and AS Rao. 1996. The lost chord: microchimerism and allograft survival. *Immunol. Today* 17:577.

146. Schlitt, HJ, J Hundrieser, B Ringe, and R Pichlmayr. 1994. Donor-type microchimerism associated with graft rejection eight years after liver transplantation. *New Engl. J. Med.* 330:646.

147. Sivasai, KS, YG Alevy, BF Duffy, DC Brennan, GG Singer, S Shenoy, JA Lowell, T Howard, and T Mohanakumar. 1997. Peripheral blood microchimerism in human liver and renal transplant recipients: rejection despite donor-specific chimerism. *Transplantation* 64:427.

148. Taniguchi, H, T Toyoshima, K Fukao, and H Nakauchi. 1996. Presence of hematopoietic stem cells in the adult liver. *Nature Med.* 2:198.

149. Murase, N, TE Starzl, Q Ye, A Tsamandas, AW Thomson, AS Rao, and AJ Demetris. 1997. Multilineage hematopoietic reconstitution of supralethally irradiated rats by syngeneic whole organ transplantation. *Transplantation* 61:1.

150. Schlitt, HJ. 1997. Is microchimerism needed for allograft tolerance. *Transplant. Proc.* 29:82.

151. Wood, KJ and DH Sachs. 1996. Chimerism and transplantation tolerance: cause and effect. *Immunol. Today* 15:584.

152. Elwood, ET, CP Larsen, DH Maurer, KL Routenberg, JF Neylan, JD Whelchel, DP O'Brien, and TC Pearson. 1997. Microchimerism and rejection in clinical transplantation. *Lancet* 349:1358.

153. Hisanaga, M, J Hundrieser, K Boker, K Uthoff, G Raddatz, T Wahlers, K Wonigeit, R Pichlmayr, and HJ Schlitt. 1996. Development, stability, and clinical correlations of allogeneic microchimerism after solid organ transplantation. *Transplantation* 61:40.

154. Schlitt, HJ, J Hindrieser, and M Hisanaga. 1994. Patterns of donor-type microchimerism after heart transplantation. *Lancet* 340:1469.

155. Bushell, A, TC Pearson, PJ Morris, and KJ Wood. 1995. Donor-recipient microchimerism is not required for tolerance induction following recipient pretreatment with donor-specific transfusion and anti-CD4 antibody. *Transplantation* 59:1367.

156. Alard, P, JA Matriano, S Socarras, MA Ortega, and JW Streilein. 1996. Detection of donor-derived cells by polymerase chain reaction in neonatally tolerant mice. Microchimerism fails to predict tolerance. *Transplantation* 60:1125.

157. Fontes, P, AS Rao, AJ Demetris, A Zeevi, M Trucco, P Carroll, W Rybka, WA Rudert, C Ricordi, F Dodson, R Shapiro, A Tzakis, S Todo, K Abu-Elmagd, M Jordan, JJ Fung, and TE Starzl. 1994. Bone marrow augmentation of donor-cell chimerism in kidney, liver, heart and pancreas islet transplantation. *Lancet* 344:151.

158. Ricordi, C, T Karatzas, J Nery, M Webb, G Selvaggi, L Fernandez, FA Khan, P Ruiz, E Schiff, L Olson, H Fernandez, J Bean, V Esquenazi, J Miller, and AG Tzakis. 1997. High-dose donor bone marrow infusions to enhance allograft survival: the effect of timing. *Transplantation* 63:7.

159. Mathew, JM, M Carreno, L Fuller, C Ricordi, V Esquenazi, and J Miller. 1997. Modulatory effects of human donor bone marrow cells on allogeneic immune responses. *Transplantation* 63:686.

160. Thomas, J, M Carver, P Cunningham, K Park, J Gonder, and F Thomas. 1987. Promotion of incompatible allograft acceptance in rhesus monkeys given post-transplant antithymocyte globulin and donor bone marrow. *Transplantation* 43:332.

161. Thomas, JM, KM Verbanac, JP Smith, J Kasten-Jolly, U Gross, LM Rebellato, CE Haisch, FM Carver, and FT Thomas. 1995. The facilitating effect of one-DR antigen sharing in renal allograft tolerance induced by donor bone marrow in rhesus monkeys. *Transplantation* 59:245.

162. Kawai, T, AB Cosimi, RB Colvin, J Powelson, J Eason, T Kozlowski, M Sykes, R Monroy, M Tanaka, and DH Sachs. 1995. Mixed allogeneic chimerism and renal allograft tolerance in cynomologous monkeys. *Transplantation* 59:256.

163. Kimikawa, M, DH Sachs, RB Colvin, A Bartholomew, T Kawai, and AB Cosimi. 1997. Modifications of the conditioning regimen for achieving mixed chimerism and donor-specific tolerance in cynomolgus monkeys. *Transplantation* 64:709.

164. Sayegh, MH, NA Fine, JL Smith, HG Rennke, EL Milford, and NL Tilney. 1991. Immunologic tolerance to renal allografts after bone marrow transplants from the same donors. *Ann. Intern. Med.* 114:954.

165. Helg, C, B Chapuis, J-F Bolle, P Morel, D Salomon, E Roux, V Antonioli, M Jeannet, and M

Leski. 1995. Renal transplantation without immunosuppression in a host with tolerance induced by allogeneic bone marrow transplantation. *Transplantation* 58:1420.

166. Sorof, JM, MA Koerper, AA Portale, D Potter, K DeSantes, and M Cowan. 1995. Renal transplantation without chronic immunosuppression after T cell-depleted, HLA-mismatched bone marrow transplantation. *Transplantation* 59:1633.
167. Nikolic, B and M Sykes. 1997. Mixed hematopoietic chimerism and transplantation tolerance. *Immunologic Research* 16:217.
168. Nikolic, B and M Sykes. 1997. Bone marrow chimerism and transplantation tolerance. *Curr. Opin. Immunol.* 9:634.
169. Owen, RD. 1945. Immunogenetic consequences of vascular anastomoses between bovine twins. *Science* 102:400.
170. Anderson, D, RE Billingham, GH Lampkin, and PB Medawar. 1951. The use of skin grafting to distinguish between monozygotic and dizygotic twins in cattle. *Heredity* 5:379.
171. Billingham, RE, GH Lampkin, PB Medawar, and HLl Williams. 1952. Tolerance to homografts, twin diagnosis, and the freemartin condition in cattle. *Heredity* 6:201.
172. Billingham, RE, L Brent, and PB Medawar. 1953. "Actively acquired tolerance" of foreign cells. *Nature* 172:603.
173. Main, JM and RT Prehn. 1955. Successful skin homografts after the administration of high dosage X radiation and homologous bone marrow. *J. Natl. Cancer Inst.* 1023.
174. Ildstad, ST and DH Sachs. 1984. Reconstitution with syngeneic plus allogeneic or xenogeneic bone marrow leads to specific acceptance of allografts or xenografts. *Nature* 307(5947):168.
175. Singer, A, KS Hathcock, and RJ Hodes. 1981. Self recognition in allogeneic radiation chimeras. A radiation resistant host element dictates the self specificity and immune response gene phenotype of T-helper cells. *J. Exp. Med.* 153:1286.
176. Sykes, M, MA Sheard, and DH Sachs. 1988. Graft-versus-host-related immunosuppression is induced in mixed chimeras by alloresponses against either host or donor lymphohematopoietic cells. *J. Exp. Med.* 168:2391.
177. Sharabi, Y and DH Sachs. 1989. Mixed chimerism and permanent specific transplantation tolerance induced by a non-lethal preparative regimen. *J. Exp. Med.* 169:493.
178. Nomoto, K, K Yung-Yun, K Omoto, M Umesue, Y Murakami, and G Matsuzaki. 1995. Tolerance induction in a fully allogeneic combination using anti-T cell receptor-αβ monoclonal antibody, low dose irradiation, and donor bone marrow transfusion. *Transplantation* 59:395.
179. Colson, YL, H Li, SS Boggs, KD Patrene, PC Johnson, and ST Ildstad. 1996. Durable mixed allogeneic chimerism and tolerance by a nonlethal radiation-based cytoreductive approach. *J. Immunol.* 157:2820.
180. Mayumi, H and RA Good. 1989. Long-lasting skin allograft tolerance in adult mice induced across fully allogeneic (multimajor H-2 plus multiminor histocompatibility) antigen barriers by a tolerance-inducing method using cyclophosphamide. *J. Exp. Med.* 169:213.
181. Ardavin, C, L Wu, C-L Li, and K Shortman. 1993. Thymic dendritic cells and T cells develop simultaneously in the thymus from a common precursor population. *Nature* 362:761.
182. Sykes, M. 1996. Chimerism and central tolerance. *Curr. Opin. Immunol.* 8:694.
183. Ruedi, E, M Sykes, ST Ildstad, CH Chester, A Althage, H Hengartner, DH Sachs, and RM Zinkernagel. 1989. Antiviral T cell competence and restriction specificity of mixed allogeneic (P1 + P2 -->0 P1) irradiation chimeras. *Cell. Immuol.* 121:185.
184. Ildstad, ST, SM Wren, JA Bluestone, SA Barbieri, and DH Sachs. 1985. Characterization of mixed allogeneic chimeras. Immunocompetence, in vitro reactivity, and genetic specificity of tolerance. *J. Exp. Med.* 162:231.
185. Tomita, Y, A Khan, and M Sykes. 1994. Role of intrathymic clonal deletion and peripheral anergy in transplantation tolerance induced by bone marrow transplantation in mice conditioned with a non-myeloablative regimen. *J. Immunol.* 153:1087.
186. Colson, YL, J Lange, K Fowler, and ST Ildstad. 1997. Mechanism of cotolerance in nonlethally conditioned mixed chimeras: negative selection of the Vbeta T-cells receptor repertoire by both host and donor bone marrow-derived cells. *Blood* 88:4601.
187. Manilay, JO, DA Pearson, JJ Sergio, KG Swenson, and M Sykes. 1998. Intrathymic deletion of alloreactive T cells in mixed bone marrow chimeras prepared with a non-myeloablative conditioning regimen. *Transplantation* 66:96.
188. Khan, A, Y Tomita, and M Sykes. 1995. Thymic dependence of loss of tolerance in mixed allogeneic bone marrow chimeras after depletion of donor antigen. Peripheral mechanisms do not contribute to maintenance of tolerance. *Transplantation* 62:380.
189. Powelson, J, M Bailin, A Bartholomew, R Colvin, HZ Hong, M Johnson, M Kimikawa, T Sablinski, SL Wee, DH Sachs, and AB Cosimi. 1996. A mixed chimerism approach to renal transplantation between concordant nonhuman primate species. *Transplant. Proc.* 28:761.
190. Tomita, Y, A Khan, and M Sykes. 1996. Mechanism by which additional monoclonal antibody

injections overcome the requirement for thymic irradiation to achieve mixed chimerism in mice receiving bone marrow transplantation after conditioning with anti-T cell mAbs and 3 Gy whole body irradiation. *Transplantation* 61:477.

190b. Wekerle, T, MH Sayegh, H Ito, J Hill, A Chandraker, DA Pearson, KG Swenson, G Zhao, and M Sykes. 1999. Anti-CD154 or CTLA4Ig obviates the need for thymic irradiation in a non-myeloablative conditioning regimen for the induction of mixed hematopoietic chimerism and tolerance. *Transplantation* 68:1348.

191. Tomita, Y, DH Sachs, A Khan, and M Sykes. 1996. Additional mAb injections can replace thymic irradiation to allow induction of mixed chimerism and tolerance in mice receiving bone marrow transplantation after conditioning with anti-T cell mAbs and 3 Gy whole body irradiation. *Transplantation* 61:469.

192. Tomita, Y, DH Sachs, and M Sykes. 1994. Myelosuppressive conditioning is required to achieve engraftment of pluripotent stem cells contained in moderate doses of syngeneic bone marrow. *Blood* 83:939.

193. Stewart, FM, RB Crittenden, PA Lowry, S Pearson-White, and PJ Quesenberry. 1993. Long-term engraftment of normal and post-5-fluorouracil murine marrow into normal non-myeloablated mice. *Blood* 81:2566.

194. Sykes, M, GL Scott, K Swenson, DA Pearson, and T Wekerle. 1998. Separate regulation of peripheral hematopoietic and thymic engraftment. *Exp. Hematol.* 26:457.

195. Sykes, M, GL Szot, K Swenson, and DA Pearson. 1997. Induction of high levels of allogeneic hematopoietic reconstitution and donor-specific tolerance without myelosuppressive conditioning. *Nature Med.* 3:783.

196. Aversa, F, A Tabilio, A Terenzi, A Velardi, F Falzetti, C Gionnoni, R Iacucci, T Zei, MP Martelli, C Gambelunghe, M Rossetti, P Caputo, P Latini, C Aristei, C Raymondi, Y Reisner, and MF Martelli. 1994. Successful engraftment of T-cell-depleted haploidentical "three-loci" incompatible transplants in leukemia patients by addition of recombinant human granulocyte colony-stimulating factor-mobilized peripheral blood progenitor cells to bone marrow inoculum. *Blood* 84:3948.

197. Emerson, SG. 1996. Ex vivo expansion of hematopoietic precursors, progenitors, and stem cells: The next generation of cellular therapeutics. *Blood* 87:3082.

198. Piacibello, W, F Sanavio, L Garetto, A Severino, D Bergandi, J Ferrario, F Fagioli, M Berger, and M Aglietta. 1997. Extensive amplification and self-renewal of human primitive hematopoietic stem cells from cord blood. *Blood* 89:2644.

199. De Vries-van der Zwan, A, AC Besseling, LP De Waal, and CJP. Boog. 1997. Specific tolerance induction and transplantation: a single-day protocol. *Blood* 89:2596.

200. Koch, U and R Korngold. 1997. A synthetic CD4-CDR3 peptide analog enhances bone marrow engraftment across major histocompatibility barriers. *Blood* 89:2880.

201. Kaufman, CL, YL Colson, SM Wren, S Watkins, RL Simmons, and ST Ildstad. 1994. Phenotypic characterization of a novel bone marrow-derived cell that facilitates engraftment of allogeneic bone marrow stem cells. *Blood* 84:2436.

202. Gandy, KL and IL Weissman. 1998. Tolerance of allogeneic heart grafts in mice simultaneously reconstituted with purified allogeneic hematopoietic stem cells. *Transplantation* 65:295.

203. Sykes, M, M Sheard, and DH Sachs. 1988. Effects of T cell depletion in radiation bone marrow chimeras. I Evidence for a donor cell population which increases allogeneic chimerism but which lacks the potential to produce GVHD. *J. Immunol.* 141:2282.

204. Sykes, M, CH Chester, TM Sundt, ML Romick, KA Hoyles, and DH Sachs. 1989. Effects of T cell depletion in radiation bone marrow chimeras: III. Characterization of allogeneic bone marrow cell populations that increase allogeneic chimerism independently of graft-vs-host disease in mixed marrow recipients. *J. Immunol.* 143:3503.

205. Martin, PJ. 1993. Donor CD8 cells prevent allogeneic marrow graft rejection in mice: potential implications for marrow transplantation in humans. *J. Exp. Med.* 178:703–712.

206. Martin, PJ. 1995. Influence of alloreactive T cells on initial hematopoietic reconstitution after marrow transplantation. *Exp. Hematol.* 23:174.

207. Lapidot, T, Y Faktorowich, I Lubin, and Y Reisner. 1992. Enhancement of T-cell-depleted bone marrow allografts in the absence of graft-versus-host disease is mediated by CD8+CD4– and not by CD8–CD4+ thymocytes. *Blood* 80:2406.

208. Wekerle, T, MH Sayegh, J Hill, Y Zhao, A Chandraker, KG Swenson, G Zhao, and M Sykes. 1998. Extrathymic T cell deletion and allogeneic stem cell engraftment induced with costimulatory blockade is followed by central T cell tolerance. *J. Exp. Med.* 187:2037.

209. Ildstad, ST and SM Wren. 1991. Cross-species bone marrow transplantation: Evidence for tolerance induction, stem cell engraftment, and maturation of T lymphocytes in a xenogeneic stromal environment (Rat --> Mouse). *J. Exp. Med.* 174:67.

210. Sharabi, Y, I Aksentijevich, TM Sundt III, DH Sachs, and M Sykes. 1990. Specific tolerance induc-

tion across a xenogeneic barrier: production of mixed rat/mouse lymphohematopoietic chimeras using a nonlethal preparative regimen. *J. Exp. Med.* 172:195.

211. Lee, LA, JJ Sergio, and M Sykes. 1995. Evidence for non-immune mechanisms in the loss of hematopoietic chimerism in ratXmouse mixed xenogeneic chimeras. *Xenotransplantation* 2:57.
212. Gritsch, HA and M Sykes. 1996. Host marrow has a competitive advantage which limits donor hematopoietic repopulation in mixed xenogeneic chimeras. *Xenotransplantation* 3:312.
213. Aksentijevich, I, DH Sachs, and M Sykes. 1992. Humoral tolerance in xenogeneic BMT recipients conditioned with a non-myeloablative regimen. *Transplantation* 53:1108.
214. Yang, Y-G, E deGoma, H Ohdan, JL Bracy, Y Xu, J Iacomini, AD Thall, and M Sykes. 1998. Tolerization of anti-galα1-3gal natural antibody-forming B cells by induction of mixed chimerism. *J. Exp. Med.* 187:1335.
215. Klinman, NR. 1996. The "clonal selection hypothesis" and current concepts of B cell tolerance. *Immunity* 5:189.
216. Khan, A, JJ Sergio, Y Zhao, DA Pearson, DH Sachs, and M Sykes. 1997. Discordant xenogeneic neonatal thymic transplantation can induce donor-specific tolerance. *Transplantation* 63:124.
217. Zhao, Y, K Swenson, JJ Sergio, JS Arn, DH Sachs, and M Sykes. 1996. Skin graft tolerance across a discordant xenogeneic barrier. *Nature Med.* 2:1211.
218. Zhao, Y, JA Fishman, JJ Sergio, JL Oliveros, DA Pearson, GL Szot, RA Wilkinson, JS Arn, DH Sachs, and M Sykes. 1997. Immune restoration by fetal pig thymus grafts in T cell-depleted, thymectomized mice. *J. Immunol.* 158:1641.
219. Zhao, Y, JJ Sergio, K Swenson, JS Arn, DH Sachs, and M Sykes. 1997. Positive and negative selection of functional mouse CD4 cells by porcine MHC in pig thymus grafts. *J. Immunol.* 159:2100.

8. XENOTRANSPLANTATION: HYPERACUTE AND DELAYED XENOGRAFT REJECTION

Kwabena Mawulawde, M.D.
and Joren C. Madsen, M.D., D.Phil.
Division of Cardiac Surgery and
Transplantation Biology Research Center,
Department of Surgery, Massachusetts General
Hospital, Harvard Medical School, Boston

INTRODUCTION

According to the United Network for Organ Sharing (UNOS), patients waiting for a heart transplant in the U.S. have over a 20% mortality rate due to the shortage of donor organs.[1] The scarcity of donor organs accounts, in part, for the strong resurgence of interest in xenotransplantation over the past decade. Although an unlimited availability of animal organs would rectify the existing crisis, there are formidable immunobiological barriers to overcome before the full potential of trans-species organ transplantation can be realized. The earliest and perhaps most devastating immunological barrier is that of hyperacute rejection, which results from the binding of natural antibody to the vascular endothelium, fixation of complement, activation of the endothelium, and finally, to the initiation of the coagulation cascade. Attempts to prevent this powerful immune response have targeted preformed natural antibodies and the complement system for intervention. The next immunological barrier, referred to as delayed xenograft rejection or acute vascular rejection, is less well understood but probably involves multiple pathways, including antibodies and/or immune cells binding to endothelium and endothelial cell activation (Figure 1). Of the last two immunological barriers, cellular rejection and chronic rejection, the former is probably best understood as it involves mechanisms which are similar in nature, albeit stronger in intensity, to those responsible for clinical allograft rejection. In contrast, the mechanisms responsible for chronic rejection remain enigmatic both in allogeneic and xenogeneic transplantation.

Address for correspondence: Joren C. Madsen, M.D., D.Phil., Department of Surgery, Massachusetts General Hospital, Boston, MA 02114, Tel. 617-724-1130, FAX 617-726-5804

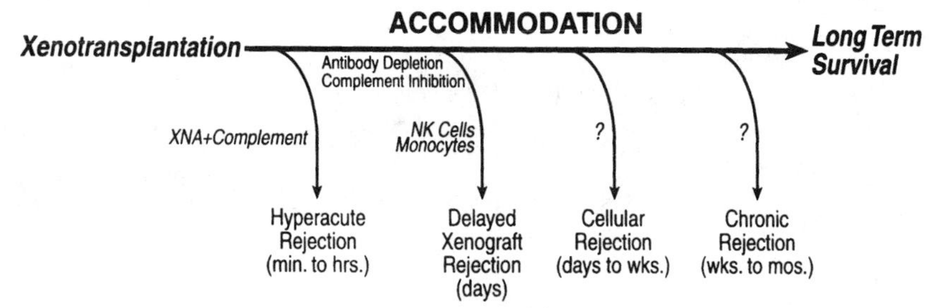

Figure 1. Possible biological outcomes of xenotransplantation. Transplantation of a discordant xenograft generally leads to hyperacute rejection. If hyperacute rejection is averted by either depletion of xenoreactive antibodies or inhibition of complement, the xenograft may fail as a result of delayed xenograft rejection. Alternatively, "accommodation" may occur wherein the vascularized graft functions without apparent injury even with the return of xenoreactive antibodies. Finally, the mechanism by which a xenograft becomes susceptible to cellular rejection and chronic rejection requires elucidation. Modified with permission from "Immunologic Barriers to Xenotransplantation", S.S. Lin, and J.L. Platt; Journal of Heart and Lung Transplantation; June 1996.

This chapter will primarily review the immunobiological mechanisms underlying hyperacute rejection and delayed xenograft rejection. In addition, the experimental strategies currently being employed to prevent these two types of xenogeneic rejection responses will be presented.

Clinical History

Clinical xenotransplantation began in 1963 when Reemtsma performed the first chimpanzee-to-human renal transplant.[2] The following year James Hardy attempted the first human cardiac xenotransplant.[3] The chimpanzee heart which Hardy grafted into his 68 year old patient dying of end-stage heart failure survived for approximately 1 hour after the cessation of cardiopulmonary bypass but was subsequently "... judged incapable of accepting the large venous return ..." due to an obvious size mismatch.[3] In retrospect, the rapidity of spontaneous cardiac dysfunction strongly implicated hyperacute rejection as the mediator of graft loss. Although others attempted cardiac xenotransplantation, none achieved patient or graft survival. These early failures, combined with the widespread acceptance of the concept of brain death in the late 1960s.[4] which resulted in a dramatic increase in available organ donors, led to a diminished interest in xenotransplantation over the next 15 years.

In 1984, clinical interest in xenotransplantation was rekindled when Bailey transplanted a baboon heart into a neonate born with hypoplastic left heart syndrome.[5] Using an intensive immunosuppression regimen, Bailey and colleagues successfully avoided hyperacute rejection but the patient succumbed to an infection on the twentieth postoperative day. Post-mortem microscopic analysis revealed a mononuclear cellular infiltrate with capillary thrombosis suggestive of delayed xenograft rejection. Since Bailey's report, there have been attempts at pig-to-human liver[6] and islet cell[7] transplantation, in addition to baboon-to-human bone marrow transplantation,[8] but none of these endeavors resulted in a clearcut clinical benefit. Perhaps the most encouraging result to date was the recent documentation that fetal pig neural cells transplanted into the brain of a patient suffering from Parkinson's disease survived over seven months with appropriate growth of non-human dopaminergic neurons using only cyclosporine for immunosuppression.[9]

Although advances in the clinical arena have been modest at best, enormous progress has been made in the scientific investigation of xenotransplantation. Not only have the immunological barriers to successful xenotransplantation been more clearly defined but also the potential solutions to these problems have increased in number and promise.

HYPERACUTE REJECTION

When a heart is transplanted from one species into a phylogenetically disparate species, i.e. pig-to-primate, an extremely fulminant immunologic reaction ensues within minutes of organ reperfusion. The once normally-appearing myocardium becomes dusky and cyanotic, with diminished, if not absent, contractility. Widespread intravascular thrombosis and interstitial hemorrhage characteristic of a hypercoagulable state mark the histology of this hyperacute rejection response (Figure 2, see color plates section, back of book). The three major physiologic components responsible for this response are 1) binding of preformed xenoreactive natural antibodies to carbohydrate moieties on the vascular endothelium of the donor organ, 2) activation of the complement cascade within the recipient, and 3) endothelial cell activation.

Early studies of xenotransplantation using a variety of different species demonstrated that hyperacute rejection did not occur in all combinations of species but only in species of great phylogenetic diversity. Realizing this, Calne suggested the terms *concordant*, to describe species combinations in which hyperacute rejection did not occur, and *discordant*, to describe combinations in which it did occur.[10] More recently, these terms have been used to distinguish between (concordant) combinations of species in which there are no preformed natural antibodies (i.e. hamster-to-rat or monkey-to-baboon) and (discordant) species combination in which natural antibodies do exist (i.e. guinea pig-to-rat or pig-to-baboon). Discordant grafts, specifically pig-to-nonhuman primates, will be the focus of this chapter.

Xenoreactive natural antibodies and the αGal epitope

It was realized as early as the mid 1960s that hyperacute rejection was due to antibody-mediated complement activation.[11] However, it was not until the early 1990s that it became clear just what porcine antigen was being targeted by human natural antibodies. Although one might imagine that human natural antibodies would recognize a wide array of antigens on pig organs, it has been documented that over 80% of human complement-fixing natural antibodies recognize a single structure—Galα1-3Gal (Figure 3), a carbohydrate which is structurally similar to blood group antigen A and B. It was the seminal work of Good and Cooper[12,13] and Galili and

B Disaccharide
αGal(1-3)βGal-R

Linear B type 2
αGal(1-3)βGal(1-4)βGlcNAc-R

Linear B type 6
αGal(1-3)βGal(1-4)βGlc-R

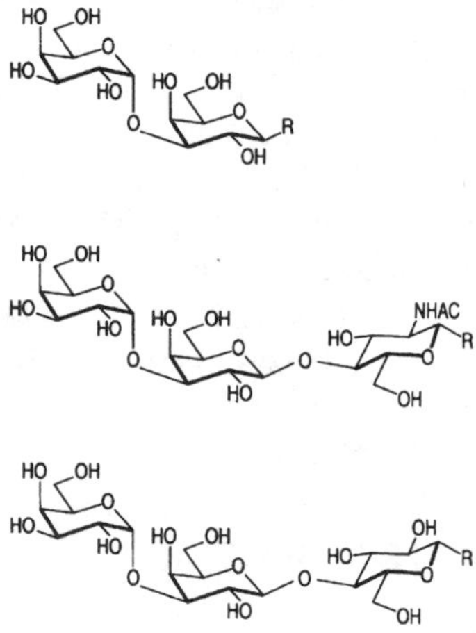

Figure 3. Synthetic oligossacharides with terminal carbohydrate structures that bind human antibodies eluded from pig heart kidney and red blood cell stroma: αGal disaccharide (*top*), αGal trisaccharide type 2 (*middle*), and αGal trisaccharide type 6 (*bottom*). R = $(CH_2)_8COOCH_3$.

colleagues[14,15] that clearly established the Galα1-3Gal terminal residue on pig endothelium as the determinant responsible for binding the major portion of preformed human natural antibodies.

Expression of the αGal epitope is governed by the presence of an α-galactosyltransferase enzyme which catalyzes the reaction:

Galβ1-4GlcNAc-R + UDP-Gal $\xrightarrow{\alpha 1,3GT}$ Galα1-3Galβ1-4GlcNAc-R + UDP.[14]

This enzyme is found in New World monkeys and all lower order mammals (including swine). As a result, these species express the αGal epitope on their vascular endothelium and do not have circulating anti-αGal antibody. In contrast, humans and all higher order primates (chimpanzees, baboons, and apes) have lost the gene for α-galactosyltransferase. The lack of constitutive αGal expression in these higher order species permits the formation of antibodies directed against the endothelial αGal determinant. These anti-αGal antibodies are not a constitutive part of the immunoglobulin repertoire of the developing fetus and, therefore, do not exist at birth. It is believed that, like the natural antibodies that bind blood group antigens, immunoglobulins that bind to the αGal epitope develop as a consequence of exposure to environmental microorganisms that express the same carbohydrate determinants.[16] Parenthetically, the loss of the α-galactosyltransferase gene during evolution may have provided a survival advantage by allowing the development of anti-αGal antibodies which could defend against environmental pathogens including viruses that express this determinant.[17]

The majority of natural antibody responsible for binding the αGal epitope on the pig endothelium is of the IgM isotype; it accounts for as much as 4% of the total circulating IgM immunoglobulin in humans.[18] It is highly likely that only IgM (but not IgG) natural antibodies can cause hyperacute rejection, probably because the greater number of receptors on the IgM compared to IgG antibodies increases its binding avidity sufficiently to trigger complement activation.[18,19] Interestingly, when humans are exposed to pig tissue, either through extracorporeal perfusion of a pig organ, pig islet cell or bone marrow transplantation, the rise in levels of anti-αGal IgG is significantly greater than the corresponding rise in anti-αGal IgM.[20] It is thought that these IgG anti-αGal antibodies may promote antibody-dependent cell-mediated cytotoxicity (ADCC) by binding NK cells and macrophages through the Fc portion of the antibody. This mechanism of xenograft destruction is probably more important in delayed xenograft rejection than in hyperacute rejection (see below). Although antibodies to foreign alloantigens may exist in prospective recipients due to prior exposure, preformed IgG antibodies directed against foreign MHC molecules do not seem to play a major role in hyperacute rejection.[21,22]

Complement Activation

The development of hyperacute rejection depends absolutely on the activation of complement. In some models of discordant xenotransplantation (i.e. guinea pig-to-rat), complement is activated through the alternative pathway in the absence of preformed antibody.[23–25] However, in what is considered the most clinically relevant model, pig-to-primate, complement is activated through the classical pathway after binding of natural antibody and formation of antigen-antibody complex (Figure 4, see color plates section, back of book).[26,27] In either case, the terminal event in the complement cascade is the formation of the membrane attack complex (MAC) which mediates cytolysis by forming pores in cell membranes.[28–30] However, the membrane attack complex is probably not the only complement component implicated in hyperacute rejection. Inflammatory mediators such as C3b and terminal complement proteins undoubtedly contribute to the process.[31]

In humans, the vigor of the complement cascade is regulated by a number of endothelial proteins including decay activating factor (DAF or CD55), membrane cofactor protein (MCP or CD46) and CD59 (Table 1). These complement regulatory proteins are membrane glycoproteins (Figure 5) that act as inhibitors at several key points in the cascade where the activation of both pathways may be halted. Of major importance in discordant xenotransplantation is the fact that these regulatory proteins function effectively only with the complement proteins of their own species.[32] Indeed, part of the reason the hyperacute rejection response is so explosive and universal in pig-to-human transplantation is that the species-specific pig complement regulatory proteins in the xenograft are unable to control human complement proteins, resulting in uncontrolled activation of the host's complement system. This concept is the basis for the creation of transgenic animals expressing human complement regulatory proteins, with the hope being that organs from such animals would resist injury by human complement (see below).

Type I Endothelial Activation

Resting endothelium and the molecules expressed on the surface of quiescent endothelial cells perform several important functions, including prevention of intravascular coagulation and platelet aggregation. The binding of xenoreactive anti-

Table 1. Regulators of Complement Activation

Proteins	Location	Target	Function
Decay Accelerating Factor (DAF)	Membrane: Blood cells, endothelial and epithelial cells	C4b2a, C3bBb	Accelerates classical and alternative pathway C3 convertases degradation
Membrane Cofactor Protein (MCP) (CD46)	Membrane: Most blood Cells (Except RBC), Fibroblast, Endothelial and Epithelial cells	C3b, C4b	Co-factor for Factor I mediated cleavage of C3, C3b, C4b
CD59 (Membrane Inhibitor of Reactive Lysis (MIRL)	Membrane: Most blood cells, platelets, endothelial, epithelial cells	C7, C8	Prevents MAC formation and lysis by blocking C9 binding to C8; action restricted to C8, C9 of same species
Complement Receptor type 1 (CR1) (CD35)	Membrane: Most blood cells, mast cells	C3b, C4b, iC3b	Co-factor for Factor I-mediated cleavage of C3b, C4b; Increases dissociation of classical and alternative pathway C3 convertase
Cl Inhibitor	Serum	Clr, Cls	Binds to Clr, Cls and blocks their activity in classical pathway
Factor H	Serum	C3b	Increases degradation of alternative pathway. C3 convertase (C3bBb)
Factor I	Serum	C4b, C3b	Cleaves and inactivates C4b and C3b using factor H, CRI, MCP as cofactors

Modified with permission from Abbas Abdul K., Lichtman Andrew H., Prober Jordans. Cellular and Molecular Immunology, p. 304. Copyright 1994, W.B. Saunders Co.

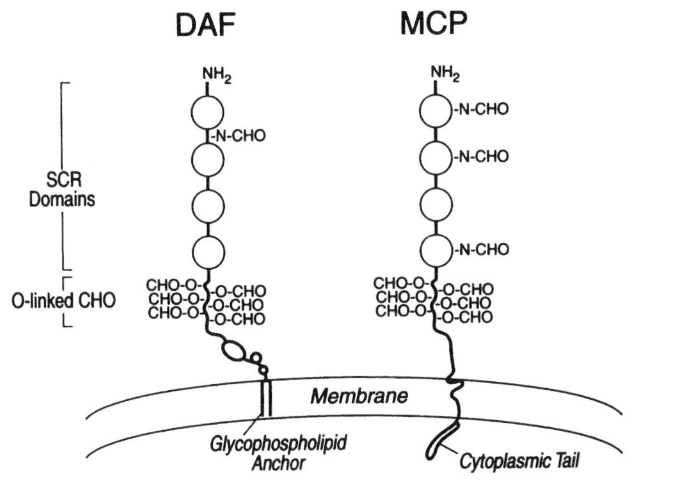

Figure 5. Structure of membrane glycoproteins decay-accelerating factor (DAF) and membrane cofactor protein (MCP) deduced from cDNA sequence and biochemical studies. The short consensus repeats (SCR) are depicted as globular structures and sites of N- and O-linked carbohydrates (CHO) are indicated.[118]

bodies and activation of complement on the endothelial surface stimulates the resting endothelium to initiate a rapid, protein-synthesis-independent response referred to as type I endothelial cell activation.[33] This response is manifested by 1) a change in endothelial cell shape,[34] 2) the loss of heparan sulfate from the cell surface,[35] and 3) the elaboration of proinflammatory cytokines, chemokines and adhesion molecules.[36] Reconfiguration of endothelial cell shape causes the cells to separate from one another, forming gaps which allow intravascular fluid to extravasate and platelets to be activated through contact with matrix. The loss of heparan sulfate increases sensitivity to oxidant-mediated injury and gives rise to procoagulant changes on the endothelial surfaces. The elaboration of inflammatory mediators also contributes to vasoconstriction and direct injury by polymorphonuclear leukocytes. Also, the attachment and activation of platelets leads to the release of a variety of vasoactive substances such as thromboxane A_2 that constrict vascular smooth muscle and alter regional blood flow. These changes account for the early intravascular thrombosis and extravascular hemorrhage observed in hyperacute rejection (Figure 6, see color plates section, back of book).

PREVENTION OF HYPERACUTE REJECTION

The pharmacologic immunosuppressive agents that are currently being used to treat allogeneic rejection have no effect in the prevention of hyperacute rejection. Therefore, new approaches have been devised to overcome early xenogeneic rejection (Table 2). Since the two principal factors that precipitate hyperacute rejection are xenogeneic antibodies and complement, both of these circulating plasma constituents have been targeted for depletion and/or inhibition in attempts to prevent hyperacute rejection.

Table 2. Methods of preventing hyperacute rejection

Directed at the Recipient
1) Depletion or inhibition of preformed natural antibody
2) Depletion or inhibition of complement
Directed at the Donor
1) Expression of human complement regulatory proteins in transgenic swine
2) Replacement of αGal with another carbohydrate in transgenic swine

Depletion or Inhibition of Anti-αGal Antibody

Four primary methods of depleting or inhibiting anti-αGal antibody and prolonging experimental xenograft survival have been described. They include 1) plasmapheresis,[37,38,39] 2) donor organ perfusion,[26,40] 3) extracorporeal immunoadsorption,[41] and 4) oligosaccharide infusion.[42] Although effective to varying degrees at removing or inactivating natural xenogeneic antibodies, none prevent their return. Xenoreactive antibodies usually return within 24–48 hours in untreated recipients and between 5 and 7 days in immunosuppressed hosts.

Plasmapheresis represents an effective, albeit nonspecific, method of removing xenogeneic antibody. In addition to preformed anti-αGal antibodies, plasmapheresis also eliminates useful proteins that contribute to hemostasis and the antimicrobial defense. Furthermore, plasma exchange can cause paradoxical thrombosis secondary to an increase in the synthesis of acute phase reactant proteins.[43] For these reasons, methods have been developed which selectively target xenogeneic antibodies for removal or inactivation.

Donor organ perfusion is more selective than plasmapheresis in removing natural antibodies directed against αGal. This technique involves connecting a vascularized organ from the prospective donor (e.g. a swine liver) to the recipient's (e.g. baboon) circulatory system through catheters that connect the organ with the recipient's circulating blood volume (Figure 7). During this process, the recipient's xenogeneic antibodies are absorbed out of the recipient's circulation and onto the vascular endothelium of the donor organ, which is discarded. A second organ from the donor swine (e.g. a heart) is then transplanted into the antibody-depleted recipient baboon. Cooper et al[40] used porcine kidneys to absorb out natural antibody in baboon recipients which subsequently received pig hearts. Survival of the cardiac xenografts was prolonged from 3 hours in untreated controls to 4–5 days in the group treated with donor organ perfusion.

Extracorporeal immunoadsorption makes use of synthetic immunoaffinity columns containing αGal oligosaccharides (Figure 8, see color plates section, back of book). When placed inline with the recipient's circulation, these highly specific immunoaffinity columns deplete only those anti-swine antibodies that are detrimental to the transplant.[41,44] Unfortunately, like donor organ perfusion, extracorporeal immunoadsorption is unable to prevent the return of the anti-αGal antibodies. Indeed, even with adjunctive therapy (i.e. pharmacologic immunosuppression and splenectomy) the reduction in natural antibody is always transient and is sometimes followed by a rebound within several days to levels of antibody higher than that observed at baseline.[31] Interestingly, in some clinical situations, the return of an anti-

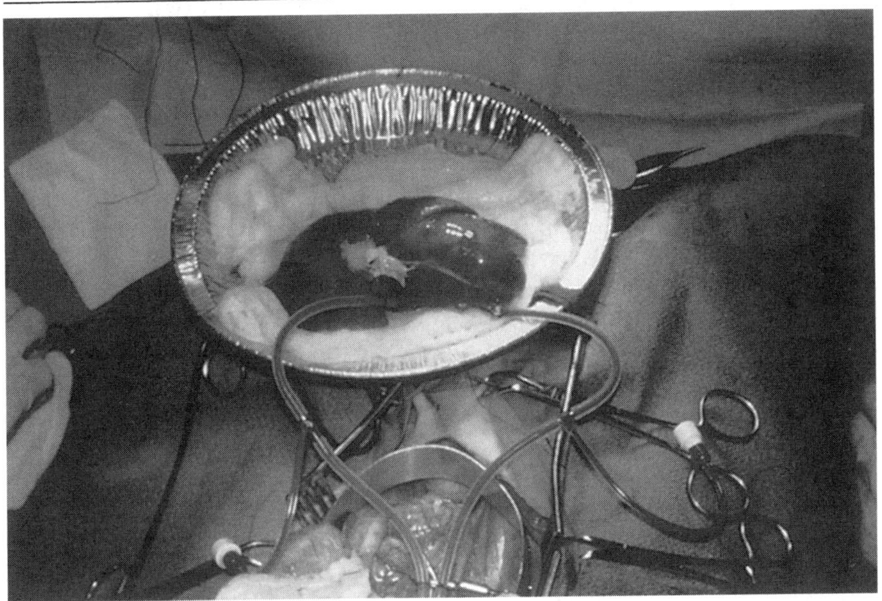

Figure 7. An isolated pig liver being perfused with baboon blood to adsorb the baboon's anti-αGal antibodies. The inflow to the pig liver is via a cannula from the femoral artery of the baboon. The outflow from the liver returns to the inferior vena cava of the baboon, thus completing the circuit without mechanical assistance.

body depleted by immunoadsorption is not always detrimental. For instance, when a transplant recipient is depleted of anti-ABO blood group antibodies and subsequently receives an ABO-incompatible organ, long-term survival of the transplanted organ can be achieved even after the return of antibody directed against the target blood group epitopes on the donor organ. The mechanism underlying this phenomenon, initially described by Guy Alexandre[45,46] and later coined "accommodation" by Bach et al,[12,47,48] is unknown and its relevance to hyperacute rejection and discordant xenografts is unclear at present.

Another experimental approach involves treating the recipient with the continuous intravenous infusion of synthetic or natural αGal oligosaccharides in order to inhibit natural antibody.[49] The infused oligosaccharides are bound by circulating anti-αGal antibodies which are no longer free to attack a subsequently transplanted organ. The infused sugar is, however, rapidly excreted making this tactic limited by the difficulty and expense of synthesizing large quantities of oligosaccharides. This problem may be solved by new enzymatic methods to produce the relevant oligosaccharides.[49] An alternative to the use of αGal oligosaccharides, either in immunoaffinity columns or as intravenous infusions, are murine-derived anti-idiotypic antibodies.[50,51] Initial studies with these murine antibodies directed against human anti-pig antibodies have shown them to be effective in temporarily inhibiting circulating anti-αGal antibodies in baboons.[51] In summary, the ideal technique to remove or inactivate preformed natural xenogeneic antibodies and prevent their return without jeopardizing the baseline immunologic properties of circulating non-xenogenic antibodies has not been achieved. More recent efforts to impact natural antibody have concentrated on attempts to eliminate or tolerize the B cells that produce the αGal antibodies.[52]

Suppression of Host Complement Activation

Attempts to control complement activation in the host have made use of systemic treatment with either purified cobra venom factor or soluble complement receptor type 1 (sCR1). By activating C3b, purified cobra venom factor is very effective in depleting complement and temporarily protecting a discordant xenograft from hyperacute rejection.[53,54] However, even concomitant pharmocologic immunosuppression, treatment with cobra venom factor typically delays rejection by only a matter of days. Within a week, xenografts usually develop the histopathological features of delayed xenograft rejection and fail. The longest survival of a pig organ in a nonhuman primate treated with cobra venom factor has been 27 days.[55]

Soluble complement receptor type 1 is also effective in suppressing complement activation and prolonging the survival of discordant xenografts.[56,57] The sCR1 molecule is a soluble form of the human complement receptor 1[58] which is found on most lymphohematopoietic cells. Complement receptor 1 controls complement activation by accelerating the dissociation of the classical pathway C3 and C5 convertases. Discordant xenografts have survived for more than three weeks in recipients treated with sCR1. Like purified cobra venom factor, the protection afforded the xenograft by sCR1 is temporary.

Genetically Engineered Donor Swine

Perhaps the most significant advances in providing long-term suppression of complement activation have been achieved through the use of genetically engineered swine. Using microinjection techniques (Figure 9, see color plates section, back of book), transgenic swine have been created which express human complement regulatory proteins on their vascular endothelium.[59,60] Since these regulatory proteins are species-specific, functioning effectively only with the complement proteins of their own species, it was hypothesized that organs from swine which express human regulatory proteins would successfully inhibit the activation of human complement.

The concept of expressing human inhibitors of complement in the pig originated with Dalmasso and colleagues[32] and was based on earlier work by Medof et al.[61] When human decay accelerating factor (hDAF or CD55) was incorporated into porcine endothelial cells in vitro, it rendered the pig endothelial cells resistant to cytotoxicity mediated by human complement in a dose-dependent fashion. Of note, the level of functional hDAF expressed on pig endothelial cells that was required to abrogate hyperacute rejection was much higher than that normally present on human endothelial cells.[62,63] However, exactly how much higher the levels of hDAF must be to prevent hyperacute rejection is unclear.

White and colleagues[59,64] have successfully bred transgenic swine that express hDAF on their vascular endothelium. When hearts from these hDAF pigs were heterotopically transplanted into non-immunosuppressed cynomolgus monkeys, hyper-

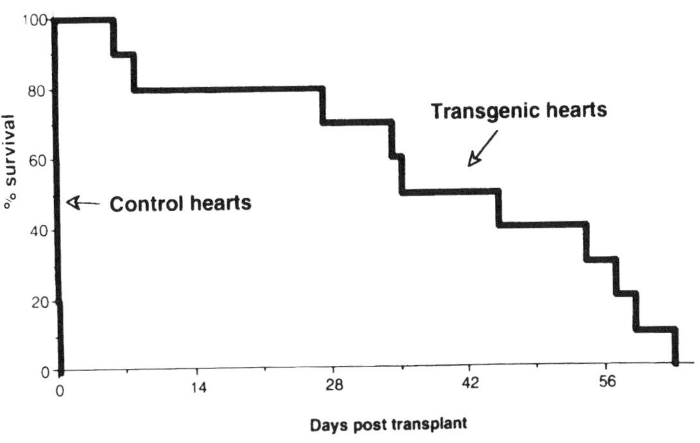

Figure 10. Survival of hearts from hDAF transgenic swine (n = 10, median survival = 40 days) and normal controls (n = 5, median survival = 55 minutes) transplanted heterotopically into immunosuppressed cynomolgus monkeys. Reproduced with permission from "Effect of Transgenic Expression of Human Decay-Accelerating on the inhibition of Hyperacute Rejection of Pig Organs". E. Cozzi, N. Yannoutos, G.A. Langford, G. Pino-Chavez, J. Wallwork, D.J.G. White, in *XENOTRANSPLANTATION: The Transplantation of Organs and Tissues between Species.* D.K.C. Cooper, E. Kemp, J.L. Platt, D.J.G. White, eds, Springer-Verlag, Heidelberg, 1997.

acute rejection was successfully avoided. The hDAF hearts survived for up to 5 days (range 97–126 hours) while control hearts from non-transgenic pigs survived for an average of 1.6 days (range 0.4–101 hours).[65] Adding cyclosporine, cyclophosphamide, and methlyprednisolone extended hDAF heterotopic cardiac xenograft survival to a median of 40 days (Figure 10).[65] More recently, White and colleagues demonstrated that hearts from hDAF transgenic pigs transplanted orthotopically into immunosuppressed baboons were capable of maintaining an adequate cardiac output for nine days.[66]

Transgenic swine have also been created which express CD59.[67] When hearts from CD59 transgenic pigs were transplanted into baboons, there was diminished complement activation as demonstrated by the markedly reduced deposition of the membrane attack complex.[67] Orthotopic transplantation of CD59-expressing pig hearts into baboons treated with plasmapheresis, steroids, and cyclosporine resulted in up to 2 week survival compared to the 24 to 30 hour survival of nonengineered control hearts.[68] Recently, transgenic swine have been produced which express both hDAF and human CD59 proteins on their vascular endothelium. Early results suggest that the survival times of hearts from these double transgenic swine do not exceed the survival times of hDAF-expressing hearts.[69] However, organ-specific expression of the transgenes in the double transgenic animals was less than that observed in human tissue and, therefore, improved results might be observed with better expression of the two transgenes.[33]

A second approach to genetic engineering donor swine is competitive glycosylation, which involves inserting a gene which competes with or masks the αGal epitope with an overabundance of another oligosaccharide epitope.[70,71] For instance, Sandrin and colleagues have transferred the α1,2 fucosyltransferase (or

H-transferase) gene, which humans use to form the blood group O antigen, into mice[72] and swine.[73] In vitro experiments confirmed that by competing more successfully for substrate than the galactosyltransferase enzyme, transfer of the H-transferase gene reduced the expression of αGal to a remarkable degree (<5% of its original expression).[72,73] However, it is unclear at present what percentage of αGal expression must be eliminated before hyperacute rejection is completely prevented.

A third approach would be to eliminate or "knock out" the gene that encodes for the galactosyltransferase enzyme. These knockout animals would be deficient in αGal epitopes, theoretically leaving no target for human anti-αGal antibodies.[74] Although knock-out animals lacking the galactosyltransferase enzyme have been produced in mice through homologous recombination,[75,76] this technology is not yet available in the pig due to the unavailability of porcine embryonic stem cells. Furthermore, some studies have suggested that eliminating the αGal epitope would expose underlying "cryptic" oligosaccharide determinants against which humans may also have preformed antibody.[77]

In summary, the most promising way of overcoming hyperacute rejection appears to involve a multifunctional approach aimed at modifying the donor organ by deleting the αGal epitope and adding one or more genes for human complement regulatory proteins in combination with treating the recipient to deplete or inhibit anti-αGal antibodies.[78]

DELAYED XENOGRAFT REJECTION

Using one or more of the methods described above, hyperacute rejection can now be prevented in discordant species combinations. Even so, a vigorous rejection still develops in these recipients days to weeks following transplantation. Histologically, this delayed rejection response is characterized by the same diffuse intravascular coagulation and lack of cellular infiltrate seen in hyperacute rejection (Figure 11, see color plates section, back of book). This immune response appears mediated by antibody which, like hyperacute rejection, targets the vascular endothelium. Less is known about this second type of xenogeneic rejection response than about hyperacute rejection. Indeed, while some refer to it as delayed xenograft rejection, others call it acute vascular rejection.

Type II Endothelial Cell Activation

The primary component in the pathophysiology of delayed xenograft rejection is endothelial cell activation, similar in many ways to hyperacute rejection. However, this activation does not appear to require complement and occurs more slowly, allowing time for new gene transcription and protein synthesis by the endothelium.[31] This delayed endothelial activation is referred to as type II activation.

The most important factor responsible for type II endothelial activation is antibody binding.[81] Like hyperacute rejection the principal antibody specificity, at least in the pig-to-primate combination, appears to be the αGal epitope; however, antibodies against other antigenic determinants may also play a role. In contrast to hyperacute rejection, IgG antibodies are as effective as IgM antibodies.[80] This has clinical implications as the level of IgG anti-αGal antibodies increases rapidly after exposure to pig tissue. In addition to antibody, there are cellular elements which can initiate type II endothelial cell activation through the elaboration of cytokines.[81] Most notable are monocytes and NK cells that activate endothelial cells through the production of TNFα and IFNγ, respectively.[82,83]

There are two predominant physiologic consequences of type II endothelial activation. One is the generation of a pro-coagulant state due to the loss of thrombomodulin and other regulators of thrombosis such as heparan sulfate.[84–86] Thrombomodulin normally binds thrombin and leads to the activation of protein C which has anticoagulant effects.[87] Down-regulation of endothelial thrombomodulin results in loss of these anticoagulant mechanisms. Heparan sulfate produces its antithrombotic effect by binding or complexing to antithrombin III and thereby interfering with thrombin activity. Loss of heparan sulfate from the endothelial cell surface results in loss of anticoagulant activity via antithrombin III inhibition of blood coagulation proteases and the induction of tissue factor activity (Figure 6).[35,87–89]

The other physiologic consequences of type II endothelial activation is the up-regulation of a large number of proinflammatory genes encoding molecules such as IL-1, E-Selectin, P-selectin, ICAM-I, and VCAM-1. In addition, the activated endothelial cells secrete IL-1, IL-6, and IL-8 as well as platelet-activating factor (PAF) and plasminogen activator inhibitor (PAI-1). IL-l is stimulatory to the endothelium and functions to activate monocytes. IL-8 is a chemoattractant for leukocytes and it also mimics some of the functions of C5a. PAF serves to activate neutrophils and platelets. Secretion of plasminogen activator inhibitor (PAI-1) inhibits the naturally occurring action of tissue plasminogen activator and results in a fall in the fibrinolytic activity on the endothelial cell surface. This provides the physiological basis for the pathologic findings of platelet aggregation and clot formation in delayed xenograft rejection (Figure 6). Of note, these events are thought to be in part, the consequence of an increase in transcriptional activity mediated by nuclear factor kappa B (NF-κB).[90–93]

PREVENTION OF DELAYED XENOGRAFT REJECTION

Due to the importance of antibody in delayed xenograft rejection, current therapies to control this immune response have been primarily directed against B cells. Treatment protocols have included cyclophosphamide, leflunomide, brequinar, 15-deoxyspergualin, and methotrexate.[31] The longest graft survival in a pig-to-primate model has been achieved using cyclophosphamide in addition to complement inhibition and anti-T cell therapy.[94] Using this regimen, hearts survived for 6 to 8 weeks without evidence of delayed xenograft rejection.[94] However, the high doses of cyclophosphamide required to obtain these results are not without substantial toxicity and mortality.

NF-κB and the Role of "Protective Genes"

Given the large number of proinflammatory genes that are up-regulated in type II endothelial activation as a consequence of the transcriptional factor NF-κB,[90–92,95]

Bach and colleagues[33] have suggested that targeting NF-κB for inhibition would be an ideal way to prevent delayed xenograft rejection. NF-κB is present in the cytoplasm of quiescent endothelial cells and is associated with an inhibitory protein, IkBα.[96,97] Upon type II endothelial activation, IkBα is degraded, which releases and activates NF-κB.[98–100] NF-κB is then translocated to the nucleus where it binds to the targeted DNA sequence and activates transcription of various proinflammatory and prothombotic genes.

In studying ways of inhibiting NF-κB, Ferran and colleagues[101] have investigated the role of anti-apoptotic genes in endothelial cells. Three genes, A20, bcl-2 and bcl-xl, not only prevented apoptosis but were also effective at blocking the up-regulation of NF-κB. The expression of these "protective" genes in endothelial cells blocked the up-regulation of the pro-inflammatory genes in vitro.[33] Further evidence that these particular genes exert a protective influence come from a hamster-to-rat cardiac xenograft model wherein recipients were treated with daily cobra venom factor and cyclosporine. All the surviving xenografts expressed the three anti-apoptotic genes in their endothelium, whereas the endothelium from hearts that were rejected did not.[102]

Based on these results, Bach and colleagues have suggested that genetic modifications of donor animals by the transgenic expression of protective genes that inhibit NF-κB and prevent apoptosis might be used to diminish type II endothelial activation.[103,104] Another genetic engineering approach to the prevention of delayed xenograft rejection would be overexpression of antithrombotic molecules on the surface of resting endothelium (i.e. thrombomodulin) of the donor so that these antithrombotic molecules would not be lost during the initial phase of endothelial cell activation.[33,36,86]

THE ROLE OF TOLERANCE INDUCTION STRATEGIES

Once hyperacute and delayed xenograft rejection can be prevented effectively, the next major obstacle to successful xenotransplantation is that of the cellular immune responses to xenografts. Cell-mediated immune responses to xenografts are stronger than the comparable responses observed in allografts since the antigenic disparity between discordant xenogeneic species is far greater than that between allogeneic individuals. For this reason, the success of clinical xenotransplantation will likely depend on developing ways to induce immunological tolerance to pig antigens in the recipient.[31] One promising means of inducing tolerance across a xenogeneic barrier is by establishing "mixed chimerism" in the host through the infusion of donor bone marrow at the time of organ transplantation (see Chapter 7). As opposed to bone marrow infusion for hematopoietic malignancies where 100% chimerism is desired and achieved by the ablation of the host hematopoietic system by lethal irradiation, in solid organ transplantation tolerance, complete chimerism is neither necessary nor desirable. Mixed chimeras possess bone marrow precursor cells of both host and donor origin.[105,106] Both types of mature T-cell populations develop in the host, and are restricted through positive selection in the thymus to the recognition of host MHC plus peptides of foreign antigens (MHC + X). Thus mixed chimeras are both immunocompetent and tolerant to both self and donor MHC.

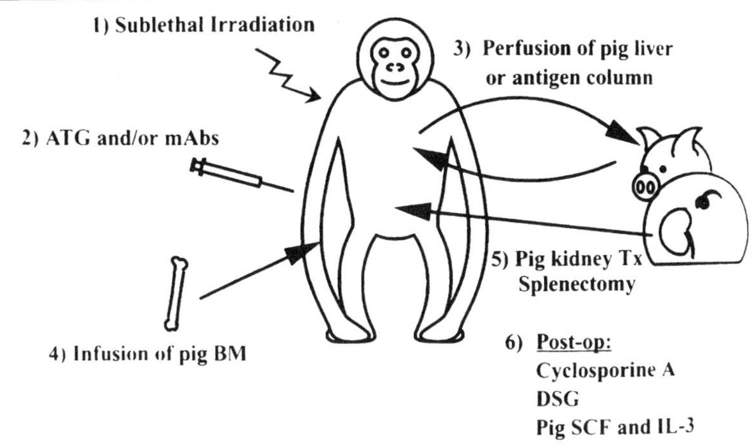

Figure 12. Protocol for xenogeneic tolerance induction through mixed chimerism. Natural antibody is depleted through the absorption of the anti-αGal antibody on a solid matrix column that bears the α1,3Gal sugar moiety. The early preparative regimen of lethal irradiation used to "make space" for the donor bone marrow has been supplanted by a less toxic nonmyeloablative regimen. Antithymocyte globulin (ATG) and/or anti-T cell monoclonal antibodies are used to remove mature T cells from the recipient. Cyclosporine is added to immunosuppress any residual T cells in the posttransplant period. On day 0, the recipient receives bone marrow (5×10^8 cells/kg) and a kidney transplant from the same donor miniature swine. Splenectomy is performed and 15-deoxyspergulin is added to diminish antibody responses. Recombinant cytokines (SCF and IL-3) are administered for 2 weeks after the preparative regimen to aid engraftment of the pig bone marrow.[26,31] Mixed chimeras possess bone marrow precursor cells of both host and donor origin.[105,106] Both types of mature T-cell populations develop in the host, and are restricted through positive selection in the thymus to the recognition of host MHC plus peptides of foreign antigens (MHC + X). Thus mixed chimeras are both immunocompetent and tolerant to both self and donor MHC.

Sachs and colleagues have investigated this strategy in the pig-to-nonhuman primate model (Figure 12).[107,108] The early preparative regimen of lethal irradiation used to "make space" for the donor marrow has been supplanted by less toxic non-myeloablative methods. One such regimen that has been successfully employed involves depleting mature host T-cells by using monoclonal antibodies against CD4 and CD8 cells. A boost of thymic irradiation of 700R was added to the regimen because depletion of T-cells with monoclonal antibodies against CD4 and CD8 was not as efficient in the thymus as in the periphery.[109]

An alternative protocol that has also been evaluated consists of a preparative regimen of sub-lethal whole body irradiation in three fractions of 1.0 Gy on days −6, −5, and along with 7.0 Gy of thymic irradiation on day −1. Splenectomy to avoid antibody responses[110,111] ATG (Upjohn) on days −2, −1, and 0 (50 mg/kg iv), followed by cyclosporine (15 mg/kg /day iv) to further suppress T cell function in the immediate post-operative period, was also a part of the protocol (Figure 12). On day 0, the recipient primates received a kidney transplant and bone marrow (5×10^8 cells/kg) harvested from the same donor miniature swine. In these experiments, the avoidance of hyperacute rejection was possible through the absorption of the anti-αGal antibody on a solid matrix column which bears the α1,3 Gal sugar moiety (Figure 8).[26,107,112,113] Using this regimen, the investigators were able to avoid hyperacute rejection in more than 20 pig-to-primate xenotransplants.[37] Invariably, however, there was return of the antibodies within 7–15 days coinciding with loss of the graft by delayed xenograft rejection. Nevertheless, it is encouraging to note that during the period between transplantation and graft loss, the pig kidney was able to maintain normal BUN, creatinine, and electrolyte balance suggesting that once the immunologic hurdles have been overcome.

The survival of pig bone marrow-derived cells in primates to achieve a satisfactory level of mixed chimerism seems to require species-specific growth factor.[46,114] Sachs and colleagues have recently demonstrated that administration of pig recombinant cytokines (SCF and IL-3) to primates for 2 weeks after the preparative regimen, enabled the survival of pig bone marrow cells for more than 6 months.

The benefits of achieving immunologic tolerance to xenografts have far reaching implications. One of the major advantages of successful application of this strategy would be the avoidance of long term immunosuppression. Loss of transplanted organs from chronic rejection would not be a significant factor, since the grafted organ would, presumably, escape the persistent immunologic bombardment implicated in chronic rejection.[115]

SUMMARY

Within a relatively short time-span, a significant number of barriers to xenotransplantation have been identified and potential solutions generated. Attempts to overcome the barriers of hyperacute and delayed xenograft rejection have included modification of the recipient by depleting or inhibiting natural antibody and complement, and modification of the donor by genetically engineering changes in the expression of relevant endothelial antigens. Attempts to overcome the barriers of cellular rejection and chronic rejection have included the induction of tolerance through bone marrow transplantation and the creation of mixed chimerism. However, there are still other issues pertinent to xenotransplantation which where not covered in this review such as 1) potential biochemical and physiologic differences between donor and recipient, 2) potential transmission of zoonoses and retrovirus transmission, and 3) ethical controversies. These issues are discussed in several excellent reviews.[31,78,116,117,119]

The diversity of the biological pathways involved in xenograft rejection make it highly likely that the clinical application of xenotransplantation will require an interdisciplinary approach that would include natural antibody depletion, gene therapy, transgenic technology, and tolerance induction. The hope is that with collaboration the barriers to xenograft survival will be overcome in the not too distant future.

ACKNOWLEDGEMENTS

The authors thank Dr. David K. C. Cooper for his critique and invaluable comments and Mrs. Laurie Neiderer for her expert assistance in the preparation of this manuscript.

REFERENCES

1. Reported deaths on the OPTN waiting List from 1988 through 1996. United Network for Organ Sharing. 1997.
2. Reemtsma K, McCracken BH, Schlegel JV, Pearl M. Heterotransplantation of the kidney: two clinical experiences. Science 1964;143:700.
3. Hardy JD, Chavez CM, Kurrus FD, et al. Heart transplantation in man. JAMA 1964;188:1132.
4. Beecher H, Adams RD, Barger AC, et al. A definition of reversible coma. JAMA 1968;205:85.
5. Bailey LL, Nehlsen-Cannarella WSL, Concepcion W, Jolley WB. Baboon-to-human cardiac xenotransplantation in a neonate. JAMA 1985;254:3321.
6. Makowka L, Cramer DV, Hoffman A, et al. The use of a pig liver xenograft for temporary support of a patient with fulminant hepatic failure. Transplantation 1995;59:1654.
7. Groth CG, Korsgren O, Wennberg L, et al. Xenoislet rejection following pig-to-rat, pig-to-primate, and pig-to-man transplantation. Transplant Proc 1996;28:538.
8. Ildstad ST. Xenotransplantation for AIDS. Lancet 1996;347:761.
9. Deacon T, Schumacher J, Dinsmore J, et al. Histological evidence of fetal pig neural cell survival after transplantation into a patient with Parkinson's disease. Nature Medicine 1997;3:350.
10. Calne RY. Organ transplantation between widely disparate species. Transplant Proc 1970;2:550.
11. Perper RJ, Najarian JS. Experimental renal heterotransplantation. I. In widely divergent species. Transplantation 1966;4:377.
12. Good AH, Cooper DKC, Malcolm AJ, et al. Identification of carbohydrate structures that bind human antiporcine antibodies: implications for discordant xenografting in humans. Transplant Proc 1992;24:559.
13. Cooper DKC, Good AH, Koren E, et al. Identification of alpha-galactosyl and other carbohydrate epitopes that are bound by human anti-pig antibodies: relevance to discordant xenografting in man. Transplant Immunology 1993;1:198.
14. Galili U, Macher BA, Buehler J, Shohet SB. Human natural anti-a-galactosyl IgG. II. The specific recognition of α(1–3) linked galactose residues. J Exp Med 1985;162:573.
15. Galili U, Rachmilewitz EA, Peleg A, Flechner I. A unique natural human IgG antibody with anti-alpha-galactosyl specificity. J Exp Med 1984;160:1519.
16. Galili U, Mandrell RE, Hamadeh RM, Shohet SB, Griffiss JM. The interaction between the human natural anti-agalactosyl IgG (anti-Gal) and bacteria of the human flora. Infectious Immunology 1988;57:1730.
17. Rother RP, Fodor WL, Springhorn JP, et al. A novel mechanism of retrovirus inactivation in human serum mediated by anti-alpha-galactosyl natural antibody. J Exp Med 1995;182:1345.
18. Parker W, Bruno D, Holzknecht ZE, Platt JL. Characterization and affinity isolation of xenoreactive human natural antibodies. J Immunol 1994;153:3791.
19. Sandrin MS, Vaughan HA, Dabkowski PL, McKenzie IF. Anti-pig IgM antibodies in human serum react predominantly with Gal(alpha 1–3)Gal epitopes. Proc Natl Acad Sci U S A 1993;90:11391.
20. Galili U, Tibell A, Samuelsson B, Rydberg L, Groth CG. Increased anti-Gal activity in diabetic patients transplanted with porcine islet cells. Transplant Proc 1996;28:564.
21. Michler RE, Shah AS, Itescu S, et al. The influence of concordant xenografts on the humoral and cell-mediated immune responses to subsequent allografts in primates. Journal of Thoracic and Cardiovascular Surgery 1996;112:1002.
22. Bartholomew A, Latinne D, Sachs DH, et al. Utility of xenografts: Lack of correlation between PRA and natural antibodies to swine. Xenotransplantation 1997;4:34.
23. Miyagawa S, Hirose H, Shirakura R, et al. The mechanism of discordant xenograft rejection. Transplantation 1988;46:825.
24. Gambiez L, Weill BJ, Chereau C, Calmus Y, Houssin D. The hyperacute rejection of guinea pig to rat heart xenografts is mediated by preformed IgM. Transplant Proc 1990;22:1058.
25. Johnston PS, Wang MW, Lim SML, Wright LJ, White DJG. Discordant xenograft rejection in an antibody-free model. Transplantation 1992;54:573.
26. Sablinski T, Latinne D, Gianello P, et al. Xenotransplantation of pig kidneys to nonhuman primates: I. Development of the model. Xenotransplantation 1995;2:264.
27. Dalmasso AP, Vercelolotti GM, Fischel RJ, Bolman RM, Bach FH, Platt JL. Mechanism of complement activation in the hyperacute rejection of porcine organs transplanted into primate recipients. Am J Pathol 1992;140:1157.
28. Müller-Eberhard HJ. Complement: chemistry and pathways. In: Inflammation. Basic Principles and Clinical Correlates, Gallin JI, Goldstein IM, Snyderman R, eds. New York, Raven Press, 1992;33.
29. Frank MM. Complement system. In: Samter's Immunological Diseases, Frank MM, Austen KF, Claman HN, Unanue ER, eds. Boston, Little, Brown and Co., 1995;331.

30. Abbas AK, Lichtman AH, Pober JS. The complement system. In: Cellular and Molecular Immunology, Abbas AK, Lichtman AH, Pober JS, eds. Philadelphia, W.B. Saunders Co., 1994;225.
31. Auchincloss H, Sachs DH. Xenogeneic Transplantation. Annu Rev Immunol 1998;16:433.
32. Dalmasso AP, Vercelolotti GM, Platt JL, Bach FH. Inhibition of complement-mediated endothelial cell cytotoxicity by decay-accelerating factor: Potential for prevention of xenograft hyperacute rejection. Transplantation 1991;52:530.
33. Bach FH. Xenotransplantation: Problems and prospects. Annual Reviews of Medicine 1998;49:301.
34. Saadi S, Platt JL. Transient peturbation of endothelial integrity induced by natural antibodies and complement. J Exp Med 1995;181:21.
35. Platt JL, Vercelolotti GM, Lindman BJ, Oegema TR, Jr., Bach FH, Dalmasso AP. Release of heparan sulphate from endothelial cells: Implications for pathogenesis of hyperacute rejection. J Exp Med 1990;171:1363.
36. Parker W, Saadi S, Lin SS, Holzknecht ZE, Bustos M, Platt JL. Transplantation of discordant xenografts: a challenge revisited. Immunology Today 1996;17:373.
37. Alexandre GPJ, Gianello P, Latinne D, et al. Plasmapheresis and splenectomy in experimental renal xenotransplantation. In: Xenograft 25, Hardy MA, ed. New York, Excerpta Medica, 1989;259.
38. Rydberg L, Hallberg E, Samuelsson B, et al. Studies on the removal of anti-pig xenoantibodies in the human by plasmapheresis/immunoadsorption. Xenotransplantation 1995;2:253.
39. Gannedahl G, Tufveson G, Sundberg B, Groth CG. The effect of plasmapheresis and deoxyspergualin or cyclophosphamide treatment on an anti-porcine Gal-a(1–3)-Gal antibody levels in humans. Xenotransplantation 1996;3:166.
40. Cooper DKC, Human PA, Lexer G, et al. Effects of cyclosporine and antibody adsorption on pig cardiac xenograft survival in the baboon. Journal of Heart Transplantation 1988;7:238.
41. Taniguchi S, Neethling FA, Korchagina EY, et al. In vivo immunoadsorption of anti-pig antibodies in baboons using a specific Galα1-3Gal column. Transplantation 1996;62:1379.
42. Kooyman DL, McClellan SB, Parker W, et al. Identification and characterization of a galactosyl peptide mimetic. Implications for use in removing xenoreactive anti-α Gal antibodies. Transplantation 1996;61:851.
43. Platt JL. Therapeutic strategies for hyperacute xenograft rejection. In: Hyperacute Xenograft Rejection, Platt JL, ed. Austin, R.J. Landes Co., 1995;161.
44. Cooper DKC, Cairns TDH, Taube DH. Extracorporeal immunoadsorption of anti-pig antibody in baboons using αGal oligosaccharide immunoaffinity columns. Xeno 1996;4:27.
45. Alexandre GPJ, Squifflet JP. Significance of the ABO antigen system. In: Organ Transplantation and Replacement, Cerilli GJ, ed. Philadelphia, J.B. Lippincott, 1988;223.
46. Alexandre GPJ, Squifflet JP, deBruyere M, et al. Present experiences in a series of 26 ABO-incompatible living donor renal allografts. Transplant Proc 1987;19:4538.
47. Platt JL, Vercelolotti GM, Dalmasso AP, et al. Transplantation of discordant xenografts: A review of progress. Immunology Today 1990;11:450.
48. Bach FH, Turman MA, Vercelolotti GM, Platt JL, Dalmasso AP. Accommodation: a working paradigm for progressing toward clinical discordant xenografting. Transplant Proc 1991;23:205.
49. Simon PM, Neethling FA, Taniguchi S, et al. Intravenous infusion of Galα1-3Gal oligosaccharides in baboons delays hyperacute rejection of porcine heart xenografts. Transplantation 1998;65:346.
50. Koren E, Milotec F, Neethling FA, et al. Murine monoclonal anti-idiotypic antibodies directed against human anti-αGal antibodies prevent rejection of pig cells in culture: implications for pig-to-human organ xenotransplantation. Transplant Proc 1996;28:559.
51. Koren E, Milotec F, Neethling FA, et al. Monoclonal anti-idiotypic antibodies neutralizes cytotoxic effects of anti-αGal antibodies. Transplantation 1996;62:837.
52. Yang YG, deGoma E, Ohdan H, et al. Tolerization of anti-Galalpha1-3Gal natural antibody-forming B cells by induction of mixed chimerism. J Exp Med 1998;187:1335.
53. Leventhal JR, Dalmasso AP, Cromwell JW, et al. Prolongation of cardiac xenograft survival by depletion of complement. Transplantation 1993;55:857.
54. Candinas D, Lesnikoski BA, Robson SC, et al. Effect of repetitive high-dose treatment with soluble complement receptor type 1 and cobra venom factor on discordant xenograft survival. Transplantation 1996;62:336.
55. Kobayashi T, Taniguchi S, Ye Y, et al. Delayed xenograft rejection in C3-depleted discordant (pig-to-baboon) cardiac xenografts treated with cobra venom factor. Transplant Proc 1996;28:560.
56. Pruitt SK, Baldwin WD, Marsh Jr HC, Linn SS, Yeh CG, Bollinger RR. The effect of soluble complement receptor type 1 on hyperacute xenograft rejection. Transplantation 1991;52:868.
57. Pruitt SK, Kirk AD, Bollinger RR, et al. The effect of soluble complement receptor type 1 on hyperacute rejection of porcine xenografts. Transplantation 1994;57:363.
58. Weisman HF, Bartow T, Leppo MK, et al. Soluble human complement receptor type 1: *in vivo* inhibitor of complement suppressing post-ischemic myocardial inflammation and necrosis. Science 1990;249:146.

59. Cozzi E, White DJG. The generation of transgenic pigs as potential organs donors for humans. Nature Medicine 1995;1:964.
60. McCurry KR, Kooyman DL, Alvarado CG, et al. Human complement regulatory proteins protect swine-to-primate cardiac xenografts from humoral injury. Nature Medicine 1995;1:423.
61. Medof ME, Kinoshita T, Nussenzweig V. Inhibition of complement activation on the surface of cells after incorporation of decay-accelerating factor (DAF) into their membranes. J Exp Med 1984;160:1558.
62. Rosengard AM, Cary NRB, Langford GA, Tucker AW, Wallwork J, White DJG. Tissue expression of human complement inhibitor, decay-accelerating factor, in transgenic pigs. Transplantation 1995;59:1325.
63. Cozzi E, Tucker AW, Langford GA, et al. Characterization of pigs transgenic for human decay-accelerating factor. Transplantation 1997;64:1383.
64. Schmoeckel M, Nollert G, Shahmohammadi M, et al. Prevention of hyperacute rejection by human decay accelerating factor in xenogeneic perfused working hearts. Transplantation 1996;62:729.
65. Cozzi E, Yannoutsos N, Langford GA, Pinto-Chavez G, Wallwork J, White DJG. Effect of transgenic expression of human decay-accelerating factor on the inhibition of hyperacute rejection of pig organs. In: Xenotransplantation, Cooper DKC, Kemp E, Platt JL, White DJG, eds. Heidelberg, Springer-Verlag, 1997;665.
66. Schmoeckel M, Bhatti FNK, Zaidi A, et al. Orthotopic heart transplantation in a transgenic pig-to-primate model. Transplantation 1998;65:1570.
67. Diamond LE, McCurry KR, Martin MJ, et al. Characterization of transgenic pigs expressing functionally active human CD59 on cardiac endothelium. Transplantation 1996;61:1241.
68. Squinto SP. Genetically modified animal organs for human transplantation. World Journal of Surgery 1997;21:939.
69. Byrne GW, McCurry KR, Martin MJ, McClellan SM, Platt JL, Logan JS. Transgenic pigs expressing human CD59 and decay-accelerating factor produce an intrinsic barrier to complement-mediated damage. Transplantation 1997;63:149.
70. Sandrin MS, Fodor WL, Mouhtouris E, et al. Enzymatic remodeling of the carbohydrate surface of a xenogeneic cell substantially reduces human antibody binding and complement-mediated cytolysis. Nature Medicine 1995;1:1261–1267.
71. Sandrin MS, Fodor WL, Cohney S, et al. Reduction of the major porcine xenoantigen Galα (1,3)Gal by expression of α (1,2) fucosyltransferase. Xenotransplantation 1996;3:134.
72. Chen C, Fisicaro N, Shinkel TA, et al. Reduction in Gal-α1,3-Gal epitope expression in transgenic mice expressing human H-transferase. Xenotransplantation 1996;3:69.
73. Koike C, Kannagi R, Takuma Y, et al. Introduction of α (1,2)-fucosyltransferase and its effect on αGal epitopes in transgenic pig. Xenotransplantation 1996;3:81.
74. Cooper DKC, Koren E, Oriol R. Genetically-engineered pigs. Lancet 1993;342:682.
75. Thall AD, Murphy HS, Lowe JB. α1,3-Galactosyltransferase-deficient mice produce naturally occurring cytotoxic anti-Gal antibodies. Transplant Proc 1996;28:556.
76. Tearle RG, Tange MJ, Zanettino ZL, et al. The α1,3-galactosyltransferase knock-out mouse. Implications for xenotransplantation. Transplantation 1996;61:13.
77. McKenzie IF, Cohney S, Vaughan HA, et al. Overcoming the anti-αGal(1–3)Gal reaction in xenotransplantation. Xenotransplantation 1995;3:86.
78. Cooper DKC. Xenoantigens and xenoantibodies. Xenotransplantation 1998;5:6.
79. Hasan R, Van den Bogaerde JB, Wallwork J, White DJG. Evidence that long-term survival of concordant xenografts is achieved by inhibition of antispecies antibody production. Transplantation 1992;54:408.
80. Minanov OP, Itescu S, Neethling FA, et al. Anti-Gal IgG antibodies in sera of newborn humans and baboons and its significance in pig xenotransplantation. Transplantation 1997;63:182.
81. Goodman DJ, Millan M, Ferran C, Bach FH. Mechanism of delayed xenograft rejection. In: Xenotransplantation: The transplantation of organs and tissues between species, Cooper DKC, Kemp E, Platt JL, White DJG, eds. Heidelberg, Springer, 1997;77.
82. Blakely ML, Van der Werf WJ, Berndt MC, Dalmasso AP, Bach FH, Hancock WW. Activation of intragraft endothelial and mononuclear cells during discordant xenograft rejection. Transplantation 1994;58:1059.
83. Robertson MJ, Ritz J. Role of IL-2 receptors in NK cell activation and proliferation. In: NK Cell-Mediated Cytotoxicity: Receptors, Signaling and Mechanism, Lotzova E, Herberman RB, eds. Boca Raton, CRC Press, 1992;183.
84. Robson SC, Siegel JB, Lesnikoski BA, et al. Aggregation of human platelets induced by porcine endothelial cells is dependent upon both activation of complement and thrombin generation. Xenotransplantation 1996;3:24.
85. Robson SC, Kaczmarek E, Siegel JB, et al. Loss of ATP diphosphohydrolase activity with endothelial cell activation. J Exp Med 1997;185:153.

86. Bach FH. Genetic engineering as an approach to xenotransplantation. World Journal of Surgery 1997;21:913.
87. Esmon CT. Cell mediated events that control blood coagulation and vascular injury. Annual Review of Cell Biology 1993;9:1.
88. Balla G, Jacob HS, Balla J, et al. Ferritin: A cytoprotective antioxidant stratagem of endothelium. Journal of Biological Chemistry 1992;267:18148.
89. Platt JL, Dalmasso AP, Lindman BJ, Ihrcke NS, Bach FH. The role of C_{5a} and antibody in the release of heparan sulfate from endothelial cells. Eur J Immunol 1991;21:2287.
90. Whelan J, Ghersa P, van Huijsduijnen RH, et al. An NFkB-like factor is essential but not sufficient for cytokine induction of endothelial leukocyte adhesion molecule 1 (ELAM-1) gene transcription. Nucleic Acids Research 1991;19:2645.
91. deMartin R, Vanhove B, Cheng Q, et al. Cytokine-inducible expression in endothelial cells of an IkBα-like gene is regulated by NFkB. EMBO Journal 1993;12:2773.
92. Cogswell JP, Godlevski MM, Wisely GB, et al. NF-kB regulates IL-1B transcription through a consensus NF-kB binding site and a nonconsensus CRE-like site. J Immunol 1994;153:712.
93 Millan MT, Geczy C, Stuhlmeier KM, Goodman DJ, Ferran C, Bach FH. Human monocytes activate porcine endothelial cells, resulting in increased E-selectin, interleukin-8, monocyte chemotactic protein-1, and plasminogen activator inhibitor-type-1 expression. Transplantation 1997;63:421.
94. Waterworth PD, Cozzi E, Tolan MJ, Langford G, Braidley P, Chavez G, Dunning J, Wallwork J, White D. Pig-to-primate cardiac xenotransplantation and cyclophosphamide therapy Transplant Proc 1997;29:899–900.
95. Voraberger G, Schäfer R, Stratowa C. Cloning of the human gene for intercellular adhesion molecule 1 and analysis of its 5′-regulatory region. J Immunol 1991;147:2777.
96. Siebenlist U, Franzoso G, Brown K. Structure, regulation and function of NF-kB. Annual Review of Cell Biology 1994;10:405.
97. Finco TS, Baldwin AS, Jr. Mechanistic aspects of NF-kB regulation: The emerging role of phosphorylation and proteolysis. Immunity 1995;3:263.
98. DiDonato J, Mercurio F, Rosette C, et al. Mapping of the inducible IkB phosphorylation sites that signal its ubiquitination and degradation. Molecular and Cellular Biology 1996;16:1295.
99. Beg AA, Finco TS, Nantermet PV, Baldwin AS, Jr. Tumor necrosis factor and interleukin-1 lead to phosphorylation and loss of IkBα: a mechanism for NF-kB activation. Molecular and Cellular Biology 1993;13:3301.
100. Henkle T, Machieldt T, Alkalay I, Krönke M, Ben-Nerial Y, Baeuerie PA. Rapid proteolysis of IkBα is necessary for activation of transcription factor NF-kB. Nature 1993;365:182.
101. Cooper JT, Stroka DM, Brostjian C, Palmetshofer A, Bach FH, Ferran C. A20 blocks endothelial cell activation through a NF-kappaB-dependent mechanism. Journal of Biological Chemistry 1996;271:18068.
102. Bach FH, Ferran C, Hechenleitner P, et al. Accommodation of vascularized xenografts: Expression of "protective genes" by donor endothelial cells in a host Th2 cytokine environment. Nature Medicine 1997;3:196.
103. Goodman DJ, von Albertini MA, McShea A, Wrighton CJ, Bach FH. Adenoviral-mediated overexpression of IkBα in endothelial cells inhibits natural killer cell-mediated endothelial cell activation. Transplantation 1996;62:967.
104. Stroka DM, Copper ML, Brostjian C, et al. Expression of a negative dominant mutant of human P55 tumor necrosis factor-receptor inhibits TNF and monocyte-induced activation in porcine aortic endothelial cells. Transplant Proc 1997;29:882.
105. Ildstad ST, Bluestone JA, Barbieri S, Sachs DH. Characterization of mixed allogeneic chimeras. Immunocompetence, in vitro reactivity, and genetic specificity of tolerance. J Exp Med 1985;162:231.
106. Sykes M, Sachs DH. Mixed allogeneic chimerism as an approach to transplantation tolerance. Immunology Today 1988;9:23.
107. Sachs DH, Sykes M, Greenstein J, Cosimi AB. Tolerance and xenograft survival. Nature Medicine 1995;969.
108. Sablinski T, Gianello PR, Bailin M, et al. Pig to monkey bone marrow and kidney xenotransplantation. Surgery 1997;121:381.
109. Sharabi Y, Sachs DH. Mixed chimerism and permanent specific transplantation tolerance induced by a nonlethal preparative regimen. J Exp Med 1989;169:493.
110. Xu Y, Lorf T, Sablinski T, et al. Removal of anti-porcine natural antibodies from human and nonhuman primate plasma in vitro and in vivo by a Galα1-3Galb1-4bGlc-X immunoaffinity column. Transplantation 1998;65:172.
111. Kozlowski T, Fuchimoto Y, Monroy R, et al. Apheresis and column absorption for specific removal of Gal-alpha-1,3 Gal natural antibodies in a pig-to-baboon model. Transplant Proc

1997;29:961.
112. Latinne D, Gianello P, Smith CV, et al. Xenotransplantation from pig to cynomolgus monkey: Approach toward tolerance induction. Transplant Proc 1993;25:336.
113. Tanaka M, Latinne D, Gianello P, et al. Xenotransplantation from pig to cynomolgus monkey: The potential for overcoming xenograft rejection through induction of chimerism. Transplant Proc 1994;26:1326.
114. Sachs DH, Sablinski T. Tolerance across discordant xenogeneic barriers. Xeno 1995;2:234.
115. Madsen JC, Yamada K, Allan JS, et al. Prevention of cardiac allograft vasculopathy across class I MHC disparities by the induction of transplantation tolerance. Transplantation 1998;65:304.
116. Platt JL. The immunological barriers to xenotransplantation. Critical Reviews in Immunology 1996;16:331.
117. Cooper DKC, Kemp E, Reemstsma K, White DJG, eds. Xeno-transplantation—The Transplantation of Organs Between Species. Berlin: Springer, 1997.
118. Atkinson JP, Oglesby TJ, White D, Adams EA, Liszewski MK. Separation of self from non-self in the complement system: a role for membrane cofactor protein and decay accelerating factor. Clin Exp Immunol 1991;86:27.
119. Lambrigts D, Sachs DH, Cooper DKC, Discordant organ xenotransplantation in primates: world experience and current status. Transplantation 1998;66:547.

Section 2. Clinical Assessment and Management of Cardiac Allograft Rejection

9. ENDOMYOCARDIAL BIOPSY DIAGNOSIS OF CARDIAC ALLOGRAFT REJECTION

Barbara Czerska, MD*, Mary E. Keohane, MD†, and Edward F. Philbin, MD**
*Section of Heart Failure and Cardiac Transplantation, Division of Cardiovascular Medicine, and †Department of Pathology, Henry Ford Health System, Detroit, MI, USA; Cardiovascular Division, Albany Medical Center, Albany, NY, USA

Sakakibara and Kono introduced a transvenous approach for endomyocardial biopsy in 1962 revolutionizing the utilization of this procedure.[1] Prior to this, myocardial samples were obtained using a transthoracic needle or during open heart surgery. More convenient access and the development of new bioptomes made endomyocardial biopsy safer and more widely used, becoming a valuable tool in the diagnosis of cardiac diseases.[2,3] It also introduced a working link between the pathologist and clinical cardiologist.[4,5]

Caves et al. at Stanford University were the first to use transvenous endomyocardial biopsy for the evaluation of allograft rejection.[6] With time, endomyocardial biopsy became the primary procedure for diagnosing cardiac rejection. The evolution of cardiac transplantation from an experimental procedure to an accepted form of therapy for end stage heart disease was facilitated by the development of new immunosuppressive agents and the availability of endomyocardial biopsy for clinical follow up of transplant recipients.[7]

The introduction of the immunosuppressive agent cyclosporine led to dramatic improvement in survival rates after cardiac transplantation, but also altered the clinical picture of acute allograft rejection.[7,8] In cyclosporine-treated patients, histologic evidence of acute rejection can be present before clinical signs or symptoms of allograft compromise. It has also been recognized that allograft failure can occur with a negative biopsy.[9] Though many noninvasive techniques have been examined and hold promise as useful diagnostic modalities,[10–14] the diagnosis of acute allograft rejection in cyclosporine-treated transplant recipients remains highly dependent on endomyocardial biopsy.

The interpretation of endomyocardial biopsy has become a crucial skill for physicians managing cardiac transplant patients. Indeed, cardiopathologists may find the interpretation of endomyocardial biopsies challenging in certain cases.[15] The introduction of new micromolecular techniques, immunohistochemistry, in situ tissue hybridization, and biopsy culture has brought new understanding of the normal and pathobiology of cardiac allografts.[15,16] Our growing knowledge has begotten more controversy regarding interpretation of biopsy findings.

PATHOLOGIC MANIFESTATIONS OF ACUTE ALLOGRAFT REJECTION

Cellular Infiltration

The histologic diagnosis of acute cellular rejection is based on the presence of lymphoid infiltrates within the myocardium. The grading of rejection is based on the location and extent of cellular infiltrates and accompanying myocyte and interstitial changes.

Focal perivascular and interstitial lymphoid infiltrates (Figure 1, see color plates section, back of book) or diffuse minimal interstitial lymphoid infiltrates (Figure 2, see color plates section, back of book) characterize mild rejection. There is no distortion or disruption of myocyte architecture.

Moderate rejection is characterized by interstitial lymphocytic infiltrate with evidence of myocyte disruption in single or multiple foci (Figure 3 and 4, see color plates section, back of book); lymphocytes surround individual myocytes causing indentation or scalloping of the edges. Accumulations of activated lymphocytes separate adjacent myocytes and may also be associated with inter-myofiber edema thereby distorting the architecture of myocardium. In cyclosporine-treated patients, the infiltrate may also contain eosinophils.

Severe rejection is recognized by the presence of aggressive, mixed inflammatory infiltrates composed of polymorphonuclear leukocytes, lymphocytes and scattered plasma cells with myocyte damage and/or necrosis. Interstitial edema, hemorrhage, and vasculitis are also seen (Figure 5, see color plates section, back of book). Cardiac transplant centers have reported variable degrees of myocyte necrosis in severe rejection that have been attributed, in part, to the different immunosuppressive protocols.[7,20–22]

Immunophenotyping studies using pan-T-cell antibodies Leu-1 or T-11 and with macrophage antibodies Leu-M3 or Leu-M5 have shown that interstitial infiltrates consist of admixtures of cytotoxic/suppressor and helper/inducer T-lymphocytes. Antibodies against T-cell subsets T-4 and T-8, and pan B-cell antibodies Leu-14 and B-1 have been used to characterize dense infiltrates. Several studies have shown no clear relationship between the proportion of lymphocyte subsets and the severity of the rejection process, although more CD8+ lymphocytes and macrophages were seen in severe rejection. It has been observed that among patients with severe rejection treated with murine monoclonal antibodies to CD3 (OKT3), a different subpopulation of lymphocytes is found.[16] Immunophenotyping is not routinely used to grade rejection.[17–19]

Myocyte Damage

Myocyte injury is seen at the periphery and within cellular infiltrates of moderate and, to a greater degree, severe rejection.[17,23] Damaged myocytes appear shrunken, frayed and occasionally vacuolated. Early myocyte injury may be difficult to evaluate on routine light microscopy—Masson's trichrome stain may be helpful—damaged myocytes appear blue-gray instead of the normal red color. Electron microscopy is not routinely used in the interpretation of endomyocardial biopsy, however, it can help in determining the extent of myocyte injury at the ultrastructural level.[23–25] Mild myocyte injury is characterized by an increase in the number of mitochondria and glycogen with separation and displacement of the contractile elements. Condensation of Z-band material into large nodular clumps or linear aggregates can be seen in more severe myocyte injury. Complete dissolution of sarcomeres with filament loss and complete Z-band loss can be seen with the most severe injury. Follow up studies have shown that myocyte injury during acute rejection may be reversible as it is in myocarditis.[23–25] The ultrastructure of regenerating myocytes morphologically resembles embryonic myocytes with prominent rough endoplasmic reticulum, free ribosomes, sarcomereogenesis, and large oval nuclei.

Vascular Changes

Vascular changes in biopsy material can be secondary to 1) reactive change, 2) drug effect, 3) severe cellular rejection, 4) acute vascular rejection, 5) hyperacute rejection, and, 6) chronic vascular rejection. Reactive endothelial cell swelling seen in the first week post-transplant may be secondary to harvesting or ischemic injury—accompanying focal myocyte necrosis, focal neutrophilic infiltrate and prominent contraction bands may also be seen. Similar findings of endothelial cell swelling with prominent nuclei can be seen in early post-transplant biopsies in patients treated with OKT3 or antilymphocyte globulin (ALG), and is thought to be secondary to endothelial cell activation.[26,27]

Acute vascular rejection is well documented, and becomes histologically evident after the first week post-transplant. The histology varies according to the severity—mild vascular rejection is characterized by endothelial cell swelling and vacuolization and/or lymphocytic endothelialitis. Moderate vascular rejection shows mural infiltrates of lymphocytes and/or neutrophils. Severe vascular rejection is evidenced by fibrinoid necrosis of the vascular wall associated with marked interstitial hemorrhage and edema with prominent myocyte necrosis. Retrospective studies have reported increased mortality among patients with histological evidence of acute vascular rejection.[28–34]

Immunofluorescence of acute vascular rejection has been outlined by Hammond et al.[28,29] Fluorescein isothiocyanate labeled antibodies directed against complement (C3, C1q) and immunoglobulins (IgG and IgM) are positive within the vessel wall. Grading of vascular rejection is based on the intensity of immunofluorescent staining relative to albumin and fluoresceinated mouse immunoglobulin controls. The scale ranges from 0 to 3+, where grade 0 indicates no reaction and grade 3+ indicates strongly positive fluorescent staining.

Fluorescein isothiocyanate labeled antibodies directed against complement, immunoglobulins and fibrinogen may also be localized in the interstitium. Immunofluorescent staining in severe cellular rejection occurs in a granular pattern between myocytes.[28,29,32] Vascular humoral rejection appears as a circular reaction surrounding vessel walls or as a linear pattern along vessels. Increased vascular endothelial expression of HLA-DR precedes histological evidence of vascular rejection by 1 to 3 weeks.[28] No correlation between the distribution of immunoflourescence and the severity of acute cellular rejection has been found.[28–32]

The distinct pattern of mixed vascular and acute cellular rejection has been described and includes the histologic picture of cellular rejection (lymphoid infiltrates) with positive vascular immunofluorescence.[28–36]

Hyperacute rejection is uncommon—it is seen immediately after transplantation in recipients with preformed anti-donor antibodies.[37,38] The pathognomonic changes consist of intravascular fibrin thrombi, interstitial hemorrhage, massive interfascicular edema and eventual neutrophilic infiltrates resulting in graft failure. The pathogenesis is due to recipient antibodies binding to donor endothelium with activation of complement and subsequent endothelial cell injury with platelet aggregation.

Chronic vascular rejection is the leading cause of graft failure after the first year following transplant. The full length of the coronary artery can be affected including small intramyocardial branches and therefore can be seen on endomyocardial biopsy. The histology is that of concentric fibrointimal proliferation with luminal compromise. The internal elastic lamina and muscular media are usually not affected.

EVOLUTION OF CLASSIFICATIONS OF PARENCHYMAL REJECTION

The first histological classification of acute allograft rejection was published by Billingham and coworkers at Stanford University in 1973[6,39] and provided the blueprint for the development of many modified grading systems reported over the next two decades.[7,18,21,40–44] Grading acute allograft rejection can be based on qualitative or quantitative histological parameters (Table 1).

The modified Stanford classification measures acute cellular rejection using five grades, i.e. mild, moderate, severe, resolving, and resolved. In the Stanford system, myocyte damage or disruption is the main criterion for distinguishing between mild and moderate/severe rejection; frank myocyte necrosis is seen in severe rejection. The qualitative classification of Pomerance and Stovin has an additional minimal rejection grade but only one resolving grade.[41] The Cleveland Clinic classification by Ratliff et al.,[18] has an additional accelerating mild rejection grade in addition to the grades proposed by Pomerance and Stovin. All of these classifications emphasize the extent of myocyte injury rather than necrosis, taking into account that myocyte injury can occur before myocyte necrosis.[45]

Because the majority of cyclosporine-treated patients present with some degree of interstitial infiltrate on biopsy, the concept of rejection as a continuing process with stable and unstable phases has been proposed.[18] Additional subclassifications

Table 1. Histologic Grading of Cardiac Allograft Rejection Using Published Qualitative and Quantitative Grading Systems

Grading System	No Rejection	Minimal Rejection	Mild Rejection	Moderate Rejection	Severe Rejection	Resolving Rejection	Resolved Rejection
		Qualitative	Grading	Systems			
Stanford			Mild	Moderate	Severe	Resolving	Resolved
Pomerance & Stovin	No	Minimal	Mild	Moderate	Severe	Resolving	
Cleveland Clinic	No	Minimal	Mild or AMR	Moderate	Severe	Resolving	
		Quantitative	Grading	Systems			
Texas Heart Institute	0	1	2 or 3	4–8	9 or 10		
Hannover	A-0		A-1 or A-2	A-3	A-4	A-5a	A-5b
Brigham & Womens	0		1–3	4–6	7		
Utah	1		2 or 2.5	3	4		
Pittsburgh	1		2	3A or 3B	4		
			ISHLT				
ISHLT	0		1A or 1B	2 or 3A	3B or 4	†	‡

* AMR indicates accelerating mild rejection; ISHLT indicates International Society for Heart and Lung Transplantation.
† Resolving rejection denoted by lesser grade.
‡ Resolved rejection denoted by grade 0.

include a stable phase when augmentation of chronic immunosuppressive therapy is unnecessary, and an unstable phase when interventions are indicated.

Each grade of rejection in the Stanford system describes a spectrum of histological abnormalities, therefore, there is subjectivity in biopsy interpretation. Furthermore, the descriptive system does not address late changes after cardiac transplantation such as graft coronary disease and does not lend itself readily to statistical analysis. The Stanford grading system is simple, comprised of five grades, each of which has implications for clinical management. The system has been used for nearly 30 years, with high reproducibility within centers.

An alternative methodology for histological grading of acute allograft rejection uses quantitative terminology. Examples include the Texas Heart Institute system proposed by McAllister,[43] the Hannover classification proposed by Kemitz,[21] and the Brigham and Womens Hospital and Utah grading systems.[44]

The most extensive numerical classification scheme is the Texas Heart Institute system which consists of 10 grades of rejection, 3 of which describe mild rejection, 5 describing moderate rejection, and 2, severe rejection (Table). Extent and location of cellular infiltrates, presence of myocyte degeneration and interstitial changes determine the assignment of rejection grade.

The advocates of quantitative scales believe that such systems provide more precise measurements of the degree of allograft rejection. Such systems potentially enhance communication between the pathologist, cardiologist, surgeon and patient, and better lend themselves to statistical analysis. Furthermore, quantitative techniques offer a level of precision that may be of value in assessing rejection patterns which emerge over time.[47]

With more than 200 cardiac transplant centers worldwide, the need to standardize grading systems has been emphasized.[46–48] In 1990 the International Society of Heart and Lung Transplantation (ISHLT) introduced a new grading system and encouraged its use.[49] This facilitated multicenter trials assessing immunosuppressive medications in the cardiac transplant population.

The ISHLT working formulation recognizes two subcategories for mild, moderate and severe rejection (Table). Thus, mild rejection was further stratified based on the pattern of inflammation into focal mild rejection and diffuse mild rejection categories (grades 1A and 1B respectively). Moderate rejection was divided into focal moderate rejection (grade 2) and multifocal moderate rejection (grade 3A). Grade 3B described diffuse, borderline severe acute rejection, and grade 4 severe acute rejection. The ISHLT grading system did not assign a separate grade for resolving or resolved rejection. The ISHLT working formulation recommends recording the number of pieces of myocardium, as well as the presence or absence of humoral changes, Quilty lesions, ischemic changes, infections and lymphoproliferative disorders.[49]

INTER- AND INTRA-OBSERVER VARIATIONS IN INTERPRETATION OF BIOPSY

The ISHLT working formulation proposed a standardization of grading systems among different transplant centers.[49] The reproducibility, feasibility and predictability of the ISHLT working formulation was confirmed within individual centers.[15,49–51]

The first available data on diagnostic consistency and inter-observer variability was reported from the Rapamycin Cardiac Rejection Treatment Trial pathologists.[52] The 16 trial pathologists independently read in randomized order, an identical series of 23 biopsies representing all ISHLT grades of rejection and other post-transplant pathologies. Their interpretations were compared to the index diagnosis which was previously determined by two independent trial pathologists with a 96% rate of agreement. A major discrepancy was defined as one which would affect clinical decisions, while a minor discrepancy was one which would not. The inter-observer agreement was assessed by weighted kappa values for major and minor discrepancies. Of 368 biopsy readings by 16 pathologists, there was exact agreement in 265 cases (72%). Of 103 discrepant readings, 50 were minor and 53 major discrepancies. Of the 53 major discrepancies, 81% involved grades 1A/1B versus 2, 2 versus 3A, and Quilty B lesions versus 2/3A rejection. In 54% of cases when readers misdiagnosed findings other than rejection as rejection, the grades assigned were sufficient to adversely alter therapy.

The inter-observer variability assessed by kappa statistics in this study achieved value of 0.67 for combined major and minor discrepancies, suggesting good inter-observer agreement. Thus, the ISHLT working formulation proved to facilitate uniformity in the interpretation of cardiac allograft biopsies. This study also helped define common problems in biopsy interpretation. The most controversial grade of rejection was 2, giving the highest disagreement rate among pathologists. In the interpretation of non-rejection pathology, Quilty B lesions proved to be the most controversial, followed by ischemic injury, biopsy site, lymphoproliferative disorders and toxoplasmosis. This study confirmed the unpublished experience of many transplant centers regarding difficulties in the diagnosis of grade 2 rejection and Quilty B lesions. Better clarification of the definition of grade 2 rejection and Quilty B lesions can further enhance diagnostic consistency in the evaluation of endomyocardial biopsies.

PATHOLOGIC CHANGES UNRELATED TO ALLOGRAFT REJECTION

Ischemic Changes

The majority of endomyocardial biopsies performed within the first week post-transplant show evidence of ischemic injury secondary to harvesting or reperfusion.[7,15,18,39,40] Ischemic change is usually focal and characterized by myocyte shrinkage, pyknotic nuclei and minimal mixed cellular infiltrate of lymphocytes and/or neutrophils (Figure 6, see color plates section, back of book). Occasionally, microinfarction can be seen which in some cases may be due to air embolism within the coronary circulation or the use of inotropic agents during the peri-transplant period.[56] Subsequent biopsies up to 4 to 6 weeks post-transplantation may show evolution of the ischemic process with granulation tissue, macrophages and scant lymphoid infiltrate with progression to fibrosis (Figure 7, see color plates section, back of book). Evolving ischemic injury may be mistaken for acute rejection.[15,18] It is helpful to remember that in ischemia myocyte damage is greater than the inflammatory infiltrate while in rejection the opposite is true.

Ischemic myocardial injury seen later in the post-transplant course suggests graft vascular disease or chronic vascular rejection.[57] Multiple pathologic studies have demonstrated intramyocardial ischemic changes in failed allografts.[55] The presence of late ischemic changes in endomyocardial biopsies carries a high positive predictive value (92%) for significant allograft vasculopathy, but a low predictive negative value of 51%.[57] Depending on the degree of ischemic insult, histological changes include myocyte vacuolization, hypereosinophilia, and myocyte coagulative necrosis with different stages of healing.[58–60]

Previous Biopsy Site

Changes secondary to a previous biopsy site are frequently encountered. Recent biopsy sites show a cup-shaped area with a superficial layer of fresh thrombus overlying inflammatory granulation tissue with acute and chronic inflammation and hemosiderin-laden macrophages (Figure 8, see color plates section, back of book). Healed biopsy sites consist of fibrous tissue with or without a mild infiltrate of lymphocytes and /or plasma cells; multinucleated giant cells of the foreign body type may also be seen. The periphery of a healed biopsy site may show disorganized myocytes. Suture granulomata may rarely be detected in myocardial samples on biopsy taken near the surgical anastomotic line.[15,18,61]

Interstitial Fibrosis

Fibrosis has been found in more than 50% of consecutive endomyocardial biopsies.[62] Two types of interstitial fibrosis have been described in cardiac allograft-replacement fibrosis and pericellular fibrosis. Experimental studies and clinical examinations of allograft specimens have identified potential factors that can induce fibrosis after transplantation[63] and include cyclosporine treatment, donor ischemic time and prior rejection episodes.[64–68]

Recent long term follow up studies of allograft recipients did not show a significant correlation between rejection and an increase in the collagen density on endomyocardial biopsies.[59–63] Endomyocardial biopsies of patients with angiographically-documented graft atherosclerosis showed a significant increase in interstitial and perivascular fibrosis.[69] Type II and type IV collagen, laminin and fibronectin were increased in areas of fibrosis and in vessel walls. Fibronectin accumulates more in the subendothelium and in the inner media of affected vessel walls. This suggests that biopsy-proven fibrosis may be an additional marker for chronic graft atherosclerosis. Moreover, fibrosis and right ventricular collagen content correlate with diastolic and systolic dysfunction of the allograft.[70]

Calcification

Dystrophic calcification has been described in the myocardium of cardiac allografts.[61,71] These changes have been observed in areas of necrosis, hemorrhage, or fibrosis with normal serum calcium and phosphate levels. A second pattern of delicate encrustation of mitochondria may represent the initial deposition of insoluble hydroxyapatite minerals in either the mitochondria or matrix vesicles. The pathogenesis and significance of these changes are not well known.[71,72]

Myocyte Hypertrophy

Several morphometric studies of biopsy specimens have described myocyte hypertrophy.[61,73] The extent of myocyte hypertrophy was shown not to be affected by different immunosuppressive therapies or by the occurrence or severity of systemic hypertension after transplantation. Several donor- and recipient-specific variables such as ischemic time and degree of HLA matching did not show significant correlation with the development of hypertrophy. Serial follow up evaluations of biopsy specimens have shown that myocyte hypertrophy occurs early after transplantation (the majority within 3 months post-transplant) and does not evolve during the subsequent follow up period. Pathologic studies of explanted failed allografts documented significant hypertrophy in the majority. Allograft hypertrophy documented by echocardiography and morphometric evaluation is associated with an increased risk of cardiovascular mortality in the cardiac transplant population.[74]

Quilty Lesions

Quilty lesions were named after the first patient in whom these changes were seen on biopsy;[15,18] their pathogenesis is uncertain. They are subendocardial collections of lymphocytes, with occasional histiocytes and plasma cells, set within a background rich in capillaries. Quilty effect can be found in up to 50% of cases, and is more common in cyclosporine-treated patients. No clear correlation between plasma cyclosporine levels and the occurrence of Quilty lesions has been noted.[75] A more recent study reported a correlation between tissue levels of cyclosporine and Quilty lesions.[76]

Quilty lesions are classified by the ISHLT working formulation as a Quilty A or non-invasive lesion when the infiltrate does not involve the underlying myocardium (Figure 9, see color plates section, back of book), or a Quilty B or invasive lesion when the infiltrate extends into the underlying myocardium (Figure 10, see color plates section, back of book). Joshi et al.,[77] reviewed ten years experience at Stanford University, and found no clinical difference between Quilty A versus Quilty B. In addition, there was no difference in the rate of viral infections and none of the Quilty positive biopsies were associated with a higher rate of severe rejection.[77] This study also found that allograft recipients who had a pre-transplant diagnosis of dilated cardiomyopathy had a higher prevalence of Quilty lesions in biopsy material than those with ischemic cardiomyopathy.

Quilty lesions are not related to post-transplant lymphoproliferative disorders and may not be recipient-specific, as these infiltrates may not recur in a second transplant. In situ hybridization shows increased expression of EBV markers in Quilty positive patients.[75–77] Immunophenotyping studies of Quilty lesions with utilization of avidin-biotin-peroxidase technique showed that these infiltrates consist of both

B- and T-lymphocytes, as well as histiocytes. Thus, it has been suggested that Quilty B lesions may represent chronic rejection with acute rejection in the adjacent myocardium.[78] A study by Fishbein et al. using step sectioning and immunohistochemical staining reported that up to 91% of biopsies previously interpreted as grade 2 rejection were Quilty B lesions.[79]

PATHOLOGIC MANIFESTATION OF DISEASES OF IMMUNOCOMPROMISE

Myocarditis

Infectious myocarditis, caused by viruses, fungi, protozoa and bacteria, is a major contributor to death in the first 3 months following transplant. The immunocompromised patient is susceptible to infections The most common infections seen on heart biopsy are toxoplasmosis and cytomegalovirus (CMV). The encysted trophozites of Toxoplasma gondii can be seen in biopsy specimens sometimes without accompanying inflammatory infiltrate (Figure 11, see color plates section, back of book). The intranuclear inclusions of CMV can rarely be seen within the myocardium (Figure 12, see color plates section, back of book).[80–82]

In situ DNA hybridization and immunoperoxidase staining are used to identify the causative agent when atypical inflammatory infiltrates are present or clinical factors raise suspicion of the diagnosis. These techniques may confirm myocarditis caused by Ebstein-Barr virus (EBV), adenovirus, CMV, and herpes simplex virus.[15,80]

Giant Cell Myocarditis

Idiopathic giant cell myocarditis is a rare disorder affecting young to middle aged patients. It presents with progressive heart failure and cardiac arrhythmias.[83] The mortality rate is high with a median survival of 5.5 months after diagnosis. Treatment of this disease remains symptomatic, though some patients respond to immunosuppressive treatment.[84,85] Cardiac transplantation can improve survival, however, giant cell myocarditis may recur in the transplanted hear.[84–90] The histologic features of giant cell myocarditis consist of diffuse and prominent interstitial infiltrates of T-lymphocytes, plasma cells and the characteristic multinucleated giant cells with areas of diffuse myocardial necrosis (Figure 13, see color plates section, back of book). Rarely, acute rejection may be represented by an infiltrate rich in giant cells resembling giant cell myocarditis.[91]

The Multicenter Giant Cell Myocarditis Study Group followed 34 patients with this disorder who underwent cardiac transplantation.[83] Nine patients (26%) had recurrence of giant cell myocarditis in the transplanted heart within 3 years (range, 3 weeks to 9 years). Three of the 9 patients had impairment of cardiac function with recurrence of giant cell myocarditis; 2 responded to increased immunosuppression. Survival after transplantation among patients with giant cell myocarditis is worse than those transplanted for lymphocytic myocarditis.[83] More frequent and longer surveillance with endomyocardial biopsy for early detection of recurrence is recommended after transplantation for giant cell myocarditis.

Post-Transplant Lymphoproliferative Disorders

It is well recognized that immunosuppressed patients are prone to develop neoplastic disorders. Powerful suppression of cell mediated immune responses enhances susceptibility to lymphomas, in particular. The incidence of lymphoproliferative disorders in cardiac transplant population is reported to be 1–2%, which represents a 30- to 50-fold increase over the general population. Cardiac transplant recipients treated with OKT3 have an 11% incidence of lymphoproliferative disorders.[18,62,92–94]

Post-transplant lymphoproliferative disease (PTLD) is a B-cell lymphoid proliferation that usually contains EBV genomic material and transformation antigens. PTLD can present with a polymorphic or monomorphic lymphoid infiltrate. The monomorphic forms are often monoclonal and usually are more aggressive, frequently requiring antineoplastic therapy.[62,93–95] PTLD can occur in a number of sites including the gastrointestinal tract, liver and brain.[94,95] PTLD involving the heart presents as a florid and dense infiltrate of atypical lymphoid cells (Figure 14, see color plates section, back of book).[62,94–95] In situ hybridization for EBV, immunohistochemistry and gene rearrangement studies can support the diagnosis.

Amyloidosis

Amyloidosis represents a group of disease processes characterized by the deposition of amorphous, proteinaceous extracellular deposits in various tissues and organs. Ultrastructurally, these deposits show a beta-pleated sheet conformation; thus, they demonstrate affinity for alkaline Congo Red histochemical stain. The biochemical composition of the deposited protein defines the major types of amyloid, i.e. AA amyloid, Asc (senile) amyloid, and AL amyloid. The heart can be involved in most forms of amyloidosis and is associated with a poor prognosis, with an average survival of 6 months after diagnosis. Amyloid deposits can be seen in the interstitium, intramyocardial vessels, conduction system, valves, and endocardium.[96,97] Amyloidosis is considered a contraindication to cardiac transplantation because of potential recurrence in the transplanted heart and the impact of immunosuppression on disease progression. According to the United Network for Organ Sharing at least 44 patients with cardiac amyloidosis have undergone heart transplantation.[96,97] Many of these patients had acceptable clinical outcomes early post-transplant.[98,99] However, long term follow up of 10 cases showed 100% mortality three years after transplant.[100] There are individual case reports of patients with systemic amyloidosis with long term survival of 69 and 118 months reported after cardiac transplant.[101–103] Frequent surveillance with endomyocardial biopsy may benefit such patients.

Sarcoidosis

Cardiac transplantation has been utilized in patients with end stage heart disease secondary to cardiac sarcoidosis.[104–106] Recurrence of sarcoidosis has been reported in cardiac allografts.[107,108] Post-transplant cardiac sarcoidosis may present as unexplained heart failure with conduction abnormalities. Sarcoidosis is characterized by well-formed, non-necrotizing epitheloid granulomata with varying numbers of multinucleated giant cells of the foreign body or Langhans type. Histologically, discrete clusters of epitheloid histiocytes with giant cells are rimmed by fibrosis with lymphocytes and plasma cells. The giant cells may contain stellate intracytoplasmic asteroid bodies or laminated calcific concretions called Schaumann bodies. The etiology of sarcoidosis remains elusive, but it is notable that transmission of sarcoidosis via a cardiac allograft has been reported, suggesting the possibility of a transmissible agent.[109]

Chronic Pathologic Manifestations of Allograft Vasculopathy

Transplant-related vasculopathy is the primary cause of graft failure after the first year.[112–114] It is usually clinically silent, although angina may occur.[110] Angiographically-defined coronary artery disease occurs in 40% of allografts at 3 years and 50% of allografts at 5 years after transplantation;[111] intravascular ultrasound is more sensitive in detecting arterial changes. Allograft vasculopathy is a dynamic process and is histologically distinct from conventional atherosclerosis in several important aspects. The full length of the coronary artery is involved including smaller intramyocardial branches unlike classical atherosclerosis which favors the proximal segments of the epicardial vessels.[112,113,115,116] Concentric fibrointimal proliferation, sparing the internal elastic lamina is seen in allograft vasculopathy which contrasts with eccentric atherosclerotic plaques with inner media involvement seen in conventional coronary artery disease (Figure 15, see color plates section, back of book). There may be evidence of a healed or active vasculitis in graft vasculopathy and the outer layer of the media may show myocytolysis. Late after transplantation, the lesions of allograft vasculopathy may appear similar to non-transplant atherosclerosis with eccentric fibrolipid plaque with clusters of foam cells, calcification, with or without disruption of the internal elastic lamina.

In patients with transplant vasculopathy, endomyocardial biopsy may show intimal proliferation within small caliber arteries and arterioles. Myocyte hypertrophy, interstitial and perivascular fibrosis have also been detected. The accumulation of collagen type III and IV, laminin and fibronectin may be seen in the subendothelium and inner media of the vessel.[69]

Immunocytochemical studies of endomyocardial biopsy show that the development of vasculopathy late post-transplantation was preceded by the appearance of ICAM-1/HLA-DR on vascular endothelium within 3 months after transplant.[118,119] This report raised speculation that endothelial activation in the early postoperative period heralds the development of allograft vasculopathy.

THERAPEUTIC INTERVENTIONS BASED ON PATHOLOGIC INTERPRETATIONS

The endomyocardial biopsy should not be the sole determinant of subsequent clinical management (see Chapter 10). Inherent problems of subjectivity in biopsy interpretation and sampling bias limits the usefulness of the biopsy as a management tool. The grading systems used are based solely on histological findings without clinical corollary. Thus, the exact point in the spectrum of histological rejection that requires additional treatment remains variable and should be decided on a case-to-case basis.[120–124] Withholding additional immunosuppression because myocyte necrosis is absent despite a prominent infiltrate is debatable. The need to treat rejection with focal myocyte damage, regardless of the extent of inflammatory infiltrates, is also controversial. Further complicating the decision-making process is the potential risk of additional immunosuppressive therapy.

Histologic criteria for grading acute rejection is based on the most severe lesions present within the endomyocardial fragments. A semiquantitative evaluation, which takes into account not only the severity of myocyte injury but the extent of the inflammatory process, may be more useful in the prediction of outcomes.[125] Thus, even low grade rejection, if observed in all pieces of biopsy specimens might be a trigger for adjunctive treatment.

Our prior comments notwithstanding, ISHLT grade 1A and 1B rejection is not treated by the majority of centers, but is usually followed with serial biopsies. However, in as many as one-third of cases, moderate rejection is observed on subsequent biopsies.[126] A randomized trial which utilized doubling of maintenance doses of cyclosporine to treat mild rejection showed a significant decrease in the incidence of progression to moderate rejection.[127]

Controversy exists regarding the clinical significance of focal moderate rejection (ISHLT grade 2) which may be histologically similar to a tangentially sectioned Quilty B lesion. It has been reported that up to 11–15% of grade 2 rejections progress to a higher grade on subsequent biopsy.[120–123] The recommended treatment of focal moderate rejection includes either an increase in the oral dose of cyclosporine or no treatment with follow up biopsy.

Multifocal moderate rejection (ISHLT grade 3A) usually requires therapy with intravenous methylprednisolone for 3 days or an oral prednisone pulse with tapering over two weeks. The oral and intravenous forms of treatment have the same efficacy and similar complication rates, however, oral therapy costs less. Increasing the dose of maintenance immunosuppression is also an option in patients who experience moderate rejection. The treatment of severe rejection (ISHLT grades 3B and 4) usually requires intravenous methylprednisolone with the addition of cytolytic therapy (OKT3 or antithymocyte globulin, ATG).

Persistent or recurrent cellular infiltrates of ISHLT grade 3A or higher have a negative impact on allograft function and are associated with development of allograft vasculopathy. The treatment of recurrent or persistent cardiac allograft rejection was recently reviewed by Kirklin and McGiffin.[128] These authors argue for examination of clinical and social factors in addition to biopsy interpretation in directing immunosuppressive therapy. These factors include the presence of hemodynamic compromise, presence of humoral rejection, time from transplantation, patient's travel distance and cost of therapy.[128] Using this paradigm, low grade infiltrates (ISHLT grades 1B and 2) might be a trigger for incremental immunosuppressive therapy within the first 6 months post-transplant based on reports that early postoperative grade 1B and 2 biopsies are associated with a 25% probability of having higher grades of rejection on a subsequent biopsy.

FALSE-POSITIVE AND FALSE-NEGATIVE DIAGNOSIS AND DIFFERENTIAL DIAGNOSIS IN BIOPSY

The interpretation of circumscribed inflammatory infiltrates associated with apparent myocyte damage represents a true challenge for cardiopathologists.[15,16,18] These changes may occur with focal ischemic injury (Figure 16, see color plates section, back of book), infections, post-transplant lymphoproliferative disorders, tangentially sectioned Quilty B lesions (Figure 17, see color plates section, back of book), and ISHLT grade 2 rejection (Figure 3). The majority of false-positive and false-negative endomyocardial biopsy readings involve focal inflammatory infiltrat.[15,16,52]

DIFFICULTY IN INTERPRETATION OF ENDOMYOCARDIAL BIOPSY AND TROUBLE-SHOOTING

The differentiation between acute allograft rejection and non-rejection pathology in cyclosporine-treated patients may be difficult.[15,16] Quilty B lesions clearly belong in this category. How can Quilty B lesions be differentiated from grade 2 acute rejection? Some authors recommend step sectioning and immunohistochemical labeling.[79] Quilty B lesions consist of B-lymphocytes centrally and T-lymphocytes at the periphery with a prominent capillary background, compared to infiltrates of acute rejection.[15] In Quilty lesions and grade 1 rejection damaged myocytes are not observed.[129]

Acute ischemic injury may be differentiated from rejection on two points—in ischemic injury myocyte damage precedes the inflammatory infiltrate and the extent of myocyte injury is greater than that of the infiltrate—the opposite is true for rejection. Healing ischemic injury shows granulation tissue with a mixed inflammatory infiltrate including lymphocytes and hemosiderin-laden macrophages.[15,16,18,125]

The presence of granulomata, clusters of epitheloid histiocytes and eosinophilic infiltrate, should prompt a search for an infectious agent with additional techniques, e.g. culture, histochemical stains for organisms, immunohistochemistry, in situ hybridization and polymerase chain reaction in order to identify causative factors.

In summary, endomyocardial biopsy remains the primary tool in the diagnosis of acute cardiac rejection. To further its diagnostic sensitivity and specificity, new micromolecular and histological techniques are encouraged, thereby providing more reliable guidance for clinical management.

REFERENCES

Introduction

1. Sakakibara S, Kono S. Endomyocardial biopsy. Jpn Heart J 1962;3:537–542.
2. Caves PK, Schultz WP, Dong E, et al. A new instrument for transvenous cardiac biopsy. Am J Cardiol 1974;33:264–267.
3. Mason JM. Techniques for right and left ventricular endomyocardial biopsy. Am J Cardiol 1978;41:887–892.
4. Laser JA, Fowles RE, Mason JW. Endomyocardial biopsy. Cardiovasc Clin 1985;15:141–163.

5. Lie JT. Diagnostic histology and myocardial disease in endomyocardial biopsy and at autopsy. Pathol Annu 1989;24:255–293.
6. Caves PK, Stinson EB, Graham AF, et al. Percutaneous transvenous endomyocardial biopsy. JAMA 1973;225:288–291.
7. Billingham ME. Endocardial biopsy detection of acute rejection in cardiac allograft recipients. Heart Vessels 1985;1:86–90.
8. Forbes RDC, Rowan RA, Billingham ME. Endocardial infiltrates in human transplants: a serial biopsy analysis comparing four immunosuppressive protocols. Human Pathology 1990;21:850–855.
9. Mills RM, Naftel DC, Kirklin JK, et al. Heart transplant rejection with hemodynamic compromise: a multiinstitutional study of the role of endomyocardial cellular infiltrate. Cardiac Transplant Research Database. J Heart Lung Transplant 1997;16:813–821.
10. Tugulea S, Ciubotariu R, Colovai AI, et al. New strategies for early diagnosis of heart allograft rejection. Transplantation 1997;64:842–847.
11. Pellicalli AM, Cosial JB, Ferranti E, et al. Alteration of left ventricular filling evaluated by Doppler echocardiography as a potential marker of acute rejection in orthotopic heart transplant. Angiology 1996;47:35–41.
12. Anderson Jr, Hossein Nia M, Brown PA, et al. Creatine kinase MB isoform: a potential predictor of acute cardiac allograft rejection. J Heart Lung Transplant 1995;14:666–670.
13. Hossein Nia M, Holt DW, Murday AJ, et al. Cardiac troponin I release in heart transplantation. Ann Thorac Surg 1996;61:277–278.
14. Benvenuti C, Bories PN, Loisance D. Increased serum nitrate concentration in cardiac transplant recipients: a marker for acute allograft cellular rejection. Transplantation 1996;61:745–749.
15. Winters GL. The challenge of endomyocardial biopsy interpretation in assessing cardiac allograft rejection. Current Opinion Cardiol 1997;12:146–152.
16. Billingham ME. Can histopathology guide immunosuppression for cardiac rejection in the light of new techniques? Transplantation Proc 1997;29:35S–36S.

Infiltrates and Myocyte Damage

17. Rose ML, Yacoub MH. Immunocytochemical analysis of transplanted heart and lung. In Rose ML, Yacoub MA (eds). Immunology of Heart and Lung Transplantation. London: Edward Arnold 1993;166.
18. Kottke Marchant K, Ratliff NB. Endomyocardial biopsy. Pathologic findings in cardiac transplant recipients. Pathol Annu 1990;25:211–244.
19. Hoshinaga K, Mohanakamur T, Goldman MH, et al. Clinical significance of in-situ detection of T-lymphocyte subsets and monocyte macrophage lineages in heart allografts. Transplantation 1984;38:634–638.
20. Myles JL, Ratliff NB, McMahon JT. Reversibility of myocyte injury in moderate and severe acute rejection in cyclosporine treated cardiac transplant patients. Arch Pathol Lab Med 1987;П1:947–952.
21. Kemmitz J, Cohnert T, Schafers HJ, et al. A classification of cardiac allograft rejection: a modification of the classificaton by Billingham. Am J Surg Pathol 1987;11:503–515.
22. Sibley RK, Olivari MT, Ring WS, et al. Endomyocardial biopsy in cardiac allograft recipient. A review of 570 biopsies. Ann Surg 1986;203:177–187.
23. McMahon JT, Ratliff NB. Regeneration of adult human myocardium after acute heart transplant rejection. J Heart Lung Transplant 1990;9:554–567.
24. Ratliff NB, Myles JL, McMahon JT, et al. Myocyte injury in acute cardiac transplant rejection and in lymphocytic myocarditis is similar and is reversible. Transplant Proc 1987;19:2568–2572.
25. McMahon JT, Ratliff NB. Endomyocardial biopsies prepared for electron microscopy are essential for evaluation of transplant rejection. Proceedings of the International Symposium on Inflammatory Heart Disease. Aspen, Colorado, 1988:566.

Humoral Rejection and Vascular Changes

26. Herskowitz A, Soule LM, Mellits E, et al. Arteriolar vasculitis on endomyocardial biopsy: a histologic predictor of poor outcome in cyclosporine treated heart transplant recipients. J Heart Transplant 1987;6:127–136.
27. Yowell RL, Hammond EH, Bristow MR, et al. Acute vascular rejection involving the major coronary arteries of a cardiac allograft. J Heart Transplant 1988;7:191–197.

28. Hammond EH, Yowell RL, Nunoda S, et al. Vascular (humoral) rejection in heart transplantation: pathologic observations and clinical implications. J Heart Transplant 1989;8:430–443.
29. Hammond EH, Hansen JK, Spencer LS, et al. Vascular rejection in cardiac transplantation: histologic, immunopathologic, and ultrastructural features. Cardiovasc Pathol 1993;2:21–34.
30. Miller LW. The diagnosis, incidence, and management of vascular rejection in heart transplantation. J Heart Lung Transplant 1993;12:S111–S112.
31. Smith SH, Kirklin JK, Geer JC, et al. Arteritis and cardiac rejection after transplantation. Am J Cardiol 1987;59:1171–1173.
32. Caple JF, McMahon JT, Myles JL, et al. Acute vascular (humoral) rejection in non OKT3-treated cardiac transplants. Cardiovasc Pathol 1995;4:13–18.
33. Bush GJ, Reynolds ES, Galvanek EG, et al. Human renal allografts. The role of vascular injury in early graft failure. Medicine 1971;50:29–84.
34. Mihatsch MJ, Thiel G, Basler V, et al. Morphological patterns in cyclosporine treated renal transplant recipients. Transplant Proc 1985;17:101–117.
35. Mass AJ, Sibley R, Mauer M, et al. The value of the needle renal allograft biopsy. Ann Surg 1993;197:226–237.
36. Bergstrand A, Bohman SO, Famsworth A, et al. Renal histopathology in kidney transplant recipients immunossupressed with cyclosporine A: results of an international workshop. Clin Nephrol 1985;24:107–119.
37. Rose AG, Cooper DKC, Human PA, et al. Histopathology of hyperacute rejection of heart: experimental and clinial observations in allografts and xenografts. J Heart Lung Transplant 1991;10:223–334.
38. Weil RR, Clark DR, Iwaki Y, et al. Hyperacute rejection of a transplanted human heart. Transplantation 1981;32:71–72.

Histologic Classification

39. Caves BC, Billingham ME, Stinson EB, et al. Serial transvenous biopsy of the transplanted human heart—improved management of acute rejection episodes. Lancet 1974;1:821–826.
40. Billingham ME. Some recent advances in cardiac pathology. Human Pathol 1979;10:367–386.
41. Pomerance A, Stovin P. Heart transplant pathology, the British experience. J Clin Pathol 1085;38:146.
42. Schoen F. Interventional and Surgical Cardiovascular Pathology, Clinical Correlations and Basic Principles. Philadelphia: WB Saunders 1989;195.
43. McAllister HA, Schnee MJ, Radovancevic B, et al. A system for grading cardiac allograft rejection. Texas Heart Institute Journal 1986;13:1–2.
44. Zebre TR, Arena V. Diagnostic reliability of endomyocardial biopsy for assessment of cardiac allograft rejection. Hum Pathol 1988;19:1307–1313.
45. Majno G, Joris I. Apoptosis, oncosis and necrosis. An overview of cell death. Am J Pathol 1995;146:3–15.
46. Billingham ME. Dilemma of variety of histopathologic grading systems for acute cardiac allograft rejection by endomyocardial biopsy. J Heart Lung Transplant 1990;9:272–276.
47. McAllister HA. Histologic grading of cardiac allograft rejection: a quantitative approach. J Heart Lung Transplant 1990;9:277–282.
48. O'Connell JB, Renlund DG. Variation in the diagnosis, treatment and prevention of cardiac allograft rejection: the need for standarization. J Heart Lung Transplant 1990;9:269–271.
49. Billingham ME, Carry NRB, Hammond ME, et al. A working formulation for the standarization of nomenclature in the diagnosis of heart and lung rejection: heart rejection study group. J Heart Transplant 1990;9:587–593.

Intra-Observer Variation

50. Nielsen H, Sorensen FB, Nielsen B, et al. Reproducibility of the acute rejection diagnosis in human cardiac allografts. The Stanford Classification and the International Grading System. J Heart Lung Transplant 1993;12:239–243.
51. Gallo P, Grillo LR, di Gioia C, et al. Working formulation nomenclature of heart transplant pathology: a retrospective evaluation of 1037 endomyocardial biopsies. Cardiovasc Pathol 1992;1: 87–92.
52. Winters GL, McManus BM. Consistencies and controversies in the International Society for Heart and Lung Transplantation working formulation for heart transplant biopsy specimen.

Rapamycin Cardiac Rejection Treatment Trial Pathologists. J Heart Lung Transplant 1996;15: 728–735.

Ischemic Changes

53. Winters GL, Davis SF, Anderson TJ, et al. Is perioperative ischemic injury a factor in early graft arteriosclerosis: evidence from endomyocardial biopsy-intravascular ultrasound correletion. J Heart Lung Transplant 1996;15:S43.
54. Day JD, Rayburn BK, Gaudin BP, et al. Cardiac allograft vasculopathy: the central pathogenetic role of ischemia-induced endothelial cell injury. J Heart Lung Transplant 1995;14:S142–S149.
55. Arbustini E, Roberts WC. Morphologic obervation in the epicardial coronary arteries and their surroundings late after cardiac transplantation (allograft vascular disease). Am J Cardiol 1996; 78:814–820.
56. Billingham ME. The postsurgical heart. The pathology of cardiac transplantation. Am J Cardiovasc Pathol 1988;1:319–324.
57. Winters GL, Schoen FJ. Graft arteriosclerosis-induced myocardial pathology in heart transplant recipients: predictive value of endomyocardial biopsy. J Heart Lung Transplant 1997;16:985–993.
58. Pirolo JS, Hutchins GM, Moore GW. Myocyte vacuolization in infarct border zones is reversible. Am J Pathol 1996;121:444–450.
59. Clausell N, Butany J, Gladstone P, et al. Myocardial vacuolization, a marker of ischemic injury, in surveilance cardiac biopsies postransplant: correlations with morphologic vascular disease and endothelial dysfunction. Cardiovascular Pathol 1996;5:29–37.
60. Neish AS, Loh E, Schoen FJ. Myocardial changes in cardiac transplant associated coronary arteriosclerosis: potential for timely diagnosis. J Am Coll Cardiol 1992;19:586–592.

Previous Biopsy Site, Fibrosis, Calcification and Hypertrophy

61. Tazelaar HD, Edwards WD. Pathology of cardiac transplantation: recipient hearts (chronic failure) and donor hearts (acute and chronic rejection). Mayo Clinic Proc 1992;67:685–696.
62. Winters GL, Constanzo-Nordin MR. Pathologic findings in 2300 consecutive endomyocardial biopsies. Mod Pathol 1991;4:441–448.
63. Kolar F, Papuosek F, Mac Naughton C, et al. Myocardial fibrosis and right ventricular function of heterotropically transplanted hearts in rats treated with cyclosporine. Mol Cell Bioch 1996; 163–164:253–260.
64. Stovin PGI, English TAH. Effects of cyclosporine on the transplanted human heart. J Heart Transplant 1987;6:180–185.
65. Tazelaar HD, Gay RE, Rowan RA, et al. Collagen profile in the transplanted hearts. Human Pathol 1990;21:424–428.
66. Winters G, Radio S, Wilson J, et al. Progression of healed rejection in human heart allografts documented by endomyocardial biopsy: exaggeration of myocardial fibrosis as compared to autopsy. Mod Pathol 1988;1:104A.
67. Pucci AM, Forbes RDC, Billingham ME. Pathologic features in long term cardiac allografts. J Heart Lung Transplant 1990;9:339–345.
68. Fornes P, Heudes D, Simon D, et al. Influence of acute or chronic rejection on myocardial collagen in serial endomyocardial biopsy specimens from cardiac allografts. J Heart Lung Transplant 1996;15:796–803.
69. Pardo-Mindan FJ, Panizo A, Lozano MD, et al. Role of endomyocardial biopsy in the diagnosis of chronic rejection in human heart transplantation. Clin Transplant 1997;11:426–431.
70. Zhuang YF, Corone-Alden S, Duval AM, et al. Right ventricular late filling termination time and its relation to intersitial collagen content in early transplanted heart: a color M-mode Doppler digital analysis. J Heart Lung Transplant 1995;14:846–855.
71. Pardo-Mindan FJ, Herreros J, Marigil MA, et al. Myocardial calcification following heart transplantation. J Heart Transplant 1986;5:332–335.
72. Cohnert TR, Kemmitz J, Heverich A, et al. Myocardial calcification after orthotopic heart transplantation. J Heart Transplant 1988;7:304–308.
73. Rowan RA, Billingham ME. Pathologic changes in long term transplanted hearts: a morphometric study of myocardial hypertrophy, vascularity and fibrosis. Human Pathol 1990;21:767–772.

74. Czerska B, McCarthy PM, Hobbs RE, et al. Hypertrophy after cardiac transplantation portends poor prognosis (abstract). Circulation 1994;90:I-420.

Quilty Lesions

75. Luthringer DJ, Yamashita JT, Czer LS, et al. Nature and significance of epicardial lymphoid infiltrates in cardiac allograft rejection. J Heart Lung Transplant 1995;14:537–543.
76. Freimark D, Czer LS, Aleksic I, et al. Pathogenesis of quilty lessions in cardiac allografts: relationship to reduced cyclosporine A. J Heart Lung Transplant 1995;14:1197–1203.
77. Joshi A, Maseka MA, Brown BW, et al. "Quilty" revisited: a 10 year perspective. Human Pathol 1995;26:547–557.
78. Kemmintz J. Grade 2 cellular heart rejection; does it exist? Yes! J Heart Lung Transplant 1995;14:800–801.
79. Fishbein MC, Bell G, Lones MA, et al. Grade 2 cellular heart rejection: does it exist? J Heart Lung Transplant 1994;13:1051–1057.

Infections and Myocarditis

80. Linder J. Infection as a complication of heart transplantation. J Heart Lung Transplant 1988;7: 390–394.
81. Dressler FA, Javier JJ, Salinas-Madrgal L, et al. Myocardial toxoplasmosis complicating cardiac transplant. Cardiovasc Pathol 1996;5:101–104.
82. Lozano MD, Pardo-Mindam J. Value of the endomyocardial biopsy in the diagnosis of toxoplasmosis after heart transplantation. Cardiovasc Pathol 1996;5:55–56.
83. Cooper LT, Berry GJ, Shabetai R. For the Multicenter Giant Cell Myocarditis Study Group Investigators. Idiopathic giant cell mycocarditis-natural history and treatment. N Engl J Med 1997;336:1860–1866.
84. Davidoff R, Palacios R, Southern J, et al. Giant cell versus lymphocytic myocarditis. A comparison of their clinical features and long term outcomes. Circulation 1991;83:953–961.
85. Cooper LT, Berry GJ, Rizeg M, et al. Giant cell myocarditis. J Heart Lung Transplant 1995;14: 394–401.
86. Cooper DK, Schlesinger RG, Shrago S, et al. Heart transplantation for giant cell myocarditis. J Heart Lung Transplant 1994;13:555.
87. Nieminen MS, Salminen US, Taskinen E, et al. Treatment of serious heart failure by transplantation in giant cell myocarditis diagnosed by endomyocardial biopsy. J Heart Lung Transplant 1994;13:543–545.
88. Gries W, Farkas D, Winters GL, et al. Giant cell myocarditis: first report of disease recurrence in the transplanted heart. J Heart Lung Transplant 1992;11:370–374.
89. Kong G, Madden B, Spyrou N, et al. Response of reccurrent giant cell myocarditis in transplanted heart to intensive immunosupression. Eur Heart J 1991;12:554–557.
90. Grant SC. Recurrent giant cell myocarditis after transplantation. J Heart Lung Transplant 1993;12:155–156.
91. Wolfson AL, Davies RA, Smith CO, et al. Giant cell myocarditis-like appearance after transplantation: an atypical manifestation of rejection? J Heart Lung Transplant 1994;13:731–733.

Lymphoproliferative Disorders

92. Fragomeni LS, Keys MP. The registry of the International Society for Heart Transplantation. J Heart Transplant 1988;7:249.
93. Cleary ML, Sklar J. Lymphoprolipherative disorders in cardiac transplant recipients are multiclonal lymphomas. Lancet 1984;489.
94. Kemmitz J, Cohnert TR. Lymphoma like lesion in human orthotopic cardiac allografts. Am J Clin Pathol 1988;89:430.
95. Eisen HJ, Hicks D, Kant JA, et al. Diagnosis of post-transplantation lymphoprolipherative disorders by endomyocardial biopsy in cardiac allograft recipients. J Heart Lung Transplant 1994;13:241–245.

Amyloidosis

96. Pelosi F Jr., Capehart J, Roberts WC. Efectivness of cardiac transplantation for primary (AL) cardiac amyloidosis. Am J Cardiol 1997;79:532–535.
97. Fernandez AL, Herreros JM, Monzonis AM, et al. Heart transplantation for Finnish type familial systemic amyloidosis. Scand Cardiovasc J 1997;31:357–359.
98. Valantine HA, Billingham ME. Recurrence of amyloid in cardiac allograft four months after transplantation. J Heart Lung Transplant 1989;8:337–341.
99. Hosenpud JD, Uretsky BF, Griffith BP, et al. Successful intermediate-term outcome for patients with cardiac amyloidosis undergoing heart transplantation: results of a multicenter survey. J Heart Lung Transplant 1990;9:346–350.
100. Hosenpud JD, DeMarco T, Frazier OH, et al. Progression of systemic disease and reduced long-term survival in patients with cardiac amyloidosis undergoing heart transplantation. Follow-up results of a multicenter survey. Circulation 1991;84:III-338–III-343.
101. Dubrey S, Simms RW, Skinner M, et al. Recurrence of primary (AL) amyloidosis in a transplanted heart with four-year survival. Am J Cardiol 1995;76:739–741.
102. Hall R, Hawkins PN. Cardiac transplantation for AL amyloidosis. BMJ 1994;309:1135–1137.
103. Deng M, Park JW, Roy-Choudury R, et al. Heart transplantation for restrictive cardiomyopathy: development of cardiac amyloidosis in preexisting monoclonal gammopathy. J Heart Lung Transplant 1992;11:139–141.

Sarcoidosis

104. Barbers RG. Role of transplantation (lung, liver, and heart) in sarcoidosis. Clin Chest Med 1997;18:865–874.
105. Shammas RL, Movahed A. Successful treatment of myocardial sarcoidosis with steroids. Sarcoidosis 1994;11:37–39.
106. Shammas RL, Movahet A. Sarcoidsis of the heart. Clin Cardiol 1993;16:462–472.
107. Oni AA, Hershberger RE, Norman DJ, et al. Recurrence of sarcoidosis in a cardiac allograft: control with augmented corticosteroids. J Heart Lung Transplant 1992;11:367–369.
108. Valantine HA, Tazelaar HD, Macoviak J, et al. Cardiac sarcoidosis: response to steroids and transplantation. J Heart Transplant 1987;6:244–250.
109. Burke WM, Keogh A, Maloney PJ, et al. Transmission of sarcoidosis via cardiac transplantation. Lancet 1990;336:1579.

Allograft Vasculopathy

110. Schroeder JS, Hunt SA. Chest pain in heart transplant recipients. N Engl J Med 1991;324: 1805–1807.
111. O'Connell JB, Bourge RC, Costanzo-Nordin MR, et al. Cardiac transplantation: recipient selection, donor procurement, and medical follow-up. A statement for health professionals from the committee on cardiac transplantation of the Council on Clinical Cardiology, American Heart Association. Circulation 1992;86:1061–1079.
112. Gao S-Z, Hunt SA, Schroeder JS, et al. Early development of accelerated graft coronary artery disease: risk factors and course. J Am Coll Cardiol 1996;28:673–679.
113. Miller LW, Wolford TL, Donohue TJ, et al. Cardiac allograft vasculopathy: new insight from intravascular ultrasound and coronary flow measurements. Transplant Rev 1995;9:77–96.
114. Topol EJ, Nissen SE. Our preocupation with coronary luminology, the dissociation between clinical and angiographic findings in ischemic heart disease. Circulation 1995;92:2333–2342.
115. Johnson DE, Gao S-Z, Schroeder JS, et al. The spectrum of coronary artery pathologic findings in human cardiac allografts. J Heart Lung Transplant 1989;8:349–359.
116. Pucci AM, Forbes RDC, Billingham ME. Pathologic features in long term cardiac allografts. J Heart Lung Transplant 1990;9:339–345.
117. Winters GL, Schoen FJ. Graft arteriosclerosis-induced myocardial pathology in heart transplant recipients: predicitve value of endomyocardial biopsy. J Heart Lung Transplant 1997;16:985–993.
118. Aretz HT, Colvin RB. Endomyocardial biopsies. An early warning system for chronic transplant arteriopathy. JAMA 1997;278:1197–1198.
119. Labarree CA, Nelson DR, Faulk WP. Endothelial activation and development of coronary artery disease in transplanted human hearts. JAMA 1997;278:1169–1175.

Therapeutic Intervention

120. Laufer G, Lackovics A, Wollenek G, et al. The progression of mild acute cardiac rejection evaluated by risk factors analysis: the impact of maintenance steroids and serum creatinine. Transplantation 1991;51:184–189.
121. Winters G, Loh E, Schoen FJ. Natural history of focal moderate cardiac allograft rejection. Is treatment warranted? Circulation 1995;91:1975–1980.
122. Brunner La Rocca HP, Sutsch G, Schneider J, et al. Natural course of moderate cardiac allograft rejection (International Society for Heart Transplantation Grade 2) early and late after transplantation. Circulation 1996;94:1334–1338.
123. White JA, Guiraudon C, Pflugfelder PW, et al. Routine surveillance endomyocardial biopsies are unnecessary beyond one year after heart transplantation. J Heart Lung Transplant 1995;14:1052–1056.
124. Sethi GK, Kosaraju S, Arabia FA, et al. Is it necessary to perform surveillance endomyocardial biopsies in heart transplant recipients. J Heart Lung Transplant 1995;14:1047–1051.
125. Frigerio M, Bonacina E, Gronda E, et al. A semiquantitative approach to the evaluation of acute cardiac rejection at endomyocardial biopsy. J Heart Lung Transplant 1997;16:1087–1098.
126. Rizeq MN, Masek MA, Billingham ME. Acute rejection: significance of elapsed time after transplantation. J Heart Lung Transplant 1994;13:862–868.
127. Kobashigawa JA. Treatment of nonhemodynamic compromising rejection: conventional approaches vs individualization /new immunosuppressive drugs. Transplant Proc 1997;29:(Suppl 8)37–39.
128. Kirklin JK, Bourge RC, McGiffin DC. Recurrent of persistent cardiac allograft rejection: therapeutic options and recommendations. Transplant Proc 1997;29:(Suppl 8)40–44.
129. Jollow KC, Sundstrom JB, Gravanis MB, et al. Apoptosis of mononuclear cell infiltrates in cardiac allograft biopsy specimens questions studies of biopsy cultured cells. Transplantation 1997;63:1482–1489.

10. CLINICAL DIAGNOSIS AND MANAGEMENT OF CARDIAC ALLOGRAFT REJECTION AND MAINTENANCE IMMUNOSUPPRESSION

Thomas G. Di Salvo, MD, MPH and
G. William Dec, MD
Heart Failure and Cardiac Transplantation Center,
Massachusetts General Hospital Boston, MA

CLINICAL DIAGNOSIS OF CARDIAC ALLOGRAFT REJECTION

Clinical Features of Acute Cellular Rejection

Early and Initial Cellular Rejection

Despite improvements in immunosuppression, cardiac rejection accounts for substantial morbidity and mortality following cardiac transplantation (Table 1). In the Cardiac Transplant Research Database (CTRD) studies, the mean cumulative number of treated rejection episodes per patient was 0.8, 1.10, and 1.3 at 3, 6, and 12 months post-transplant, repectively (Figure 1A).[1,2] Actuarial freedom from first treated rejection episode was 39% at 6 months and 37% at 12 months (Figure 1B). Overall, more than 90% of all rejection episodes occur in the first six months post-transplant.[3]

In a CTRD study, younger recipient age and female donor gender were the only independent predictors of early treated rejection episodes.[1] In a separate CTRD study, rejection within six months post-transplant was more frequent in white recipients with a higher number of HLA mismatches.[2] In smaller studies, other factors associated with increased risk of rejection have included human leukocyte antigen mismatch,[4] non-O blood types, panel reactive antibody screen >10%, positive donor specific crossmatch, OKT3 murine monoclonal antibody sensitization, cytomegalovirus infection,[5] other infections,[6] the presence of anti-HLA antibodies,

Address for correspondence: Thomas G. Di Salvo, MD, MPH, MGH Heart Failure Center, Massachusetts General Hospital, 55 Fruit St., Boston, MA 02114, Phone: 617-726-9230, Fax: 617-726-4105,
Email: tdisalvo@partners.org

Table 1. Epidemiology of Cardiac Allograft Rejection

Timing of Rejection
90% occur in the first six months post-transplant
Rare beyond 12 months post-transplant without decrement in immunosuppression
Risk Factors for Rejection
Factors which increase risk of rejection:
Female gender
High titer PRA pre- or post-transplant
Positive donor-specific crossmatch
Preoperative myocarditis
Factors which decrease risk of rejection:
Recipient >55 years of age
Triggers of Rejection
Tapering of immunosuppressive therapy
CMV Infection
Other infections

preoperative biopsy-proven myocarditis, and younger repicient age.[7] Due to the risk of sensitization during pregnancy, multiparous females have an increased risk of antibody-mediated rejection.[2] Acute rejection is less common in recipients over the age of 55, probably due to age-dependent modulation of immune reactivity.[2,8]

Late and Recurrent Rejection

A multicenter study of late recurrent rejection demonstrated that only 3% and 2% of patients had their first rejection episodes in the second or third post-transplant years, respectively.[9] By two years post-transplant, 33% of patients will not have experienced any rejection.[2] During the second through fourth years, the mean rejection episodes per patient were 0.18, 0.13, and 0.002 episodes, repectively. The highest likelihood for recurrent rejection occured within 2 months after a preceding rejection episode (Figure 2). Independent risk factors for recurrent rejection during the first year post-transplant include younger recipient age, female recipient gender, positive CMV serology, female donor, use of OKT3 induction therapy, earlier time since transplantation or previous rejection therapy, and greater number of previous infections. Independent risk factors for recurrent rejection after the first year post-transplant included female recipient, black recipient, use of OKT3 induction therapy, greater number of rejections, and prior CMV infections. Rejection beyond five years post-transplant is distinctly unusual without preceeding change in immunsuppression.[10]

Possible Triggers

The triggers precipitating cellular rejection remain speculative. Based on prior studies, however, clinical vigilance should be exercised in patients with recent rejection or recent decrement in immunosuppressive therapy. Recipients with gender-recipient mismatch, HLA mismatch and new or reactivated CMV infection (and other infection) appear to be at greater cumulative risk of rejection.

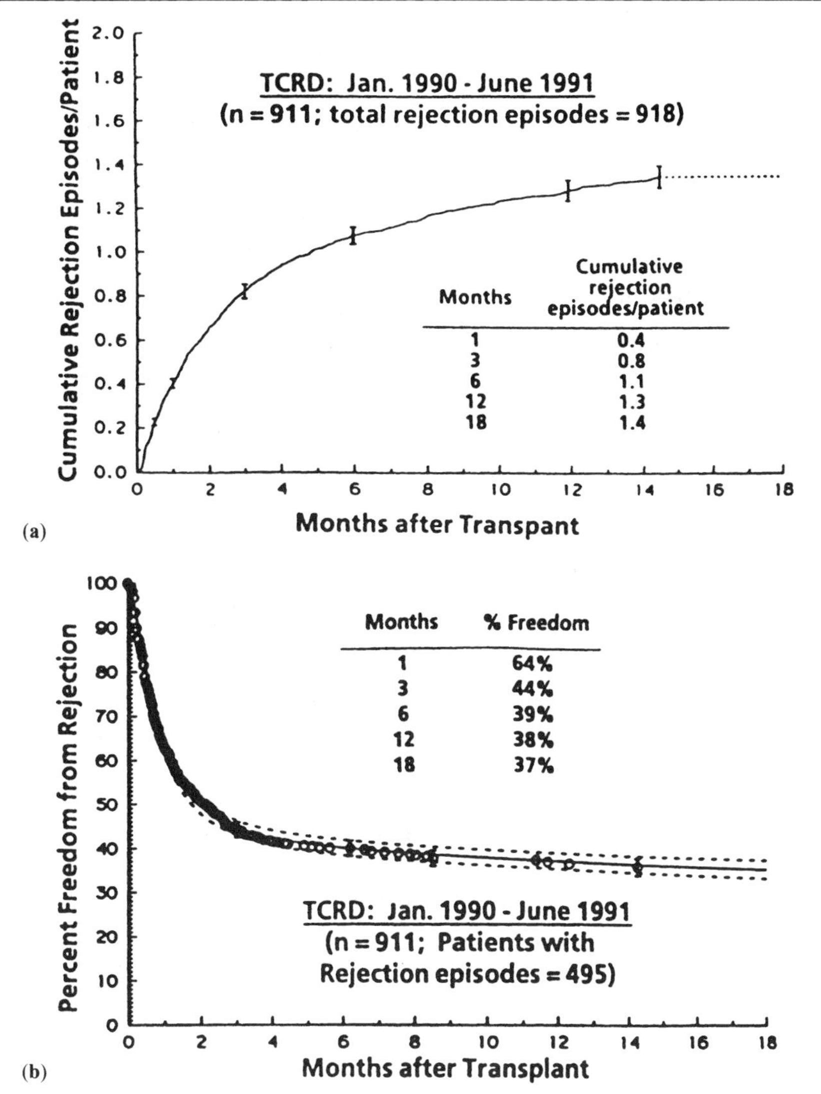

Figure 1. Panel A: Kaplan-Meier estimate of actuarial freedom from first rejection from the TCRD database January 1990 through June 1991. The bars represent 70% confidence limits. Panel B: Cumulative distribution frequency for the cumulative number of rejection episodes per patient over time from the TCRD database January 1990 through June 1991. The dashed lines enclose the 70% confidence limits. From Kobishigawa et al. Pretransplantation Risk Factors for Acute Rejection after Heart Transplantation: A Multiinstitutional Study. J Heart Lung Transplant 1993;12:355–66, reprinted by permission.

Rejection as a Cause of Death

Mortality from rejection has decreased in the current era of more effective immunosuppressive therapy. From 1980 to 1990, rejection accounted for 30% of post-transplant mortality.[11] Between 1990 and 1996, rejection accounted for approx-

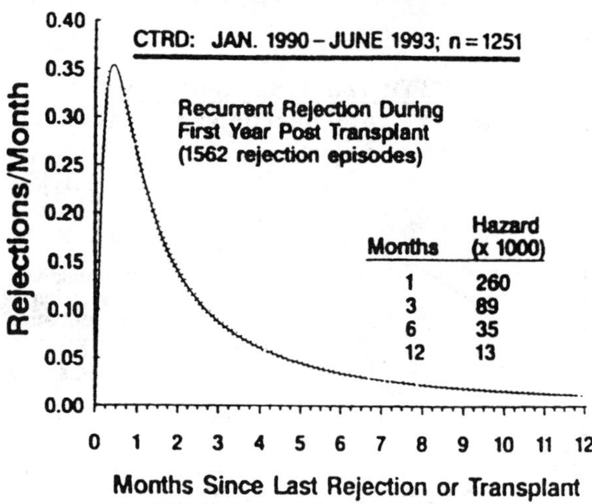

Figure 2. Hazard function for subsequent rejection after either heart transplantation or any rejection episode during the first year after heart transplantation. From Kubo et al., Risk factors for late recurrent rejection after heart transplantation: A multiinstitutional multivariate analysis. J Heart Lung Transplant 1995;14:409–18, reprinted by permission.

imately 15–26% of post-transplant mortality.[1,12,13] The risk of mortality from rejection is greatest in the first two months following transplantation.[13,14] Rejection may also result in late mortality. In recent ISHLT registries, the most common causes of death beyond the first year were cardiac allograft vasculopathy, malignancy, and rejection (Figure 3).[12] There is a low but constant hazard of mortality from rejection beyond the first transplant year.[10,13] By multivariable analysis, female and black recipients are at highest risk of death from rejection.[2]

Diagnosis of Acute Allograft Rejection

Clinical Symptoms and Signs

In the cyclosporine era, most rejection episodes are asymptomatic.[1,15] Symptoms of rejection, when present, tend to be non-specific and often subtle deriving from either systemic or pulmonary congestion (edema or right upper quadrant tenderness due to hepatomegaly and orthopnea, cough or exertional dyspnea, repectively), a systemic low-output state (fatigue, orthostasis, anorexia or post-prandial nausea), or ventricular arrhythmias (palpitations, dizziness, syncope). Atrial and ventricular arrhythmias are unreliably related to rejection as they may occur in up to 55–79% of recipients during initial hospitalization and in up to 39–43% of recipients during long-term follow-up.[16] In particular, atrial arrhythmias occur not infrequently in the denervated transplanted heart, often in the absence of significant rejection.[17] New-onset atrial flutter,[18,19] bradyarrhythmias,[20] or ventricular arrhythmias[19,21] should always heighten the clinical suspicion of acute rejection, however. Signs of rejec-

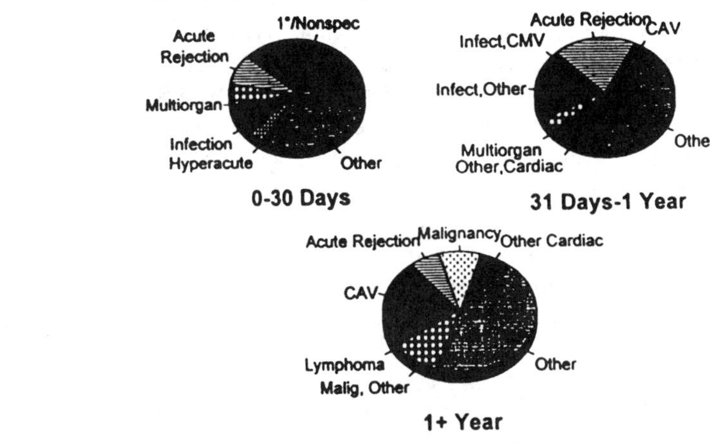

Figure 3. Heart transplantation cause of death by time after transplantation. CMV, Cytomegalovirus, CAV, cardiac allograft vasculopathy. From Hosenpud J et al., The registry of the International Society for Heart and Lung Transplantation: Fourteenth Official Report-1997. J Heart Lung Transplant 1997;16:691–712, reprinted by permission.

tion-related alterations in allograft function are typically absent in mild to moderate rejection. New findings on examination of tachycardia (heart rate >15 bpm above usual resting rate), relative hypotension (systolic blood pressure <20 mmHg less than prior values), orthostasis, jugular venous distension, a left ventricular third sound, AV regurgitant murmurs, hepatomegaly or edema should always raise the possibility of acute rejection.

Non-invasive Testing: Cardiac Functional Assessment

Currently available non-invasive modalities cannot reliably diagnose allograft cellular rejection. In the pre-cyclosporine era, a decrease in summated surface 12-lead ECG R wave amplitude resulting from myocardial edema was a reasonably reliable sign of acute allograft rejection.[15,22] Loss of R-wave amplitude is uncommon in cyclosporine-treated patients, however, and the ECG in rejection is often unchanged or non-specifically abnormal. The chest x-ray as a rule does not evidence cardiomegaly, interstitial or alveolar edema, or pleural effusion. Two-dimensional echocardiography is insensitive for mild rejection,[23,24] and may be falsely reassuring even in moderate to severe cellular rejection.[25] In the occasional patient with moderate to severe rejection, significant increase in myocardial wall thickness (>2 mm), decline in ejection fraction (>10%), or new segmental wall motion abnormalities[26] may occur. Pericardial effusion is a less specific echocardiographic sign of rejection.[27] No single conventional echocardiographic parameter has sufficient sensitivity or specificity for routine clinical decision-making purposes (see Chapter 14).[28,29]

Given the limitations of currently available non-invasive diagnostic modalities, much research has focused on the development of more sensitive modalities (see

Chapter 13).[30] Spectral frequency analysis of of the amplified surface electrocardiogram after fast Fourier transformation detects rejection better than analysis of QRS amplitude.[31] Significant decreases in paced epimyocardial electrogram amplitude have been reported with a sensitivity and specificity of 80–85% of detecting ISHLT grade 2 or greater rejection.[32] Intramyocardial electrograms may be useful in the detection of rejection.[33–35] Signal-averaged electrocardiography has a reported sensitivity of 69% and specificity of 71% for the detection of clinically relevant rejection[36] and may show a relative decrease in the high-frequency components of the signal-averaged electrocardiogram.[37] In animal models, high-resolution atrial electrocardiography for the detection of conduction disturbances[38] and intramyocardial leads measuring changes in unipolar peak-to-peak amplitude appear to be accurate means of detecting rejection.[39] Several novel doppler[28,36,40–44] and tissue acoustical characterization techniques[28–29,45–47] may enhance the sensitivity of echocardiography in the diagnosis of rejection. None of these promising techniques is readily or widely available in human recipients, however.

Non-invasive Testing: Myocardial Imaging

Indium 111-labeled antimyosin antibody scintigraphy appears to be a promising non-invasive technique in routine rejection surveillance (see Chapter 20).[48–53] Myocardial uptake of antimyosin antibodies parallels rejection activity by biopsy.[53] Given its reported negative predictive value of 98%, antimyosin scinitgraphy may be especially useful in avoiding biopsy following the first transplant year.[50,53–55] During the first year post-transplant, however, antimyosin scintigraphy has a high false-positive rate, and may be less clinically useful.[55] Dipyridamole stress testing with thallium scinitigraphy reported sensitivity of 72% in the detection of rejection.[56] Thallium uptake decreases during rejection episodes but thallium imaging may be insensitive in the detection of modest degrees of rejection.[57] In experimental animals rejection has been associated with abnormal myocardial bioenergetics, perfusion, and T2 relaxation times by magnestic resonance spectroscopy.[58–61]

Non-invasive Testing: Biochemical and Immunologic Assays

There are currently no reliable biochemical or immunologic assays reliable enough for clinical use in the diagnosis of acute cellular rejection. Neither characterization of T-cell subsets[62] nor cytoimmunologic monitoring of peripheral blood for the presence of activated lymphocytes[63] is sufficiently sensitive or specific enough to influence treatment. Although certain cytokines may be elevated in coronary sinus effluent during rejection,[64] there is no consistent relationship between serum levels of Il-2, 4, 6, 10, soluble-interleukin-2-receptor, TNF-alpha, and IFN-gamma and biopsy-proven cellular rejection.[65–67] In a preliminary study, soluble vascular adhesion molecule-1 levels increased prior to biopsy-proven rejection.[65] Plasma endothelin levels are not a reliable marker of rejection.[68] Other modalities or serologic assays, including indium-111-labeled lymphocyte migration studies,[69] neopterine levels,[70] transferrin receptors,[71] hypoxanthine guanine phosphoribosyltransferase activity in

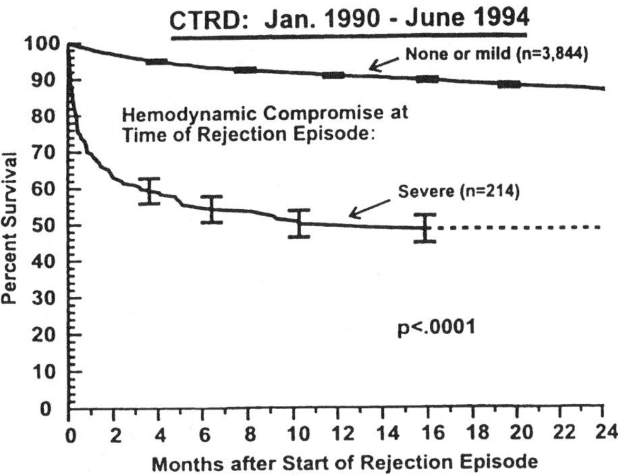

Figure 4. Actuarial survival after rejection episode. Upper curve indicates rejection with no or mild hemodynamic compromise, and lower curve rejection with severe hemodynamic compromise. Error bars enclose 70% confidence limits. From Mills et al. Heart transplant rejection with hemodynamic compromise: A multiinstitutional study of the role of endomyocardial cellular infiltrate. J Heart Lung Transplant 1997;16:813–21, reprinted by permission.

T cells,[72] breath pentane levels,[73] urinary polyamines,[74] serum prolactin levels,[75] IL-2 receptors,[76] beta-2 microglobulin levels,[77] antimyolemma/antisarcolemmma antibodies, troponin-T,[78] creatine kinase MB isoforms,[79] or serum myoglobin[80] are neither sufficiently sensitive nor specific for the diagnosis of cardiac rejection. Indium111 labeled anti-MHC class II antigen antibody imaging has shown promise in experimental animal models of rejection.[81]

Hemodynamics

Hemodynamic abnormalities do not correlate well with the histologic grade of cellular rejection.[82] Significant elevation of right or left ventricular filling pressures or decline in cardiac output are unusual during mild to moderate rejection, but are not infrequent during severe rejection. Acute diastolic dysfunction may occur during moderate rejection, and place recipients at risk for late restrictive-constrictive physiology.[83]

Rejection with hemodynamic compromise (defined as a change in echocardiographic left ventricular systolic function or the need for pharmacologic inotropic support) accounts for 5% of treated rejection episodes.[84] Multivariable recipient risk factors for its occurrence include recipient black race, female gender and diabetes mellitus. Outcome remains poor, with 3-month actuarial survival of only 60% (Figure 4). Among survivors, patients with lesser grades of ISHLT rejection on endomyocardial biopsy generally have lower two year mortality rates than patients with higher grades of ISHLT rejection (46% vs 84% survival, respectively).

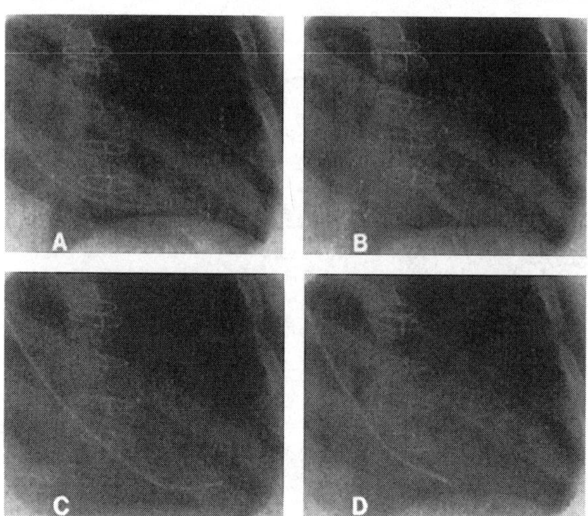

Figure 5. The technique of endomyocardial biopsy with a 45 cm sheath. A pigtail catheter is placed into the right ventricle (A). The sheath is advanced over the catheter into the right ventricle and the pigtail catheter is removed (B). The bioptome is passed through the sheath, and the jaws are opened as the tip of the bioptome emerges. The bioptome is advanced until contact with the ventricular septum is made ©. After the sample is taken the bioptome is withdrawn, leaving the sheath in the right ventricle in position for subsequent biopsies (D). From Williams et al. Biopsy-induced flail tricuspid leaflet and tricuspid regurgitation following orthotopic cardiac transplantation. Am J Cardiol 1996;7:1339–44, reprinted by permission.

Pediatric Considerations

Surveillance endomyocardial biopsy in children remains controversial given the morbidity of biopsies in children.[85,86] In most centers, serial echocardiography is used to detect rejection, particularly in infants and younger children.[86] Unfortuantely, systolic echocardigraphic indices in children correlate poorly with degree of rejection by biopsy.[86,87] Although no gold standard exists, better methods of echocardiographic edge detection[88] or ultrasonic tissue characterization hold promise.[47]

Endomyocardial Biopsy

Percutaneous endomyocardial biopsy was first described by Caves in 1973.[89] At the Massachusetts General Hospital, endomyocardial biopsy is performed by percutaneous entry of the internal jugular vein with a 45 cm 8FR sheath inserted over a guidewire and dilator.[90] After removal of the dilator, a 8FR pigtail catheter is advanced flouroscopically over a guidewire through the sheath to the RV apex (Figure 5). The sheath is advanced over the pigtail catheter into the right ventricle and the pigtail catheter is removed. After aspitation and flushing of the sheath, a 50 cm 7Fr bioptome is inserted through the sheath and at four to six tissue myocar-

Table 2. Indications for Non-Scheduled Biopsies

Clinical Features
New or suspected allograft dysfunction
Pulmonary or systemic congestion
Tachycardia
Hypotension
Fatigue
Dizziness or orthostasis
Arrhythmias
New atrial or ventricular
Echocardiographic Features
10% of greater decline in ejection fraction
2 mm or greater increase in left ventricular wall thickness
Significant left ventricular dilation (>5 mm)
New pericardial effusion
New segmental wall motion abnormalities
Hemodynamics
8–10 mm Hg increase in pulmonary capillary wedge pressure
>25% decline in cardiac output

dial tissue specimens are obtained from the right ventrciular septum endomyocardium. Percutaneous transvenous biopsy may also be performed from femoral vein,[91] external jugular vein,[92] and left subclavian vein.[93] In selected instances, left ventricular biopsy by using longer sheaths and bioptomes can be performed.[93]

Adult recipients undergo scheduled endomyocardial biopsies. Biopsies are initially performed weekly in adults for the first month and then every 2–4 weeks over the next two months. Biopsy frequency is decreased to every 3–4 months for the remainder of the first year and to every six months during the second year in non-rejectors.

Non-scheduled biopsies are indicated for clinically suspected rejection (Table 2). Such indications include new or suspected symptomatic heart failure, arrhythmias, unexplained tachycardia or hypotension, and echocardiographic abnormalties as discussed above.

Complications of Biopsy

The rate of serious complications following percutaneous transvenous endomyocardial biopsy in transplant recipients is 0.3–0.7%.[94,95] Complications include carotid artery puncture, pneumothorax, right ventricular perforation, supraventricular or ventricular arrhythmias, embolization, formation of coronary artery-right ventricular fistulae at biopsy sites,[96] vasovagal reactions, prolonged bleeding, and fibrosis at prior skin puncture sites.[97] Flail tricuspid valve leaflet resulting in significant tricuspid regurgitation occurs with use of a shorter 10 cm and is reduced by use of a longer 45 cm sheath placed across the tricuspid which directs the bioptome away from the tricuspid valve appartatus.[90]

ISHLT Grading Scheme

The International Society of Heart and Lung Transplantation working formulation for biopsy interpretation was adopted in 1990[98,99] (see Chapter 9). The purpose of the working formulation was to provide a simple and reproducible grading system for cellular allograft rejection. The two most significant histopathologic findings are 1) the extent, type, and location of inflammatory cell infiltrate and 2) the presence and degree of associated myocyte necrosis. Controversy continues as to whether endocardial infiltrates (so-called "Quilty" lesions) are associated with rejection.[100] The Loyola experience suggests that endocardial infiltrates are not only associated with biopsy-proven rejection but also predict future rejection episodes.[101] The Zurich experience reported that Quilty lesions were independent predictors of progression of grade 2 biopsies to higher degress of rejection.[102] Other studies have not observed such an association.[103]

According to the ISHLT grading schema, biopsy interpretation concordance between experienced pathologists is seen in about 85% of biopsies; 81% of discrepancies arise in distinguishing grade 1A/B vs 2, grade 2 vs 3A, and 2/3A vs Quilty B.[104] In particular, greater precision in the diagnosis of grade 2 rejection is necessary.[100,105] In the first four to six weeks following transplantation, distinguishing rejection from perioperative ischemic myocardial injury remains challenging, especially since the two may coexist.[106]

A close correlation exists between right ventricular biopsy results and the autopsy grade of rejection (r = 0.86, Table 5).[107] Specificity is high for all ISHLT grades of rejection, but sensitivity is much less for mild to moderate grades of rejection. There appears to be no advantage to routine sampling of left ventricular myocardium. At least four fragments of myocardium at a minimum are required to exclude rejection with greater than 95% certainty.[108] If all four myocardial fragments are negative, there is only a 0.02% probability of missing clinically significant rejection. However, when mild rejection is present on one of four fragments, there is a 2% chance of underlying moderate to severe rejection; when all four fragments show mild rejection, there is a 28% chance of underlying moderate-severe rejection.

Role of Annual Biopsy

Several studies have reported a low yield of routine surveillance endomyocardial biopsies, particularly after the first post-transplant year. Sethi reported no difference in actuarial survival or freedom from rejection in patients who did not have surveillance biopsies beyond six months.[109] In another retrospective study, White reported that only 0.6% of 1,123 surveillance biopsies performed in 235 patients 1 year or more after transplantation revealed ISHLT grade 2 or greater rejection and that no late deaths were predicted on the basis of routine surveillance biopsy results.[103] Based on larger multicenter reports of the low but constant hazard of late cellular rejection and risk of late rejection mortality,[12] many centers continue to perform 6 to 12 month routine surveillance biopsies indefinitely after transplantation.

Evaluation for Suspected Allograft Rejection: The Complementary Role of Echocardiographic and Endomyocardial Biopsy Findings and the Integration of Clinical Information

Echocardiographic assessment of allograft left ventricular wall thickness, chamber dimension, and systolic and diastolic function may provide important ancillary information in the clinical decision-making process in patients with mild to moderate grades of cellular rejection. This is particularly true when significant changes in allograft dimensions or function are discovered. In such instances, therapy of otherwise mild to moderate grades of cellular rejection should be carefully considered. Although echocardiography is not performed routinely at the time of every endomyocardial biopsy at our center, it is utilized when new or worsening symptoms or signs of allograft dysfunction or arrhythmias occur or when routine right heart catheterization reveals a 7–10 mmHg or greater increase in the pulmonary capillary wedge pressure or a 25% or greater decline in cardiac output.

All available clinical information should be considered when cellular rejection is suspected. Factors which should be considered include the prior history of rejection, time since transplantation, adequacy of current immunosuppressive therapy, clinical presentation, presence or absence of hemodynamic or echocardiographic abnormalities and the risk to the patient and the allograft of undiagnosed cellular rejection. Given the inherent limitations of all non-invasive modalities in the diagnosis of cellular rejection, the findings at endomyocardial biopsy must be heavily relied upon to establish the correct diagnosis. Occasionally, a significant decline in allograft function by echocardiography or right heart catheterization occurs despite the absence of cellular or vascular rejection or angiographically apparent allograft vasculopathy. Enhanced immunosuppression should be considered only after more detailed evaluation for rejection (repeat biopsy), coronary allograft vasculopathy (intracoronary ultrasound or assessment of coronary flow reserve by position emission tomography), and constrictive pericardial disease (magnetic resonance imaging of the pericardium) has been performed.[110]

MANAGEMENT OF CARDIAC ALLOGRAFT REJECTION

The Decision to Treat Cardiac Allograft Rejection

There is wide variation from center to center in the management of acute cellular rejection (Table 3).[7,111] Factors to consider in the management of acute cellular rejection include the clinical presentation, histologic severity of rejection, time since transplantation, prior history of rejection, allograft function, and morbidity of planned immunosuppressive therapy.

Significance of Mild Rejection (Grade 1A and 1B)

Approximately 80% of episodes of mild rejection resolve without treatment.[23,112] Long-term survival does not appear to be affected adversely by not treat-

Table 3. When to Treat Cardiac Allograft Rejection

Biopsy positive for cellular rejection:
ISHLT grade 3A or greater biopsy result
ISHLT grade 2 biopsy result associated with one of the following*:
10% fall in echocardiographic ejection fraction
New echocardiographic segmental wall motion abnormalities
25% or greater fall in cardiac output
Otherwise unexplained hypotension or tachycardia
New atrial of ventricular arrhythmias
Biopsy negative for cellular rejection, positive for vascular rejection
10% fall in echocardiographic ejection fraction
New echocardiographic segmental wall motion abnormalities
25% or greater fall in cardiac output
Otherwise unexplained hypotension or tachycardia
New atrial of ventricular arrhythmias
Biopsy negative for cellular rejection and vascular rejection:*
Otherwise unexplained hypotension
Clinically apparent heart failure
>15% fall in echocardiographic ejection fraction
New echocardiographic segmental wall motion abnormalites
Alloantibody demonstrated and decline in allograft function

* in the absence of progressive coronary allograft vasculopathy.

ing mild rejection.[112] Presently, only episodes of grade 1A or 1B rejection associated with allograft dysfunction are treated with enhanced immunosuppression. Although up to 37% of patients with mild rejection may evidence clinical or echocardiographic signs of some aspect of allograft dysfunction, signs of severe allograft dysfunction or arrhythmias warranting therapy occur in only approximately 10% of patients.[23] Approximately 30% of episodes with some sign of allograft dysfunction progress to higher histologic grades of rejection compared to 10% of episodes without signs of dysfunction.[23] Thus, untreated mild rejection episodes associated with some sign of allograft dysfunction necessitates increased surveillance at a minimum. Biopsy-proven myocardial necrosis is not requisite for immune-mediated impairment of allograft function.[23,110]

Signficance of Moderate Rejection (Grade 2 and 3A)

Grade 2 and 3A rejection may also resolve spontaneously without specific treatment in 80%–85% of cases.[102,112–114] Progression is more likely earlier within the post-transplant first year.[102,114] In the Zurich experience, repeat endomyocardial biopsy routinely performed 7–10 days following an ISHLT grade 2 biopsy revealed progression to grade 3A or greater rejection in 18.7%, grade 2 rejection in 21.9%, resolution of rejection in 59.4%.[102] Independent predictors of progression to grade 3A or greater included shorter period of time since transplant, lower cyclosporine level, blood group type B, "Quilty" lesions on prior biopsies, HLA mismatch, and younger recipient age. Risk of progression was greatest in the first few months after transplant, but progression could occur even late, prompting the authors to argue that ISHLT grade 2 rejection is not benign. Survival data was not presented. In the Padova experience, 256 ISHLT grade 2 biopsies progressed in 17.2%, remained unchanged in 16.8%, and resolved in 66%.[114] In the Brigham and Women's hospital experience in 208 consecutive recipients where grade 2/3A rejection was not routinely treated in the absence of hemodynamic compromise, there was no difference in long-term survival in patients with grade 2–3A rejection.[113] Based upon these findings, "early" grade 2 and grade 3A rejection (occurring within the first 6 months post-transplant) is treated in our center unless the level of maintenance immunosuppression is clearly inadequate at the time. "Late" grade 2 rejection (occurring after the first 6 months post-transplant) is treated if accompanied by any signs of hemodynamic or echocardiographic allograft dysfunction. "Late" grade 2 rejection unaccompanied by hemodynamic or echocardiographic signs of allograft dysfunction is not usually treated unless the recipient has a history of frequent or severe rejection. Repeat biopsy should always be performed within 14 days in untreated patients. Lack of resolution of rejection on a follow-up biopsy mandates treatment at our center. Grade 3A and higher grades of rejection are always treated.

Relation to Coronary Allograft Vasculopathy and Ventricular Dysfunction

The relation of the frequency or severity of cellular rejection episodes to coronary allograft vasculopathy remains controversial.[115–117] Most but not all retrospective studies have failed to find a relationship between either the frequency or severity of early or late rejection episodes and subsequent coronary allograft vasculopathy.[111,112,114,118–123] There appears to be no association between acute rejection and allograft myocardial collagen density[124] or coronary vascular reserve.[125] However, in several retrospective studies, repetitive nontreated episodes of grade 1B or 2 acute rejection have been reported to impair long-term allograft systolic[126] and diastolic function.[83] In a retrospective study, progression of grade 2 biopsies to higher degrees of rejection was associated with a greater risk of long-term cardiac allograft systolic dysfunction.[114] Prospective randomized trials of treatment of moderate grades of rejection are necessary to resolve the conflicting observations from these retrospective studies.[126]

Decision to Treat Biopsy-Negative "Rejection"

Allograft left ventricular dysfunction may occur in the absence of histologic rejection or angiographically apparent coronary allograft vasculopathy.[110] In a small series from our center, enhanced immunosuppression resulted in improvement in left ventricular function in seven of ten such patients, raising the possibility that immune-mediated phenomena in the absence of histologic rejection may result in reversible allograft dysfunction. Prior to empiric therapy with enhanced immunosuppresion, however, other causes of biopsy-negative allograft left ventricular dysfunction such as coronary allograft vasculopathy, cytomegalovirus infection and constrictive pericarditis must be excluded.

Available Therapeutic Agents and Protocols

Steroids

In histologically moderate to moderately severe rejection (ISHLT grade 2/3A) without hemodynamic compromise, an intravenous pulse of 500–1,000 mg of methylprednisolone daily for 3 days is successful in 85% of cases.[127,128] Of the non-responders, approximately half respond to a second course of intravenous steroids and the rest to antilymphocyte globulin.[127] Following an intravenous pulse, a steroid taper does not appear beneficial in decreasing subsequent rejection.[129] At our center, following an intravenous steroid pulse, the daily maintenance prednisone dose is usually doubled with subsequent tapering guided by the results of subsequent endomyocardial biopsies.

Oral prednisone may also be effective in treating moderate rejection.[130] Oral pulses of prednisone 500–1,000 mg total dose divided over seven to ten days, are successful in 65% of patients with acute rejection in the absence of hemodynamic compromise.[131] In a randomized trial of patients with asymptomatic moderate rejection (ISHLT grade 3A) without hemodynamic compromise, a seventeen day course of oral prednisone (100 mg daily for three days, followed by a taper to the previous maintenance dose of prednisone over 14 days) was as effective as 3 days of 1,000 mg of intravenous methylprednisolone.[132] For patients with asymptomatic moderate rejection (ISHLT grade 3A), 100 mg of prednisone for three days without a taper may also be effective in up to 75% of patients particularly if the rejection occurs more than 60 days after transplantation.[133] Oral prednisone treatment is especially useful in asymptomatic moderate rejection after the initial 3–6 posttransplant months.

Anti-lymphocyte Therapy

Histologically severe rejection (ISHLT grade 3B/4), rejection associated with hemodynamic compromise, and rejection refractory to steroids is usually treated with antilymphocyte antibody therapy.[7] OKT3, a murine monoclonal antibody specific for the T lymphocyte CD3 cell surface receptor, is effective in 90% of instances of hemodynamically significant or refractory rejection.[134–139] OKT3 5 mg per day is administered intravenously for 10–14 days. Adverse effects include a self-limited lymphokine-mediated systemic reaction (fever, nausea, malaise, headache, diarrhea), hypotension, bronchospasm, pulmonary edema, and aseptic meningitis.[137] Pretreatment with steroids, acetaminophen and diphenhydramine decreases the initial systemic reaction.[140] Longer-term risks include cytomegalovirus reactivation and post-transplant lymphoproliferative disease.

Cyclosporine, Tacrolimus, and Mycophenolate

The role of therapy with cyclosporine, tacrolimus, and mycophenolate in treating acute rejection is evolving. In a randomized trial of patients with mild acute rejection (ISHLT grade 1A and 1B), high dose oral cyclosporine aimed to increase the cyclosporine trough whole blood level 50% successfully resolved rejection in the majority of cases on repeat biopsy in 7–10 days and reduced the progression of mild to moderate rejection.[141] Tacrolimus and mycophenolate have been largely studied as "rescue" therapies for recurrent rejection (see below).

Selection of Appropriate Therapy and Specific Recommendations for Treatment of Acute Cellular Rejection

The selection of appropriate therapy for acute cellular rejection depends on the following factors in approximate order of clinical priority: 1) the histologic grade of rejection, 2) presence of absence of hemodynamic compromise, 3) presence or absence of allograft dysfunction by echocardiography, 4) adequacy of current immunosuppresive therapy, 5) level of current immunosuppression, 6) time since transplantation, 7) number and frequency of prior rejection episodes, 8) morbidity of therapy, 9) available immunosuppressive agents.

Table 4 outlines the approach to early and late cellular rejection. In most instances, early rejection (within the first 6 months post transplant) should be treated with a pulse of 500–1,000 mg of methylprednisolone intravenously daily for 3 days with re-biopsy in 7–10 days. This approach will reverse moderate to moderately severe early rejection in 85% of cases.[3] Early rejection that is more histologically severe (ISHLT grade 3B or 4), refractory to several courses of steroids, or associated with hemodynamic compromise should be treated with antilymphocyte antibody therapy. OKT3 is successful in nearly 90% of cases.[142] After the initial 6 months, moderate rejection without hemodynamic compromise can be safely and effectively treated with an oral "pulse" of prednisone.[132]

Recurrent or Refractory Cellular Rejection

Cellular rejection may recur despite enhanced immunosuppression or fail to respond to corticosteroids. *Persistent steroid-resistant rejection* has been defined as a course of rejection in which a biopsy grade 3A or greater is present on two or more successive biopsies 7 to 10 days apart, each treated with augmented IV or oral steroids.[143] *Recurrent steroid-resistant rejection* has been defined as three or more rejection episodes treated with augmented immunosuppression within a 2-month period.[143] Recipients with persistent or recurrent steroid-resistant rejection have usually received several courses of intravenous corticosteroids and a course of anti-lymphocyte antibody following intravenous corticosteroids. Enhanced maintenance immunosuppression is necessary in such recipients to prevent ongoing or future rejection. Options for enhanced immunosuppression include tacrolimus, mycophe-olate, methotrexate, total lymphoid irradiation, dactinomyin, plasmapheresis and photopheresis.

Table 4. Management of Cellular Rejection: MGH Protocol

Clincal/Histologic Situation	Agent	Protocol
Acute Cellular Rejection		
Mild (ISHLT < 2) rejection at any time post-transplant	Maintenance combination therapy	1. Rebiopsy per biopsy schedule 2. If suspect symptoms/signs develop, rebiopsy with echo
Moderate (ISHLT = 2) rejection within initial 3 months	IV Methylprednisolone	1. 500–1,000 mg daily for 3 days 2. Increase oral prednisone to 5 mg above prior dose 3. Rebiopsy in 10–14 days
Moderate rejection (ISHLT = 2) within initial 3–6 months	Prednisone	1. 1.5 mg/kg daily for 3 days 2. Taper over 14 days to 5 mg/kg above prior dose 3. Rebiopsy following taper
Moderate rejection (ISHLT = 2) beyond 6 months	Prednisone *or* maintenance combination therapy in selected patients	1. 1.0 mg/kg daily for 3 days 2. Taper beyond over 14 days to 5–10 mg above prior dose 3. Rebiopsy following taper 4. If elect to continue maintenance combination therapy only, re-biopsy in 10 days
Moderate rejection (ISHLT 3A, 3B) within initial 6 months	IV Methylprednisolone	1. 1,000 mg for 3 days 2. Increase prednisone to 5 mg/kg above prior dose 3. Rebiopsy in 7–10 days
Moderate or severe rejection (ISHLT 2–4) with hemodynamic compromise	Methylprednisolone + OKT3	1. Methyprednisolone 500–1,000 mg daily for 3 days 2. OKT3 5 mg/d for 7–10 days 3. Rebiopsy 7–10 days after completion of OKT3
Recurrent or Refractory Acute Cellular Rejection		
Moderate rejection (ISHLT 2, 3A, 3B)		1. Methylprednisolone 1 gram IV daily for 3 days 2. Increase cyclosporine to a achieve a trough level of 250 ng/dl *plus either* 3. Replacing azathioprine with mycophenolate 1 gram po bid or adding a fourth immunosuppresive agent (methotrexate, dactinomycin) *and considering* 4. Replacing cyclosporin with tacrolimus
Severe rejection (ISHLT 4) or moderate rejection (ISHLT 2, 3A, 3B) with hemodynamic compromise		1. Methylprednisolone 1 gram IV daily for 3 days 2. OKT3 5 mg/day for 10–14 days (or ATG if OKT3 has been recently given or CD3+ cell clearance is inadequate) 3. Replace cyclosporine with tacrolimus *plus either* 4. Replacing azathioprine with mycophenolate 1 gram po bid or adding a fourth immunosuppresive agent (methotrexate, dactinomycin) *and considering* 5. Total lymphoid irradiation or retransplantation for progressive left ventricular dysfunction

Tacrolimus

Tacrolimus (FK506) is a macrolide antibiotic with an immunosuppressive potency 100-fold greater than that of cyclosporine in vitro.[144] In small prospective controlled studies of tacrolimus compared to cyclosporine as maintenance immunosuppression in heart transplant recipients, tacrolimus resulted in a decreased rate or rejection and a steroid-sparinng effect.[145–147] Tacrolimus is also effective as "rescue" therapy in patients with recurrent or refractory rejection when substituted for cyclosporine as baseline immunosuppression.[144,148–150] Oupatient conversion from cyclosporine to tacrolimus (initial dose 0.1 mg/kg/day subsequently adjusted to a trough level of 15–20 ng/ml) has been reported to be safe in a relatively small cohort of patients with recent steroid-resistant cellular rejection.[150] At our center, tacrolimus is substituted for cyclosporine in patients with recurrent or refractory rejection and in selected patients following a single severe episode of rejection.

Mycophenolate

Mycophenolate mofetil (MMF), a morpholinoethyl ester of mycophenolic acid, is a semisynthetic fungal product which inhibits de novo purine biosynthesis by reversible, noncompetitive inhibition of inosine monophosphate dehydrogenase and guanylate synthase.[151,152] Unlike azathioprine, MMF is relatively selective for activated lymphocytes since activated lymphocytes are dependent on the de novo purine biosynthesis pathway for full expression of their prolierative response.

In preliminary non-randomized studies, MMF (1,000–1,500 mg twice daily) substituted for azathioprine was effective in the treatment of recurrent or persistent rejection.[151,153] In non-randomized high-risk patients at Utah, MMF was associated with low rates of recurrent rejection; resolution of 68% of episodes of mild (ISHLT grade 1B or 2) rejection was achieved by an increase in the dose of MMF alone.[152] As discussed below, MMF is now used in place of azathioprine in virtually all newly transplanted patients at our center. In addition, MMF is substituted for azathioprine in patients with a single episode of severe rejection and in most patients with more than one treated episode of moderate cellular rejection. Adverse effects common with MMF include nausea, dyspepsia, diarrhea, and leukopenia.[152]

Methotrexate

Methotrexate, an analogue of folic acid, competitively inhibits the enzyme deydro-folic reductase thereby inhibiting DNA synthesis and cellular proliferative responses to immune stimuli.[154] Methotrexate has been used effectively in cases of rejection refractory to standard triple-drug maintenance therapy in intravenous doses ranging from 10–50 mg weekly for 1–5 weeks[154] and in oral doses of 2.5–15 mg 1 day/week for three consecutive weeks[155] and doses of 5 mg on two successive days per week (10 mg/week) for a total of 6 weeks.[156] In a retrospective review from Stanford, methotrexate appeared as effective as total lymphoid radiation for patients with persistent or recurrent cellular rejection.[157] Although patients with recurrent rejection treated with methotrexate experience a decrease in rejection rates compared to untreated patients, their overall rates of rejection remain higher than in non-rejecting patients.[158] Methotrexate has also been successfully used as rescue and adjuvant immunotherapy in children.[159] An increased incidence of leukopenia (which may be delayed for several weeks following methotrexate) and infection have been reported.

Total Lymphoid Irradiation

Total lymphoid irradiation (TLI) is low-dose radiotherapy directed at major lymph node chains and immune effector organs, including cervical, axillary, mediastinal, periaortic and iliofemoral lymph nodes and the thymus and spleen.[160] TLI has been used as rescue therapy in selected recipients with refractory rejection unresponsive to pulse corticosteroids and cytolytic therapy.[160–163] Typically, both an upper mantle field and lower inverted Y field are employed.[161] Treatment protocols vary, with fractions of 80 cGy delivered twice weekly for a total dose of 640–800 cGy.[161] Leukopenia and thrombocytopenia, which appear in the majority of patients,[160] may interrupt or abort the planned dosing schedule and appear following completion of therapy.[161] TLI appears effective in reversing histologic rejection in 40–80 % cases, but may not reverse ventricular dysfunction.[161,162] Since histologic rejection may recur after cessation of TLI,[161,162] enhanced immunosuppression therapy is required. The long-term risk of leukemia or lymphoma is not yet known.

Datinomycin

Actinomycin D, a crystalline chromopeptide antibiotic, inhibits lymphocyte proliferation and is a potent antitumor agent.[164] Actinomycin D was used in the early days of cardiac transplantation in the therapy of acute rejection.[165] In a more recent report in patients with recurrent cellular or humoral rejection, intravenous actinomycin 5 micrograms per kilogram every 6 weeks decreased the number of ISHLT grade 2 or higher endomyocardial biopsies and treated rejection episodes with a steroid-sparing effect and a paucity of significant adverse effects.[164] Its role in the current era of tacrolimus and mycophenolate is uncertain.

Plasmapheresis

Plasmapheresis, usually reserved for cases of proven or presumed vascular rejection, has been used in severe steroid-resistant mixed cellular and vascular rejection[166a] (see Chapter 12). Plasmapheresis is likely most effective when donor-specific anti-HLA class I or II antibodies are detected. Cyclophosphamide or MMF may be effective adjunctive agents given their potent B-cell suppressive effects (Table 5).

Table 5. Management of Vascular Rejection: MGH Protocol

Clinical/Histologic Situation	Protocol
Moderate Rejection	1. Plasmapheresis 3× weekly for 3 weeks 2. Methylprednisolone 1,000 mg IV qd × 3 days followed by an oral prednisone pulse with taper over 14 days 3. Increase cyclosporine dosing to achieve a trough level of >250 ng/dl 4. Replace azathioprine with cyclophosphamide 1–2 mg/kg daily or mycophenolate mofetil 1–2 grams/day 5. Consider replacement of cyclosporine with tacrolimus
Severe rejection	1. Plasmapheresis 3× weekly for 3 weeks 2. OKT3 5 mg/day for 10–14 days (or ATG if OKT3 has been recently given and CD3+ cell clearance is inadequate 3. Methylprednisolone 1,000 mg IV qd × 3 days followed by an oral prednisone pulse with taper over 14 days 4. Increase cyclosporine dosing to achieve a trough level of >250 ng/dl 5. Replace azathioprine with cyclophosphamide 1–2 mg/kg daily or mycophenolate mofetil 1–2 grams daily. 6. Replacement of cyclosporine with tacrolimus 7. Retransplantation for progressive left ventricular dysfunction

Phototherapy

The technique of phototherapy involves in vivo treatment of mononuclear cells with oral 8-methoxypsoralen, ex vivo exposure of selected treated cells to ultraviolet-A light via selective lymphocytapheresis, and subsequent in vivo reinfusion of the photoactivated cells.[167] The reinfusion of 8-methoxypsoralen treated photoactivated mononuclear cells results in a downregulation of immune responsiveness toward the graft by an as yet poorly understood mechanism. Phototherapy has been used sucessfully in highly sensitized patients at risk of rejection,[168] as therapy of non-hemodynamically significant moderate rejection,[167] as adjunctive therapy in the first six months following transplantation,[169] and as adjunctive therapy in patients with recurrent rejection.[170] When used as adjuntive therapy in patients with recurrent rejection, phototherapy reduces the histologic severity of rejection and may permit the reduction in the doses of cyclosporine, prednisone, and azathioprine.[170]

Retransplantation

Recurrent or refractory rejection is a controversial indication for retransplantation. Mortality following retransplantation is high with a one-year survival rate of only 40% and a five year survival of only 33%.[171,172] In a multicenter report, rejection as the reason for retransplantation was a predictor of mortality following retransplantation.[172] In the Stanford experience, the 1 year survival for patients retransplanted for rejection was only 33% compared to 69% for patients retransplanted for coronary allograft vasculopathy.[171] Thus, retransplantation for allograft loss due to rejection is usually not recommended.

Evolving Therapies

Evolving therapies for recurrent or refractory allograft rejection under investigation include novel monoclonal antibodies, rapamycin (in conjunction with tacrolimus), leflunimide, mizoribine, brequinar sodium, and 15-deoxyspergualin. These agents are discussed in detail in Chapter 11.

MAINTENANCE IMMUNOSUPPRESSION

Combination Immunosuppressive Maintenance Therapy

Combination maintenance therapy has been used since the initial days of cardiac transplantation as it affords appropriately potent immunosuppression while minimizing the adverse effects associated with individual immunosuppressive agents themselves.[165,7,173] Prior to the introduction of cyclosporine, most cardiac transplant recipients were treated with a chronic oral double-drug regimen of azathioprine and prednisone[165] with high rates of mortality and frequent rejection. The introduction of cyclosporine in 1981 ushered in the current era of combination maintenance immunosuppressive therapy and impressive declines in mortality and rejection.[174–176] The triple drug combination of 1) cyclosporine, 2) azathioprine or mycophenolate mofetil, and 3) prednisone remains the current standard maintenance immunosuppressive regimen for most heart transplant recipients.[7] Data supporting the efficacy of cyclosporine-based triple drug maintenance immunosuppression is based largely on retrospective studies, however.[175,177,178] Few randomized prospective trials of triple-drug versus double-drug immunosuppressive therapy have been performed. An Australian study randomized 112 patients to low-dose cyclosporine, azathioprine, and prednisolone versus cyclosporine and azathioprine.[179,180] Patients randomized to double-drug maintenance immunosuppression experienced signficantly more rejection and 47% of patients experienced sufficient rejection (four treated rejection episodes) to warrant cross-over to the triple-drug arm. In this small study, there was no difference in rates of 5-year survival infection, systolic function, or allograft coronary vasculopathy.

Triple-drug Maintenance Immunosuppressive Therapy

At our institution, virtually all recipients receive triple-drug maintenance immunosuppressive therapy (Table 6). Cyclosporine is a lipophilic, cyclic endecapeptide extracted from the fungus *Tolypocladium inflatum Gams*.[181] After entering the cell, cyclosporine binds to cyclophilin, an intracellular immunophilin.[182] The cyclosporin-cyclophilin complex then inhibits calcineurin, a calcium-dependent intracellular serine phosphatase pivotal in the signal transduction pathways leading to activation of multiple cytokine gene promoters. Inhibition of calcineurin activity results in diminished activation of transcription factors critical to the activation of transciption of T-cell modulatory cytokines such as IL-2, INF-g, IL-4, TNF-a, and

Table 6. MGH Immunosuppressive Protocol

Intraop:	Solumedrol 500 mg IV off bypass Azathioprine 5 mg/kg IV
Postop:	Post-op days 1–2: Solumedrol 125 mg IV q8 hrs Post-op day 3: start prednisone 80 mg bid Post-op days 4–7: taper prednisone to 40 mg qd Post-op days 7–14: taper prednisone to 30 mg qd As directed by biopsy results thereafter: decrease prednisone 2.5 mg if biopsy < ISHLT 2; once prednisone dose reaches 15 mg, taper more slowly by alternating present dose with 2.5 mg less than present dose; taper until prednisone dose reaches 5 mg/day. Cyclosporine: 5 mg/kg in divided doses bid; target trough level 250 ng/dl for first year, 150–200 ng/dl second year, 100–150 ng/dl subsequent years or Tacrolimus: adjusted to maintain trough levels of 10–12 ng/dl Azathioprine: 2 mg/kg po daily, adjusted to maintain WBC >4,000 mm^3 or Mycophenolate: 1 gram po bid, adjusted to maintain WBC >4,000 mm^3

CD40 ligand. In the absence of these T-cell modulatory cytokines, diminished T cell activation and proliferation result. The degree of immunosuppressive effect is correlated with the cyclosporine trough level.[183]

Individual patients may exhibit up to three-fold differences in the relative bioavailability of the same dose of cyclosporine.[184] The relative bioequivalence of intravenous to oral cyclosporine dosages is approximately 1 : 3.[181] Cyclosporine is metabolized by the hepatic cytochrome P-450 enzyme system. Drugs which inhibit the cytochrome P-450 enzyme system (ketoconazole, erythromycin, oral contraceptives, androgens, methylprednisolone, diltiazem, and verpamil) increase cyclosporine plasma levels and drugs which induce the cytochrome P-450 enzyme system (rifampin, phenobarbital, phenytoin, carbamazepine, valproate) decrease cyclosporine levels.[181] Whole blood levels of cyclosporine may be measured by either radioimmunoassay or high-performance liquid chromatography techniques.[181] Ketoconazole,[185] diltiazem, and verapamil[186] may permit smaller daily doses and promote renal-sparing effects.

The microemulsion cyclosporine preparation (Neoral, Novartis) improves absorption of cyclosporine from the promixmal small intestine and results in a 24% increase in cyclosporine exposure with little change in trough levels.[187,188] In a randomized trial of the newer microemulsion cyclosporine preparation versus the oil based formulation (Sandimmune) in over 380 patients at 24 centers, there was no difference in allograft or patient survival or renal dysfunction; less severe rejection (e.g., in particular rejection requiring antibody therapy) was noted in women treated with the microemulsion preparation.[189]

A large "head-to-head" comparison of cyclosporine and tacrolimus as maintenance immunosuppressive regimen has not been performed to date. A trial of tacrolimus (0.10–0.15 mg/kg/day in divided doses with a target trough level of 5–10 ng/ml) versus cyclosporine (6–8 mg/kg/day in divided doses with a target trough level of 150–250 ng/ml) in 85 patients at 6 centers showed no significant differences at 12 months in survival, incidence of rejection, renal function, hyperglycemia or kyperkalemia.[190] The incidence of hypertension requiring pharmacologic treatment (71% vs 48%, $p = 0.05$) and mean serum cholesterol at 3, 6 and 12 were both higher in the cyclosporine treated patients, however.

Adverse effects of cyclosporine include nephrotoxicity[191] leading to end-stage renal disease in up to 6% of transplant recipients who survive greater than 3 years,[192] hypertension due to sympathetic activation,[193] neurotoxicity,[194–197] tremor, hypertrichosis, gum hypertrophy, hyperuricemia due to decreased urate clearance,[198] hyperkalemia, hyperlipidemia, hyperlycemia, and hepatotoxicity.

Myocphenolate Mofetil (MMF)

In an ongoing 5-year, randomized, double-blind, active-controlled trial of 650 patients in 28 centers, MMF (3,000 mg/day) is being compared to azathioprine (1.5–3 mg/kg/day).[199] Approximately 11% of randomized, enrolled patients withdrew from the study prior to receiving study drug, primarily because of inability to extubate by post-transplant day two as specified in the study protocol. The one year study results have been reported for all randomized patients (enrolled patients) and for patients who actually received study medications (treated patients). Survival and rejection were similar in the enrolled patients (MMF, n = 337; azathioprine, n = 323). In the treated cohort (MMF, n = 289; azathioprine, n = 289), there were significant reductions in one year mortality (6.2% vs 11.4%, p = 0.031) and treated rejection episodes (65.7% vs 73.7 %, p = 0.026) in the MMF patients. In addition, there were trends in the treated MMF patients toward fewer grade 3A rejections (45% vs 52.9%, p = 0.055) and treatment with cytolytic therapy (15.2% vs 21.1%, p = 0.061). Opportunistic infections, predominantely herpes simplex, were more common in the MMF treated patients (53.3% vs 43.6%, p = 0.025). The three-year results in the treated patients continue to show improved graft survival (88.1% vs 81.6%, p = 0.029) without an increase in malignancy.[200] The importance of routine monitoring of MMF drug levels remains controversial. Some studies have reported a significantly decreased incidence of rejection when MMR trough levels are greater than 2–3 mg/l.[201,202] In addition, one observational, retrospective study reported that conversion from MMF to azathioprine late after transplantation resulted in both an increase in mean biopsy scores and episodes of rejection.[203]

Azathioprine

Azathioprine is a purine analogue which inhibits DNA synthesis and non-specifically suppresses the function of activated T and B cells, monocytes, and other immune effector cells.[204] A pro-drug, azathioprine is converted in the liver to the active metabolite 6-mercaptopurine which is in turn converted to the active metabolite thioinosinic acid. The major toxicity of azathioprine is bone marrow suppression. Any or all of the three major hematopoietic cell lines may be affected. Other adverse effects include hepatoxicity, alopecia, stomatitis, and acute pancreatitis. Due to its photosensitizing effects, azathioprine may increase the incidence of skin cancers post-transplantation. An important drug interaction may occur with allopurinol, an inhibitor of xanthine oxidase which also inhibits the metabolism of azathioprine. When given concurrently with allopurinol, the dose of azathioprine should be reduced by 25–33% to avoid excessive accumulation and toxicity. Azathioprine may also enhance the hematopoietic suppressive effects of ganciclovir and trimethoprim-sulfamethoxazole.

Prednisone

The exact immunosuppressive mechanism of corticosteroids remains obscure.[204] Corticosteroids likely work by inhibiting the activiation of transcription factors such as activator protein-1 (AP-1) and nuclear factor kappa b (NF-kB) which regulate the rate of transcription of the genes for multiple immune regulatory proteins. The immunosuppressive effects of corticosteroids are pleiotropic and include the suppression of macrophage function, inhibition of T cell proliferation, inhibition of cytokine and adhesion molecule production, alteration of leukocyte trafficking, and reduction of major HLA expresssion. In addition to these immunosuppressive effects, corticosteroids are also anti-inflammatory, likely due to the production of lipocortin, a protein inhibitor of phospholipase A2.

The adverse effects of steroids are often although not invariably dose-dependent and include glucose intolerance and diabetes, hypertension, increased appetite, fluid retention, Cushingoid features, mood alterations, acne, cataracts, avascular necrosis, osteoporosis, and myopathy.

Controversy Over Prophylactic Induction Cytolytic Therapy

At present, approximately 30% of transplant centers advocate routine use of induction cytolytic therapy with either OKT3 or ATG (antithymocyte globulin) following cardiac transplantation. The role of routine induction cytolytic therapy remains controversial and preferential, given the lack to date of a large prospective multicenter randomized controlled clinical trial of its efficacy.[140,205] OKT3 is a murine monoclonal antibody against the T cell surface CD3+ molecule complex.[140] The immunosuppressive effects of OKT3 result from both depletion of CD3+ positive T cells via opsonization and modulation and/or removal of CD3+ molecules from the T cell surface. OKT3 is usually administered as a 5 mg intravenous dose daily for 7 to 14 days. A 2.5 mg intravenous dose daily for 7 days may also be efficacious.[206] Efficacy of therapy is monitored by daily determinations of the concentration of circulating CD3 positive cells, which should be fewer than 25 cells per mm^3. In early single center reports, use of either OKT3[207–212] or ATG[213] induction therapy decreased the incidence of early rejection but did not decrease the cumulative incidence of rejection at six months.[208] When not used routinely, OKT3 is often used selectively to spare recipients the nephrotoxic effects of cyclosporine.[208]

Adverse effects of OKT3 include a cytokine release syndrome, the development of anti-murine antibodies, and an increased risk of infection and post-transplant lymphoproliferative disease (PTLD). The cytokine release syndrome is due to massive release of TNF and IFN-g. This syndrome, which typically commences within 15 to 30 minutes after administration of the first or second dose, usually results in a serum-sickness syndrome of fever, chills, nausea, diarrhea, headache, myalgia, and weakness. With more severe and fortunately less common reactions, acute bronchospasm, non-cardiogenic pulmonary edema, hypotension, and renal dysfunction may occur. Premedication with intravenous corticosteroids, diphenhydramine, and acetaminophen helps to minimize but not necessarily abrogate the reaction. Anti-murine antibodies develop in 14–27% of patients and should be measured 2–4 weeks after therapy particularly in patients in whom repeat treatment may be necessary. Low titers (<1 : 100) of such antibodies may not preclude re-treatment with OKT3.[214,215] However, titers in excess of 1 : 1,000, even if decreased in titer on subsequent determinations, preclude readministration of OKT3. In the Utah experience, sensitization as denoted by the formation of antimurine antibodies in excess of 1 : 100 has been associated with more frequent vascular rejection and early allograft loss due to rejection.[214] The incidence of infection, particularly reactivation of CMV infection, is increased.[216] The risk of CMV reactivation mandates antiviral chemotherapy with intravenous ganciclovir during the course of OKT3. Finally, the use of OKT3 in many, but not all reports, has been linked to an increase in risk of PTLD.[217] Doses in excess of 75 mg carry the greatest risk.

ATG is polyclonal anti-lymphocyte globulin prepared in rabbits or horses.[182,213,216] The immunosuppressive effects of ATG derive from opsonization of T cells and subsequent complement-mediated cytolysis and modulation of the activation responses of T cell surface molecules to proliferative stimuli. ATG is usually administered as a 10–15 mg per kg intravenous infusion over 24 hours. A cytokine release syndrome may occur after administration of ATG, but is usually milder than that seen with OKT3. Monitoring with peripheral blood lymphocyte counts or T cell subsets by flow cytometry is usual.

Major disadvantages of the use of induction cytolytic therapy include cost, the logistical problems of administration and increased incidence of infections and PTLD.[140,205] Major advantages include a lower incidence of early rejection and the need for lower doses of maintenance immunosuppressives.[205] The later is particularly appealing in patients with impaired renal function.

The role of newer, more targeted monoclonal antibodies is evolving. Daclizumab is a molecularly engineered human IgG1 monoclonal antibody that binds to but does not activate the high-affinity interleukin-2 receptor.[218] In a promising recent study, daclizumab given as induction therapy (1.0 mg/kg within 24 hours of transplantation and every two weeks thereafter for a total of 5 doses) reduced the frequency or rejection, (63% vs 18%, relative risk 2.8, 95% confidence interal 1.1–7.4, p = 0.04), severity of rejection and time to first rejection. Other antibodies are also under development. In a pilot study of 60 patients, the monoclonal interleukin-2 receptor antibody (BT563) was as effective as OKT3 in the prevention of acute rejection.[219] The effects of monoclonal antibodies targeted against various "accessory" T cell ligands (CD2, CD4, CD8, CD11a, CD18, CD28, CD5), antigen presenting cell ligands (CD58, MCH class II and I, CD54, B7-1, B7-2, CD72), adhesion molecules (LFA-1, ICAM-1), activated lymphocyte ligands (IL-2 receptor), T-cell costimulatory activation pathway components[220] in addition to immunoglobulin fusion proteins (CTLA4Ig) await future studies.[220,221]

Controversy Over Steroid-free Protocols

The role of steroid-free protocols in maintenance immunosuppression continues to be controversial.[222] Advantages of steroid-free protocols include a lower incidence of infections, lesser weight gain, fewer Cushingoid effects, and less hypercholesterolemia. Disadvantages include the increased vigilance required in rejection surveillance, the enhanced compliance required of the patient, enhanced toxicity of other immunosuppressives and uncertain effects on expense, late rejection and late coronary allograft vasculopathy.

In an early retrospective non-randomized report in 46 recipients, successful discontinuation of steroids was achieved in 52% of recipients who were maintained on cyclosporine and azathioprine following induction therapy with high-dose cyclosporine or ATG.[223] Patients weaned from steroids had later and less frequent rejection, less weight gain and a 54% reduction in infections. Weaning was less likely to be successful in women, patients with preoperative positive cross-match and prior cardiac surgery. In a later retrospective report of the cumulative experience in 416 recipients, 30% of patients had early (within 3 months of transplant) successful withdrawl of steroids.[224] Male gender was the only independent predictor of successful early corticosteroid withdrawl. The incidence of late rejection (greater than 1 year after transplant) was significantly less in patients withdrawn from corticosteroids. In multivariate analysis, independent predictors of mortality included the frequency of infections, older age, failed early corticosteroid withdrawal, and female gender. The Utah group concluded that successful early corticosteroid withdrawal identifies a subgroup of "immunologically privileged" recipients at low risk of late rejection and mortality. Several smaller single-center reports corroborate the Utah experience.[225–228]

One prospective randomized trial of corticosteroid withdrawal has been reported.[229] Of the 53 patients randomized to corticosteroid withdrawl, 47% were converted to maintenance steroids for resistant rejection.[180] Rejection was more frequent in the corticosteroid withdrawl group. The incidence of hyperlipidemia and hypertension were higher in the triple-agent group, but the incidence of steroid-related morbidity (diabetes, bone complications, cataracts, obesity) was not different. In a retrospective review of the cumulative experience at the same institution, a success rate of 69% was reported during initial withdrawal with no adverse effects. The authors concluded that 50% of recipients can be safely weaned from steroids but that predictive markers for likely success of steroid withdrawal are needed. The protocol for steroid withdrawal at the MGH appears in Table 7. Steroid withdrawal protocols should be individualized based on the frequency and severity of previous rejection episodes.

Novel Agents: HMG-CoA Reductase Inhibitors

Pravastatin, a HMG-CoA reductase inhibitor, reduces hypercholesterolemia following transplantation.[230] In a prospective, randomized, open-label trial, pravastatin therapy (daily dose 40 mg) resulted in a significantly lower mean cholesterol level (196 ± 36 vs 248 ± 49 mg/dL), less frequent rejection accompanied by hemodynamic

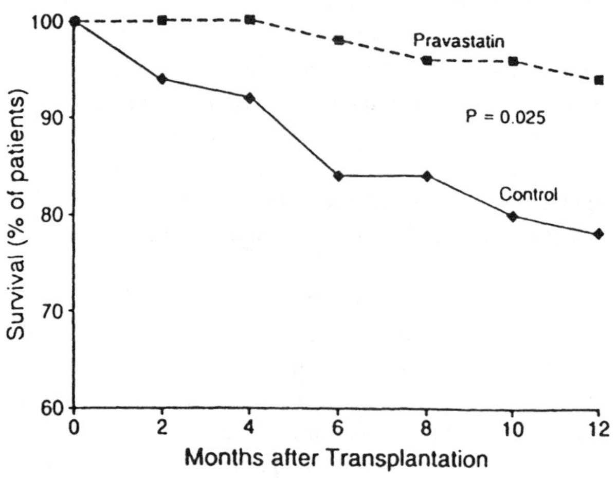

Figure 6. Survival during the first year after cardiac transplantation in the study patients (hatched line, pravastatin patients; solid line, control patients). From Kobashigawa et al. Effect of pravastatin on outcomes after cardiac transplantation. N Engl J Med 1995;333:621–7, reprinted by permission.

Table 7. Steroid Withdrawal Protocol

Immunosuppression Protocol for Steroid Withdrawal

		Months Posttransplant				
	Pretransplant	1	2	3	4	5
Steroid*	10	0.3	0.2	0.1	0.05	off
Cyclosporine*	1–3 IV	4.4	3.9	3.7	3.6	3.7
Azathioprine*	2	1.9	1.8	1.8	1.7	1.7

* mg/kg

Biopsy Schedule

Routine	SW (Late)
Weekly × 4	5 mg
Bi-weekly × 3	2.5 mg
Monthly × 6	0
Bi-monthly × 2	Monthly × 3
Every 3 mo × 4	Every 3 mo × 6
Yearly	Every 4 mo

Reprinted with premission from Handbook of Transplantation, Belfus and Hanley publishers, 1996. St. Louis, Mo.

compromise, improved survival (Figure 6) and a lower incidence of coronary vasculopathy by angiography.[230] In selected subgroups of patients, pravastatin therapy was associated with less progression of maximal intimal thickening and the intimal index by intracoronary ultrasound and diminished cytotoxicity of natural killer cells by specific lysis assay. In a rat heterotopic cardiac transplant model, pravastatin inhibits coronary allograft vasculopathy by inhibiting the synthesis and degradation of extracellular matrix proteins and macrophage infiltration.[231] In a recent 12-month open-label observational trial, pravastatin and simvistatin resulted in comparable reductions in lipids but pravastatin-treated patients had significantly less rhabdomylolyisis or myositis and nonsignificant trends toward better survival and fewer immunosuppression-related deaths.[232] Until larger and appropriately powered trials comparing different statins are available, however, the preferred statin for transplant recipients remain uncertain.[233]

Future Options

Despite impressive recent achievements in the understanding of T-cell biology and the recipient immune response, the diagnosis and management of acute cellular rejection following cardiac transplantation remains challenging. More reliable methods of non-invasive assessment of cellular rejection are needed given the expense and limitations of endomyocardial biopsy. Better and more precisely targeted immunosuppressive agents are necessary for both acute and chronic maintenance therapy. Modulation of the recipient immune response to facilitate allograft tolerance rather than enhanced non-specific immunosuppressive therapy will likely provide better protection against cellular rejection with less long-term morbidity.

REFERENCES

1. Kobashigawa J, Kirklin J, Naftel D, et al. Pretransplantation Risk Factors for Acute Rejection after Heart Transplantation: A Multiinstitutional Study. J Heart Lung Transplant 1993;12:355–66.
2. Jarcho J, Naftel D, Shroyer T, et al. Influence of HLA mismatch on rejection after heart transplantation: A multiinstitutional study. J Heart Lung Transplant 1994;13:583–96.
3. Miller L. Long-term complications of cardiac transplantation. Prog Cardiovasc Dis 1991;33:229–82.
4. Zerbe T, Arena V, Kormos R, Griffith B, Hardesty R, Duquesnoy R. Histocompatibility and other risk factors for histological rejection of human cardiac allografts during the first three months following transplantation. Transplantation 1991;52:485–90.
5. Grattan M, Moreno-Cabral C, Starnes V, Oyer P, Stinson E, Shumway N. Cytomegalovirus infection is associated with cardiac allograft rejection and atherosclerosis. JAMA 1989;261:3561–6.
6. Winters G, Costanzo-Nordin M, O'Sullivan E, et al. Predictors of late acute orthotopic heart transplant rejection. Circulation 1989;80 (suppl III):III-106–III-110.
7. Miller L, Schlant R, Kobashigawa J, Kubo S, Renlund D. Task Force 5: "Complications" in 24th Bethesda Conference, Cardiac Transplantation. J Amer Coll Cardiol 1993;22:41–54.
8. Renlund D, Gilbert E, O'Connell J, et al. Age-associated decline in cardiac allograft rejection. Am J Med 1987;83:391–8.
9. Kubo S, Naftel D, Mills R, et al. Risk factors for late recurrent rejection after heart transplantation: A multiinstitutional, multivariable analysis. J Heart Lung Transplant 1995;14:409–18.
10. Gallo P, Agozzino L, Angelini A, et al. Causes of late failure after heart transplantation: A ten-year survey. J Heart Lung Transplant 1997;16:1113–21.
11. Hosenpud JD, Bennett LE, Keck BM, Boucek MM, Novick RJ. The Registry of the International Society for Heart and Lung Transplantation: Seventeenth Official Report-2000. J Heart Lung Transplant 2000;19:909–31.
12. Hosenpud J, Bennett L, Keck B, Fiol B, Novick R. The registry of the International Society for Heart and Lung Transplantation: Fourteenth Official Report-1997. J Heart Lung Transplant 1997;16:691–712.
13. McGriffin D, Kirklin J, Naftel D, Bourge R. Competing outcomes after heart transplantation: a comparison of eras and outcomes. J Heart Lung Transplant 1997;16:190–8.
14. Bourge R, Naftel D, Costanzo-Nordin M, et al. Pretransplantation risk factors for death after heart transplantation: A multiinstitutional study. J Heart Lung Transplant 1993;12:549–62.

15. Stevenson L, Miller L. Cardiac transplantation as therapy for heart failure. Current Problems in Cardiology 1991;April:221–305.
16. Little R, Kay G, Epstein A, et al. Arrhythmias after orthotopic cardiac transplantation: Prevalence and determinants during initial hospitalization and late follow-up. Circulation 1989;80 (suppl III):III-140–III-146.
17. Pavri B, O'Nunain S, Newell J, Ruskin J, Dec G. Prevalence and prognostic significance of atrial arrthythmias after orthotopic cardiac transplantation. J Amer Coll Cardiol 1995;25:1673–80.
18. Scott C, Dark J, McComb J. Arrhythmias after cardiac transplantation. Am J Cardiol 1992;70:1061–3.
19. Park J, Hsu D, Hordof A, Addonizion L. Arrhythmias in pediatric heart transplant recipients: Prevalence and association with death, coronary artery disease, and rejection. J Heart Lung Transplant 1993;12:956–64.
20. Blanche C, Czer L, Trento A, et al. Bradyarrhythmias requiring pacemaker implantation after orthotopic heart transplantation: Association with rejection. J Heart Lung Transplant 1992;11:446–52.
21. de Jonge N, Jambroes G, Lahpor J, Woolley S. Ventricular fibrillation during acute rejection after heart transplantation. J Heart Lung Transplant 1992;11:797–8.
22. Stinson E, Dong E, Bieber C, Schroeder J, Shumway N. Cardiac transplantation in man: Early rejection. J Amer Med Assoc 1969;207:2233–42.
23. Yeoh T, Frist W, Eastburn T, Atkinson J. Clinical significance of mild rejection of the cardiac allograft. Circulation 1992;86 (suppl II):II-267–II-271.
24. Cilberto G, Mascarello M, Gronda E, et al. Acute rejection after heart transplantation: Noninvasive echocardiographic evaluation. J Am Coll Cardiol 1994;23:1156–61.
25. Gill E, Borrego C, Bray B, Renlund D, Hammond E, Gilbert E. Left ventricular mass increases during cardiac allograft vascular rejection. J Amer Coll Cardiol 1995;25:922–6.
26. Cilberto G, Cataldo G, Cipriani M, et al. Echocardiographic assessment of cardiac allograft rejection. European Heart Jour 1989;10:400–8.
27. Hauptman P, Couper G, Aranki S, Kartashov A, Mudge G, Loh E. Pericardial effusions after cardiac transplantation. J Am Coll Cardiol 1994;23:1625–9.
28. Dodd D, Brady L, Carden K, Frist W, Boucek M, Boucek R. Pattern of echocardiographic abnormalities with acute cardiac allograft rejection in adults: Correlation with endomyocardial biopsy. J Heart Lung Transplant 1993;12:1009–18.
29. Angermann C, Nassau K, Stempfle H, et al. Recognition of acute cardiac allograft rejection from serial integrated backscatter analyses in human orthotopic heart transplant recipients: Comparison with conventional echocardiography. Circulation 1997;95:140–50.
30. Kemkes B, Schutz A, Engelhardt M, Brandl U, Breuer M. Noninvasive methods of rejection diagnosis after heart transplantation. J Heart Lung Transplant 1992;11:S211–31.
31. Haberl R, Weber M, Reichenspurner H, et al. Frequency analysis of the surface electrocardiogram for recognition of acute rejection after orthotopic cardiac transplantation in man. Circulation 1987;76:101–8.
32. Auer T, Schreier G, Hutten H, et al. Paced epimyocardial electrograms for noninvasive rejection monitoring after heart transplantation. J Heart Lung Transplant 1996;15:993–8.
33. Wahlers T, Haverich A, Schafers H, et al. Changes of the intramyocardial electrogram after orthotopic heart transplantation. J Heart Lung Transplant 1986;5:450–6.
34. Warnecke H, Schuler S, Goetze H, et al. Noninvasive monitoring of cardiac allograft rejection by intramyocardial electrogram recordings. Circulation 1986;74 (suppl III):III-72–III-76.
35. Grauhan O, Muller J, Pfitzmann R, et al. Humoral rejection after heart transplantation: reliability of intramyocardial electrogram recordings (IMEG) and myocardial biopsy. Transplant International 1997;10:439–45.
36. Morocutti G, Di Chiara A, Proclemer A, et al. Signal-averaged electrocardiography and doppler echocardiographic study in predicting acute rejection in heart transplantation. J Heart Lung Transplant 1995;14:1065–72.
37. Graceffo M, O'Rourke R. Cardiac transplant rejection is associated with a decrease in the high-frequency components of the high-resolution, signal-averaged electrocardiogram. American Heart J 1996;132:820–6.
38. Babuty D, Aupart M, Machet M, Rouchet S, Cosnay P, Barnier D. Detection of acute cardiac allograft rejection with high resolution electrocardiography: experimental study in rats. J Heart and Lung Transplant 1996;15:1120–9.
39. Everett J, Palmer M, Jessurun J, Shumway S. Noninvasive diagnosis of cardiac allograft rejection in an orthotopic canine model. Ann Thorac Surg 1996;62:1337–40.
40. Valantine H, Yeoh T, Gibbons R, et al. Sensitivity and specificity of diastolic indexes for rejection surveillance: temporal correlation with endomyocardial biopsy. J Heart Lung Transplant 1991; 10:757–65.

41. Desruennes M, Corcos T, Cabrol A, et al. Doppler echocardiography for the diagnosis of acute cardiac allograft rejection. J Am Coll Cardiol 1988;12:63–70.
42. St. Goar F, Gibbons R, Schnitter I, Valantine H, Popp R. Left ventricular diastolic function: Doppler echocardiographic changes soon after cardiac transplantation. Circulation 1990;82:872–8.
43. Valantine H. Rejection surveillance by doppler echocardiography. J Heart Lung Transplant 1993;12:422–6.
44. Hosenpud J. Noninvasive diagnosis of cardiac allograft rejection: Another of the many searches for the grail. Circulation 1992;85:368–71.
45. Stempfle H, Angermann C, Kraml P, Schutz A, Kemkes B, Theisen K. Serial changes during acute allograft rejection: quantitative ultrasound tissue analysis versus myocardial histologic findings. J Amer Coll Cardiol 1993;1:310–7.
46. Masuyama T, Valantine H, Gibbons R, Schnittger I, Poop R. Serial measurement of integrated-ultrasonic backscatter in human cardiac allografts for the recognition of acute rejection. Circulation 1990;81:829–39.
47. Gotteiner N, Vonesh M, Crawford S, et al. Myocardial acoustics in pediatric allograft rejection. J Heart Lung Transplant 1996;15:596–604.
48. Frist W, Yasuda T, Segall G, et al. Noninvasive detection of human cardiac transplant rejection with indium-111 antimyosin (Fab) imaging. Circulation 1987;76 (suppl V):V-81–V-85.
49. Schuetz A, Fritsch S, Kemkes B, et al. Antimyosin monoclonal antibodies for early detection of cardiac allograft rejection. J Heart Lung Transplant 1990;9:654–61.
50. Ballester M, Carrio I. Noninvasive detection of acute heart rejection: the quest for the perfect test. J Nucl Cardiol 1997;4:249–55.
51. Schuetz A, Breuer M, Kemkes B. Antimyosin antibodies in cardiac rejection. Ann Thorac Surg 1997;63:578–81.
52. Obrador D, Ballester M, Carrio I, et al. The diagnosis of rejection activity in the heart transplant by monoclonal antimyosin antibodies. Revista Espanola de Cardiologia 1995;48 Suppl 7:92–5.
53. Ballester M, Obrador D, Carrio I, et al. Early postoperative reduction of monoclonal antimyosin antibody uptake is associated with absent rejection-related complications after heart transplantation. Circulation 1992;85:61–8.
54. Hesse B, Mortensen S, Folke M, Brodersen A, Aldershvile J, Pettersson G. Ability of antimyosin scintigraphy monitoring to exclude acute rejection during the first year after heart transplantation. J Heart Lung Transplant 1995;14:23–31.
55. De Nardo D, Scibilia G, Macchiarelli A, et al. The role of indium-111 antimyosin (Fab) imaging as a noninvasive surveillance method of human heart transplant rejection. J Heart Lung Transplant 1989;8:407–12.
56. Picano E, De Pieri G, Salerno J, et al. Electrocardiographic changes suggestive of myocardial ischemia elicited by dipyridamole infusion in acute rejection early after heart transplantation. Circulation 1990;81:72–7.
57. Richter J, Herreros J, Serena A, Domper M, Ramirez J, Arcas R. Thallium scintigraphy in human transplants: A way to detect myocardial damage. J Heart Lung Transplant 1991;10:33–7.
58. Canby R, Evanochko W, Barrett L, et al. Monitoring the bioenergetics of cardiac allograft rejection using in vivo P-31 nuclear magnetic resonance spectroscopy. J Am Coll Cardiol 1987;9:1067–74.
59. Konstam M, Aronovitz M, Runge V, et al. Magnetic resonance imaging with gadolinium-DPTA for detecting cardiac transplant rejection in rats. Circulation 1988;78 (suppl III):III-87–III-94.
60. Eugene M, Lechat P, Hadjiisky P, Teillac A, Grosgogeat Y, Cabrol C. Nuclear magnetic resonance and proton relaxation times in experimental hetertopic heart transplantation. J Heart Lung Transplant 1986;5:39–45.
61. Aherne T, Tscholakoff D, Finkbeiner W, et al. Magnetic resonance imaging of cardiac transplants: the evaluation of rejection of cardiac allografts with and without immunosuppression. Circulation 1986;74:11–22.
62. May R, Cooper C, Du Toit E, Reichart B. Cytoimmunologic monitoring after heart and heart-lung transplantation. J Heart Lung Transplant 1990;9:133–5.
63. Hanson C, Bolling S, Stoolman L, et al. Cytoimmunologic monitoring and heart transplantation. J Heart Lung Transplant 1988;7:424–9.
64. Fyfe A, Daly P, Galligan L, Pirc L, Feindel C, Cardella C. Coronary sinus sampling of cytokines after heart transplantation: Evidence for macrophage activation and interleukin-4 production within the graft. J Am Coll Cardiol 1993;21:171–6.
65. George J, Kirklin J, Naftel D, et al. Serial measurements of interleukin-6, interleukin-8, tumor necrosis factor-alpha, and soluble vascular cell adhesion molecule-1 in the peripheral blood plasma of human cardiac allograft recipients. J Heart Lung Transplant 1997;16:1046–53.
66. Grant S, Lamb W, Brooks N, Brenchley P, Hutchinson I. Serum cytokines in human heart transplant recipients: Is there a relationship to rejection? Transplantation 1996;62:480–91.

67. Deng M, Erren M, Kammerling L, et al. The relation of interleukin-6, tumor necrosis factor-alpha, IL-2, and IL-2 receptor levels to cellular rejection, allograft dysfunction, and clinical events after cardiac transplantation. Transplantation 1995;60:1118–23.
68. Dengler T, Zimmermann R, Tiefenbacher C, Braun K, Sack F, Kubler W. Endothelin plasma levels in acute graft rejection after heart transplantation. J Heart Lung Transplant 1995;14:1057–64.
69. Eisen H, Eisenberg S, Saffitz J, Bolman R, Sobel B, Bergmann S. Noninvasive detection of rejection of transplanted hearts with indium-111-labeled lymphocytes. Circulation 1987;75:868–76.
70. Volk H, Schuler S, Czerlinsi S, et al. Serum levels of soluble interleukin-2 receptor C-reactive protein, neopterin, myoglobin and light chains of cardiac myosin fail to correlate with the occurence of rejection in long-term renal and heart transplant patients. Clin Transplant 1992;6:21–6.
71. Hoshinga K, Wood N, Wolfgang T. Clinical usefulness of monitoring for transferrin receptor-positive circulatin lymphocytes in cardiac transplant recipients. Transplant Proc 1986;18:743–4.
72. Ansari A, Mayne A, Sundstrom J, et al. Frequency of hypoxanthine guanine phosphoribosyltransferase (HPRT(-)) T cells in the peripheral blood of cardiac transplant recipients: a noninvasive technique for the diagnosis of allograft rejection. Circulation 1995;92:862–74.
73. Sobotka P, Gupta D, Lansky D, Costanzo M, Zarling E. Breath pentane is a marker of acute cardiac allograft rejection. J Heart Lung Transplant 1994;13:224–9.
74. Carrier M, Russell D, Wild J, Emery R, Copeland J. Urinary polyamines as markers of cardiac allograft rejection: a clinical evaluation. J Thorac Cardiovasc Surg 1987;96:806–10.
75. Carrier M, Russell D, Wild J, Emery R, Copeland J. Prolactin as a marker of rejection in human heart transplantation. J Heart Lung Transplant 1987;6:290–2.
76. Roodman S, Miller L, Tsai C. Role of interleukin 2 receptors in immunologic monitoring following cardiac transplantation. Transplantation 1988;45:1050–6.
77. Goldman M, Lippman R, Landwehr D, et al. Beta 2 microglobulin and the diagnosis of cardiac transplant rejection. Transplantation 1983;36:209–11.
78. Zimmermann R, Baki S, Dengler T, et al. Troponin T release after heart transplantation. Br Heart J 1993;69:395–8.
79. Anderson J, Hossein-Nia M, Brown P, Corbishley C, Murday A, Holt D. Creatine kinase MB isoforms: a potential predictor of acute cardiac allograft rejection. J Heart Lung Transplant 1995;14:666–70.
80. Gash A, Kayne F, Morely D, Fitzpatrick J, Alpern J, Brozena S. Serum myoglobin does not predict cardiac allograft rejection. J Heart Lung Transplant 1994;13:451–4.
81. Isobe M, Narula J, Soughern J, Strauss H, Khaw B, Haber E. Imaging the rejecting heart: In vivo detection of major histocompatibility complex class II antigen induction. Circulation 1992;85: 738–46.
82. von Scheidt W, ziegler U, Kemkes B, Erdmann E. Heart transplantation: Hemodynamics over a five-year period. J Heart Lung Transplant 1991;10:342–50.
83. Valantine H, Appleton C, Hatle L, et al. A hemodynamic and doppler echocardiographic study of ventricular function in long-term cardiac allograft recipients: Etiology and prognosis of restrictive-constrictive physiology. Circulation 1989;79:66–75.
84. Mills R, Haftel D, Kirklin J, et al. Heart transplant rejection with hemodynamic compromise: A multiinstitutional study of the role of endomyocardial cellular infiltrate. J Heart Lung Transplant 1997;16:813–21.
85. Zales V, Crawford S, Backer C, et al. Role of endomyocardial biopsy in rejection surveillance after heart transplantation in neonates and children. J Am Coll Cardiol 1994;23:766–71.
86. Santos-Ocampo S, Sekarski T, Saffitz J, et al. Echocardiographic characteristics of biopsy-proven cellular rejection in infant heart transplant recipients. J Heart Lung Transplant 1996;15:25–34.
87. Neuberger S, Vincent R, Doelling N, et al. Comparison of quantitative echocardiography with endomyocardial biopsy to define myocardial rejection in pediatric patients after cardiac transplantation. American Journal of Cardiology 1997;79:447–50.
88. Kimball T, Semler D, Witt S, Khoury P, Daniels S. Noninvasive markers for acute heart transplant rejection in children with the use of automatic border detection. Journal of the American Society of Echocardiography 1997;10:964–72.
89. Caves P, Stinson E, Billingham M, Shumway N. Percutaneous transvenous endomyocardial biopsy in human heart recipients. Ann Thorac Surg 1973;15:325–35.
90. Williams M, Lee M, DiSalvo T, et al. Biopsy-induced flail tricuspid leaflet and tricuspid regurgitation following orthotopic cardiac transplantation. Am J Cardiol 1996;77:1339–44.
91. Anderson J, Marshall H. The femoral venous approach to endomyocardial biopsy: comparison with internal jugular and transarterial approaches. Am J Cardiol 1984;53:833–7.
92. Anderson A, Levin T, Feldman T. External jugular vein approach for percutaneous right ventricular biopsy. J Heart Lung Transplant 1997;16:576–8.

93. Mills R, Young J. Chapter 35: Evaluation for cardiac transplantation and follow-up of the cardiac transplant recipient. In Diagnostic and Therapeutic Cardiac Catheterization, Second Edition, Edited by Carl Pepine, Williams and Wilkins, 1994.
94. Fowles R, Mason J. Endomyocardial biopsy. Ann Intern Med 1982;97:885–94.
95. Bhat G, Burwig S, Walsh R. Morbidity of endomyocardial biopsy in cardiac transplant recipients. Am Heart J 1993;125:1180–1.
96. Fitchett D, Forbes C, Guerraty A. Repeated endomyocardial biopsy causing coronary arterial-right ventricular fistula after cardiac transplantation. Am J Cardiol 1988;62:829–31.
97. Deckers J, Hare J, Baughman K. Complications of transvenous right ventricular endomyocardial biopsy in adult patients with cardiomyopathy: A seven-year survey of 546 consecutive diagnostic procedures in a tertiary referral center. J Am Coll Cardiol 1992;19:43–7.
98. Billingham M, Cary N, Hammond M, et al. A working formulation for the standardization of nomenclature in the diagnosis of heart and lung rejection: Heart rejection study group. J Heart Lung Transplant 1990;9:587–93.
99. Billingham M. Dilemma of variety of histopathologic grading systems for acute cardiac allograft rejection by endomyocardial biopsy. J Heart Lung Transplant 1990;9:272–6.
100. Fishbein M, Bell G, Lones M, et al. Grade 2 cellular heart rejection: does it exist? J Heart Lung Transplant 1994;13:1051–7.
101. Constanzo-Nordin M, Winters G, Fisher S, et al. Endocardial infiltrates in the transplanted heart: Clinical significance emerging form the analysis of 5,026 endomyocardial biopsy specimens. J Heart Lung Transplant 1993;12:741–7.
102. Brunner-La Rocca H, Sutsch G, Schneider J, Follath F, Kiowski W. Natural course of moderate cardiac allograft rejection (International Society for Heart Transplantation Grade 2) early and late after transplantation. Circulation 1996;94:1334–8.
103. White J, Guiraudon C, Pflugfelder P, Kostuk W. Routine surveillance myocardial biopsies are unnecessary beyond one year after heart transplantation. J Heart Lung Transplant 1995;14: 1052–6.
104. Winters G, McManus B, Pathologists RCRTT. Consistencies and controversies in the application of the International Society for Heart and Lung Transplantation working formulation for heart transplant biopsy specimens. J Heart Lung Transplant 1996;15:728–35.
105. Nielsen H, Sorensen F, Nielsen B, Bagger J, Thayssen P, Baandrup U. Reproducibility of the acute rejection diagnosis in human cardiac allografts: The Stanford classification and the International grading system. J Heart Lung Transplant 1993;12:239–43.
106. Fyfe B, Loh E, Winters G, Couper G, Kartashov A, Schoen F. Heart transplantation-associated perioperative ischemic myocardial injury: Morphological features and clinical significance. Circulation 1996;93:1133–40.
107. Nakhleh R, Jones J, Goswitz J, Anderson E, Titus J. Correlation of endomyocardial biopsy findings with autopsy findings in human cardiac allografts. J Heart Lung Transplant 1992;11:479–85.
108. Sharples L, Cary N, Large S, Wallwork J. Error rates with which endomyocardial biopsy specimens are graded for rejection after cardiac transplantation. Am J Cardiol 1992;70:527–30.
109. Sehti G, Kosaraju S, Arabia F, Roasdo L, McCarthy M, Copeland J. Is it necessary to perform surveillance endomyocardial biopsies in heart transplant recipients? J Heart Lung Transplant 1995;14:1047–51.
110. McNamara D, Di Salvo T, Mathier M, Keck S, Semigran M, Dec G. Left ventricular dysfunction after heart transplantation: incidence and role of enhanced immunosuppression. J Heart Lung Transplant 1996;15:506–15.
111. O'Connell J, Renlund D. Variations in diagnosis, treatment, and prevention of cardial allograft rejection: the need for standardization? J Heart Lung Transplant 1990;9:269–71.
112. Lloveras J, Escourrou G, Delisle M, et al. Evolution of untreated mild rejection in heart transplant recipients. J Heart Lung Transplant 1992;11:751–6.
113. Winter G, Loh E, Schoen F. Natural history of focal moderate cardiac allogaft rejection: Is treatment warranted? Circulation 1995;91:1975–80.
114. Milano A, Caforio A, Livi U, et al. Evolution of focal moderate (International Society for Heart and Lung Transplantation Grade 2) rejection of the cardiac allograft. J Heart Lung Transplant 1996;15:456–60.
115. Costanzo-Nordin M. Cardiac allograft vasculopathy: Relationship with acute cellular rejection and histocompatibility. J Heart Lung Transplant 1992;11:S90–103.
116. Hauptman P, Nakagawa T, Tanaka H, Libby P. Acute rejection: Culprit of coincidence in the pathogenesis of cardiac graft vascular disease? J Heart Lung Transplant 1995;14:S173–80.
117. Weis M, von Scheidt W. Cardiac allograft vasculopathy. Circulation 1997;96:2069–77.
118. Gao S, Schroeder J, Alderman E, et al. Clinical and laboratory correlates of accelerated coronary artery disease in the cardiac transplant patient. Circulation 1987;76 (suppl V):V-56–V-61.

119. Uretsky B, Murali S, Reddy P, et al. Development of coronary artery disease in cardiac transplant patients receiving immunosuppressive therapy with cyclosporine and prednisone. Circulation 1987;76:827–34.
120. Olivari M, Homan D, Wilson R, Kubo S, Ring W. Coronary artery disease in cardiac transplant patients receiving triple-drug immunosuppression. Circulation 1989;80 (suppl III):III-111–III-115.
121. Gao S, Schroeder J, Hunt S, Valantine H, Hill I, Stinson E. Influence of graft rejeciton on incidence of accelerated graft coronary artery disease: A new approach to analysis. J Heart Lung Transplant 1993;12:1029–35.
122. Stovin P, Sharples L, Schofield P, et al. Lack of association between endomyocardial evidence of rejection in the first six months and the later development of transplant-related coronary artery disease. J Heart Lung Transplant 1993;12:100–6.
123. Hornick P, Smith J, Pomerance A, et al. Influence of acute rejection episodes, HLA matching, and donor/recipient phenotype on the development of "early" transplant-associated coronary artery disease. Circulation 1997;96 (suppl II):II-148–II-153.
124. Fornes P, Heudes D, Simon D, Guillemain R, Amrein C, Bruneval P. Influence of acute or chronic rejection on myocardial collagen density in serial endomyocardial biopsy specimens from cardiac allografts. J Heart Lung Transplant 1996;15:796–803.
125. Nitenberg A, Aptecard E, Benvenuti C, et al. Effects of time and previous acute rejection episodes on coronary vascular reserve in human heart transplant recipients. J Am Coll Cardiol 1992;20: 1333–8.
126. Anguita M, Lopez-Rubio F, Arizon J, et al. Repetitive nontreated episodes of grade 1B or 2 acute rejection impair long-term cardiac graft function. J Heart Lung Transplant 1995;14:452–60.
127. Miller L. Treatment of cardiac allograft rejection with intravenous corticosteroids. J Heart Lung Transplant 1990;9:283–7.
128. Heublein B, Wahlers T, Haverich A. Pulsed steroids for treatment of cardiac rejection after transplantation: What dosage is necessary? Circulation 1989;80 (suppl III):III-97–III-99.
129. Lonquist J, Radovancevic B, Vega J, et al. Reevaluation of steroid tapering after steroid pulse therapy for heart rejection. J Heart Lung Transplant 1992;11:913–19.
130. Michler R, Smith C, Drusin R, et al. Reversal of cardiac transplant rejection without massive immunosuppression. Circulation 1986;74 (suppl III):III-68–III-71.
131. Hosenpud J, Norman D, Pantely G. Low-dose oral prednisone in the treatment of acute cardiac allograft rejection not associated with hemodynamic compromise. J Heart Lung Transplant 1990;9: 292–6.
132. Kobashigawa J, Stevenson L, Moriguchi J, et al. Is intravenous glucocorticoid therapy better than an oral regimen for asymptomatic cardiac rejection? A randomized trial. J Am Coll Cardiol 1993;21:1142–4.
133. Park M, Starling R, Ratliff N, et al. Oral steroid pulse without taper for the treatment of asymptomatic moderate cardiac allograft rejection. J Heart Lung Transplant 1999;18:1224–7.
134. Costanzo-Nordin M, O'Sullivan E, Hubbell E, et al. Long-term follow-up of heart transplant recipients treated with murine antihuman mature T cell monoclonal antibody (OKT3): The Loyola experience. J Heart Lung Transplant 1989;8:288–95.
135. Macris M, Frazier O, Lammermeier D, Radovancevic B, Duncan J. Clinical experience with muromonab-CD3 monoclonal antibody (OKT3) in heart transplantation. J Heart Lung Transplant 1989;8:281–7.
136. Sweeney M, Sinnott J, Cullison J, Weinstein S, Cardiac Transplant Team. The use of OKY3 for stubborn heart allograft rejection: An advance in clinical immunotherapy? J Heart Lung Transplant 1987;6:324–8.
137. Bristow M, Gilbert E, Renlund D, DeWitt C, Buronw N, O'Connell J. Use of OKT3 monoclonal antibody in heart transplantation: Review of the initial experience. J Heart Lung Transplant 1988;7:1–11.
138. Costanzo-Nordin M, Silver m, O'Connell J, et al. Successful reversal of acute cardiac allograft rejection with OKT3 monoclonal antibody. Circulation 1987;76 (suppl V):V-71–V-80.
139. Gilbert E, Dewitt C, Eiswirth C, et al. Treatment of refractory cardiac allograft rejeciton with OKT3 monoclonal antibody. Am J Med 1987;82:202–6.
140. Taylor D, Kfoury A, Pisani B, Hammond E, Renlund D. Antilymphocyte-antibody prophylaxis: Review of the adult experience in heart transplantation. Transplant Proc 1997;29 (suppl 8A): 13S–15S.
141. Kobashigawa J, Stevenson L, Moriguchi J, et al. Randomized study of high dose oral cyclosporine therapy for mild acute cardiac rejection. J Heart Lung Transplant 1989;8:53–8.
142. Haverty T, Sanders M, Sheahan M. OKT3 treatment of cardiac allograft rejection. J Heart Lung Transplant 1993;21:591–8.
143. Kirklin J, Bourge R, McGiffin D. Recurrent of persistent cardiac allograft rejection: Therapeutic options and recommendations. Transplant Proc 1997;29 (suppl 8A):40S–44S.

144. Mentzer R, Jahania M, Lasley R, US Multicenter FK506 Study Group. Tacrolimus as a rescue immunosuppression after heart and lung transplantation. Transplantation 1998;65:109–13.
145. Pham S, Kormos R, Hattler B, et al. A prospective trial of tacrolimus (FK506) in clinical heart transplantation: intermediate-term results. J Thorac Cardiovasc Surg 1996;111:764–72.
146. Armitage J, Dormos R, Fung J, et al. Preliminary experience with FK506 in thoracic transplantation. Transplantation 1990;52:164–7.
147. Rinaldi M, Pellegrini C, Martinelli L, et al. FK506 effectiveness in reducing acute rejection after heart transplantation: A prospective randomized study. J Heart Lung Transplant 1997;16:1001–10.
148. Meiser B, Uberfuhr P, Fuchs A, et al. Tacrolimus: A superior agent to OKT3 for treating cases of persistent rejection after intrathoracic transplantation. J Heart Lung Transplant 1997;16:795–800.
149. Asante-Korang A, Boyle G, Webber S, Miller S, Fricker F. Experience of FK506 immune suppression in pediatric heart transplantation: A study of long-term adverse effects. J Heart Lung Transplant 1996;15:415–22.
150. Yamani M, Starling R, Pelegrin D, et al. Efficacy of tacrolimus in patients with steroid-resistant cardiac allograft cellular rejection. J Heart Lung Transplant 2000;19:337–42.
151. Kirklin J, Bourge R, Naftel D, et al. Treatment of recurrent heart rejection with mycophenolate mofetil (RS-61443): Initial clinical experience. J Heart Lung Transplant 1994;13:444–50.
152. Taylor D, Ensley R, Olsen S, Dunn D, Renlund D. Mycophenolate mofetil (RS-61443): Preclinical, clinical, and three-year experience in heart transplantation. J Heart Lung Transplant 1994;13: 571–82.
153. Ensley R, Bristow M, Olsen S, et al. The use of mycophenolate mofetil (RS-61443) in human heart transplant recipients. Transplantation 1993;56:75–82.
154. Costanzo-Nordin M, Grusk B, Silver M, et al. Reversal of recalcitrant cardiac allograft rejection with methotrexate. Circulation 1988;78 (suppl III):III-47–III-57.
155. Bourge R, Kirklin J, White-Williams C, et al. Methotrexate pulse therapy in the treatment of recurrent acute heart rejection. J Heart Lung Transplant 1992;11:1116–24.
156. Hosenpud J, Hershberger R, Ratkovec R, et al. Methotrexate for the treatment of patients with multiple episodes of acute cardiac allograft rejection. J Heart Lung Transplant 1992;11:739–45.
157. Ross H, Gullestad L, Pak J, Slauson S, Valantine H, Hunt S. Methotrexate of total lymphoid radiation for treatment of persistent or recurrent allograft cellular rejection: A comparative study. J Heart Lung Transplant 1997;16:179–89.
158. Costanzo M, Koch D, Fisher S, Heroux A, Kao W, Johnson M. Effects of methotrexate on acute rejection and cardiac allograft vasculopathy in heart transplant recipients. J Heart Lung Transplant 1997;16:169–78.
159. Bouchart F, Gundry S, Schaack-Gonzales J, et al. Methotrexate as rescue/adjunctive immunotherapy in infant and adult heart transplantation. J Heart Lung Transplant 1993;12:427–33.
160. Salter M, Kirklin J, Bourge R, et al. Total lymphoid irradiation in the treatment of early or recurrent heart rejection. J Heart Lung Transplant 1992;11:902–12.
161. Hunt S, Strober S, Hoppe R, Stinson E. Total lymphoid irradiation for treatment of intractable cardiac allograft rejection. J Heart Lung Transplant 1991;10:211–16.
162. Keogh A, Morgan G, Macdonald P, Spratt P, Mundy J, McCosker C. Total lymphoid irradiation for resistant rejection after heart transplantation: Only moderate success medium-term. J Heart Lung Transplant 1996;15:231–3.
163. Madden B, Backhouse L, McClosky D, Reynolds L, Tait D, Murday A. Total lymphoid irradiation as rescue therapy after heart transplantation. J Heart Lung Transplant 1996;15:234–8.
164. Di Salvo T, Narula J, Cosimi A, Keck S, Dec G, Semigran M. Actinomycin D is an effective adjunctive immunosuppressive agent in recurrent cardiac allograft rejection. J Heart Lung Transplant 1995;14:955–62.
165. Stinson E, Dong E, Bieber C, Popp R, Shumway N. Cardiac transplantation in man II. Immunosuppressive therapy. J Thor Cardiovasc Surg 1969;58:326–43.
166. Partanen J, Nieminen M, Krogerus L, Harjula A, Mattila S. Heart transplant rejection treated with plasmapheresis. J Heart Lung Transplant 1992;11:301–5.
166a. Grauhan O, Knosalla C, Ewert R, et al. Plasmapheresis and cyclosphosphamide in the treatment of humoral rejection after heart transplantation. J Heart Lung Transplant 2001;20:316–21.
167. Costanzo-Nordin M, Hubbell E, O'Sullivan E, et al. Successful treatment of heart transplant rejection with photophoresis. Transplantation 1992;53:808–15.
168. Rose E, Barr M, Xu H, et al. Photochemotherapy in human heart transplant recipients at high risk for fatal rejection. J Heart Lung Transplant 1992;11:746–50.
169. Meiser B, Kur F, Reichenspurner H, et al. Reduction of the incidence of rejection by adjunct immunosuppression with photochemotherapy after heart transplantation. Transplantation 1994; 57:563–8.
170. Dall'Amico R, Livi U, Milano A, et al. Extracorporeal photochemotherapy as adjuvant treatment of heart transplant recipients with recurrent rejection. Transplantation 1995;60:45–9.

171. Smith J, Ribakove G, Hunt A, et al. Heart retransplantation: the 25-year experience at a single institution. J Heart Lung Transplant 1995;14:832–9.
172. Ensley R, Hunt S, Taylor D, et al. Predictors of survival after repeat heart transplantation. J Heart Lung Transplant 1992;11:S142–S158.
173. McGoon M, Frantz R. Techniques of immunosuppression after cardiac transplantation. Mayo Clin Proc 1992;67:586–95.
174. Griffith B, Hardesty R, Deeb G, Starzl T, Bahnson H. Cardiac transplantation with cyclosporin A and prednisone. Ann Surg 1982;196:324–9.
175. Kahan B. Immunosuppressive therapy with cyclosporine for cardiac transplantation. Circulation 1987;75:40–56.
176. Trento A, Griffith B, Hardesty R, Kormos R, Thompson M, Bahnson H. Cardiac transplantation: improved quality of survival with a modified immunosuppressive protocol. Circulation 1987;76 (suppl V):V-48–V-51.
177. Yacoub M, Alivizatos P, Khaghani A, Mitchell A. The use of cyclosporine, azathioprine and anithymocyte globulin with or without low-dose steroids for immunosuppression of cardiac transplant patients. Transplant Proc 1985;17:221–2.
178. Grattan M, Moreno-Cabral C, Starnes V, Oyer P, Stinson E, Shumway N. Eight-year results of cyclosporine-treated patients with cardiac transplants. J Thor Cardiovasc Surg 1990;99:500–9.
179. Esmore D, Spratt P, Keogh A, Chang V. Cyclosporine and azathioprine immunosuppression without maintenance steroids: A prospective randomized trial. J Heart Lung Transplant 1989; 8:194–9.
180. Keogh A, Macdonald P, Mundy J, Chang V, Harvison A, Spratt P. Five-year follow-up of a randomized double-versus triple-drug therapy immunosuppressive trial after heart transplantation. J Heart Lung Transplant 1992;11:550–6.
181. Kahan B. Cyclosporine. New Engl J Med 1989;321:1725–38.
182. Halloran P, Lui S. Chapter 12, Approved Immunosuppresants in *Primer on Transplantation*, DJ Norman and WN Suki, eds, The American Society of Transplant Physicians. 1998.
183. El Gamel S, Keevil B, Rhaman A, Campbell C, Derianiya A, Yonan A. Cardiac allograft rejection: Do trough cyclosporine levels correlate with the grade of histologic rejection? J Heart Lung Transplant 1997;16:268–74.
184. Best N, Trull A, Tan K, Spiegelhalter D, Cary N, Wallwork J. Pharmacodynamics of cyclosporine in heart and heart-lung transplant recipients. Transplantation 1996;62:1429–35.
185. Keogh A, Spratt P, McCosker C, Macdonald P, Mundy J, Kaan A. Ketoconazole to reduce the need for cyclosporine after cardiac transplantation. N Engl J Med 1995;333:628–33.
186. Chan C, Maurer J, Cardella C, Cattran D, Pei Y. A randomized controlled trial of verapamil on cyclosporine nephrotoxicity in heart and lung transplant recipients. Transplantation 1997;63: 1435–40.
187. White M, Pelletier G, Tan A, Jesina C, Carrier M. Pharmacokinetic, hemodynamic, and metabolic effects of cyclosporine: Sandimmune versus the microemulsion Neoral in heart transplant recipients. J Heart Lung Transplant 1997;16:787–94.
188. Valantine H. Neoral use in the cardiac transplant recipient. Transplant Proc 2000;32(3A suppl): 27S–44S.
189. Eisen H, Hobbs R, Davis S, G, et al. Safety, tolerability and efficacy of cyclosporine microemulsion in heart transplant recipients: a randomized, multicenter, double-blind comparison with the oil based formulation of cyclosporine-results at six months after transplantation. Transplantation 1999;68:663–71.
190. Taylor D, Barr M, Radonvancevic B, et al. A randomized, multicenter comparison of tacrolimus and cyclosporine immunosuppressive regimens in cardiac transplantation: Decreased hyperlipidemia and hypertension with tarcolimus. J Heart Lung Transplant 1999;18:336–45.
191. Myers B, Ross J, Newton L, Leutscher J, Perlroth M. Cyclosporine-associated chronic nephropathy. N Engl J Med 1984;311:699–705.
192. Goldstein D, Zuech N, Sehgal V, Weinber A, Drusin R, Cohen D. Cyclosporine-associated endstage nephropathy after cardiac transplantation. Transplantation 1997;63:664–8.
193. Scherrer U, Vissing S, Morgan B, et al. Cyclosporine-induced sympathetic activation and hypertension after heart transplantation. New Engl J Med 1990;323:693–9.
194. de Groen P, Aksamit A, Rakela J, Forbes G, Krom R. Central nervous system toxicity after liver transplantation: The role of cyclosporine and cholesterol. New Engl J Med 1987;317:861–6.
195. Adams D, Gunson B, Honigsberger L, et al. Neurological complications following liver transplantation. Lancet 1987;I:949–51.
196. Lane R, Roche S, Leung A, Greco A, Lange L. Cyclosporine neurotoxicity in cardiac transplant recipients. J Neurol, Neurosurg, and Psych 1988;51:1434–7.
197. Cooper D, Novitzky D, Davis L, et al. Does central nervous system toxicity occur in transplant

patients with hypocholesterolemia receiving cyclosporine? J Heart Lung Transplant 1989;8: 211–14.
198. Lin H, Rocher L, McQuillan M, Schmaltz S, Palella T, Fox I. Cyclosporine-induced hyperuricemia and gout. New Engl J Med 1989;321:287–92.
199. Kobashigawa J, Miller L, Renlund D, et al. A randomized, active-controlled trial of mycophenolate mofetil in heart transplant recipients. Transplantation 1999;66:507–15.
200. Keogh A, Bourge R, Costanzo M, et al. Three year results of the double-blind randomized multicenter trial of mycophenolate mofetil in heart transplant patients (abstract). J Heart Lung Transplant 1999;18:53.
201. Meiser B, Pfeiffer M, Schmidt D, et al. Combination therapy with tracrolimus and mycophenolate mofetil following cardiac transplantation: importance of mycophenolic acid therapeutic drug monitoring. J Heart Lung Transplant 1999;18:143–9.
202. Yamani M, Starling R, Goormastic M, et al. The impact of routine mycophenolate mofetil drug monitoring on the treatment of cardiac allograft rejection. Transplantation 2000;69:2326–30.
203. Taylor D, Sharma R, Kfoury A, Renlund D. Increased incidence of allograft rejection in stable heart transplant recipients after late conversion from mycophenolate mofetil to azathioprine. Clin Transplant 1999;13:296–9.
204. Halloran P, Lui S. Approved Immunosuppressants. Chapter 12 in Primer on Transplantation, DJ Norman and WN Suki, eds. American Society of Transplant Physicians. 1998.
205. Renlund D, O'Connell J, Bristow M. Early rejection prophylaxis in heart transplantation: Is cytolytic therapy necessary? J Heart Lung Transplant 1989;8:191–3.
206. Alonso-Poupon L, Serrano-Fiz S, Rubio J, et al. Efficacy of low-dose OKT3 as cytolytic induction therapy in heart transplantation. J Heart Lung Transplant 1995;14:136–42.
207. Mentis A, Powell A, Novick R, et al. A prospective randomized controlled trial of initial immunosuppression with ALG versus OKT3 in recipients of cardiac allografts. J Heart Lung Transplant 1992;11:569–76.
208. Kobashigawa J, Stevenson L, Brownfield E, et al. Does short-course induction with OKT3 improve outcome after heart transplantation? A randomized trial. J Heart Lung Transplant 1993;12:250–8.
209. Griffith B, Kormos R, Armitage J, Dummer J, Hardesty R. Comparative trial of immunoprophylaxis with RATG versus OKT3. J Heart Transplant 1990;9:301–5.
210. Kormos R, Herlan D, Armitrage J, et al. Monoclonal versus polyclonal antibody therapy for prophylaxis against rejection after heart transplantation. J Heart Transplant 1990;9:1–10.
211. Hegewald M, O'Connell J, Renlund D, et al. OKT3 monoclonal antibody given for ten versus fourteen days as immunosuppressive prophylaxis in heart transplantation. J Heart Lung Transplant 1989;8:303–10.
212. Starnes V, Oyer P, Steinson E, Dein J, Shumway N. Prophylactic OKT3 used as induction therapy for heart transplantation. Circulation 1989;80(suppl III):III-79–III-83.
213. Kawaguchi A, Szentpetery S, Mohanakumar T, Barnhart G, Lower R. Effects of prophylactic rabbit anithymocyte globulin in cardiac allograft recipients treated with cyclosporine. J Heart Lung Transplant 1987;6:214–17.
214. O'Connell J, Renlund D, Hammond E, et al. Sensitization to OKT3 monoclonal antibody in heart transplantation: Correlation with early allograft loss. J Heart Lung Transplant 1991;10:217–22.
215. Schroeder T, First M, Hurtubise P, et al. Immunologic monitoring with orthoclone OKT3 therapy. J Heart Lung Transplant 1989;8:371–80.
216. Costanzo-Nordin M, O'Sullivan J, Johnson M, et al. Prospective randomized trial of OKT3-versus horse antithymocyte globulin-based immunosuppressive prophylaxis in heart transplantation. J Heart Lung Transplant 1990;9:306–15.
217. Swinnen L, Costanzo-Nordin M, Fisher S, et al. Increased incidence of lymphoproliferative disorder after immunosuppression with the monoclonal antibody OKT3 in cardiac transplant recipients. N Engl J Med 1990;323:1723–8.
218. Beniaminovitz A, Itsecu S, Lietz K, et al. Prevention of rejection in cardiac transplantation by blockade of the interleukin-2 receptor with a monclonal antibody. New Engl J Med 2000;342: 613–19.
219. Van Gelder T, Balk A, Jonkman F, et al. A randomized trial comparing safety and efficacy of OKT3 and a monoclonal anti-interleukin-2 receptor antibody (BT563) in the prevention of acute rejection after heart transplantation. Transplantation 1996;62:51–5.
220. Sayegh M, Turka L. The role to T-cell costimulatory activation pathways in transplant rejection. N Engl J Med 1998;338.
221. Strom T, Ettenger R. Investigational immunosuppressants: Biologics. Chapter 14 in Primer on Transplantation, DJ Norman and WN Suki, eds. American Society of Transplant Physicians. 1998.
222. Miller L. Steroid withdrawl in heart transplantation: Editorial. J Heart Lung Transplant 1992; 11:410–13.

223. Renlund D, O'Connell J, Gilbert E, Watson F, Bristow M. Feasibility of discontinuation of corticosteroid maintenance therapy in heart transplantation. J Heart Transplant 1987;6:71–8.
224. Taylor D, Bristow M, O'Connell J, et al. Improved long-term survival after heart transplantation predicted by successful early withdrawal from maintenance corticosteroid therapy. J Heart Lung Transplant 1996;15:1039–46.
225. Pritzker M, Lake K, Reutzel T, et al. Steroid-free maintenance immunotherapy: Minneapolis Heart Institute experience. J Heart Lung Transplant 1992;11:415–20.
226. Kobashigawa J, Stevenson L, Brownfield E, et al. Initial success of steroid weaning late after heart transplantation. J Heart Lung Transplant 1992;11:428–30.
227. Miller L, Wolford T, McBride L, Peigh P, Pennington D. Successful withdrawal of corticosteroids in heart transplantation. J Heart Lung Transplant 1992;11:431–4.
228. Olivari M, Jessen M, Baldwin B, et al. Triple-drug immunosuppression with steroid discontinuation by six months after heart transplantation. J Heart Lung Transplant 1995;14:127–35.
229. Keogh A, Macdonald P, Narvison A, Richens D, Mundy J, Spratt P. Initial steroid-free versus steroid-based maintenance therapy and steroid withdrawal after heart transplantation: Two views of the steroid question. J Heart Lung Transplant 1992;11:421–7.
230. Kobashigawa J, Katznelson S, Laks H, et al. Effect of pravastatin on outcomes after cardiac transplantation. N Engl J Med 1995;333:621–7.
231. Maggard M, Ke D, Want T, et al. Effects of pravastatin on chronic rejection of rat cardiac allografts. Transplantation 1998;65:149–55.
232. Keogh A, Macdonald P, Kann A, Aboyoun C, Spratt P, Mundy J. Efficacy and safety of pravastatin vs simvastatin after cardiac transplantation. J Heart Lung Transplant 2000;19:528–37.
233. Ballantyne C. Statins after cardiac transplantation: Which statin, what dose, and how low should we go? J Heart Lung Transplant 2000;19:515–17.

11. NEW IMMUNOSUPPRESSIVE AGENTS

J.F. Gummert[1,3], T. Ikonen[2,3], R.E. Morris[3]
Stanford University School of Medicine, Stanford, California USA

INTRODUCTION

In the 1990's, many new small and large molecules have been discovered and developed for use as immunosuppressants in transplantation. This chapter focuses on those small molecules that have shown to have immunosuppressive activity in patients[1,2] (Figure 1). Two monoclonal antibodies are also included as examples of a resurgence of development in this area.

Conventional wisdom has held that the price for reducing the incidence of allograft rejection by improved immunosuppressants is a proportional increase in the incidence of infection and malignancy. When the data from Phase III trials of new immunosuppressants are analyzed, however, the statistically significant reduction in the incidence of acute rejection produced by these new drugs has not been accompanied by increases in infection and malignancy rates in the first year post transplantation.

Since each of the new immunosuppressants reviewed in this chapter differs in its mechanisms of action (Figure 2), and since its toxicities are mechanism-based, the wide array of new drugs offers the opportunity to use combinations that block different pathways of immune activation while at the same time selecting combinations with non-overlapping toxicity profiles so that doses of each drug can be reduced below toxic levels.

The development of so many novel and very different small molecule and monoclonal antibody immunosuppressants will enable the clinician to tailor therapy for individual patients more precisely than ever before. Designing individualized regimens, however, presumes that the clinician understands the many facets of this new world of immunosuppression. This chapter has been prepared to provide a foundation for this understanding.

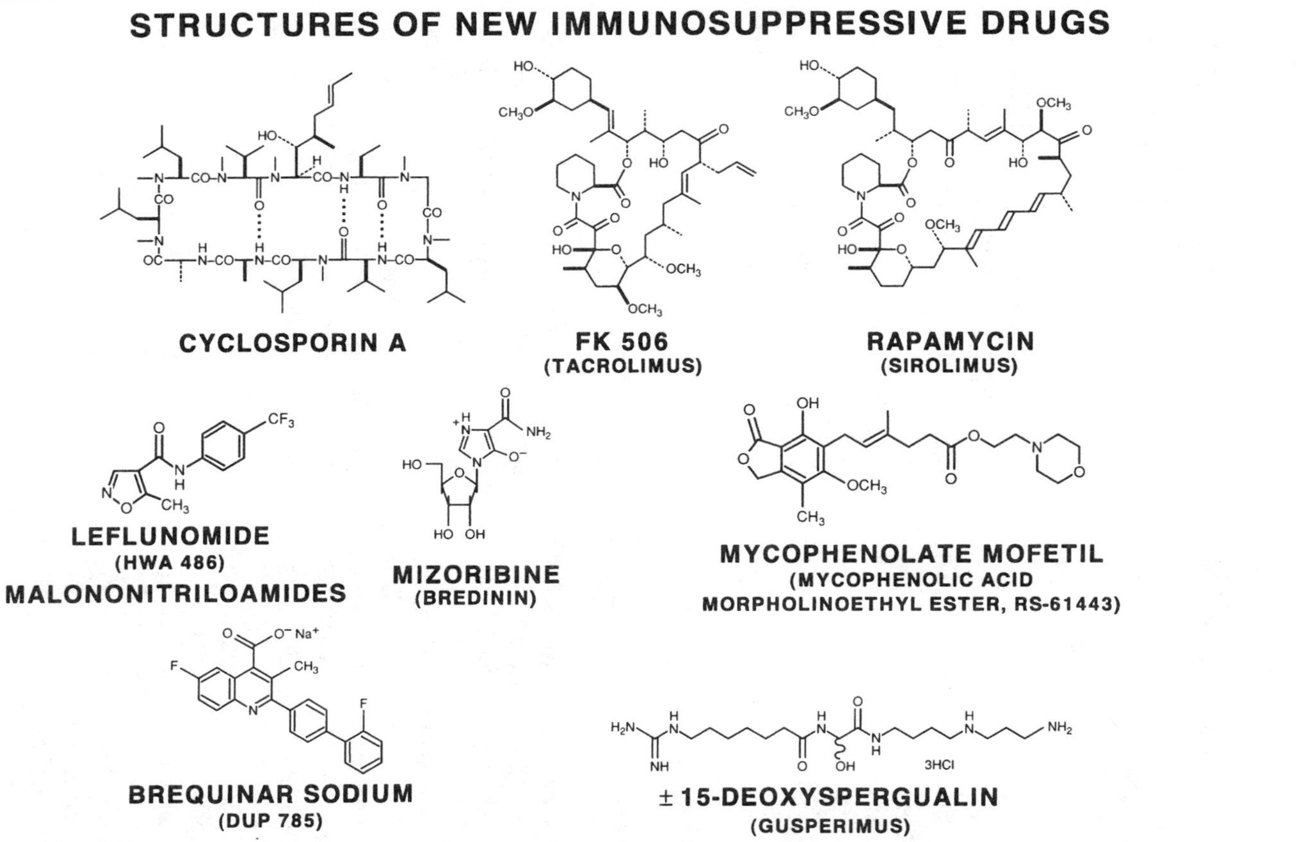

STRUCTURES OF NEW IMMUNOSUPPRESSIVE DRUGS

CYCLOSPORIN A

FK 506
(TACROLIMUS)

RAPAMYCIN
(SIROLIMUS)

LEFLUNOMIDE
(HWA 486)
MALONONITRILOAMIDES

MIZORIBINE
(BREDININ)

MYCOPHENOLATE MOFETIL
(MYCOPHENOLIC ACID
MORPHOLINOETHYL ESTER, RS-61443)

BREQUINAR SODIUM
(DUP 785)

± 15-DEOXYSPERGUALIN
(GUSPERIMUS)

Figure 1. Chemical structures of new immunosuppressive drugs (Used with permission; Morris RE: New immunosuppressive drugs. In: Busuttil RW, Klintmalm GB. *Transplantation of the Liver*, Philadelphia, PA, WB Saunders Company, 1996).

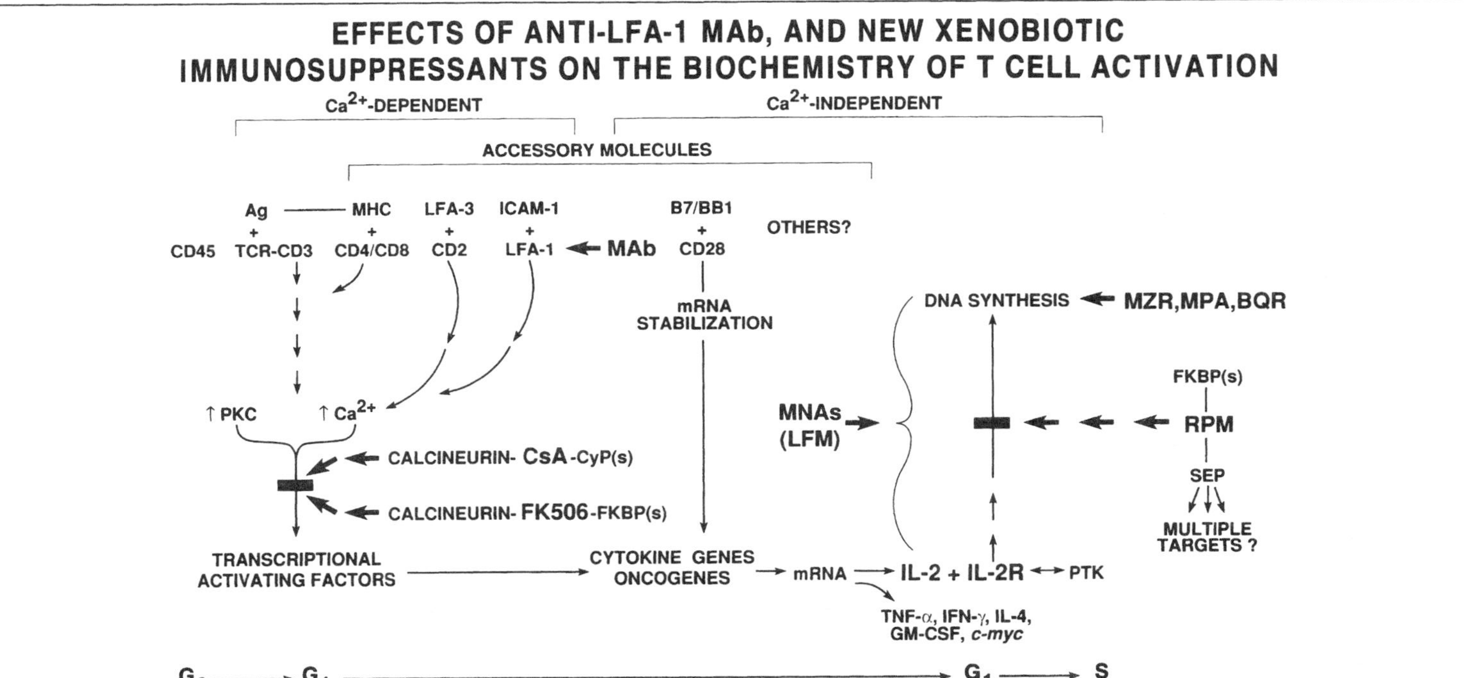

Figure 2. Schematic representation of site of action of new immunosuppressants in T cell. MHC = major histocompatibility complex; PTK = protein tyrosine kinase; PLC = phospholipase; CyP = cyclophlin; FKBP = FK506 binding protein; CsA = cyclosporine; MPA = mycophenolic acid; RPM = rapamycin; BQR = breqinar; DSG = deoxyspergualin (gusperimus); MZR = mizobine; LFM = leflunomide; Ca^{+2} = calcium ion; Ag = antigen; LFA = lymphocyte function-associated antigen; IL = interleukin; TN-alpha = tumor necrosis factor-alpha; GM-CSF = granulocyte-macrophage colony-stimulating factor; IFN-gamma = interferon gamma; mRNA = messenger RNA; Pase = phosphatase; PKC = protein kinase C; TCR = T cell receptor complex; ICAu = intercellular adhesion molecule; PLC = phospholipase C. (Used with permission; Morris RE: New immunosuppressive drugs. In: Busuttil RW, Klintmalm GB. *Transplantation of the Liver*, Philadelphia, PA, WB Saunders Company, 1996).

BREQUINAR SODIUM

Brequinar (brequinar sodium) is a substituted 4-quinolinecarboxylic acid analogue produced by total organic synthesis and was originally developed as a new anticancer agent. Several phase II trials have been conducted.[3–6] Because its low efficacy in cancer patients the development of this drug shifted in the direction of a immunosuppressant. Brequinar was first shown to suppress graft rejection in mice by Morris and Murphy.[7] Pioneering studies with this drug were performed by Jaffee at DuPont Merck.[8,9] Cramer and Makowka[10,11] at Cedars Sinai in Los Angeles began to investigate brequinar in many preclinical transplantation models.

Brequinar is a reversible, noncompetitive inhibitor of dihydroorotate dehydrogenase (DHODH), a key enzyme in the *de novo* pyrimidine synthesis pathway. Activated lymphocytes need both the salvage pathway and the *de novo* pathways since high levels of RNA and DNA synthesis in proliferating lymphocytes require a large amount of pyrimidines. By selectively blocking the *de novo* pathway, lymphocyte proliferation is inhibited.

Brequinar is water soluble and has a bioavailability >90% after oral administration. It is highly protein bound in plasma. The primary site of metabolism is the liver (P450 cytochrome oxidase) and the kidney. Clearance will be reduced by liver and kidney dysfunction. The drug is found in tissues even after it has been eliminated from the blood, which may be a further potential problem for clinical use. *In vitro* data have shown the inhibition of T and B cell proliferation in different species. The sensitivity to the inhibitory effect depends on the cell type, species and the strength of the mitogenic stimulus.[12] *In vivo*, prolongation of heart, liver, kidney and small bowel allografts in rats has been demonstrated.[10] Brequinar also suppresses the production of donor antibodies. In animal models, the primary toxicities are leukopenia, thrombocytopenia and diarrhea.

The phase I clinical trials of brequinar with liver, kidney and heart allograft patients have shown a high interindividual variation in drug plasma levels. The oral clearance was reduced in all 3 patient populations (12–19 mL/min) compared to previous trials with cancer patients (30 mL/min). The terminal half life was 13–18 h.[13] Further trials in kidney allograft recipients comparing brequinar with azathioprine have shown a narrow therapeutic window. Acute rejection episodes were not reduced in patients receiving 100 mg every other day whereas treatment with 200 mg every other day resulted in a decrease of rejection episodes but toxic side effects became clinically apparent.[14]

The extended plasma half-life may be responsible for the relatively low therapeutic index of this drug compared to other new immunosuppressants.

Its use in transplant patients is challenging. The future development of this compound is uncertain. Modification of brequinar to improve the therapeutic index may be necessary to warrant further clinical trials.[15]

GUSPERIMUS (15-DEOXYSPERGUALIN)

Gusperimus is an analog of the parent drug spergualin (anti-cancer drug) extracted from the culture filtrate of *Bacillus laterosporus* and was isolated by

Takeuchi in 1981. In 1985 the immunosuppressive activities were demonstrated in skin allografts in mice.[16] A thorough review has been published and should be used for primary reference.[17] In 1994, gusperimus was approved in Japan for clinical use as a treatment for acute rejection in renal transplant patients. In western Europe and in North America, pilot studies have been conducted in the setting of kidney allograft rejection.

Gusperimus is highly unstable in aqueous solution and the oral bioavailability is very low (<5%).[18] Therefore it is only available in a parenteral formulation. The drug displays a biexponential decay in plasma and has an initial half-life of approximately 5 to 60 minutes and a terminal half life of 2 hours.[19]

The proposed mechanism of action involves inhibition of nuclear translocation of NF-kappaB. The translocation of NF-kappaB into the nucleus is facilitated by chaperone proteins like Hsc70. The cytosolic protein Hsc70 is a member of the heat shock protein (Hsp) family. Gusperimus binds to Hsc70, which is then unavailable for translocation resulting in inhibition of the transcription of NF-kappaB dependent cytokines.[19]

In vivo, prolongation of allograft and xenograft survival in different species has been reported. These experiments are summarized in a review by Kaufman.[20]

In murine heart allograft recipients, gusperimus was shown to prevent and treat acute rejection as well as to prevent accelerated rejection in presensitized animals. These studies also showed that gusperimus and cyclosporine synergize to suppress rejection.[21] The combination of gusperimus and cyclosporine was also synergistic in a rat heterotopic allograft model.[22] Gusperimus has been particularly effective for the control of ongoing rejection in several animal models, which may be due to its ability to inhibit macrophage proliferation within grafts.[23] In the rat aorta allograft model, gusperimus effectively inhibited intimal thickening.[24] In a murine model gusperimus suppressed antibody production when given at the time of the antigen challenge.[25]

The clinical experience with gusperimus was reviewed by Gores.[26] Many clinical trials have been conducted in renal transplant patients in Japan. The trials have focused primarily on its use for the treatment of ongoing rejection.[27-29] A pilot study of gusperimus at the University of Minnesota addressed the use of gusperimus in patients with acute refractory renal allograft rejection.[30] Three out of 6 patients showed improved serum creatinine concentrations after gusperimus treatment. Based on the animal data showing the ability to suppress humoral immunity, studies have been done with patients receiving ABO incompatible renal allografts. In addition, these patients were treated with a conditioning protocol including plasmapheresis and immunoabsorption. At the time of transplantation, splenectomy was performed and after transplantation the graft was irradiated, 80% 3 year survivals were achieved.[31] However, the contribution of gusperimus is unclear since other groups have reported similar results using the same conditioning protocol without gusperimus.[32] Side effects include leukopenia, thrombocytopenia, gastrointestinal disturbances, reversible hypotension and transient perioral numbness. In contrast to other immunosuppressants DSG has no diabetogenic properties and is not nephro- or hepatotoxic.[26,27,29,33]

To summarize, in clinical studies DSG has demonstrated a favorable safety profile with only temporary and mild side effects. In pilot studies it has shown to be able to reverse acute renal allograft rejection but those studies are preliminary. The mechanism of action is different from other immunosuppressive drugs, which could be a useful attribute for combination regiments. Due to the pharmacokinetic properties (only parenteral application possible), DSG has currently no role in maintenance immunosuppressive therapy.

MIZORIBINE (BREDININ)

Mizoribine (bredinin, MZR) is an imidazole nucleoside and was first isolated from the culture filtrates of *Eupenicillium brefeldianum* by Mizuno in Japan in 1974.[34] Five years after its discovery MZR was reported to be an effective immunosuppressant in renal allograft patients and in 1984 it was approved for use in transplant recipients in Japan. Outside Japan MZR is not well known and remains unapproved and investigational, whereas in Japan it has replaced azathioprine for use in immunosuppressive protocols.

MZR, soluble in water and stable at acid and alkaline pH, is a prodrug and converted by intracellular phosphorylation to mizoribine 5′-monophosphate, which is a competitive inhibitor of inosine monophosphate dehydrogenase (IMPDH) and guanosine-monophosphate synthetase (GMPs).[35] Primarily responsible for its pharmacodynamic properties is the inhibition of IMPDH. The active drug is not incorporated into DNA or RNA and leaves the cell after dephosphorylation when the extracellular concentration decreases.[35]

In vitro, MZR inhibits human T—cell proliferation and the expression of T-cell surface antigens following allostimulation. Under the same conditions, mycophenolic acid (MPA) was 1000 fold more potent.[36] *In vivo*, MZR minimally prolongs skin and heterotopic heart allografts in rodents.[37]

The European MZR clinical trial compared MZR to azathioprine in triple immunosuppressive regimens in cadaveric kidney allograft recipients. MZR was well tolerated. Leukopenia occurred only in 10% of the patients compared to 45% in the azathioprine group. The incidence of rejection was 20% (per 32.8 patient-month) in the MZR group compared to 65% (per 16.9 patient-month) in the azathioprine group.[38]

The half-life of MZR is 2–3 hours in patients with normal renal function, but is markedly prolonged in patients with renal dysfunction. The correlation between AUC and dose is poor in those patients, which may be considered a disadvantage compared to MMF.[39]

The main adverse effects in clinical studies have been gastrointestinal side effects and leukopenia associated with high blood levels.[39]

TACROLIMUS (FK506)

History

Tacrolimus, a metabolite of an actinomycete *Streptomyces tsukubaensis* was first demonstrated to be immunologically effective *in vivo* in rat heart allograft recipients.[40,41] It was soon found a potent alternative to cyclosporine (CsA) in several experimental models; in the mid-1990s, it gained world-wide approval for clinical use in liver transplant recipients.

Medicinal chemistry

Being a hydrophobic macrolactam, tacrolimus is structurally unrelated to CsA, although these two molecules share similarities in their mechanism of action.[42] Tacrolimus differs from other macrolactams, except sirolimus, by carrying a hemiketal-masked, alpha, beta-diketoamide incorporated into its 23-membered ring.[43] Since tacrolimus is minimally soluble in aqueous solvents, it is formulated in alcohol and a surfactant for continuous intravenous administration.[43] The oral formulation is composed of capsules of a solid dispersion of tacrolimus in hydroxypropyl methylcellulose.[44]

Pharmacology

Absorption of tacrolimus is incomplete after oral administration. Its bioavailability ranges from 10 to 60% with peak blood levels after 1 to 2 hours and half life of 8 to 24 hours.[45–47] Bile salts do not play a central role in the oral bioavailabilty of tacrolimus. The oral dose of tacrolimus needs to be higher than intravenous doses. Administration of tacrolimus by the intravenous route leads to a rapid distribution of the drug reflected as a rapid decline of the initial peak concentration, followed by a slower decline over the next 24 hours.[48] Tacrolimus is highly bound to plasma proteins, e.g. albumin, and to red blood cells and lymphocytes.[49,50] Most of the solid organs exhibit a high concentration of tacrolimus, particulary the lungs, heart, kidney, pancreas, spleen, and liver.

The major part of the metabolism takes place in the intestinal wall and in the liver by the cytochrome P450 system.[51,52] At least 15 metabolites have been detected, and some of them show pharmacological activity.[53,54]

Drug level monitoring is required, because tacrolimus has high inter- and intraindividual variability and narrow therapeutic index.[47] Drug levels can be monitored by an enzyme-linked immunoabsorbent assay or by a radioreceptor assay from whole blood.[55,56] For clinical heart transplantation target trough levels are generally 10–20 ng/ml for the first 30 days after transplantation, after 90 days the target levels are 5–10 ng/ml.

Mechanism of Action

The intracellular pathways that lead to immunosuppression are believed to be similar for tacrolimus and CsA, which might offer one explanation for the observed antagonism of these two drugs.[57–59] The process is initiated by binding of the tacrolimus molecule to cytoplasmic immunophilins, FK506-binding proteins

(FKPBs), of which the isoform FKBP12 seems to be involved in the immunosuppressive effect caused by tacrolimus.[60–62]

The tacrolimus-FKBP complex inhibits the activity of calcineurin, a serine-threonine phosphatase that regulates Interleukin 2 (IL-2) promoter induction after T-cell activation.[63,64] Inhibition of calcineurin impedes calcium-dependent signal transduction, and inactivates transcription factors (NF-AT) that promote cytokine gene activation, because they are direct or indirect substrates of calcineurin's serine-threonine phosphatase activity.[65,66] As a consequence, the transcription of cytokines IL-2, IL-3, Il-4, IL-5, IFN-gamma, TNF-apha, and GM-CSF, and IL-2 and IL-7 receptors is suppressed by tacrolimus.[67–70]

Tacrolimus inhibits lymphocyte activation *in vitro* 10 to 100 times more potently than CsA.[70] One explanation might be the higher binding affinity of tacrolimus to FKPB compared to the binding of CsA to its immunophilin called cyclophilin.[61] Other immunosuppressive effects of tacrolimus include the inhibition of T cell proliferation and the inhibition of primary or secondary cytotoxic cell proliferation *in vitro*, whereas direct cytotoxicicity and calcium-independent T cell stimulation are not affected.[71,72] Tacrolimus also suppresses B cell activation *in vitro*: both induced immunoglobulin production by B cells and the proliferation of stimulated B cells.[73] Although the exact mode of action is still uncertain, inhibition of T cell-dependent B cell activation offers one plausible explanation. *In vivo*, tacrolimus inhibits proliferative and cytotoxic responses to alloantigens and suppresses primary antibody responses to T cell-dependent antigens, whereas secondary antibody responses, IL-2 stimulated cell proliferation, natural killer or antibody-dependent cytotoxic cell function are not inhibited.[74–76]

Animal Studies

Tacrolimus was first described as a promising immunosuppressive agent to control acute rejection in experimental heart transplantation in rats.[77] Later studies showed its efficacy for suppression of heart allograft rejection in non-human primates.[78,79–81] Controversial results have been published concerning the role of tacrolimus in prevention of chronic rejection. In a heterotopic rat cardiac transplant model high dose tacrolimus treatment reduced the incidence of cardiac allograft vascular disease,[82] whereas other studies show that tacrolimus was not able to prevent GVD.[81,83] In a rat hind limb transplant model, tacrolimus was superior to sirolimus or CsA in prolongation of allograft survival.[84]

A new field of interest in the applications of tacrolimus immunosuppression is xenotransplantation. Tacrolimus has been shown to prolong the survival of concordant heart xenografts in a hamster to rat model when combined with antiproliferative drugs or splenectomy,[85–87] as well as in a concordant model in primates.[88]

Clinical trials

Tacrolimus has been investigated in clinical transplantation of all solid organs, and it has been approved as an immunosuppressant agent for primary therapy for patients with liver and kidney transplants. In prospective trials in heart transplant recipients, 1-year and 5-year survival rates did not differ significantly between tacrolimus and cyclosporine based regimens.[89] However, tacrolimus seemed to be associated with a lower number of acute rejection episodes.[89,90] Similarly, tacrolimus treatment of acute rejection refractory to CsA has been reported to be successful[90–92,92,93] and recently the superiority of tacrolimus over OKT3 for treating persistent rejection after intrathoracic organ transplantation has been described.[93] The percentage of patients without coronary angiopathy did not differ between tacrolimus and cyclosporine. Tacrilomus has recently been shown effective as manotherapy in a cohort of stable adult heart transplant recipients.[93a]

In a limited number of studies on pediatric heart transplantation, the beneficial effects of tacrolimus seemed to be more evident than in adults.[94] Unlike cyclosporine regimens, most of the children on tacrolimus-based immunosuppression could be weaned from steroids, and the rate of freedom from acute rejection was higher with tacrolimus.[95]

Adverse Effects and Toxicity

Significant nephro- and neurotoxicity has been reported in patients receiving tacrolimus treatment.[89,96,97] One mechanism for the neurotoxicity appears to be related to the inhibition of calcineurin phosphatase, but the etiology of its renal vasculopathic effects is unclear. Reduced renal glomerular and cortical blood flow and increased renal vascular resistance are generally associated with increased thromboxane A2, endothelin production or stimulated intrarenal renin production.[96] Cardiomyopathy, anemia, chronic diarrhea, onset of diabetes and allergies have been reported in patients receiving tacrolimus.[97,98] Compared to cyclosporine, hypercholesteremia and hypertension is less common, and gingival hyperplasia and hirsutism are notably absent in patients receiving chronic tacrolimus.[89,96,98] Lymphoproliferative disease and infections are associated with tacrolimus based immunosuppressive protocols.[98,99]

MYCOPHENOLATE MOFETIL

History

Mycophenolic acid (MPA) was initially derived from cultures of Penicillium spp. by Gosio[100] in 1896 and purified by Alsberg and Black in 1913. Antibacterial and antifungal activities were recognized in the 1940s. Antitumor activity was described in 1968,[101] MPA was further studied for psoriasis,[102] but did not gain clinical use. Mitsui and Suzuki[103] demonstrated potential immunosuppressive properties, but the failure to prolong mouse skin graft survival substantially delayed its further studies as an immunosuppressant. The rapid metabolism of MPA in mice in contrast to other species (e.g. rats) accounted for its early experimental failure. These species differences in half lives led to its reevaluation in rats as an immunosuppressant for allograft recipients and prompted the first studies to show its efficacy for this indication.[104,105–107]

Further developmental work produced an ester prodrug of MPA, mycophenolate mofetil (MMF), which demonstrated a higher bioavailability in cynomolgus monkey than MPA.[108] Further clinical studies in cadaveric kidney[109] and liver transplantation[110] showed promising results. In 1995 MMF was approved by the US Food and Drug Administration for prevention of acute renal allograft rejection. In 1998 approval was granted for its use in heart transplant patients. Despite the variety of other novel purine (mizoribine) and pyrimidine (leflunomide, brequinar) inhibitors recently developed for transplantation, MMF is currently the leading candidate for replacement of azathioprine.

Medicinal Chemistry

MMF, the 2-morpholinoethyl ester of MPA, can be considered a prodrug. It is rapidly and completely hydrolyzed into its active metabolite MPA after oral administration by plasma esterases. The parent compound is not measurable in plasma.[108] MMF is only slightly soluble in water.

Pharmacology

The volume of distribution of MPA in healthy volunteers is 3.6 L/kg[111] after oral or intravenous administration. The ratio of the oral and intravenous area under the curve is 94%.[111] At clinically relevant concentrations MPA is almost completely (>99%) bound to plasma albumin.[112] Therefore, plasma is the matrix of choice for measurement of MPA concentrations.[113] MPA is metabolized to mycophenolic acid glucuronide (MPAG) by UDP-glucuronosyl transferase in the liver and MPAG is the primary urinary excretion product of the drug. Approximately 87% of the drug is eliminated in urine; 6% is eliminated in the faeces.[111,113]

MPAG is only a weak IMPDH inhibitor. The MPAG inhibitory concentrations (IC_{50}) with recombinant IMPDH were found to be 532- to 1022-fold higher than those for MPA.[114] However, in another study MPAG IC_{50}'s for inhibition of human lymphocyte IMPDH were only 10-fold higher compared to MPA.[115] Other unidentified metabolites are suspected to be pharmacologically active.[114,116] MPA undergoes substantial enterohepatic circulation; MPAG is converted by mucosal enzymes and gut flora to MPA and is reabsorbed. This results in secondary peaks in pharmacokinetic studies after 6–12 and 24 h.[113]

For clinical use, MPA plasma concentrations are measured by EMIT. The necessity of therapeutic drug monitoring is still under investigation.[117]

Mechanism of Action

MPA is a highly selective non-competitive and reversible inhibitor of IMPDH type II. IMPDH is a crucial enzyme in the *de novo* biosynthesis of guanosine. Inhibition of IMPDH causes a depletion of guanine nucleotides.[118] Proliferating lymphocytes differ from most other cells in that they are fully dependent on both the *de novo* pathway and the salvage pathway of purine biosynthesis. Most other cell lines can maintain their function with the salvage pathway alone. Due to this property of lymphocytes and the high specificity of MPA for IMPDH compared with other nicotinamide adenine dinucleotides,[119] MPA is a very specific lymphocyte inhibitior. MPA inhibits proliferation of both T and B lymphocytes[120] in response to mitogenic and allospecific stimulation. The inhibitory effect can be reversed *in vitro* (peripheral human blood lymphocytes and lymphoma cell lines) by adding guanosine or desoxyguanosine.[118]

Antibody formation in humans to horse antilymphocyte globulin is also inhibited by MMF.[121] In human spleen cells stimulated by tetanus toxoid, antibody formation is inhibited even after adding MPA at day 3.[120,122]

Guanosine nucleotides are necessary for glycosylation of lymphocyte and monocyte glycoproteins; by inhibiting guanosine nucleotide synthesis, glycosylation of adhesion molecules is suppressed. The inhibition of migration to sites of rejection or inflammation may be impaired. *In vitro* studies in human cell lines have shown that MPA inhibits the incorporation of mannose and fucose into cellular glycoproteins.[123] Human monocytes exposed to MPA demonstrate decreased adherence to endothelial cells or extracellular protein matrix.[124]

Animal Studies

The first promising animal study of MMF was in the heterotopic heart transplantation rat model. MMF at 40 mg/kg/day administered over 50 days post transplant resulted in indefinite survival of the graft, 20 mg/kg/day resulted in a 50 day survival.[104,107] In the same model the combination of cyclosporine (0.75 mg/kg/day) and MMF (10 mg/kg/day) produced at least an additive effect with a graft survival over 50 days. Either drug alone resulted in a graft survival of only 10–11 days.[106,107] In a cynomolgus monkey heart allograft model with MMF doses between 70 and 175 mg/kg/day prolongation of graft survival could be achieved (19–62 days compared to 9 days in controls).[106] Ongoing rejection could also be reversed when MMF was given at the time of rejection.[107]

MMF decreased graft vascular disease in a chronic heterotopic heart rat model.[106] In renal[125] and aortic[126] transplantation models chronic rejection was reduced. Further, MMF was effective in reducing antibody mediated rejection in the rat heterotopic heart model.[127]

In animal models of concordant cardiac xenotransplantation MMF showed only a very limited improvement in graft survival[87] while in discordant xenotransplant MMF had no beneficial effect.[128]

Clinical Trials

The first clinical studies were done in 1992 (safety and efficacy phase I trials).[129] The studies showed that oral doses of MMF from 100 mg/day to 3500 mg/day were well tolerated. There was a significant correlation between rejection episodes and low MPA blood levels. In 1995, results were published from the first placebo controlled study of this agent. In Europe MMF was combined with CSA and steroids for prevention of acute rejection in cadaveric renal transplantation. 491 patients were enrolled in this multicenter trial with three treatment arms (placebo, MMF 2 g/d and MMF 3 g/d). This study showed that MMF significantly reduced the rate of biopsy proven rejection or other treatment failure during the first six months after transplantation. Overall, the frequency of adverse events was similar in all treatment groups. Gastrointestinal problems, leukopenia and opportunistic infections were more common in the MMF groups and there was a trend toward more events with higher doses.[130] The results from a US study with 499 renal transplant patients were comparable. Biopsy proven acute rejection episodes or treatment failure occurred in 47.6% of patients in the azathioprine group compared with 31.1% in the 2 g MMF and 3 g MMF group.[109] The tricontinental (Australia, Europe, US) study in cadaver kidney transplant recipients showed that MMF significantly reduced the incidence of rejection episodes in the first 6 months after transplantation. Significant improvement in graft survival could not be demonstrated.[131] A pooled analysis of all 3 studies together showed a significant decrease in acute rejection episodes: 40.8% (placebo/azathioprine) vs. 16.9% (2 g MMF) and 16.5% (3 g MMF) but no significant improvement in 1 year graft survival: 90.4% (2 g MMF) and 89.2% (3 g MMF) compared with 87.6% (placebo/azathioprine).[132]

In a non-randomized study by Kirklin, MMF substituted for azathioprine has been shown effective in treating recurrent or persistent cardiac allograft rejection. Frequency of rejection decreased from 0.67 rejection episodes per patient per month before MMF treatment to 0.27 rejection episodes per patient per month after initiating MMF therapy.[133] Similar results were reported by Taylor.[134] In the most recent multicenter heart trial, 28 centers enrolled 650 patients. MMF (3 g/day) was tested vs. azathioprine (1.5–3 mg/kg/day). Because 11% of the patients withdrew from the study before receiving study drug, the data were analyzed on all randomized patients (enrolled patients) and on treated patients (n = 578). Comparing treated patients, in the MMF group the 1-year mortality was 6.2% vs. 11.4% in the azathioprine group. The requirement for rejection treatment was significantly reduced in the MMF group (65.7% vs. 73.7%). However, opportunistic infections were more common in the MMF group (mostly herpes simplex).[135]

Currently, MMF is used in patients who have contraindications for azathioprine (such as the need for allopurinol) or as the primary choice of an antimetabolite. Based on the experience in clinical trials the recommended initial dose is 2 g/day divided in two doses.

Adverse Side Effects and Drug Toxicity

The most common side effects of MMF in humans are diarrhea, vomiting, opportunistic infections and leukopenia. The mechanism of myelotoxicity is not well understood: Because of selective inhibition of the *de novo* pathway of purine synthesis, MPA should affect only proliferating lymphocytes. In contrast to transplant recipients, the patients treated with MMF for psoriasis or autoimmune diseases rarely develop leukopenia.

SIROLIMUS

History

Sirolimus (rapamycin), a microbial product isolated from the actinomycete *Streptomyces hygroscopicus* was initially discovered as an antifungal agent in the mid-1970's.[136] Because of its immunological side-effects, it was never considered seriously for clinical use as an antibiotic, until the advent of tacrolimus and the recognition of the structural similarities between these two drugs led two research groups independently to study its immunosuppressive properties in experimental organ transplantation.[137,138] Based on the findings of these two groups and subsequent preclinical studies, sirolimus is considered a promising immunosuppressive agent which is presently undergoing several controlled clinical trials in organ transplantation.

Medicinal chemistry

Structurally resembling tacrolimus, sirolimus contains the same tricarbonyl region including an amide, a ketone and a hemiketal, but a triene segment in sirolimus differentiates these two drugs. Because of this structural difference, sirolimus is a hydrophobic drug that has low stability in aqueous solutions.

A new sirolimus derivative SDZ-RAD has been developed with approximately two- to three-fold lower *in vitro* potency, but *in vivo* potency not different from that of sirolimus.[139]

Pharmacology

When administered orally to human kidney recipients, sirolimus was absorbed rapidly with a peak blood concentration at 1.4 hours.[140] Oral bioavailability of sirolimus is 15% in kidney transplant recipients, and the mean half life about 60 hours.[141,142] In the blood, more than 95% of the drug is bound to red blood cells.[143] The drug is widely distributed into tissue stores.[144] Sirolimus is metabolized by cytochrome P450 system and more than 10 metabolites have been identified, some of them with low immunosuppressive activity *in vitro*.[145,146]

In experimental studies, sirolimus is often administered on a dose weight basis. However, therapeutic monitoring of the drug and administration based on effective blood concentrations might be more useful in the clinical setting.[143,147,148] The best method to assess sirolimus from the blood is based on HPLC (high-performance liquid chromatography), because of the assay's sensitivity to detect low concentrations.[149,150] HPLC can detect sirolimus concentrations in the ng/mL range, and newly developed HPLC/mass spectroscopy methods can detect concentrations as low as 0.25 ng/L.[151]

Mechanism of Action

Being lipophilic, sirolimus passes through cell membranes easily, whereafter the segment of the macrolactam ring identical to tacrolimus binds to cytosolic FKBPs. The consequent mechanisms of action for tacrolimus-FKBP12 and sirolimus-FKBP complexes differ in several ways.[152,153] Unlike tacrolimus, sirolimus does not inhibit calcineurin phosphatase, but its molecular targets include RAFT1/FRAP proteins in mammalian cells (homologs with yeast TOR1 and TOR2), associated with cell cycle progression through G1, but the exact mechanism of inhibition of cell cycle progression through these proteins is still unknown.[154–157]

Another, possibly even more effective, way to prolong the cell cycle at G1/S interface is sirolimus' ability to selectively inhibit the synthesis of ribosomal proteins and to inhibit the induction of mRNA for new ribosomal proteins. These effects are mediated by inactivation of p70 s6 kinase ($p70^{s6k}$), specifically the sites of action associated with phosphorylation.[153,158–161] In addition, sirolimus inhibits IL-2 induced binding of transcription factors in the PCNA (proliferating cell nuclear antigen) promoter, thus inhibiting progression to DNA synthesis and S phase. As a consequence of its inability to interfere with early events after T cell activation, sirolimus is a less effective inhibitor of cytokine synthesis than CsA and tacrolimus.[162,163]

On the other hand, sirolimus inhibits several of the CsA resistant pathways in both T and B cell stimulation.[164] Sirolimus inhibits B cell immunoglobulin synthesis and antibody dependent cellular cytotoxicity, as well as lymphocyte activated killer cells and natural killer cells.[165,166] A characteristic feature of sirolimus is its ability to inhibit growth factor signaling for both immune and nonimmune cells.[167–169] This antiproliferative effect includes at least fibroblasts, endothelial cells, hepatocytes, and smooth muscle cells. This antiproliferating effect of sirolimus renders it (at least theoretically) as a promising compound for the prevention of chronic rejection.[167,168,170]

Slight interaction between prednisolone and sirolimus has been observed in stable human kidney transplant recipients and potent interaction between sirolimus and cyclosporine during *in vivo* animal studies.[59,171] Sirolimus and cyclosporine show synergism in immunosuppression both in vitro and in vivo.[59,172–175] There might also be interaction in absorption and transport in intestinal tract.[176]

Animal Studies

Efficacy of sirolimus has been proven in several animal models.[136] It prolonged graft survival in mouse heart graft recipients, heterotopic rat[177] and rabbit cardiac allograft models as monotherapy. In rats, sirolimus acts synergistically in combination with CsA.[178–181] Transplant vasculopathy is significantly inhibited in a heterotopic rat cardiac transplant model and in transplanted femoral artery allografts in a dose dependent manner.[81,169,182] In another studies, sirolimus was able to prevent accelerated cardiac rejection in presensitized mice[136] and rats,[183,184] but did not prevent the development of transplant vasculopathy.[163]

Sirolimus has proven effective in large animal kidney allograft models, but reports of toxicity have been more frequent compared to rodent models.[185–188]

In cynomolgus monkeys, abdominal heart allograft survival is prolonged by sirolimus monotherapy. The median graft survival was 36–45 days compared to 8 days in vehicle controls.[136,189]

Sirolimus effectively reverses ongoing allograft rejection in several solid organs including the heart.[183] Sirolimus can also induce strain specific long-term tolerance in the rat.[190,191] In xenografting, sirolimus alone has only a limited effect on prevention of hyperacute or acute xenograft rejection, but it appears to potentiate the effect of other drugs when used in combination by inhibiting immunoglobulin production and reducing xenoreactive antibodies.[192–194]

Clinical trials

Clinical trials with sirolimus immunosuppression have mainly been published from kidney transplant recipients.[141,142,195] Sirolimus when added to maintenance immunosuppression was effective treatment of acute cardiac rejection in a dose dependent manner in a series of heart transplant recipients.[196] Clinical trials examining sirolimus in heart transplant patients are now ongoing in the United States and Europe.

Adverse Effects and Toxicity

The current profile of adverse effects in humans is mainly based on preclinical studies and Phase I and II studies in stable kidney recipients.[141,197] Headache, nausea, dizziness, changes in blood glucose level, epistaxis, infection, and decrease in platelets and white blood cells have been described in association with short term sirolimus administration.[141,196,198]

The nephrotoxicity associated with tacrolimus and cyclosporine was avoided by sirolimus in several studies in rats and in pigs possibly due to the lack of effect on calcineurin.[199–202] However, hypomagnesemia and tubular injury were side-effects in normal rats receiving sirolimus, and progression of kidney failure in spontaneously hypertensive rats has been described.[203] Myocardial and retinal infarctions have been described in rats after a high dosage of sirolimus.[202,204] In dogs, severe gastrointestinal toxicity with mucosal necrosis and submucosal vasculitis has been described.[185,205] Severe vasculitis was also seen in primates.[186] As with other immunosuppressive drugs, infectious complications occur in animals treated with sirolimus.[179,187]

LEFLUNOMIDE AND MNA'S

History

Leflunomide and the malononitriloamides (MNA) are a new class of immunomodulating drugs, which are currently undergoing investigation for use in transplantation. In 1985 Schleierbach and Bartlett first recognized the antiinflammatory and immunomodulating properties of leflunomide, which differ from classical antiinflammatory and immunosuppressive drugs. The immunosuppressive effects of leflunomide have been investigated extensively in animal-models of transplantation. Because of its long half-life (11–16 days) in humans, the clinical development of leflunomide is restricted to the use in patients with autoimmune disease such as rheumatoid arthritis.

A large preclinical program has started to evaluate the potential use of the leflunomide analogues HMR 715 and HMR 279. These analogues, malononitriloamides (MNAs), are very similar in structure to the active metabolite of leflunomide, A77 1726 and may have a more favorable pharmacokinetic profile. One of these analogues will probably undergo clinical trials if the preclinical testing establishes their safety and efficacy.

Medicinal Chemistry

Leflunomide [N-(4-trifluoro-methylphenyl)-5-methylisoxazol-4-carboxamide] is a synthetic isoxazole derivative that is metabolized in the gut and liver to its active form, the malononitriloamide A77 1726. This metabolite is stable and represents more than 90% of the metabolites in the serum in animals and humans. It is hydrophilic and readily soluble in water.

Pharmacology

There is still little information about the pharmacology of leflunomide and no data about MNA's in humans. Most data have been derived from animal experiments. The bioavailability of leflunomide in rabbits is close to 100% after oral administration, plasma to whole blood ratio is one. A77 1726 is primarily associated (95%) with the lipoprotein free fraction of plasma.[206]

In rats, the peak drug level is reached after 8 to 12 hours. In humans, leflunomide has a half-life between 5 and 18 days[207] and the plasma clearance rate is 0.3 mL/kg/hour. There are several catabolic pathways for A77 1726. For therapeutic drug monitoring in animal models, HPLC methods are available for leflunomide (A77 1726) and the MNA's.

Mechanism of Action

Leflunomide is considered a prodrug because it is readily metabolized to the main metabolite A77 1726 that is pharmocologically active. The effects of the other MNA's appear to be identical to those of A77 1726.[208] Leflunomide suppresses T-cell and B-cell proliferation in vitro[209] and inhibits the proliferation of smooth muscle cells in vitro.[210,211]

The primary known effect of the MNA's is the inhibition of protein tyrosine kinases and dihydroorotate dehydrogenase (DHODH).

Protein tyrosine kinases play a critical role at various steps in the signal transduction pathways, including mitogenesis and transformation.[212] Much higher concentrations of A 77 1726 are needed to block the tyrosine kinase activity than to inhibit lymphocyte proliferation in vitro. In addition, flow cytometric studies demonstrate that A77 1726 blocks the cell cycle progression from G1 to S phase. This suggests that protein tyrosine kinase activity which is necessary for the early phases of cell cycle progression is not inhibited by A 77 1726.

DHODH is a critical enzyme for *de novo* pyrimidine synthesis. Rapidly proliferating cells, like lymphocytes, need both "de novo" pathway and salvage pathway for their nucleotide requirements. Therefore the inhibition of the "de novo" purine pathway is an excellent target for immunosuppressive drugs.

In vitro, DHODH is inhibited by A 77 1726 in the nanomolar or low micromolar range.[213] At concentrations that block cell proliferation, A77 1726 inhibits DHODH; the antiproliferative effects can be antagonized by pyrimidine nucleotides. Addition of uridine or cytidine, but not adenosine or guanosine can antagonize the effect of A77 1726.[209]

The antiproliferative potency of A77 1726 differs, depending on the species and the cell type. Rat lymphocytes are the most sensitive and human lymphocytes are the least sensitive.

More direct evidence that A77 1726 interferes with the 'de novo' pyrimidine biosynthetic pathway *in vivo* comes from murine studies. Treatment of mice with leflunomide, but not cyclosporine reduces DHODH activity in lymphocytes infiltrating heart allograft.[214] Although the administration of 20 mg/kg leflunomide prolonged nonvascularized heart to ear transplants in mice, the coadministration of leflunomide with high doses of uridine resulted in mean survival times similar to untreated control animals.

In vitro and in vivo experiments in allotransplantation and xenotransplantation showed that A 77 1726 prevents antibody production.[211,215–217]

The effects of A77 1726 on cytokine synthesis or growth factor receptor expression are contradictory and are dependent on the cell line, the type of mitogen and A77 1726 concentration. Most studies have shown that A77 1726 has a minimal effect in antiproliferative concentrations on cytokine production and cytokine receptor expression.[218–220]

Animal Studies

Leflunomide has been extensively investigated in numerous animal models of transplantation and autoimmune diseases, such as tubulointerstitial nephritis in rats.[221] The prevention of acute allograft rejection has been tested in mice (heart), rats (heart, skin, intestine, lung, myocutaneous), dogs (kidney) and monkeys (heart).

When administered for 7 days in the heterotopic rat heart model (BN to Lewis), leflunomide prolonged graft survival with doses as low as 0.63 mg/kg. Administration of 5 mg/kg over 21 days resulted in a 50% rate of indefinite graft survival.[222]

Prolonged graft survival (36 days) was achieved in a dose range finding study in cynomolgus monkeys with heterotopic heart transplants,[211] when leflunomide was given in a daily dose of 15 mg/kg. Ongoing acute rejection in heterotopic heart transplants between different rat strains was successfully treated with leflunomide doses between 5 and 20 mg/kg.[223]

In rat models for prevention and treatment of chronic rejection, leflunomide inhibited graft vascular disease in heart, aorta and femoral vessel allografts. The delayed treatment with leflunomide halted the progression of preexisting graft vascular disease.[208,223–226]

Leflunomide has been tested in several models for concordant and discordant xenotransplantation. In the hamster to rat heart-transplant model, graft survival up to 76 days was achieved with a dose of 15 mg/kg.[227] In the guinea pig to rat heterotopic heart transplantation model, leflunomide in combination with cobra venom factor resulted in the longest graft survival (129 hr) reported in this model.[228]

Clinical Trials

Available data from human trials with leflunomide are entirely from phase I and II trials in rheumatoid arthritis. Oral doses between 10 and 25 mg/kg per day were effective compared to placebo. 402 patients were enrolled in the phase II prospective randomized trial to access the safety and effectiveness of leflunomide. A dose dependent improvement in the primary and secondary outcome measures was observed.[207] For the MNA's, clinical data are not available.

Adverse Effects and Toxicity

The most important side effect in cynomolgus monkeys was anemia.[211] In the phase II leflunomide study, adverse effects included gastrointestinal symptoms, rash and allergic reactions, weight loss and reversible alopecia. The incidence of infections in the leflunomide group was not increased; decreases in hematocrit and hemoglobin were observed in all groups.

Toxicity data are not yet available for MNA's in humans.

MONOCLONAL ANTIBODIES

History

In the late 1960's the introduction of polyclonal T-cell antibodies (ALG, ATS, ATG) led to prolonged graft survival. Because of the nonspecific immunosuppression achieved with polyclonal antibodies and the increased knowledge about rejection and T-cell activation, specific monoclonal T-cell antibodies were developed. Monoclonal antibodies provide more selective immunosuppression and are often cheaper to produce than polyclonal antibodies. Several target categories for monoclonal antibodies emerged.

The first commercially available monoclonal antibody was OKT3 (murine CD3) which was introduced in 1981. It is routinely used for both induction therapy

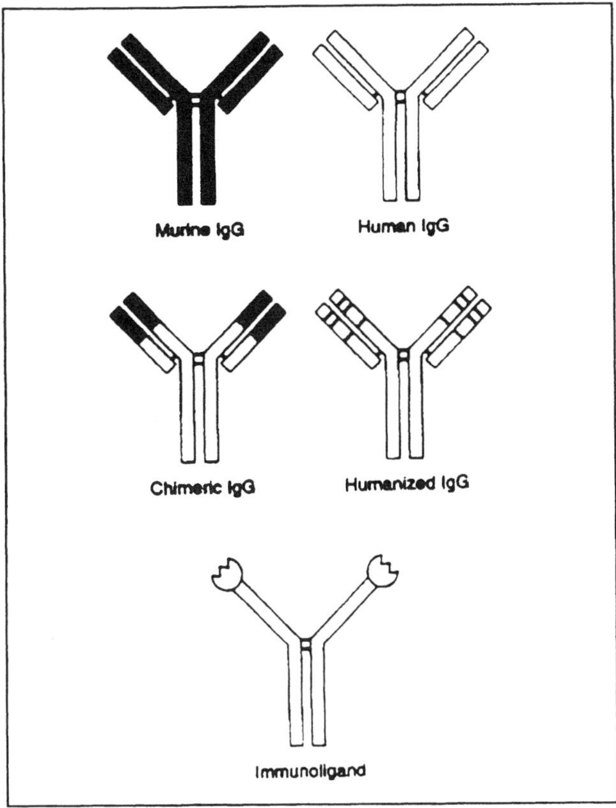

Figure 3. Murine (black) and human (white) IgG molecules are shown in the upper left and right illustrations. To convert a murine antibody into an antibody capable of activating human Fc receptor-positive phagocytes and human complement, the genes for murine heavy and light chains are fused to human Fc cDNA. The product of this fusion gene is a chimeric antibody (murine sequences shown in black and human sequences shown in white). A humanized IgG antibody is constructed by splicing murine complementarily detemining region, i.e. antigen binding DNA into a human cDNA backbone. Immunoligands are constructed by replacing human heavy chain variable cDNA sequences with a selected targeting sequence, i.e. cytokine, cell surface receptor ectodomain, etc. The entire resultant protein is composed entirely of human sequences. (Used with permission; Morris RE: New immunosuppressive drugs. In: Busuttil RW, Klintmalm GB. *Transplantation of the Liver*, Philadelphia, PA, WB Saunders Company, 1996).

and rejection treatment. Because OKT3 is a non-human protein and because of its interaction with all lymphocytes, there are significant side effects in patients treated with OKT3, including cytokine release syndrome and increased risk of malignancies.[229]

Recent studies have been focusing on more specific monoclonal antibodies targeted to regulate the immune response to the transplant, thereby reducing side effects.[230-232] Another major achievement has been the development of chimeric and humanized monoclonal antibodies (Figure 3) which reduce immunogenicity and better support human immune effector functions.[233]

INTERLEUKIN 2—RECEPTOR MONOCLONAL ANTIBODIES

The important role of the IL-2/IL-2 receptor system in lymphocyte proliferation and the selective expression of this receptor on activated T-lymphocytes lead to investigation of the IL-2 receptor as a target for monoclonal antibody therapy.

Mechanism of Action

The high-affinity interleukin—2 receptor consists of three noncovalently bound chains: a 55-kd α-chain (CD 25, Tac), a 75 kd β-chain and a 64 kd γ-chain.[234] The α-chain is only expressed on activated T-lymphocytes. Theoretically, the clonal proliferation of activated T-cells is suppressed by blocking this receptor, but the exact mechanism of action of IL-2 receptor antibodies is not known.

Hypothetically, by binding of the antibody with the expressed IL2–receptor the receptor cannot be activated by free interleukin-2. The expression of the interleukin-2 receptor may be down regulated.

There are two reasons for the weak performance of specific murine monoclonal antibodies. First, there is a rapid development of neutralizing antibodies against the monoclonal antibodies in about 80% of the recipients, thus limiting the therapeutic use of MAbs.[232] Second, the ability of murine antibodies to interact with the human complement system to lyse cells can be impaired. Humanized or chimeric antibodies could overcome this limitation. They do not elicit an antibody reaction and are able to interact with the human complement system.

Animal Studies

Kirkman et al. demonstrated in 1987 a prolongation of murine cardiac allograft survival by the anti-interleukin-2 receptor monoclonal antibody AMT-13.[235] In 1989 a prolongation of murine cardiac allograft survival by IL-2 toxin was described.[236] Prolongation of kidney allograft survival in cynomolgus monkeys has been achieved with use of an anti-Tac monoclonal antibody.[237]

Clinical trials

A variety of IL-2 receptor antibody studies have been performed in humans with kidney or heart transplantation. 33B3.1, a rat IgG2a monoclonal antibody prevented renal allograft rejection as effectively as ATG, but with better tolerance.[231]

Anti—Tac, a murine IgG2a monoclonal antibody directed against the α-chain of human IL-2 receptors, combined with standard cyclosporine therapy showed a marked reduction in the incidence of early renal graft rejection. However, no improvement in either graft or patient survival could be demonstrated.[238,239] BT 563, a murine IgG1 anti-IL-2 receptor antibody, showed in an open label liver transplant study of 19 patients a reduced incidence of rejection[240,241] and 10 mg/day prevented rejection without apparent side effects.[242] BT 563 has also been shown to effectively prevent rejection after kidney transplantation without infectious complications or side effects.[243] BT 563 has also been used in an open label randomized study in heart transplant recipients. In this study, 10 mg BT 563 was given intravenously from day 0 to day 6. Cyclosporine therapy was started on day 3. The rejection incidence after week 1 was as high as 50%. These disappointing results were attributed to the late onset of cyclosporine therapy and to the redundancy of the cytokine network.[244,245]

A new generation of humanized IL2—receptor antibodies has recently been introduced. Daclizumab, (HAT (humanized anti Tac) or Zenapax®) is a genetically engineered humanized IgG that binds to the α-chain of the interleukin-2 receptor. Results from phase I and III trials in kidney transplant are encouraging: daclizumab significantly reduced the incidence of acute rejection in kidney transplant patients.[246]

Another antibody used for prophylaxis in a phase III clinical trial of cadaver—kidney transplant patients[247] is basiliximab (Simulect®), a chimeric (human and mouse) monoclonal antibody directed against the α-chain of the interleukin-2 receptor. It is produced in vitro by continuous culture fermentation of a murine-myeloma cell-line transfected with plasmid-borne recombinant gene construct coding for murine variable regions and human constant regions. Basiliximab—given on day 1 and 4 (20 mg) was tested against placebo. There was a significantly lower rejection rate in the basiliximab group and the steroid dosage could be reduced. Both agents are now being prospectively studied in heart transplant patients.

Adverse Side Effects and Drug Toxicity

IL-2 receptor antibodies were well tolerated and have almost no side effects compared to OKT3. No evidence of cytokine release syndrome has been seen. The infection rate was comparable with the placebo group and no significant difference regarding malignancies was observed in these short-term studies.

ANTI-LFA-1 AND ANTI-ICAM-1 MONOCLONAL ANTIBODIES

History

The concept of potential ability of anti-LFA-1 mAb therapy to prolong allograft survival was raised in mid 1980's when experiments in mice injected with allogenic tumors showed delayed rejection in treatment group.[248] The first studies to show its efficacy for suppression of rejection were performed in murine heart transplant recipients.[249,250] Better understanding of the role of cellular interactions in the development of immunity and inflammation and recognition of the pivotal role of adhesion molecules, especially lymphocyte function-associated antigen-1 (LFA-1 or CD11a/CD18) and its counter receptors, intercellular adhesion molecules ICAM-1, ICAM-2 and ICAM-3, further encouraged research into the inhibition of costimulatory signals of T-cell activation as one possibility for induction of allograft tolerance.[251] LFA-1 is a key member of the beta 2 integrin family and serves an important role in facilitating leukocyte adhesion to the endothelium.

ICAM-1 is a membrane glycoprotein and constitutively expressed on the surface of 20% of mononuclear cells, 25% of B cells, and on the vascular endothelium. ICAM-1 is highly inducible on multiple cell surfaces by activation or transformation. Once expressed, ICAM-1 functions in antigen-dependent T cell adhesion as a ligand for LFA-1 molecules expressed on the T cell surface.

Mechanism of Action

Monoclonal antibodies against LFA-1 and its ligands inhibit many T-cell dependent immune functions *in vitro* including T-cell activation, lysis of target cells and adhesion to endothelium.[252,253] Both the alpha (CD11a) and beta (CD18) chains of LFA-1 mediate cell signaling through the tyrosine kinase—phosphatidylinositol pathway.[254]

In vitro and *in vivo* studies suggest that early interruption of LFA-signaling is critical for the immunosuppressive and antiproliferative effect of LFA-1 and ICAM-1 inhibition. In experimental studies, pretreatment of the recipient followed by a short course of posttransplant treatment has been shown effective in improving allograft survival.[255] In addition to early initiation of treatment, the efficacy of anti-LFA-1 is dependent on complete saturation of receptors with high dose of antibody.

Animal Studies

A variety of animal studies using anti-LFA-1 mAb alone or in combination with anti-ICAM-1 mAb have been performed in mice, rats and primates. In the primarily unvascularized heart to ear allograft model in mice, anti-CD11a mAb monotherapy was able to prolong graft survival indefinitely when given over a period of 14 weeks.[250,255]

Other studies of vascularized heart allografts in mice and rats have shown that brief combination therapy after transplantation with anti-CD11a mAb and either anti-ICAM-1 mAb or ICAM-1 antisense oligonucleotide induces long-term graft acceptance. In contrast, short-term treatment of these agents as monotherapy only provided minimal prolongation of graft survival.[256–260] In fully incompatible rats, anti-LFA-1 and anti ICAM-1 mAbs combined with mycophenolate mofetil synergistically prolonged graft survival.[260] Early short-term therapy with combination of mAbs has recently been demonstrated to inhibit accelerated graft vasculopathy in heterotopically transplanted mice hearts.[261]

In non-human primate studies using cynomolgus monkeys, both renal and cardiac allograft rejection was delayed by anti-ICAM-1 mAb treatment from 9 days to 24 days.[262,263]

Clinical Trials

No studies of anti-LFA-1 mAb treatment have been published in human heart recipients. In renal transplant recipients anti-CD11a mAb failed to reverse acute renal allograft rejection,[264] emphasizing the importance of early interrupting the immune response. The results for prevention of acute renal rejection by anti-CD11a mAb treatment administered for ten days after transplantation was equal to the outcome after OKT3 or ATG induction protocols.[265,266] Favorable results have also been reported after bone marrow transplantation in children.[267,268]

Adverse Effects and Toxicity

Severe adverse effects during anti-LFA-1 or anti ICAM-1 mAb administration have not been reported, except one case of Quincke's edema during intravenous infusion. Fever of short duration and mild to moderate transient increase in liver enzymes have been the commonest side-effects.[269,270] It remains unanswered if these mAbs tend to increase long-term susceptibility to lymphoproliferative disease.

CONCLUSION

Rejection, infection and malignancies remain the leading causes of death following heart transplantation. Immunosuppressive therapy can currently not prevent or treat graft vascular disease. To further improve long-term graft survival and to reduce the unacceptable high morbidity due to infections and malignancies, more effective and specific immunosuppressive therapy is needed. Two different approaches to improve immunosuppression are currently underway—the development of new small molecules as immunosuppressants and the development of targeted monoclonal antibodies. Another strategy currently investigated is the monitoring of immunosuppressive therapy by pharmacodynamic markers. The ultimate goal of immunosuppressive therapy, its elimination through the development of allograft specific tolerance, has not been reproducibly achieved and may never be realized for all patients. Perhaps the immune systems of most patients will be able to be regulated by a more sophisticated combination of several immunosuppressive drugs, antibodies and donor cells to become specifically hyporesponsive. By reducing the need of nonspecific immunosuppressants the frequency of infections, malignancies and drug toxicity can be diminished and a clinically acceptable and more realistic alternative to complete "tolerance" may become available.

ACKNOWLEDGEMENTS

1) Deutsche Forschungsgemeinschaft grants Gu 472/1-1
2) The Jalmari and Rauha Ahokas Foundation and the Academy of Finland
3) Ralph and Marian Falk Trust

REFERENCES

1. Morris RE: New immunosuppressive drugs. In: Busuttil RW, Klintmalm GB, eds. Transplantation of the liver. 1 ed. W.B. Saunders Company, 1995:750–786.

2. Brazelton TR, Morris RE: Molecular mechanisms of action of new xenobiotic immunosuppressive drugs: tacrolimus (FK506), sirolimus (rapamycin), mycophenolate mofetil and leflunomide. Curr. Opin. Immunol. 1996;8:710–720.
3. Natale R, Wheeler R, Moore M, et al.: Multicenter phase II trial of brequinar sodium in patients with advanced melanoma. Ann. Oncol. 1992;3:659–660.
4. Urba S, Doroshow J, Cripps C, et al.: Multicenter phase II trial of brequinar sodium in patients with advanced squamous-cell carcinoma of the head and neck. Cancer Chemother. Pharmacol. 1992;31:167–169.
5. Cody R, Stewart D, De Forni M, et al.: Multicenter phase II study of brequinar sodium in patients with advanced breast cancer. Am. J. Clin. Oncol. 1993;16:526–528.
6. Moore M, Maroun J, Robert F, et al.: Multicenter phase II study of brequinar sodium in patients with advanced gastrointestinal cancer. Invest. New Drugs 1993;11:61–65.
7. Murphy MP, Morris RE: Brequinar sodium is a highly potent antimetabolite immunosuppressant that suppresses heart allograft rejection. Med. Sci. Res. 1991;19:835–836.
8. Jaffee BD, Jones EA, Zajac I, Magolda RL, Cramer DV, Makowka L: Effects of brequinar sodium on cynomolgus monkeys: immunosuppression and pharmacokinetics. Transplant. Proc. 1993; 25:710–711.
9. Jaffee BD, Jones EA, Loveless SE, Chen SF: The unique immunosuppressive activity of brequinar sodium. Transplant. Proc. 1993;25:19–22.
10. Cramer DV, Chapman FA, Jaffee BD, et al.: The effect of a new immunosuppressive drug, brequinar sodium, on heart, liver, and kidney allograft rejection in the rat. Transplantation 1992;53:303–308.
11. Cramer DV, Chapman FA, Makowka L: Prevention of vascularized allograft and xenograft rejection in rodents by brequinar sodium. Transplant. Proc. 1993;25:23–28.
12. Simon P, Townsend RM, Harris RR, Jones EA, Jaffee BD: Brequinar sodium: inhibition of dihydroorotic acid dehydrogenase, depletion of pyrimidine pools, and consequent inhibition of immune functions in vitro. Transplant. Proc. 1993;25:77–80.
13. Joshi AS, King SY, Zajac BA, et al.: Phase I safety and pharmacokinetic studies of brequinar sodium after single ascending oral doses in stable renal, hepatic, and cardiac allograft recipients. J. Clin. Pharmacol. 1997;37:1121–1128.
14. Dunn JF, Hatch J, Precht A, Hart M, Li S: Brequinar sodium significantly reduces the incidence of steroid-resistant rejection and resource utilization in primary renal transplant patients compared with azathioprine. Transplant. Proc. 1996;28:955–957.
15. Cramer DV: Brequinar sodium. Transplant. Proc. 1996;28:960–963.
16. Umezawa H, Ishizuka M, Takeuchi T, et al.: Suppression of tissue graft rejection by spergualin. J. Antibiot. (Tokyo.) 1985;38:283–284.
17. Yuh DD, Morris RE: The immunopharmacology of immunosuppression by 15-deoxyspergualin. Transplantation 1993;55:578–591.
18. Thomas FT, Tepper MA, Thomas JM, Haisch CE: 15-Deoxyspergualin: a novel immunosuppressive drug with clinical potential. Ann. N.Y. Acad. Sci. 1993;685:175–192.
19. Ramos EL, Nadler SG, Grasela DM, Kelley SL: Deoxyspergualin: mechanism of action and pharmacokinetics. Transplant. Proc. 1996;28:873–875.
20. Kaufman DB: 15-Deoxyspergualin in experimental transplant models: a review. Transplant. Proc. 1996;28:868–870.
21. Yuh DD, Morris RE: 15-Deoxyspergualin is a more potent and effective immunosuppressant than cyclosporine but does not effectively suppress lymphoproliferation in vivo. Transplant. Proc. 1991;23:535–539.
22. Kaji H, Chou DT, Sutherland DE, Stephanian E, Gores PF: Synergistic effect of 15-deoxyspergualin and cyclosporine in prolonging survival of rat cardiac allografts. Transplant. Proc. 1994;26:869–870.
23. Kerr PG, Nikolic-Paterson DJ, Lan HY, Tesch G, Rainone S, Atkins RC: Deoxyspergualin suppresses local macrophage proliferation in rat renal allograft rejection. Transplantation 1994; 58:596–601.
24. Raisanen-Sokolowski A, Yilmaz S, Tufveson G, Hayry P: Partial inhibition of allograft arteriosclerosis (chronic rejection) by 15-deoxyspergualin. Transplantation 1994;57:1772–1777.
25. Alegre ML, Sattar HA, Herold KC, Smith J, Tepper MA, Bluestone JA: Prevention of the humoral response induced by an anti-CD3 monoclonal antibody by deoxyspergualin in a murine model. Transplantation 1994;57:1786–1794.
26. Gores PF: Deoxyspergualin: clinical experience. Transplant. Proc. 1996;28:871–872.
27. Amemiya H, Suzuki S, Ota K, et al.: Multicentre clinical trial of antirejection pulse therapy with deoxyspergualin in kidney transplant patients. Int. J. Clin. Pharmacol. Res. 1991;11:175–182.
28. Amemiya H, Dohi K, Otsubo O, et al.: Markedly enhanced therapeutic effect of deoxyspergualin on acute rejection when combined with methylprednisolone in kidney recipients. Transplant. Proc. 1991;23:1087–1089.

29. Amemiya H: Deoxyspergualin: clinical trials in renal graft rejection. Japan Collaborative Transplant Study of Deoxyspergualin. Ann. N.Y. Acad. Sci. 1993;685:196–201.
30. Matas AJ, Gores PF, Kelley SL, et al.: Pilot evaluation of 15-deoxyspergualin for refractory acute renal transplant rejection. Clin. Transplant. 1994;8:116–119.
31. Takahashi K, Yagisawa T, Sonda K, et al.: ABO-incompatible kidney transplantation in a single-center trial. Transplant. Proc. 1993;25:271–273.
32. Alexandre GP, Squifflet JP, De Bruyere M, et al.: Present experiences in a series of 26 ABO-incompatible living donor renal allografts. Transplant. Proc. 1987;19:4538–4542.
33. Gerber DA, Bonham CA, Thomson AW: Immunosuppressive agents: recent developments in molecular action and clinical application. Transplant. Proc. 1998;30:1573–1579.
34. Mizuno K, Tsujino M, Takada M, Hayashi M, Atsumi K: Studies on bredinin. I. Isolation, characterization and biological properties. J. Antibiot. (Tokyo.) 1974;27:775–782.
35. Kusumi T, Tsuda M, Katsunuma T, Yamamura M: Dual inhibitory effect of bredinin. Cell Biochem. Funct. 1989;7:201–204.
36. Thomson AW, Woo J, Yao GZ, Todo S, Starzl TE, Zeevi A: Effects of combined administration of FK506 and the purine biosynthesis inhibitors mizoribine or mycophenolic acid on lymphocyte DNA synthesis and T cell activation molecule expression in human mixed lymphocyte cultures. Transpl. Immunol. 1993;1:146–150.
37. Tanabe M, Todo S, Murase N, et al.: Combined immunosuppressive therapy with low dose FK506 and antimetabolites in rat allogeneic heart transplantation. Transplantation 1994;58: 23–27.
38. Lee HA, Slapak M, Raman GV, Mason JC, Digard N, Wise M: Mizoribine as an alternative to azathioprine in triple therapy immunosuppressant regimens in cadaveric renal transplantation: two successive studies. Transplant. Proc. 1995;27:1050–1051.
39. Sonda K, Takahashi K, Tanabe K, et al.: Clinical pharmacokinetic study of mizoribine in renal transplantation patients. Transplant. Proc. 1996;28:3643–3648.
40. Goto T, Kino T, Hatanaka H, et al.: Discovery of FK-506, a novel immunosuppressant isolated from Streptomyces tsukubaensis. Transplant. Proc. 1987;19:4–8.
41. Ochiai T, Nakajima K, Nagata M, et al.: Effect of a new immunosuppressive agent, FK506, on heterotopic cardiac allotransplantation in the rat. Transplant. Proc. 1987;19:1284–1286.
42. Schreiber SL, Crabtree GR: The mechanism of action of cyclosporin A and FK506. Immunol. Today 1992;13:136–142.
43. Tanaka H, Kuroda A, Marusawa H, et al.: Physicochemical properties of FK-506, a novel immunosuppressant isolated from Streptomyces tsukubaensis. Transplant. Proc. 1987;19:11–16.
44. Honbo T, Kobayashi M, Hane K, Hata T, Ueda Y: The oral dosage form of FK-506. Transplant. Proc. 1987;19:17–22.
45. Venkataramanan R, Warty VS, Zemaitis MA, et al.: Biopharmaceutical aspects of FK-506. Transplant. Proc. 1987;19:30–35.
46. Christians U, Braun F, Schmidt M, et al.: Specific and sensitive measurement of FK506 and its metabolites in blood and urine of liver-graft recipients. Clin. Chem. 1992;38:2025–2032.
47. Jusko WJ, Piekoszewski W, Klintmalm GB, et al.: Pharmacokinetics of tacrolimus in liver transplant patients. Clin. Pharmacol. Ther. 1995;57:281–290.
48. Jusko WJ: Analysis of tacrolimus FK506 in relation to therapeutic drug monitoring. Ther. Drug Monit. 1995;17:596–601.
49. Machida M, Takahara S, Ishibashi M, Hayashi M, Sekihara T, Yamanaka H: Effect of temperature and hematocrit on plasma concentration of FK506. Transplant. Proc. 1991;23:2753–2754.
50. Piekoszewski W, Jusko WJ: Plasma protein binding of tacrolimus in humans. J. Pharm. Sci. 1993;82:340–341.
51. Sattler M, Guengerich FP, Yun CH, Christians U, Sewing KF: Cytochrome P-450 3A enzymes are responsible for biotransformation of FK506 and rapamycin in man and rat. Drug Metab. Dispos. 1992;20:753–761.
52. Lampen A, Christians U, Guengerich FP, et al.: Metabolism of the immunosuppressant tacrolimus in the small intestine: cytochrome P450, drug interactions, and interindividual variability. Drug Metab. Dispos. 1995;23:1315–1324.
53. Iwasaki K, Shiraga T, Matsuda H, et al.: Further metabolism of FK506 (tacrolimus). Identification and biological activities of the metabolites oxidized at multiple sites of FK506. Drug Metab. Dispos. 1995;23:28–34.
54. Iwasaki K, Shiraga T, Nagase K, et al.: Isolation, identification, and biological activities of oxidative metabolites of FK506, a potent immunosuppressive macrolide lactone. Drug Metab. Dispos. 1993;21:971–977.
55. Murthy JN, Chen Y, Warty VS, et al.: Radioreceptor assay for quantifying FK-506 immunosuppressant in whole blood. Clin. Chem. 1992;38:1307–1310.

56. Tamura K, Kobayashi M, Hashimoto K, et al.: A highly sensitive method to assay FK-506 levels in plasma. Transplant. Proc. 1987;19:23–29.
57. Wiederrecht G, Lam E, Hung S, Martin M, Sigal N: The mechanism of action of FK-506 and cyclosporin A. Ann. N.Y. Acad. Sci. 1993;696:9–19.
58. Vathsala A, Goto S, Yoshimura N, Stepkowski S, Chou TC, Kahan BD: The immunosuppressive antagonism of low doses of FK506 and cyclosporine. Transplantation 1991;52:121–128.
59. Kahan BD: Cyclosporin A, FK506, rapamycin: the use of a quantitative analytic tool to discriminate immunosuppressive drug interactions. J. Am. Soc. Nephrol. 1992;2:S222–S227
60. Griffith JP, Kim JL, Kim EE, et al.: X-ray structure of calcineurin inhibited by the immunophilin-immunosuppressant FKBP12-FK506 complex. Cell 1995;82:507–522.
61. Schreiber SL: Chemistry and biology of the immunophilins and their immunosuppressive ligands. Science 1991;251:283–287.
62. Kaye RE, Fruman DA, Bierer BE, et al.: Effects of cyclosporin A and FK506 on Fc epsilon receptor type I-initiated increases in cytokine mRNA in mouse bone marrow-derived progenitor mast cells: resistance to FK506 is associated with a deficiency in FK506-binding protein FKBP12. Proc. Natl. Acad. Sci. U.S.A. 1992;89:8542–8546.
63. Liu J, Farmer JJ, Lane WS, Friedman J, Weissman I, Schreiber SL: Calcineurin is a common target of cyclophilin-cyclosporin A and FKBP-FK506 complexes. Cell 1991;66:807–815.
64. Clipstone NA, Fiorentino DF, Crabtree GR: Molecular analysis of the interaction of calcineurin with drug-immunophilin complexes. J. Biol. Chem. 1994;269:26431–26437.
65. Timmerman LA, Clipstone NA, Ho SN, Northrop JP, Crabtree GR: Rapid shuttling of NF-AT in discrimination of Ca2+ signals and immunosuppression. Nature 1996;383:837–840.
66. Clipstone NA, Crabtree GR: Calcineurin is a key signaling enzyme in T lymphocyte activation and the target of the immunosuppressive drugs cyclosporin A and FK506. Ann. N.Y. Acad. Sci. 1993;696:20–30.
67. Hanke JH, Nichols LN, Coon ME: FK506 and rapamycin selectively enhance degradation of IL-2 and GM-CSF mRNA. Lymphokine Cytokine. Res. 1992;11:221–231.
68. Wang SC, Jordan ML, Tweardy DJ, Wright J, Hoffman RA, Simmons RL: FK-506 inhibits proliferation and IL-4 messenger RNA production by a T-helper 2 cell line. J. Surg. Res. 1992;53: 199–202.
69. Tocci MJ, Matkovich DA, Collier KA, et al.: The immunosuppressant FK506 selectively inhibits expression of early T cell activation genes. J. Immunol. 1989;143:718–726.
70. Kino T, Inamura N, Sakai F, et al.: Effect of FK-506 on human mixed lymphocyte reaction in vitro. Transplant. Proc. 1987;19:36–39.
71. Andersson J, Nagy S, Groth CG, Andersson U: FK506 and cyclosporine inhibit antigen- or mitogen-induced monokine and lymphokine production in vitro. Transplant. Proc. 1992;24:321–325.
72. Yoshimura N, Matsui S, Hamashima T, Oka T: Effect of a new immunosuppressive agent, FK506, on human lymphocyte responses in vitro. I. Inhibition of expression of alloantigen-activated suppressor cells, as well as induction of alloreactivity. Transplantation 1989;47:351–356.
73. Morikawa K, Oseko F, Morikawa S: The distinct effects of FK506 on the activation, proliferation, and differentiation of human B lymphocytes. Transplantation 1992;54:1025–1030.
74. Maruyama M, Suzuki H, Yamashita N, Yano S: Effect of FK506 treatment on allocytolytic T lymphocyte induction in vivo: differential effects of FK506 on L3T4+ and Ly2+ T cells. Transplantation 1990;50:272–277.
75. Karlsson H, Truedsson L, Nassberger L: The immunosuppressive agent FK506 inhibits in vitro expression of membrane-bound and soluble interleukin-2 receptors on resting but not on activated human lymphocytes. Immunol. Lett. 1991;30:129–132.
76. Minoda M, Ohno M, Tomioka Y, et al.: Effects of gamma-interferon and FK506 on resting B cell proliferation of New Zealand black/white F1 mice. Microbiol. Immunol. 1992;36:885–894.
77. Ochiai T, Nakajima K, Nagata M, Hori S, Asano T, Isono K: Studies of the induction and maintenance of long-term graft acceptance by treatment with FK506 in heterotopic cardiac allotransplantation in rats. Transplantation 1987;44:734–738.
78. Flavin T, Ivens K, Wang J, et al.: Initial experience with FK506 as an immunosuppressant for nonhuman primate recipients of cardiac allografts. Transplant. Proc. 1991;23:531–532.
79. Suzuki S, Kanashiro M, Hayashi R, Kenmochi T, Fukuoka T, Amemiya H: In vivo 31P nuclear magnetic resonance findings on heterotopically allografted hearts in rats treated with a novel immunosuppressant, FK506. Heart Vessels 1990;5:224–229.
80. Murase N, Kim DG, Todo S, Cramer DV, Fung JJ, Starzl TE: Suppression of allograft rejection with FK506. I. Prolonged cardiac and liver survival in rats following short-course therapy. Transplantation 1990;50:186–189.
81. Meiser BM, Billingham ME, Morris RE: Effects of cyclosporin, FK506, and rapamycin on graft-vessel disease [see comments]. Lancet 1991;338:1297–1298.

82. Hisatomi K, Isomura T, Ohashi M, et al.: Effect of dose of cyclosporine or FK506 and antithrombotic agents on cardiac allograft vascular disease in heterotopically transplanted hearts in rats. J. Heart Lung Transplant. 1995;14:113–118.
83. Arai S, Teramoto S, Senoo Y: The impact of FK506 on graft coronary disease of rat cardiac allograft—a comparison with cyclosporine. J. Heart Lung Transplant. 1992;11:757–762.
84. Fealy MJ, Umansky WS, Bickel KD, Nino JJ, Morris RE, Press BH: Efficacy of rapamycin and FK506 in prolonging rat hind limb allograft survival. Ann. Surg. 1994;219:88–93.
85. Hayashi S, Ito M, Yasutomi M, et al.: Evidence that donor pretreatment with FK506 has a synergistic effect on graft prolongation in hamster-to-rat heart xenotransplantation. J. Heart Lung Transplant. 1995;14:579–584.
86. Yoshida Y, Kitamura S, Kawachi K, Taniguchi S, Kondo Y: Comparison of cardiac rejection in heart and heart-lung concordant xenotransplantation. J. Heart Lung Transplant. 1994;13:325–331.
87. Murase N, Starzl TE, Demetris AJ, et al.: Hamster-to-rat heart and liver xenotransplantation with FK506 plus antiproliferative drugs. Transplantation 1993;55:701–707.
88. Kawauchi M, Gundry SR, de Begona JA, et al.: Prolonged survival of orthotopically transplanted heart xenograft in infant baboons. J. Thorac. Cardiovasc. Surg. 1993;106:779–786.
89. Pham SM, Kormos RL, Hattler BG, et al.: A prospective trial of tacrolimus FK506 in clinical heart transplantation: intermediate-term results. J. Thorac. Cardiovasc. Surg. 1996;111:764–772.
90. Rinaldi M, Pellegrini C, Martinelli L, et al.: FK506 effectiveness in reducing acute rejection after heart transplantation: a prospective randomized study. J. Heart Lung Transplant. 1997;16:1001–1010.
91. Armitage JM, Kormos RL, Morita S, et al.: Clinical trial of FK506 immunosuppression in adult cardiac transplantation. Ann. Thorac. Surg. 1992;54:205–210.
92. Mentzer RMJ, Jahania MS, Lasley RD: Tacrolimus as a rescue immunosuppressant after heart and lung transplantation. The U.S. Multicenter FK506 Study Group. Transplantation 1998;65:109–113.
93. Meiser BM, Uberfuhr P, Schulze C, et al.: Tacrolimus FK506 proves superior to OKT3 for treating episodes of persistent rejection following intrathoracic transplantation. Transplant. Proc. 1997;29:605–606.
93a. Baran DA, Segura L, Kushwaha S, et al. Tacrolimus monotherapy in adult cardiac transplant recipients: Intermediate-term results. J. Heart Lung Transplant. 2001;20:59–70.
94. Armitage JM, Fricker FJ, del Nido P, Starzl TE, Hardesty RL, Griffith BP: A decade 1982 to 1992 of pediatric cardiac transplantation and the impact of FK506 immunosuppression. J. Thorac. Cardiovasc. Surg. 1993;105:464–472.
95. Swenson JM, Fricker FJ, Armitage JM: Immunosuppression switch in pediatric heart transplant recipients: cyclosporine to FK506. J. Am. Coll. Cardiol. 1995;25:1183–1188.
96. Textor SC, Wiesner R, Wilson DJ, et al.: Systemic and renal hemodynamic differences between FK506 and cyclosporine in liver transplant recipients. Transplantation 1993;55:1332–1339.
97. Abu-Elmagd K, Fung JJ, Alessiani M, et al.: The effect of graft function on FK506 plasma levels, dosages, and renal function, with particular reference to the liver. Transplantation 1991;52:71–77.
98. Atkison P, Joubert G, Barron A, et al.: Hypertrophic cardiomyopathy associated with tacrolimus in paediatric transplant patients [see comments]. Lancet 1995;345:894–896.
99. Griffith BP, Bando K, Hardesty RL, et al.: A prospective randomized trial of FK506 versus cyclosporine after human pulmonary transplantation. Transplantation 1994;57:848–851.
100. Gosio B: Ricerche batteriologiche e chimiche sulle alterazoni del mais. Rivista d'Igiene e Sanita Publica Ann. 1896;7:825–868.
101. Williams RH, Lively DH, De LD, Cline JC, Sweeny MJ: Mycophenolic acid: antiviral and antitumor properties. J. Antibiot. (Tokyo.) 1968;21:463–464.
102. Jones EL, Epinette WW, Hackney VC, Menendez L, Frost P: Treatment of psoriasis with oral mycophenolic acid. J. Invest. Dermatol. 1975;65:537–542.
103. Mitsui A, Suzuki S: Immunosuppressive effect of mycophenolic acid. J. Antibiot. (Tokyo.) 1969;22:358–363.
104. Morris RE, Hoyt EG, Eugui EM, Allison AC: Prolongation of rat heart allograft survival by RS-61443. Surgical Forum 1989;40:337–338.
105. Sweeney MJ, Hoffman DH, Esterman MA: Metabolism and biochemistry of mycophenolic acid. Cancer Res. 1972;32:1803–1809.
106. Morris RE, Wang J, Blum JR, et al.: Immunosuppressive effects of the morpholinoethyl ester of mycophenolic acid (RS-61443) in rat and nonhuman primate recipients of heart allografts. Transplant. Proc. 1991;23:19–25.
107. Morris RE, Hoyt EG, Murphy MP, Eugui EM, Allison AC: Mycophenolic acid morpholinoethylester (RS-61443) is a new immunosuppressant that prevents and halts heart allograft rejection by selective inhibition of T- and B-cell purine synthesis. Transplant. Proc. 1990;22:1659–1662.

108. Lee WA, Gu L, Miksztal AR, Chu N, Leung K, Nelson PH: Bioavailability improvement of mycophenolic acid through amino ester derivatization. Pharm. Res. 1990;7:161–166.
109. Sollinger HW: Mycophenolate mofetil for the prevention of acute rejection in primary cadaveric renal allograft recipients. U.S. Renal Transplant Mycophenolate Mofetil Study Group. Transplantation 1995;60:225–232.
110. Klupp J, Bechstein WO, Platz KP, et al.: Mycophenolate mofetil added to immunosuppression after liver transplantation—first results. Transpl. Int. 1997;10:223–228.
111. Fulton B, Markham A: Mycophenolate mofetil. A review of its pharmacodynamic and pharmacokinetic properties and clinical efficacy in renal transplantation. Drugs 1996;51:278–298.
112. Nowak I, Shaw LM: Mycophenolic acid binding to human serum albumin: characterization and relation to pharmacodynamics. Clin. Chem. 1995;41:1011–1017.
113. Shaw LM, Sollinger HW, Halloran P, et al.: Mycophenolate mofetil: a report of the consensus panel. Ther. Drug Monit. 1995;17:690–699.
114. Nowak I, Shaw LM: Effect of mycophenolic acid glucuronide on inosine monophosphate dehydrogenase activity. Ther. Drug Monit. 1997;19:358–360.
115. Griesmacher A, Weigel G, Seebacher G, Muller MM: IMP-dehydrogenase inhibition in human lymphocytes and lymphoblasts by mycophenolic acid and mycophenolic acid glucuronide. Clin. Chem. 1997;43:2312–2317.
116. Schutz E, Shipkova M, Armstrong VW, et al.: Therapeutic drug monitoring of mycophenolic acid: comparison of HPLC and immunoassay reveals new MPA metabolites. Transplant. Proc. 1998;30:1185–1187.
117. Shaw LM, Nicholls A, Hale M, Armstrong VW, Oellerich M, Yatscoff R, Morris RE, Holt DW, Venkataramanan R, Haley J, Halloran P, Ettenger R, Keown P, Morris RG: Therapeutic monitoring of mycophenolic acid: A consensus panel report. Clin. Biochem. 1998;31:317–321.
118. Ransom JT: Mechanism of action of mycophenolate mofetil. Ther. Drug Monit. 1995;17:681–684.
119. Sintchak MD, Fleming MA, Futer O, et al.: Structure and mechanism of inosine monophosphate dehydrogenase in complex with the immunosuppressant mycophenolic acid. Cell 1996;85:921–930.
120. Grailer A, Nichols J, Hullett D, Sollinger HW, Burlingham WJ: Inhibition of human B cell responses in vitro by RS-61443, cyclosporine A and DAB486 IL-2. Transplant. Proc. 1991;23:314–315.
121. Kimball JA, Pescovitz MD, Book BK, Norman DJ: Reduced human IgG anti-ATGAM antibody formation in renal transplant recipients receiving mycophenolate mofetil. Transplantation 1995; 60:1379–1383.
122. Burlingham WJ, Grailer AP, Hullett DA, Sollinger HW: Inhibition of both MLC and in vitro IgG memory response to tetanus toxoid by RS-61443. Transplantation 1991;51:545–547.
123. Sokoloski JA, Sartorelli AC: Effects of the inhibitors of IMP dehydrogenase, tiazofurin and mycophenolic acid, on glycoprotein metabolism. Mol. Pharmacol. 1985;28:567–573.
124. Laurent AF, Dumont, Poindron: Inhibition of mannosylation on human monocyte surface glycoprotein could explain some of the anti-inflammatory effects of mycophenolate mofetil. Clin. Exp. Rheumatol. 1994;12 Suppl 11:110:(Abstract).
125. Azuma H, Binder J, Heemann U, Schmid C, Tullius SG, Tilney NL: Effects of RS61443 on functional and morphological changes in chronically rejecting rat kidney allografts. Transplantation 1995;59:460–466.
126. Steele DM, Hullett DA, Bechstein WO, et al.: Effects of immunosuppressive therapy on the rat aortic allograft model. Transplant. Proc. 1993;25:754–755.
127. Knechtle SJ, Wang J, Burlingham WJ, Beeskau M, Subramanian R, Sollinger HW: The influence of RS-61443 on antibody-mediated rejection. Transplantation 1992;53:699–701.
128. Yatscoff RW, Wang S, Keenan R, Chackowsky P, Lowes N, Koshal A: Efficacy of rapamycin, RS-61443 and cyclophosphamide in the prolongation of survival of discordant pig to rabbit cardiac xenografts. Can. J. Cardiol. 1994;10:711–716.
129. Sollinger HW, Deierhoi MH, Belzer FO, Diethelm AG, Kauffman RS: RS-61443—a phase I clinical trial and pilot rescue study. Transplantation 1992;53:428–432.
130. Anonymous Placebo-controlled study of mycophenolate mofetil combined with cyclosporin and corticosteroids for prevention of acute rejection. European Mycophenolate Mofetil Cooperative Study Group [see comments]. Lancet 1995;345:1321–1325.
131. Mathew TH: A blinded, long-term, randomized multicenter study of mycophenolate mofetil in cadaveric renal transplantation: results at three years. Tricontinental Mycophenolate Mofetil Renal Transplantation Study Group. Transplantation 1998;65:1450–1454.
132. Halloran P, Mathew T, Tomlanovich S, Groth C, Hooftman L, Barker C: Mycophenolate mofetil in renal allograft recipients: a pooled efficacy analysis of three randomized, double-blind, clinical studies in prevention of rejection. The International Mycophenolate Mofetil Renal Transplant Study Groups [published erratum appears in Transplantation 1997 Feb 27; 63(4):618]. Transplantation 1997;63:39–47.

133. Kirklin JK, Bourge RC, Naftel DC, et al.: Treatment of recurrent heart rejection with mycophenolate mofetil (RS-61443): initial clinical experience. J. Heart Lung Transplant. 1994;13:444–450.
134. Taylor DO, Ensley RD, Olsen SL, Dunn D, Renlund DG: Mycophenolate mofetil (RS-61443): preclinical, clinical, and three-year experience in heart transplantation. J. Heart Lung Transplant. 1994;13:571–582.
135. Kobashigawa JA, Miller L, Renlund DG, Mentzer RM Jr, Alderman E, Bourge RC, Costanzo M, Eisen H, Dureau G, Ratkovec R, Hummel M, Ipe D, Johnson J, Keogh A, Mamelok R, Mancini D, Smart F, Valantine H: A randomized active-controlled trial of mycophenolate mofetil in heart transplant recipients. Transplantation 1999;66(4), 507–515.
136. Morris RE: Rapamycins: Antifungal, antitumor, antiproliferative, and immunosuppressive macrolides. Transplantation Reviews 1992;6:39–87.
137. Calne RY, Collier DS, Lim S, et al.: Rapamycin for immunosuppression in organ allografting [letter] [see comments]. Lancet 1989;2:227.
138. Morris RE, Meiser BM: Identification of a new pharmacologic action for an old compound. Med. Sci. Res. 1989;17:609–610.
139. Schuler W, Sedrani R, Cottens S, et al.: SDZ RAD, a new rapamycin derivative: pharmacological properties in vitro and in vivo [see comments]. Transplantation 1997;64:36–42.
140. Zimmerman JJ, Kahan BD: Pharmacokinetics of sirolimus in stable renal transplant patients after multiple oral dose administration. J. Clin. Pharmacol. 1997;37:405–415.
141. Brattstrom C, Sawe J, Tyden G, et al.: Kinetics and dynamics of single oral doses of sirolimus in sixteen renal transplant recipients. Ther. Drug Monit. 1997;19:397–406.
142. Ferron GM, Mishina EV, Zimmerman JJ, Jusko WJ: Population pharmacokinetics of sirolimus in kidney transplant patients. Clin. Pharmacol. Ther. 1997;61:416–428.
143. Yatscoff RW, Wang P, Chan K, Hicks D, Zimmerman J: Rapamycin: distribution, pharmacokinetics, and therapeutic range investigations. Ther. Drug Monit. 1995;17:666–671.
144. Napoli KL, Wang ME, Stepkowski SM, Kahan BD: Distribution of sirolimus in rat tissue. Clin. Biochem. 1997;30:135–142.
145. Christians U, Sattler M, Schiebel HM, et al.: Isolation of two immunosuppressive metabolites after in vitro metabolism of rapamycin. Drug Metab. Dispos. 1992;20:186–191.
146. Goodyear N, Murthy JN, Gallant HL, Yatscoff RW, Soldin SJ: Comparison of binding characteristics of four rapamycin metabolites to the 14 and 52 kDa immunophilins with their pharmacologic activity measured by the mixed-lymphocyte culture assay. Clin. Biochem. 1996;29:309–313.
147. Kahan BD, Murgia MG, Slaton J, Napoli K: Potential applications of therapeutic drug monitoring of sirolimus immunosuppression in clinical renal transplantation. Ther. Drug Monit. 1995; 17:672–675.
148. Yatscoff RW, Legatt DF, Kneteman NM: Therapeutic monitoring of rapamycin: a new immunosuppressive drug. Ther. Drug Monit. 1993;15:478–482.
149. Napoli KL, Kahan BD: Routine clinical monitoring of sirolimus rapamycin whole-blood concentrations by HPLC with ultraviolet detection. Clin. Chem. 1996;42:1943–1948.
150. Svensson JO, Brattstrom C, Sawe J: Determination of rapamycin in whole blood by HPLC. Ther. Drug Monit. 1997;19:112–116.
151. Streit F, Christians U, Schiebel HM, et al.: Sensitive and specific quantification of sirolimus rapamycin and its metabolites in blood of kidney graft recipients by HPLC/electrospray-mass spectrometry. Clin. Chem. 1996;42:1417–1425.
152. Chen J, Zheng XF, Brown EJ, Schreiber SL: Identification of an 11-kDa FKBP12-rapamycin-binding domain within the 289-kDa FKBP12-rapamycin-associated protein and characterization of a critical serine residue. Proc. Natl. Acad. Sci. U.S.A. 1995;92:4947–4951.
153. Marx SO, Jayaraman T, Go GL, Marks AR: Rapamycin-FKBP inhibits cell cycle regulators of proliferation in vascular smooth muscle cells. Circ. Res. 1995;76:412–417.
154. Hultsch T, Martin R, Hohman RJ: The effect of the immunophilin ligands rapamycin and FK506 on proliferation of mast cells and other hematopoietic cell lines. Mol. Biol. Cell 1992;3:981–987.
155. Koser PL, Eng WK, Bossard MJ, et al.: The tyrosine89 residue of yeast FKBP12 is required for rapamycin binding. Gene 1993;129:159–165.
156. Sabatini DM, Pierchala BA, Barrow RK, Schell MJ, Snyder SH: The rapamycin and FKBP12 target RAFT displays phosphatidylinositol 4-kinase activity. J. Biol. Chem. 1995;270:20875–20878.
157. Sabers CJ, Martin MM, Brunn GJ, et al.: Isolation of a protein target of the FKBP12-rapamycin complex in mammalian cells. J. Biol. Chem. 1995;270:815–822.
158. Diggle TA, Moule SK, Avison MB, et al.: Both rapamycin-sensitive and -insensitive pathways are involved in the phosphorylation of the initiation factor-4E-binding protein 4E-BP1 in response to insulin in rat epididymal fat-cells. Biochem. J. 1996;316 Pt 2:447–453.
159. Graves LM, Bornfeldt KE, Argast GM, et al.: cAMP- and rapamycin-sensitive regulation of the

association of eukaryotic initiation factor 4E and the translational regulator PHAS-I in aortic smooth muscle cells. Proc. Natl. Acad. Sci. U.S.A. 1995;92:7222–7226.

160. Sadoshima J, Izumo S: Rapamycin selectively inhibits angiotensin II-induced increase in protein synthesis in cardiac myocytes in vitro. Potential role of 70-kD S6 kinase in angiotensin II-induced cardiac hypertrophy. Circ. Res. 1995;77:1040–1052.
161. Sugiyama H, Papst P, Gelfand EW, Terada N: p70 S6 kinase sensitivity to rapamycin is eliminated by amino acid substitution of Thr229. J. Immunol. 1996;157:656–660.
162. Hamashima T, Yoshimura N, Ohsaka Y, Oka T, Stepkowski SM, Kahan BD: In vivo use of rapamycin suppresses neither IL-2 production nor IL-2 receptor expression in rat transplant model. Transplant. Proc. 1993;25:723–724.
163. Wasowska B, Wieder KJ, Hancock WW, et al.: Cytokine and alloantibody networks in long-term cardiac allografts in rapamycin-treated sensitized rat recipients. Transplant. Proc. 1995;27:423–426.
164. Kay JE, Kromwel L, Doe SE, Denyer M: Inhibition of T and B lymphocyte proliferation by rapamycin. Immunology 1991;72:544–549.
165. Chen H, Luo H, Daloze P, et al.: Long-term in vivo effects of rapamycin on humoral and cellular immune responses in the rat. Immunobiology 1993;188:303–315.
166. Thomson AW, Propper DJ, Woo J, Whiting PH, Milton JI, Macleod AM: Comparative effects of rapamycin, FK506 and cyclosporine on antibody production, lymphocyte populations and immunoglobulin isotype switching in the rat. Immunopharmacol. Immunotoxicol. 1993;15: 355–369.
167. Cao W, Mohacsi P, Shorthouse R, Pratt R, Morris RE: Effects of rapamycin on growth factor-stimulated vascular smooth muscle cell DNA synthesis. Inhibition of basic fibroblast growth factor and platelet-derived growth factor action and antagonism of rapamycin by FK506. Transplantation 1995;59:390–395.
168. Francavilla A, Carr BI, Starzl TE, Azzarone A, Carrieri G, Zeng QH: Effects of rapamycin on cultured hepatocyte proliferation and gene expression. Hepatology 1992;15:871–877.
169. Gregory CR, Huie P, Billingham ME, Morris RE: Rapamycin inhibits arterial intimal thickening caused by both alloimmune and mechanical injury. Its effect on cellular, growth factor, and cytokine response in injured vessels. Transplantation 1993;55:1409–1418.
170. Poon M, Marx SO, Gallo R, Badimon JJ, Taubman MB, Marks AR: Rapamycin inhibits vascular smooth muscle cell migration. J. Clin. Invest. 1996;98:2277–2283.
171. Jusko WJ, Ferron GM, Mis SM, Kahan BD, Zimmerman JJ: Pharmacokinetics of prednisolone during administration of sirolimus in patients with renal transplants. J. Clin. Pharmacol. 1996; 36:1100–1106.
172. Andoh TF, Lindsley J, Franceschini N, Bennett WM: Synergistic effects of cyclosporine and rapamycin in a chronic nephrotoxicity model. Transplantation 1996;62:311–316.
173. Granger DK, Cromwell JW, Canafax DM, Matas AJ: Combined rapamycin and cyclosporine immunosuppression in a porcine renal transplant model. Transplant. Proc. 1996;28:984.
174. Knight RJ, Polokoff EG, Martinelli GP: Rapamycin, cyclosporine, and perioperative donor-specific transfusions induce prolongation of cardiac allograft survival in the rat. Transplantation 1994; 58:1014–1020.
175. Schuurman HJ, Cottens S, Fuchs S, et al.: SDZ RAD, a new rapamycin derivative: synergism with cyclosporine [comment]. Transplantation 1997;64:32–35.
176. Dias VC, Yatscoff RW: Investigation of rapamycin transport and uptake across absorptive human intestinal cell monolayers. Clin. Biochem. 1994;27:31–36.
177. Meiser BM, Wang J, Morris RE: Rapamycin: A new and highly active immunosuppressive macrolide with an efficacy superior to cyclosporine. In: Melchers F, ed. Progress in Immunology, Proceedings of the 7th International Congress of Immunology. Springer Verlag, Berlin, Germany, 1989:1195.
178. Davies CB, Madden RL, Alexander JW, Cofer BR, Fisher RA, Anderson P: Effect of a short course of rapamycin, cyclosporin A, and donor-specific transfusion on rat cardiac allograft survival. Transplantation 1993;55:1107–1112.
179. Fryer J, Yatscoff RW, Pascoe EA, Thliveris J: The relationship of blood concentrations of rapamycin and cyclosporine to suppression of allograft rejection in a rabbit heterotopic heart transplant model. Transplantation 1993;55:340–345.
180. Stepkowski SM, Chen H, Daloze P, Kahan BD: Rapamycin, a potent immunosuppressive drug for vascularized heart, kidney, and small bowel transplantation in the rat. Transplantation 1991; 51:22–26.
181. Thliveris JA, Solez K, Yatscoff RW: A comparison of the effects of rapamycin and cyclosporine on kidney and heart morphology in a rabbit heterotopic heart transplant model. Histol. Histopathol. 1995;10:417–421.
182. Schmid C, Heemann U, Azuma H, Tilney NL: Rapamycin inhibits transplant vasculopathy in long-surviving rat heart allografts. Transplantation 1995;60:729–733.
183. Chen H, Wu WJ, Xu XD, Luo H, Daloze PM: Reversal of ongoing heart, kidney, and pancreas

allograft rejection and suppression of accelerated heart allograft rejection in the rat by rapamycin. Transplantation 1993;56:661–666.
184. Wieder KJ, Hancock WW, Schmidbauer G, et al.: Rapamycin treatment depresses intragraft expression of KC/MIP-2, granzyme B, and IFN-gamma in rat recipients of cardiac allografts. J. Immunol. 1993;151:1158–1166.
185. Collier DS, Calne R, Thiru S, et al.: Rapamycin in experimental renal allografts in dogs and pigs. Transplant. Proc. 1990;22:1674–1675.
186. Collier DS, Calne RY, Pollard SG, Friend PJ, Thiru S: Rapamycin in experimental renal allografts in primates. Transplant. Proc. 1991;23:2246–2247.
187. Granger DK, Cromwell JW, Chen SC, et al.: Prolongation of renal allograft survival in a large animal model by oral rapamycin monotherapy. Transplantation 1995;59:183–186.
188. Hartner WC, Van der Werf W, Lodge JP, et al.: Effect of rapamycin on renal allograft survival in canine recipients treated with antilymphocyte serum, donor bone marrow, and cyclosporine. Transplantation 1995;60:1347–1350.
189. Morris RE, Wang J, Gregory CR: Initial studies of th efficacy and safety of rapamycin (RPM) administered to cynomolgus monkey recipients of heart allografts. J. Heart Lung Transplant. 1991; 10:182–182. (Abstract)
190. Chen H, Luo H, Daloze P, Xu XD, Wu WJ: Rapamycin-induced long-term allograft survival depends on persistence of alloantigen. J. Immunol. 1994;152:3107–3118.
191. Goggins WC, Fisher RA, Dattilo JB, et al.: Analysis of functional renal allograft tolerance with single-dose rapamycin based induction immunosuppression. Transplantation 1997;63:310–314.
192. Hale DA, Gottschalk R, Fukuzaki T, Wood ML, Maki T, Monaco AP: Superiority of sirolimus rapamycin over cyclosporine in augmenting allograft and xenograft survival in mice treated with antilymphocyte serum and donor-specific bone marrow. Transplantation 1997;63:359–364.
193. Reichenspurner H, Soni V, Nitschke M, et al.: Obliterative airway disease after heterotopic tracheal xenotransplantation: pathogenesis and prevention using new immunosuppressive agents. Transplantation 1997;64:373–383.
194. Yatscoff RW, Wang S, Keenan R, Chackowsky P, Lowes N, Koshal A: Efficacy of rapamycin, RS-61443 and cyclophosphamide in the prolongation of survival of discordant pig to rabbit cardiac xenografts. Can. J. Cardiol. 1994;10:711–716.
195. Slaton JW, Kahan BD: Case report—sirolimus rescue therapy for refractory renal allograft rejection. Transplantation 1996;61:977–979.
196. Miller L, Brozena S, Valantine H: Treatment of acute cardiac allograft rejection with rapamycin: a multicenter dose ranging study. J. Heart Lung Transplant. 1997;16:44–44. (Abstract)
197. Almond PS, Moss A, Nakhleh RE, et al.: Rapamycin: immunosuppression, hyporesponsiveness, and side effects in a porcine renal allograft model. Transplantation 1993;56:275–281.
198. Yocum DE: Cyclosporine, FK-506, rapamycin, and other immunomodulators. Rheum. Dis. Clin. North Am. 1996;22:133–154.
199. Andoh TF, Burdmann EA, Fransechini N, Houghton DC, Bennett WM: Comparison of acute rapamycin nephrotoxicity with cyclosporine and FK506. Kidney Int. 1996;50:1110–1117.
200. DiJoseph JF, Sharma RN, Chang JY: The effect of rapamycin on kidney function in the Sprague-Dawley rat. Transplantation 1992;53:507–513.
201. Golbaekdal K, Nielsen CB, Djurhuus JC, Pedersen EB: Effects of rapamycin on renal hemodynamics, water and sodium excretion, and plasma levels of angiotensin II, aldosterone, atrial natriuretic peptide, and vasopressin in pigs. Transplantation 1994;58:1153–1157.
202. Whiting PH, Woo J, Adam BJ, Hasan NU, Davidson RJ, Thomson AW: Toxicity of rapamycin—a comparative and combination study with cyclosporine at immunotherapeutic dosage in the rat. Transplantation 1991;52:203–208.
203. DiJoseph JF, Mihatsch MJ, Sehgal SN: Renal effects of rapamycin in the spontaneously hypertensive rat. Transpl. Int. 1994;7:83–88.
204. Chan CC, Martin DF, Xu XD, Roberge FG: Side effects of rapamycin in the rat. J. Ocul. Pharmacol. Ther. 1995;11:177–181.
205. Ochiai T, Gunji Y, Nagata M, Komori A, Asano T, Isono K: Effects of rapamycin in experimental organ allografting. Transplantation 1993;56:15–19.
206. Lucien J, Dias VC, Le Gatt DF, Yatscoff RW: Blood distribution and single-dose pharmacokinetics of leflunomide. Ther. Drug Monit. 1995;17:454–459.
207. Mladenovic V, Domljan Z, Rozman B, et al.: Safety and effectiveness of leflunomide in the treatment of patients with active rheumatoid arthritis. Results of a randomized, placebo-controlled, phase II study. Arthritis Rheum. 1995;38:1595–1603.
208. Morris RE, Huang X, Gregory CR, et al.: Studies in experimental models of chronic rejection: use of rapamycin (sirolimus) and isoxazole derivatives (leflunomide and its analogue) for the suppression of graft vascular disease and obliterative bronchiolitis. Transplant. Proc. 1995;27:2068–2069.

209. Cao WW, Kao PN, Chao AC, Gardner P, Ng J, Morris RE: Mechanism of the antiproliferative action of leflunomide. A77 1726, the active metabolite of leflunomide, does not block T-cell receptor-mediated signal transduction but its antiproliferative effects are antagonized by pyrimidine nucleosides. J. Heart Lung Transplant. 1995;14:1016–1030.
210. Nair RV, Cao W, Morris RE: The antiproliferative effect of leflunomide on vascular smooth muscle cells in vitro is mediated by selective inhibition of pyrimidine biosynthesis. Transplant. Proc. 1996;28:3081.
211. Morris RE, Huang X, Cao W, Zheng B, Shorthouse RA: Leflunomide (HWA 486) and its analog suppress T- and B-cell proliferation in vitro, acute rejection, ongoing rejection, and antidonor antibody synthesis in mouse, rat, and cynomolgus monkey transplant recipients as well as arterial intimal thickening after balloon catheter injury. Transplant. Proc. 1995;27:445–447.
212. Shimokado K, Umezawa K, Ogata J: Tyrosine kinase inhibitors inhibit multiple steps of the cell cycle of vascular smooth muscle cells. Exp. Cell Res. 1995;220:266–273.
213. Davis JP, Cain GA, Pitts WJ, Magolda RL, Copeland RA: The immunosuppressive metabolite of leflunomide is a potent inhibitor of human dihydroorotate dehydrogenase. Biochemistry 1996; 35:1270–1273.
214. Silva HT, Cao W, Shorthouse R, Morris RE: Mechanism of action of leflunomide: in vivo uridine administration reverses its inhibition of lymphocyte proliferation. Transplant. Proc. 1996;28: 3082–3084.
215. Siemasko KF, Chong AS, Williams JW, Bremer EG, Finnegan A: Regulation of B cell function by the immunosuppressive agent leflunomide. Transplantation 1996;61:635–642.
216. Lin Y, Vandeputte M, Waer M: Effect of leflunomide on T-independent xenoantibody formation in rats receiving hamster heart xenografts. Transplant. Proc. 1996;28:952.
217. Lin Y, Waer M: In vivo mechanism of action of leflunomide: selective inhibition of the capacity of B lymphocytes to make T-independent xenoantibodies. Transplant. Proc. 1996;28:3085.
218. Chong AS, Finnegan A, Jiang X, et al.: Leflunomide, a novel immunosuppressive agent. The mechanism of inhibition of T cell proliferation. Transplantation 1993;55:1361–1366.
219. Lang R, Wagner H, Heeg K: Differential effects of the immunosuppressive agents cyclosporine and leflunomide in vivo. Leflunomide blocks clonal T cell expansion yet allows production of lymphokines and manifestation of T cell-mediated shock. Transplantation 1995;59:382–389.
220. Zielinski T, Muller HJ, Bartlett RR: Effects of leflunomide (HWA 486) on expression of lymphocyte activation markers. Agents Actions 1993;38 Spec No:C80–C82.
221. Bartlett RR, Schleyerbach R: Immunopharmacological profile of a novel isoxazol derivative, HWA 486, with potential antirheumatic activity—I. Disease modifying action on adjuvant arthritis of the rat. Int. J. Immunopharmacol. 1985;7:7–18.
222. Williams JW, Xiao F, Foster P, et al.: Leflunomide in experimental transplantation. Control of rejection and alloantibody production, reversal of acute rejection, and interaction with cyclosporine. Transplantation 1994;57:1223–1231.
223. D'Silva M, Candinas D, Achilleos O, et al.: The immunomodulatory effect of leflunomide in rat cardiac allotransplantation. Transplantation 1995;60:430–437.
224. MacDonald AS, Sabr K, MacAuley MA, McAlister VC, Bitter-Suermann H, Lee T: Effects of leflunomide and cyclosporine on aortic allograft chronic rejection in the rat. Transplant. Proc. 1994;26:3244–3245.
225. Swan SK, Crary GS, Guijarro C, O'Donnell MP, Keane WF, Kasiske BL: Immunosuppressive effects of leflunomide in experimental chronic vascular rejection. Transplantation 1995;60:887–890.
226. Xiao F, Chong A, Shen J, et al.: Pharmacologically induced regression of chronic transplant rejection. Transplantation 1995;60:1065–1072.
227. Xiao F, Chong AS, Foster P, et al.: Leflunomide controls rejection in hamster to rat cardiac xenografts. Transplantation 1994;58:828–834.
228. Hancock WW, Miyatake T, Koyamada N, et al.: Effects of leflunomide and deoxyspergualin in the guinea pig—rat cardiac model of delayed xenograft rejection: suppression of B cell and C-C chemokine responses but not induction of macrophage lectin. Transplantation 1997;64:696–704.
229. Swinnen LJ, Costanzo-Nordin MR, Fisher SG, et al.: Increased incidence of lymphoproliferative disorder after immunosuppression with the monoclonal antibody OKT3 in cardiac-transplant recipients [see comments]. N. Engl. J. Med. 1990;323:1723–1728.
230. Kupiec-Weglinski JW, Diamantstein T, Tilney NL: Interleukin 2 receptor-targeted therapy—rationale and applications in organ transplantation. Transplantation 1988;46:785–792.
231. Soulillou JP, Peyronnet P, Le MB, et al.: Prevention of rejection of kidney transplants by monoclonal antibody directed against interleukin 2. Lancet 1987;1:1339–1342.
232. Soulillou JP, Cantarovich D, Le MB, et al.: Randomized controlled trial of a monoclonal antibody against the interleukin-2 receptor (33B3.1) as compared with rabbit antithymocyte globulin for

prophylaxis against rejection of renal allografts [see comments]. N. Engl. J. Med. 1990;322:1175–1182.
233. Strom TB, Ettenger RB: Investigational Immunosuppressants: Biologics. In: Norman DJ, Suki WN, eds. Primer on Transplantation. 1 ed. American Society of Transplant Physicians, 1998:113–122.
234. Taniguchi T, Minami Y: The IL-2/IL-2 receptor system: a current overview. Cell 1993;73:5–8.
235. Kirkman RL, Barrett LV, Koltun WA, Diamantstein T: Prolongation of murine cardiac allograft survival by the anti-interleukin-2 receptor monoclonal antibody AMT-13. Transplant. Proc. 1987; 19:618–619.
236. Kirkman RL, Bacha P, Barrett LV, Forte S, Murphy JR, Strom TB: Prolongation of cardiac allograft survival in murine recipients treated with a diphtheria toxin-related interleukin-2 fusion protein. Transplantation 1989;47:327–330.
237. Reed MH, Shapiro ME, Strom TB, et al.: Prolongation of primate renal allograft survival by anti-Tac, an anti-human IL-2 receptor monoclonal antibody. Transplantation 1989;47:55–59.
238. Carpenter CB, Kirkman RL, Shapiro ME, et al.: Prophylactic use of monoclonal anti-IL-2 receptor antibody in cadaveric renal transplantation. Am. J. Kidney Dis. 1989;14:54–57.
239. Kirkman RL, Shapiro ME, Carpenter CB, et al.: A randomized prospective trial of anti-Tac monoclonal antibody in human renal transplantation. Transplantation 1991;51:107–113.
240. Otto G, Thies J, Kraus T, et al.: Monoclonal anti-CD25 for acute rejection after liver transplantation [letter]. Lancet 1991;338:195.
241. Otto G, Thies J, Kabelitz D, et al.: Anti-CD25 monoclonal antibody prevents early rejection in liver transplantation—a pilot study. Transplant. Proc. 1991;23:1387–1389.
242. Nashan B, Schwinzer R, Schlitt HJ, Wonigeit K, Pichlmayr R: Immunological effects of the anti-IL-2 receptor monoclonal antibody BT 563 in liver allografted patients. Transpl. Immunol. 1995;3:203–211.
243. van Gelder T, Zietse R, Mulder AH, et al.: A double-blind, placebo-controlled study of monoclonal anti-interleukin-2 receptor antibody (BT563) administration to prevent acute rejection after kidney transplantation. Transplantation 1995;60:248–252.
244. van Gelder T, Mulder AH, Balk AH, et al.: Intragraft monitoring of rejection after prophylactic treatment with monoclonal anti-interleukin-2 receptor antibody (BT563) in heart transplant recipients. J. Heart Lung Transplant. 1995;14:346–350.
245. van Gelder T, Baan CC, Balk AH, et al.: Blockade of the interleukin (IL)-2/IL-2 receptor pathway with a monoclonal anti-IL-2 receptor antibody (BT563) does not prevent the development of acute heart allograft rejection in humans. Transplantation 1998;65:405–410.
246. Vincenti F, Kirkman R, Light S, et al.: Interleukin-2-receptor blockade with daclizumab to prevent acute rejection in renal transplantation. Daclizumab Triple Therapy Study Group. N. Engl. J. Med. 1998;338:161–165.
247. Nashan B, Moore R, Amlot P, Schmidt AG, Abeywickrama K, Soulillou JP: Randomised trial of basiliximab versus placebo for control of acute cellular rejection in renal allograft recipients. CHIB 201 International Study Group. Lancet 1997;350:1193–1198.
248. Heagy W, Walterbangh C, Martz E: Potent ability of anti-LFA-1 monoclonal antibody to prolong allograft survival. Transplantation 1984;37:520–523.
249. Nakakura EK, Jardieu PM, Zheng B, Morris RE: An anti-adhesion molecule (FLA-1, CD11a) monoclonal antibody suppresses ongoing rejection and prolongs heart allograft survival indefinitly without lymphocyte depletion. J. Heart Lung Transplant. 1992;11:223–223. (Abstract)
250. Nakakura EK, Mccabe SM, Zheng B, et al.: Potent and effective prolongation by anti-LFA-1 monoclonal antibody monotherapy of non-primarily vascularized heart allograft survival in mice without T cell depletion. Transplantation 1993;55:412–417.
251. Fischer A: Anti-LFA-1 antibody as immunosuppressive reagent in transplantation. Chem. Immunol. 1991;50:89–97.
252. Dustin ML, Springer TA: Lymphocyte function-associated antigen-1 LFA-1 interaction with intercellular adhesion molecule-1 ICAM-1 is one of at least three mechanisms for lymphocyte adhesion to cultured endothelial cells. J. Cell Biol. 1988;107:321–331.
253. Springer TA, Dustin ML, Kishimoto TK, Marlin SD: The lymphocyte function-associated LFA-1, CD2, and LFA-3 molecules: cell adhesion receptors of the immune system. Annu. Rev. Immunol. 1987;5:223–252.
254. Kanner SB, Grosmaire LS, Ledbetter JA, Damle NK: Beta 2-integrin LFA-1 signaling through phospholipase C-gamma 1 activation. Proc. Natl. Acad. Sci. U.S.A. 1993;90:7099–7103.
255. Nakakura EK, Shorthouse RA, Zheng B, Mccabe SM, Jardieu PM, Morris RE: Long-term survival of solid organ allografts by brief anti-lymphocyte function-associated antigen-1 monoclonal antibody monotherapy. Transplantation 1996;62:547–552.
256. Kameoka H, Ishibashi M, Tamatani T, et al.: Comparative immunosuppressive effect of anti-CD18

and anti-CD11a monoclonal antibodies on rat heart allotransplantation. Transplant. Proc. 1993; 25:833–836.

257. Komori A, Nagata M, Ochiai T, et al.: Role of ICAM-1 and LFA-1 in cardiac allograft rejection of the rat. Transplant. Proc. 1993;25:831–832.
258. Paul LC, Davidoff A, Benediktsson H, Issekutz TB: The efficacy of LFA-1 and VLA-4 antibody treatment in rat vascularized cardiac allograft rejection. Transplantation 1993;55:1196–1199.
259. Isobe M, Yagita H, Okumura K, Ihara A: Specific acceptance of cardiac allograft after treatment with antibodies to ICAM-1 and LFA-1. Science 1992;255:1125–1127.
260. Stepkowski SM, Tu Y, Condon TP, Bennett CF: Blocking of heart allograft rejection by intercellular adhesion molecule-1 antisense oligonucleotides alone or in combination with other immunosuppressive modalities [published erratum appears in J Immunol 1995 Feb 1;154 3:1521]. J. Immunol. 1994;153:5336–5346.
261. Suzuki J, Isobe M, Yamazaki S, Horie S, Okubo Y, Sekiguchi M: Inhibition of accelerated coronary atherosclerosis with short-term blockade of intercellular adhesion molecule-1 and lymphocyte fuction-associated antigen-1 in a heterotopic murine model of heart transplantation. J. Heart Lung Transplant. 1997;16:1141–1148.
262. Cosimi AB, Conti D, Delmonico FL, et al.: In vivo effects of monoclonal antibody to ICAM-1 CD54 in nonhuman primates with renal allografts. J. Immunol. 1990;144:4604–4612.
263. Flavin T, Ivens K, Rothlein R, et al.: Monoclonal antibodies against intercellular adhesion molecule 1 prolong cardiac allograft survival in cynomolgus monkeys. Transplant. Proc. 1991;23:533–534.
264. Le Mauff B, Hourmant M, Rougier JP, et al.: Effect of anti-LFA1 CD11a monoclonal antibodies in acute rejection in human kidney transplantation. Transplantation 1991;52:291–296.
265. Hourmant M, Bedrossian J, Durand D, et al.: Multicenter comparative study of an anti-LFA-1 adhesion molecule monoclonal antibody and antithymocyte globulin in prophylaxis of acute rejection in kidney transplantation. Transplant. Proc. 1995;27:864.
266. Hourmant M, Bedrossian J, Durand D, et al.: A randomized multicenter trial comparing leukocyte function-associated antigen-1 monoclonal antibody with rabbit antithymocyte globulin as induction treatment in first kidney transplantations. Transplantation 1996;62:1565–1570.
267. Fischer A, Friedrich W, Fasth A, et al.: Reduction of graft failure by a monoclonal antibody anti-LFA-1 CD11a after HLA nonidentical bone marrow transplantation in children with immunodeficiencies, osteopetrosis, and Fanconi's anemia: a European Group for Immunodeficiency/European Group for Bone Marrow Transplantation report. Blood 1991;77:249–256.
268. Ohashi Y, Tsuchiya S, Fujie H, Minegishi M, Konno T: Anti-LFA-1 antibody treatment of a patient with steroid-resistant severe graft-versus-host disease. Tohoku. J. Exp. Med. 1992;167:297–299.
269. Haug CE, Colvin RB, Delmonico FL, et al.: A phase I trial of immunosuppression with anti-ICAM-1 CD54 mAb in renal allograft recipients. Transplantation 1993;55:766–772.
270. Hourmant M, Le Mauff B, Le Meur Y, et al.: Administration of an anti-CD11a monoclonal antibody in recipients of kidney transplantation. A pilot study. Transplantation 1994;58:377–380.

12. TREATMENT OF ACUTE VASCULAR REJECTION IN CARDIAC ALLOGRAFTS

Ilan S. Wittstein, M.D. and Edward K. Kasper, M.D.
Division of Cardiology, Department of Medicine, The Johns Hopkins University School of Medicine, Baltimore, Maryland

INTRODUCTION AND DEFINITIONS

Since the introduction of endomyocardial biopsy for routine rejection surveillance, the diagnosis of acute rejection has been based primarily on the presence and extent of lymphocytic infiltration.[1,2] Acute cardiac allograft rejection has been considered primarily a T cell phenomenon mediated by the cellular arm of the immune system. In recent years, however, several centers have reported patients with hemodynamic compromise and cardiac allograft dysfunction who have minimal evidence of lymphocytic infiltration on biopsy.[3–5] There is increasing evidence that these cases illustrate a distinct form of rejection mediated primarily by the humoral immune system in which the allograft vasculature is the primary target of injury.[4,6–10] The idea of an antibody mediated vascular rejection is supported by the kidney transplant literature where the role of humoral immunity in acute allograft rejection has been recognized for almost 30 years,[11–18] and where antibody mediated vascular injury in the absence of interstitial infiltrates has been well described.[19,20]

In 1989, Hammond et al. were the first to report a series of patients with acute humoral or vascular rejection.[6] The diagnosis was based on the demonstration by immunofluorescent staining of immunoglobulin and complement on coronary vascular endothelium in addition to light microscopic evidence of endothelial cell swelling and activation. Since that time, other investigators have reported this pattern of rejection in heart transplant recipients, and it has become increasingly clear that rejection targeting the allograft vasculature is a complex process that likely involves both humoral and cellular mechanisms. While it is now appreciated that acute

Reprints to: Ilan S. Wittstein, M.D., Division of Cardiology, The Johns Hopkins Hospital, 568 Carnegie, 600 N. Wolfe St., Baltimore, MD 21287

vascular rejection (AVR) has unique clinical characteristics and important prognostic implications, much remains unknown about the underlying pathogenesis of this condition, and effective treatment strategies remain obscure. This chapter will focus on humorally mediated AVR and will attempt to review treatment options currently available for this unique form of rejection. While the emphasis will be primarily on treatment of AVR in human cardiac allografts, some of the promising treatment strategies being used in cardiac xenograft models will be discussed as well.

PROGNOSTIC IMPLICATIONS OF AVR

There is now significant evidence to support that AVR in cardiac allografts has prognostic importance with respect to clinical course and allograft survival and is not simply an interesting histopathologic observation. Early retrospective studies demonstrated that arteriolar vasculitis seen on endomyocardial biopsy was predictive of decreased allograft and patient survival.[21,22] Several investigators have since reported the association of AVR with diminished systolic function,[4,6–9] hemodynamic instability,[4,6–9,23] and decreased graft survival.[6–8,24–26] In their initial series, Hammond et al. looked at biopsies from 36 cardiac allografts and identified three distinct rejection patterns. Fifty-six percent of the allografts exhibited cellular rejection, 19% showed pure vascular rejection, and 25% had a mixed rejection pattern.[6] Significant systolic dysfunction was more frequently seen in the patients with AVR compared to those with cellular rejection. Furthermore, 100% of patients with AVR experienced hemodynamic compromise necessitating increased immunosuppression compared to 25% of patients with cellular rejection. At 3 year follow-up, the survival rate of grafts with AVR was 57% compared to 95% with cellular rejection. The survival rate for the mixed rejection group was intermediate between cellular and vascular rejection (89%). In a follow-up study looking at a larger cohort of patients (n = 186), AVR was again more frequently associated with systolic dysfunction and hemodynamic instability.[7] Only 2% of patients with cellular rejection required inotropic support compared with 42% of the vascular rejection group. Actuarial survival at 2 years was 55% in patients with AVR and 92% in those with cellular rejection. One group has reported improved graft survival rates when AVR is treated aggressively with therapies targeting the humoral immune response.[9] Others, however, have reported rates of graft loss due to AVR to be as high as 23% even with the addition of humorally targeted treatment strategies.[8]

Several investigators have argued that an attempt to diagnose AVR with immunofluorescent staining should be standard procedure in the early post-transplant period.[6,7] Efforts to make the diagnosis in some centers have illustrated that a humorally mediated form of vascular rejection may be more common than was once believed, and one series has reported an incidence as high as 52%.[23] AVR occurs earlier after transplantation than cellular rejection,[5,7,9,23] and it can often be detected histopathologically long before clinical evidence of rejection becomes apparent. Thus, immunofluorescent staining of immunoglobulin and complement to vascular endothelial cells and light microscopic evidence of endothelial cell swelling may frequently be the only reliable ways to diagnose AVR in the early post-transplant period.

Given the strong association of this type of rejection with allograft dysfunction and loss, the argument to aggressively pursue this diagnosis seems justified. Whether histopathologic evidence of AVR in the absence of clinical rejection should be treated remains a point of debate and will be discussed later in this chapter.

HUMORAL IMMUNITY IN THE PATHOGENESIS OF AVR

Much of our understanding of the pathogenesis of AVR has come from xenograft models where the principal forms of rejection are known to be humorally mediated. In hyperacute rejection (HAR), preformed xenoreactive antibodies bind to donor endothelial cells with subsequent activation of complement. Complement-mediated endothelial injury induces procoagulant changes in the cell membrane resulting in platelet binding and fibrin deposition. The end result is thrombosis of blood vessels and loss of the graft within minutes.[27] If HAR is averted, the xenograft may develop AVR that typically occurs several days after engraftment. AVR is believed to also result from binding of anti-donor antibodies to donor endothelial cells. Activation of sublytic amounts of complement ultimately leads to a state of persistent endothelial cell activation. Several important changes in endothelial cell function occur that result in impaired anticoagulation and fibrinolysis. In addition, there is increased expression of cell surface adhesion molecules which promotes leukocyte binding to the vasculature, and potent vasoconstrictors such as endothelin-1 are secreted.[28] Together, these changes lead to fibrin deposition and accumulation that result in vascular thrombosis and xenograft loss.

In human cardiac allografts demonstrating AVR, the localization of immunoglobulin and complement primarily in the vasculature suggests that these deposits may represent binding of donor-specific antibodies to in situ allograft antigens, or alternatively may be due to preformed immune complexes. The specific antigens that are involved in AVR have not yet been identified, but there is evidence that the HLA antigen system may play an important role. Both class I and class II (HLA-DR) antigens are expressed on human vascular endothelial cells,[11] and HLA-DR expression is amplified during periods of rejection.[6] The development of antibody to donor class I HLA antigens following kidney transplantation has resulted in a vascular form of rejection characterized by complement deposition, polymorphonuclear infiltration, and endothelial injury in the microvasculature.[17] Similarly, the presence of an elevated panel of reactive antibodies (PRA) and/or a positive lymphocytotoxic crossmatch prior to heart transplantation has been associated with subsequent development of AVR.[5,6,7,24] Ratkovec et al. reviewed 328 cardiac allograft recipients and identified 11 with an IgG positive crossmatch. All 11 developed histopathologic evidence of AVR that occurred relatively early after transplant and was characterized clinically by frequent episodes of hemodynamic compromise.[5]

The appearance of anti-HLA antibodies in the post-transplant period has also been associated with AVR.[4,29,30] Costanzo-Nordin et al. reported 11 patients with acute allograft dysfunction who had no evidence of cellular rejection on EMB. Though immunofluorescence was not performed in this study, six of eleven patients (54%) developed a significant increase in levels of anti-HLA antibodies in close temporal proximity with the episode of acute allograft dysfunction.[4] Cherry et al. studied 46 biopsy specimens from 16 patients; and of the twenty-one cases of AVR identified, 67% were associated with circulating anti-HLA antibody.[30] This study also demonstrated that anti-HLA antibody was more likely to precede histopathologic evidence of AVR than it was to follow it, suggesting that anti-HLA antibody may play a role in the pathogenesis of AVR and not simply be a response to it.

Non-HLA antigen systems may also be involved in the pathogenesis of AVR. This is supported by the fact that AVR has been reported in the absence of a positive lymphocytotoxic crossmatch and elevated PRA.[9,10] There is evidence to suggest that the vascular endothelial cell (VEC) antigen system may be important in humorally mediated rejection. This antigen system, originally described by Moraes and Stastny,[31] is expressed on the surface of vascular endothelial cells and peripheral blood monocytes and is known to be an important immunogen in renal transplantation.[32–35] Cerilli et al. have shown that approximately 80% of rejections that occur after transplants from HLA-identical related kidney donors are secondary to a humoral response to donor VEC-specific antigens.[36] In addition, anti-VEC antibody is often the only donor-specific antibody that can be detected in the sera of recipients who reject their HLA-identical renal allografts.

A hyperacute form of vascular rejection in cardiac allografts attributed to the VEC antigen system has now been reported. Brasile et al. described four cardiac allograft recipients who developed acute allograft dysfunction shortly after transplant.[37] All four patients had a negative lymphocytotoxic crossmatch, and immunofluorescence revealed deposition of immunoglobulin and complement on vascular endothelium. Anti-VEC antibody was found in the sera of each patient. In one case where donor tissue was available, anti-VEC antibody from recipient serum bound to the endothelium of donor aorta and vena cava suggesting a causal relationship between the anti-VEC antibody and the episode of hyperacute rejection. Similar findings were reported in a larger series by Trento et al. in which 11 cardiac allograft recipients demonstrated histopathologic evidence of hyperacute rejection despite a compatible direct lymphocytotoxic crossmatch.[38] Circulating anti-VEC antibodies were detected in all of the patients, and immunofluorescent staining revealed immunoglobulin on the surface of the endothelium. In a control group of 18 patients who had no evidence of hyperacute rejection, cytotoxic anti-VEC antibodies could not be detected. While no human study to date has shown a causal relationship between anti-VEC antibodies and AVR, the above data strongly implicate the VEC-monocyte antigen system in humorally mediated vascular rejection in cardiac allografts.

The use of prophylactic OKT3 cytolytic therapy post-transplant has also been associated with the development of AVR.[23–25,39,40] In a series of twenty cardiac allograft recipients receiving either 14 or 21 day rejection prophylaxis with OKT3, six patients developed OKT3 sensitization characterized by declining OKT3 levels and the presence of human anti-mouse antibody (HAMA).[25] All six patients developed AVR which was coincident with HAMA production. The incidence of AVR in the non-sensitized group was considerably lower (29%). These findings were confirmed by a larger cohort of patients in which 12 patients with OKT3 sensitization were identified. Eight of the 12 patients developed AVR and the remaining four had a mixed rejection pattern.[40] Ma et al. reported that OKT3 sensitization was positively correlated with duration of prophylaxis.[24] The incidence of AVR was 7-fold higher in patients receiving a 21 day course of OKT3 compared with those treated for only 7 days.

It has been suggested that the association between OKT3 sensitization and the development of AVR may result from immune complex formation.[6,8,24,25,39] The formation of host antibodies to highly immunogenic proteins such as OKT3 could lead to deposition of immune complexes in the microvasculature with subsequent complement and neutrophil activation. Indeed, the light microscopic and immunofluorescent patterns seen with serum sickness closely resemble AVR.[25,39] Complexes of HAMA and mouse OKT3 resulting in temporal artery vasculitis have previously been reported in one cardiac allograft recipient.[41] Similarly, the use of the monoclonal anti-TCR antibody BMA-031 in kidney transplant patients has been associated with a higher incidence of AVR.[42] It is important to note that AVR has been shown to occur even in the absence of OKT3 prophylaxis.[9] Nonetheless, the above observations lend strong support to the argument that humoral responses are central to the pathogenesis of AVR.

An understanding of the pathogenesis of AVR (Table 1) and an appreciation for its prognostic implications should influence post-transplant management in several ways. First, because patients with an elevated PRA and/or lymphocytotoxic crossmatch appear to be at higher risk for developing AVR, an aggressive attempt at making the diagnosis with immunofluorescent staining is warranted in this group of patients. Secondly, the above observations suggest that cytolytic prophylaxis with monoclonal/polyclonal antibodies should be used judiciously, and a prolonged course of treatment should be avoided. Finally, when prophylaxis is given, careful monitoring for HAMA formation and falling OKT3 level should be performed so that the immunogenic stimulus can be discontinued if sensitization occurs. This strategy has been effective in one center's experience where discontinuation of OKT3 prophylaxis in the setting of documented sensitization has dramatically increased allograft survival.[40]

TREATMENT OF AVR IN HUMAN CARDIAC ALLOGRAFTS

Identification of effective treatment options for AVR in human cardiac allografts has been limited for several reasons. First, the diagnosis of vascular rejection can be difficult to establish and will frequently be missed unless immunofluorescent studies are performed in the early post-transplant period. Second, the diagnostic criteria for vascular rejection have not been standardized, and while some investigators have argued that AVR in cardiac allografts can be detected reliably with light microscopy and routine histologic preparation,[43] others have stressed the importance of both light microscopy and immunofluorescent staining in making the diagnosis.[44] Third, despite mounting evidence, there is still some skepticism within the transplant community that humoral rejection truly requires specialized treatment beyond standard immunosuppressive therapy. Finally, effective treatment options have been limited by a relatively poor understanding of the underlying pathogenesis of AVR.

Treatment of vascular rejection in cardiac allografts has relied primarily on augmentation of standard immunosuppressive therapy. (Table 2) As the pathogenesis of

AVR has become better understood, therapeutic modalities specifically targeting the humoral immune system have been introduced. The use of novel immunosuppressive agents that more specifically target B cell activity and antibody production, and techniques such as plasma exchange and immunoadsorption that decrease or remove circulating antibody, are two strategies that have prolonged graft survival in xenotransplantation and appear to also hold promise for the treatment of AVR in human allografts. The identification of effective treatments for AVR, however, is still in its early stages and well designed prospective clinical trials are desperately needed.

Cyclosporine/Corticosteroids/Azathioprine

The role of cyclosporine in the treatment of vascular rejection is controversial. There is evidence to support that cyclosporine has a toxic effect on allograft endothelial cells and can result in injury to the microvasculature. An association between cyclosporine and arterial vasculitis has been described in cardiac,[21,22] renal,[45,46] hepatic,[47] and bone marrow transplantation.[48] Others have reported that in kidney allografts, cyclosporine can cause a dose-dependent vasculopathy that is similar to hemolytic uremic syndrome and can result in increased graft loss.[49] The precise mechanism of injury is incompletely understood, but the above observations suggest that cyclosporine may alter allograft vessels and render them more susceptible to vascular rejection.

In contrast to these findings, there is support from the kidney transplant literature that cyclosporine may actually be beneficial in the prevention and treatment of AVR. Wilczek et al. found that renal allograft recipients treated with higher doses of cyclosporine were at decreased risk of developing both acute and chronic vascular rejection compared with patients receiving lower doses.[50] Similarly, in a large study from the Netherlands, the risk of developing AVR was decreased significantly in patients who received cyclosporine instead of azathioprine.[51] Ballardie et al. examined renal allograft recipients who had steroid-resistant acute vascular rejection confirmed by percutaneous needle biopsy.[52] Fourteen of these patients were treated with steroids and azathioprine and were compared to eight patients given cyclosporine instead of azathioprine. Graft survival was significantly better in the cyclosporine treated group (75%) compared to the control group (21%). Others have reported similar improvement in renal allograft function when patients with steroid-resistant AVR were converted from azathioprine to cyclosporine.[53] Thomas et al. studied the synergistic effect of cyclosporine and azathioprine in 21 renal allograft recipients with biopsy proven AVR.[54] In the control group treated with only steroids and azathioprine, stabilization or improvement in graft function was seen in 44% of patients. In the group given additional immunosuppression with cyclosporine, graft function improved or stabilized in 83% of cases.

Triple drug therapy with cyclosporine, corticosteroids, and azathioprine has become widely accepted for rejection prophylaxis in cardiac transplantation. Standard treatment of acute rejection episodes, which frequently includes augmentation of corticosteroids and addition of cytolytic therapy with monoclonal or polyclonal antibodies, targets primarily the cellular immune system and therefore may be less effective in treating humorally mediated vascular rejection. In the initial series by Hammond et al.,[6] increased immunosuppression including cytolytic therapy improved allograft function in all patients with refractory cellular rejection and hemodynamic compromise. In contrast, increased immunosuppression for patients with pure AVR still resulted in graft loss in 43% of cases. In the larger series from Ensley et al., patients with AVR were more resistant to augmented immunosuppression than were patients with cellular rejection.[7] Retreatment with antilymphocyte preparations was required more frequently in patients with AVR (57% vs 19%) and rate of allograft loss was significantly higher in this group. One center, however, has reported success in treating humorally mediated rejection with only standard immunosuppressive therapy.[4] Of 11 patients with acute allograft dysfunction and minimal cellular infiltrate on EMB, allograft function improved in all patients with increased corticosteroids with or without OKT3 therapy. This study, however, is not directly comparable to the larger Utah experience since immunofluorescence to document immunoglobulin and complement deposition was not performed.

Monoclonal/Polyclonal Antibody Therapy

Cytolytic therapy utilizing monoclonal or polyclonal antibodies targets primarily T cell activity and its efficacy in treating vascular rejection in renal allografts has historically been poor.[55] There have been reports, however, in both renal and cardiac allografts where antibody therapy has been used successfully to treat vascular rejection. Delaney et al. reported three renal allograft recipients who had biopsy proven severe vascular rejection resistant to pulse corticosteroids.[56] All three patients showed rapid clinical improvement after treatment with OKT3, and there was histologic improvement of the vascular rejection in the two patients who underwent a follow up biopsy. Immunofluorescence for immunoglobulin and complement was positive in only one of the three patients, and acute rejection was characterized histologically by transmural infiltration of both arteries and veins by predominantly T cells. This may explain, in part, why OKT3 had such a dramatic effect in this small series. Schroeder et al. compared the efficacy of OKT3 in 29 patients with acute vascular and cellular rejection versus 32 patients with only cellular rejection.[57] The rate of rejection reversal with OKT3 therapy was very high in both groups (86% for AVR and 91% for cellular rejection), but the rate of allograft loss at both 6 and 12 months was higher in the group with AVR.

Successful treatment of AVR with cytolytic therapy has also been described in cardiac allograft recipients. Ballester et al. reported four patients who developed coronary obstruction or ischemia shortly after transplantation.[58] The coronary lesions were felt to be secondary to vasculitis, and they resolved after vigorous treatment with corticosteroids and antithymocyte globulin. In a more recent series from Costanzo-Nordin et al., all three patients who received combination therapy with steroids and OKT3 demonstrated improvement in cardiac allograft function.[4] Hammond et al. treated 7 patients with pure AVR with either OKT3 or ATG and observed recovery in 4 of these patients. Three patients with mixed vascular and cellular rejection also recovered after receiving cytolytic therapy.[6] In a series of pediatric allograft recipients, Zales et al. reported two patients with humoral rejection who received cytolytic therapy.[10] One patient was treated with OKT3 and showed clinical and echocardiographic improvement. In the second patient who received a 10-day course of ATGAM, clinical improvement was noted, but follow up biopsies revealed persistent vascular rejection. In one series, OKT3 or antilymphocyte globulin (ALG) has been used to treat AVR in combination with corticosteroids, cyclophosphamide, and plasmapheresis with a high rate of rejection reversal and allograft recovery.[8]

Cyclophosphamide

Cyclophosphamide has been shown to be a potent suppressor of humoral immunity,[59,60] and the evidence suggests that it may be effective both in the prevention and treatment of AVR. To determine the safety and efficacy of cyclophosphamide in maintenance immunosuppression, Wagoner et al. retrospectively reviewed the records of 320 cardiac allograft recipients over a six year period and identified 28 patients in whom cyclophosphamide had been substituted for azathioprine because of recalcitrant allograft rejection.[61] The introduction of cyclophosphamide in these patients was associated with a reduction in treated rejection episodes from 0.37 to 0.10 episodes per patient-month for the 14 patients who had hemodynamically significant vascular rejection, and the total number of treated rejection episodes fell from 17 while on azathioprine to just 2 on cyclophosphamide (0.34 to 0.13 episodes per patient-month). Corticosteroid dose was significantly reduced while on cyclophosphamide, and there was no associated increase in risk of infection. The authors concluded that cyclophosphamide could be safely substituted for azathioprine in maintenance immunosuppression in patients with recurrent rejection, and that it may be efficacious in preventing episodes of both vascular and cellular rejection.

In a separate study, heart transplant recipients receiving a 14 day course of OKT3 prophylaxis were prospectively randomized to receive cyclophosphamide or azathioprine to determine if early rejection prophylaxis with cyclophosphamide would decrease the incidence of AVR.[62] There was no difference between the two groups in the number of patients who developed AVR, the number of hemodynamically significant episodes of AVR, the histopathologic severity of the vascular rejection, or the one year survival rate. There was, however, a significant decrease in OKT3 sensitization in the group treated with cyclophosphamide, a humorally mediated process that has been shown by some investigators to be associated with the development of AVR.

The treatment of AVR with cyclophosphamide has now been reported by several centers.[5,8,9,10,23] In most of these studies, cyclophosphamide has been used in combination with plasmapheresis and monoclonal/polyclonal antibody therapy. In a series from Olsen et al., 13 patients with acute vascular rejection were treated with cyclophosphamide, plasmapheresis, and high-dose corticosteroids.[8] Eight patients also received therapy with either OKT3 or ALG. Resolution of the acute rejection and normalization of left ventricular function was seen in 92% of these patients within seven days. Allograft survival was significantly higher at one to two years post transplant than in the group of patients with AVR from this same center treated with standard immunosuppressive therapy.[6,7] Miller et al. treated seven patients with AVR with corticosteroids, plasmapheresis, and cyclophosphamide instead of azathioprine.[9] Six of these seven patients survived and experienced no further episodes of vascular or cellular rejection. In a larger series, Lones et al. identified 42 patients with histologic and immunofluorescent evidence of AVR.[23] All patients were treated with intravenous cyclophosphamide, with or without plasmapheresis, and only three patients died of humoral rejection. Observations from these studies suggest that in combination with plasmapheresis and standard immunosuppressive therapy, cyclophosphamide may have an important role in the treatment of AVR.

Plasmapheresis

Strategies designed to remove circulating antibody such as plasmapheresis and immunoadsorption have been used to successfully treat vascular rejection in both renal and cardiac allografts. Franco et al. looked at 188 renal allograft recipients and identified 34 patients (18%) with histologic evidence of vascular rejection.[63] Plasma exchange resulted in improvement in allograft function in 83% of the patients with acute endovasculitis. There was no improvement in patients with chronic vascular changes or in patients who had chronic lesions with superimposed acute changes. Actuarial graft survival rates in patients with acute endovasculitis were 66% and 60% at 6 and 12 months, respectively. This was significantly better than graft survival rates in a control group with acute endovasculitis treated only with methylprednisolone (6 and 12 month survival rates of 7%).

Grandtnerova et al. reported 5 cadaveric renal transplant recipients with deteriorating graft function not responsive to standard immunosuppression.[64] The deterioration was felt to be secondary to AVR based on the appearance of donor-specific anti-HLA antibodies, a positive crossmatch and/or rising PRA post transplant, and increased vascular impedance. All 5 patients underwent plasmapheresis with disappearance of the antidonor antibodies and rapid improvement in graft function. Four of the five grafts were still functioning at 6 to 23 months post-transplant. In a study from Austria, 28 renal allograft recipients with histologically proven AVR were treated with plasmapheresis with improvement in graft function in 78% of cases.[65] There have been several other reports describing the potential benefit of plasmapheresis in treating renal allograft AVR, and most report higher graft survival rates than historical controls treated with standard immunosuppression.[66–68] Some studies, however, have found plasmapheresis to be of no added benefit when compared with standard therapy.[69]

Plasmapheresis has also been used to treat AVR in cardiac allograft recipients. Partanen et al. reported a case in which steroid resistant vascular rejection resolved after initiation of plasmapheresis.[70] Catalan et al. have recently reported the use of plasmapheresis to treat rejection in a patient more than 18 months post-transplant.[71] Though immunofluorescence was not performed, the episode was felt to represent AVR because acute allograft dysfunction occurred in the setting of positive lymphocytotoxic antibodies, a PRA above 85%, and no evidence of cellular rejection on biopsy. Following plasmapheresis, there was marked clinical improvement, resolution of rejection, and negative lymphocytotoxic antibodies. In a report from Sweden, five patients with allograft vasculitis on biopsy were treated with plasmapheresis as a last resort after failure with conventional therapy.[72] Clinical improvement was seen in all cases after the first few plasma exchanges and all patients were alive at 2–3.5 years post-transplant. Finally, as we have previously discussed, several centers have treated AVR with a combination of corticosteroids, cyclophosphamide, and plasmapheresis with improved graft survival rates compared to patients given conventional immunosuppressive therapy.[5,8,9,23,72a]

Another strategy intended to remove or reduce circulating immunoglobulin is extracorporeal immunoadsorption. This technique uses staphylococcal protein A to selectively remove IgG and has been used to treat AVR in both renal[73] and cardiac allografts.[74] Olivari et al. used this technique with three cardiac allograft recipients who had immunofluorescent and light microscopic evidence of AVR and graft dysfunction unresponsive to pulse corticosteroids and cyclophosphamide. In all three cases, AVR was associated with a marked increase in PRA, and specific anti-HLA class I antibodies were identified in two of the patients. Immunoadsorption was performed until PRA decreased to <5%. Removal of circulating antibody was associated with improvement in ventricular function and normalization of the endomyocardial biopsy in all three cases. The precise mechanism of action of plasmapheresis and immunoadsorption is unclear, but removal of lymphocytotoxic antibodies, immune complexes, immunoglobulins, or circulating lymphokines such as IL-1, IL-2, and B-cell differentiation factor have all been proposed.[63,72,74] Regardless of the exact mechanism, these techniques appear to hold promise for the treatment of AVR and further clinical trials are warranted.

Newer Immunosuppressive Agents for the Treatment of AVR

In the past several years, increased efforts have been made to identify new immunosuppressive agents that have greater efficacy and fewer side effects than conventional therapy. These drugs include the xenobiotic molecules such as FK506 (tacrolimus) and rapamycin, antimetabolites such as mycophenolate mofetil, mizoribine, and brequinar sodium, and even newer agents such as leflunomide and 15-deoxyspergualin. While many of these agents are showing promise in animal models in treating both acute and chronic vascular rejection, their use in humans specifically for the treatment of AVR has been limited.

FK506 has been shown in vitro to inhibit B cell activity and immunoglobulin production,[75,76] and there are now preliminary reports that it is an effective rescue agent in humans with AVR. Woodle et al. reported 16 liver transplant patients with corticosteroid and OKT3 resistant rejection.[77] Two of these patients had AVR as demonstrated immunohistologically by endothelial injury and vascular deposition of IgM and complement. Both of these patients experienced rejection reversal within four weeks of beginning FK506 therapy, and rejection did not recur in either patient. FK506 has also been used successfully as rescue therapy in renal transplant patients with AVR[78] and antibody mediated acute glomerular rejection.[79] In a large series from Jordan et al., FK506 was used in renal allograft recipients who had failed conventional immunosuppression.[80] Twenty patients were found to have elements of acute vascular rejection on biopsy, and successful rescue with FK506 was achieved

Table 1. Factors Associated with Acute Vascular Rejection

- Elevated panel reactive antibodies (PRA) prior to transplant
- Positive lymphocytotoxic crossmatch prior to transplant
- Appearance of anti-HLA antibodies post-transplant
- Appearance of anti-VEC antibodies post-transplant
- Prophylactic OKT3 therapy post-transplant
  - OKT3 sensitization (HAMA formation and falling OKT3 level)
  - Longer duration of OKT3 treatment

Table 2. Treatment Options for Acute Vascular (Humoral) Rejection

- Augmentation of standard immunosuppression
  - (cyclosporine/corticosteroids/azathioprine)
- Monoclonal/polyclonal antibody therapy (e.g. OKT3, ATG, ALG)
- Cyclophosphamide
- Newer immunosuppressive agnets
  - Tacrolimus (FK-506)
  - Mycophenolate mofetil
  - 15-deoxyspergualin
  - Rapamycin
  - Actinomycin D
- Removal of circulating antibody
  - Plamapheresis
  - Extracoporeal immunoadsoption
- Local graft irradiation

in 65% of these cases. The use of FK506 to treat AVR in cardiac allograft recipients has now also been described. Woodle et al. reported a case where the recipient had significant humoral presensitization with anti-class I antibody.[81] B cell crossmatch titers following transplant continued to rise despite OKT3 induction and daily plasmapheresis, and EMB revealed immunohistologic evidence of AVR. When FK506 was substituted for OKT3 and plasmapheresis, there was a marked decrease in B cell crossmatch titers and improvement of AVR on biopsy within seven days. By four months post-transplant, ventricular function was normal and rejection had not recurred. This report was important because it demonstrated the ability of FK506 to reverse AVR even in the presence of pre-existing, donor-specific, anti-HLA antibody, and to prevent episodes of recurrent humoral rejection.

Mycophenolate mofetil (MMF) is another new agent that may hold promise for the treatment of AVR. Its efficacy in treating AVR may result from its ability to inhibit both B and T cell proliferation and to inhibit antibody formation.[82] In the hamster-to-rat cardiac xenograft model, combination therapy with MMF, cyclosporine, and brequinar sodium resulted in suppression of cytotoxic antibody titers, a marked reduction in acute vascular injury, and prolongation of xenograft survival.[83] Inhibition of chronic vascular rejection with MMF has also been reported in a primate model of heart xenotransplantation.[84] MMF has also been shown to down regulate the expression of leukocyte adhesion molecules, thus impairing binding of inflammatory cells to vascular endothelium.[85] This may play a potentially important role in the treatment of AVR since human cardiac allograft recipients with immunohistologic evidence of vascular rejection are known to have increased capillary expression of intercellular adhesion molecule-1 (ICAM-1).[86] Further support for this mechanism of action comes from a rabbit heart transplant model in which blocking leukocyte adhesion molecule receptors with monoclonal antibodies has resulted in a decrease in vascular rejection.[87] The use of MMF to treat AVR in human studies has been limited. Ahsan et al. used MMF and FK506 as primary immunotherapy to successfully reverse AVR in a renal transplant patient.[88] In a second report, renal allograft AVR was treated with a combination of MMF and high dose steroids.[89] To our knowledge, there are no case reports where MMF has been used as primary or rescue therapy to treat AVR in cardiac allografts.

The new agent 15-deoxyspergualin (DOSP) has been shown in vitro to have suppressive effects on B cell differentiation[90] and antibody formation[91] and thus may have a role in the treatment of AVR. Deoxyspergualin has been shown by several investigators to prolong cardiac xenograft survival in a hamster-to-rat model.[92,93] Marchman et al. reported that the combination of DOSP and total lymphoid irradiation (TLI) prolonged cardiac xenograft survival in the same animal model.[94] This combined therapy also lowered anti-donor lymphocytotoxic antibody titers and decreased the incidence of vascular rejection compared with controls. In a canine kidney transplant model where donor-specific blood transfusions were given to enhance vascular rejection, DOSP treated animals demonstrated markedly reduced histologic evidence of AVR compared with untreated controls or those treated with cyclosporine.[95] Reports of DOSP being used to treat AVR in human allograft rejection are very limited. Two cases from Sweden have been reported in which renal allograft recipients developed acute graft dysfunction and a positive lymphocytotoxic crossmatch within the first week after transplant.[96] Both episodes of rejection were felt to be humorally mediated, but biopsy proven vascular rejection was only demonstrated in one patient. Treatment with a combination of DOSP and plasmapheresis resulted in improvement in allograft function, and the crossmatch and PRA status became negative in both cases. A repeat biopsy in the patient with AVR showed improvement in the vascular lesions.

Finally, other novel strategies that have been used clinically to treat AVR include actinomycin D (ACD) and local graft irradiation (LGI). ACD inhibits lymphocyte proliferation by inducing single strand breaks in DNA and blocking DNA transcription. DiSalvo et al. found ACD to be an effective adjunctive immunosuppressive agent in three heart transplant patients with AVR.[97] The use of ACD was associated with a decrease in number of rejection episodes per patient, a decrease in required steroid dose, and an increase in ventricular function. LGI has been effective in treating humoral rejection in some xenograph models, but its use in treating AVR in human graft recipients is very limited. In one report, LGI was used in 6 renal graft recipients when all efforts with standard immunosuppression had failed.[98] Five of the six patients had evidence of AVR, and LGI resulted in clinical or histologic improvement in 50% of the cases. Treatment of AVR in cardiac allograft recipients with LGI has not been reported.

HEPARIN IN THE TREATMENT OF AVR

Evidence from xenograft models has shown that several important changes in endothelial cell function occur during AVR that result in the conversion of its

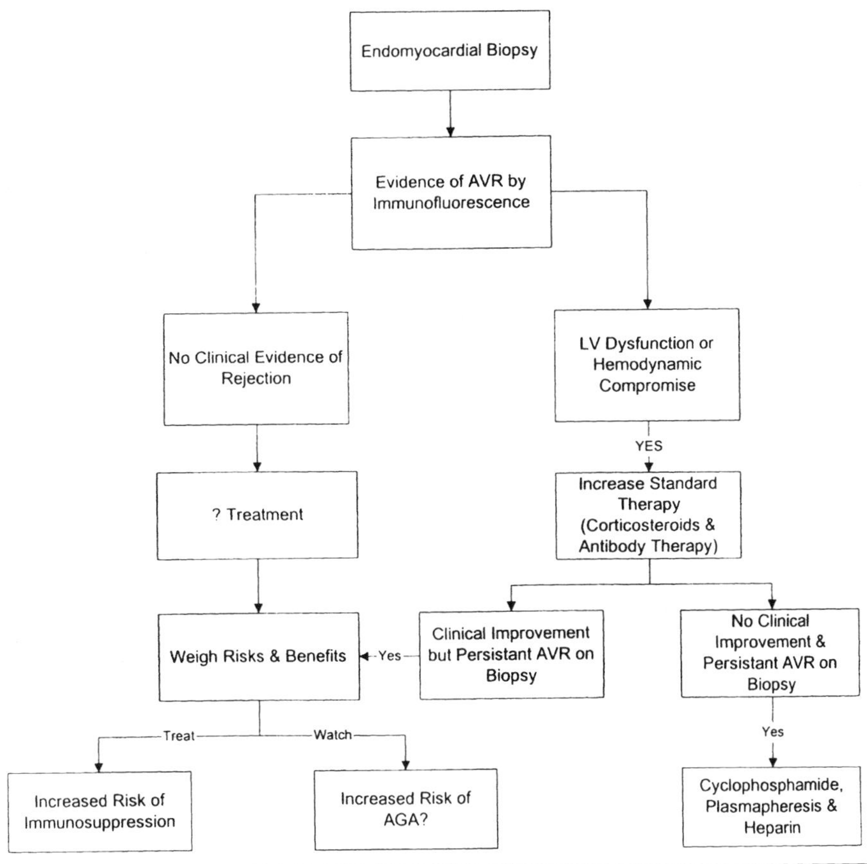

Figure 1. Treatment algorithm for asymptomatic vascular rejection.

normally thromboresistant cell surface to a thrombogenic one. These changes include induction of tissue factor, release of heparin sulfate from the cell surface, down-regulation of thrombomodulin (TM), and a decrease in endogenous tissue plasminogen activator.[28] The supportive effect that heparin has on both the fibrinolytic and antithrombin III (ATIII) anticoagulant pathways suggests a theoretic benefit in this form of vascular injury. In addition, immunocytochemical studies on endothelium from human cardiac allografts have suggested that the ATIII and TM pathways may have independent roles in the pathogenesis of cellular versus vascular rejection.[99] While down-regulation of endothelial TM was associated with cellular rejection, vascular rejection was accompanied primarily by down-regulation of ATIII. The administration of heparin could theoretically support the ATIII pathway and enable the endothelium to maintain a state of thromboresistance during an episode of AVR. While there are no clinical data that definitively support the use of anticoagulation for humoral rejection, heparin use has become standard practice in some centers for the treatment of AVR.[8,9]

THE ROLE OF AVR IN THE PATHOGENESIS OF ACCELERATED GRAFT ATHEROSCLEROSIS

Accelerated graft atherosclerosis (AGA) remains a major cause of mortality in patients surviving one year after heart transplant, and there is increasing evidence to suggest that AVR may play an important role in its pathogenesis. Rose et al. demonstrated a relationship between the presence of serum cytotoxic anti-HLA antibodies and an increased frequency of graft coronary artery disease in 118 cardiac allograft recipients.[100] Similarly, Hess et al. showed an association between circulating anti-B-cell antibodies and the development of lethal coronary disease.[101] In a large series, Hammond et al. found that patients with immunohistologic evidence of pure vascular rejection or mixed vascular rejection were at increased risk of developing coronary disease compared to patients with cellular rejection.[26]

It is not known at this time whether aggressive treatment of AVR will reduce the incidence of AGA. In clinical studies to date, the treatment of AVR has been restricted primarily to patients demonstrating both immunohistologic and clinical evidence of vascular rejection (Figure 1). Given the observed relationship between AVR and the subsequent development of coronary disease, it may be prudent to initiate therapy even in asymptomatic patients who demonstrate histologic evidence of vascular rejection. Randomized clinical trials will be necessary to determine if early treatment of asymptomatic AVR will impact favorably on the development of AGA and overall graft survival.

CONCLUSION

Two of the greatest challenges facing cardiac transplantation as it moves into the twenty-first century include the management of acute vascular rejection and the prevention and treatment of accelerated graft atherosclerosis. The humoral immune response appears to play a fundamental role in each of these processes, and while AVR is the result of antibody and complement mediated vascular injury in the early post-transplant period, AGA may in part represent the chronic sequelae of on-going humorally mediated vascular injury. Observations from clinical studies during the past ten years have left little doubt that AVR is a real and unique form of rejection that differs from cellular rejection in its underlying pathogenesis and response to standard immunosuppressive therapy. Finding effective treatment strategies for AVR has been slow due to a lack of standardized diagnostic criteria and a relatively limited understanding of the underlying pathophysiology. The time has come to initiate multicenter clinical trials designed to identify effective treatment modalities for AVR and to determine whether targeting acute humoral responses will impact favorably on AGA and long-term allograft survival.

REFERENCES

1. Hosenpud JD, Bennett LE, Keck BM, et al. The registry of the International Society for Heart and Lung Transplantation: Seventeenth official report-1997. J Heart Lung Transplant 2000;19:909–31.
2. Billingham ME. Diagnosis of cardiac rejection by endomyocardial biopsy. J Heart Transplant 1981;1:25–30.
3. Heroux A, Costanzo-Nordin MR, Radvany R, et al. Acute cardiac allograft dysfunction without cellular rejection: clinical features and role of humoral immunity. Circulation 1992;86(suppl):I-628.
4. Costanzo-Nordin MR, Heroux AL, Radvany R, et al. Role of humoral immunity in acute cardiac allograft dysfunction. J Heart Lung Transplant 1993;12:S143–6.
5. Ratkovec RM, Hammond EH, O'Connell JB, et al. Outcome of cardiac transplant recipients with a donor specific crossmatch-preliminary results with plasmapheresis. Transplantation 1992;54:651–5.
6. Hammond EH, Yowell RL, Nunoda S, et al. Vascular (humoral) rejection in heart transplantation: Pathologic observations and clinical implications. J Heart Transplant 1989;8:430–43.
7. Ensley RD, Hammond EH, Renlund RL, et al. Clinical manifestations of vascular rejection in cardiac transplantation. Transplant Proc 1991;23:1130–2.
8. Olsen SL, Wagoner LE, Hammond EH, et al. Vascular rejection in heart transplantation: Clinical correlation, treatment options, and future considerations. J Heart Lung Transplant 1993;12:S135–42.
9. Miller LW, Wesp A, Jennison SH, et al. Vascular rejection in heart transplant recipients. J Heart Lung Transplant 1993;12:S147–52.
10. Zales VR, Crawford S, Backer CL, et al. Spectrum of humoral rejection after pediatric heart transplantation. J Heart Lung Transplant 1993;12:563–72.
11. Colvin RB. The pathogenesis of vascular rejection. Transplant Proc 1991;23:2052–5.
12. Jeannet M, Pinn VW, Flax MH, et al. Humoral antibodies in renal allotransplantation in man. N Eng J Med 1970;282:111–17.
13. Najarian JS, Foker JE. Mechanism of kidney allograft rejection. Transplant Proc 1969;1:184–93.
14. Porter KA. Rejection in treated renal allografts. J Clin Path 1967;20:518–34.
15. Lordon RE, Wilson RL, Shield CF, et al. Humoral immunity in renal transplantation. Transplantation 1981;32:286–90.
16. Cerilli J, Clarke J, Doolin T, et al. The significance of a donor-specific vessel crossmatch in renal transplantation. Transplantation 1988;46:359–61.
17. Halloran PF, Wadgymar A, Ritchie S, et al. The significance of the anti-class I antibody response. Transplantation 1990;49:85–91.
18. Halloran PF, Srinivasa NS, Solez K, Williams GM. The roles of antibody in clinical rejection syndromes. In: Kidney Transplant Rejection Diagnosis and Treatment. Burdick JF, Racusen LC, Solez K, Williams GM eds. New York: Marcel Dekker 1992:359–71.
19. Busch GJ, Reynolds ES, Galvanek EG, et al. Human renal allografts: The role of vascular injury in early graft failure. Medicine 1971;50:29–83.
20. Paul LC, Baldwin WM, VanEs LA. Vascular endothelial alloantigens in renal transplantation. Transplantation 1985;40:117–23.
21. Herskowitz A, Soule LM, Ueda K, et al. Arteriolar vasculitis on endomyocardial biopsy: a histologic predictor of poor outcome in cyclosporine-treated heart transplant recipients. J Heart Transplant 1987;6:127–36.
22. Smith SH, Kirklin JK, Geer JC, et al. Arteritis in cardiac rejection after transplantation. Am J Cardiol 1987;59:1171–3.
23. Lones MA, Czer LSC, Trento A, et al. Clinical-pathologic features of humoral rejection in cardiac allografts: A study in 81 consecutive patients. J Heart Lung Transplant 1995;14:151–62.
24. Ma H, Hammond EH, Taylor DO, et al. The repetitive histologic pattern of vascular cardiac allograft rejection. Transplantation 1996;62:205–10.
25. Hammond EH, Wittwer CT, Greenwood J, et al. Relationship of OKT3 sensitization and vascular rejection in cardiac transplant patients receiving OKT3 rejection prophylaxis. Transplantation 1990;50:776–82.
26. Hammond EH, Yowell RL, Price GD, et al. Vascular rejection and its relationship to allograft coronary artery disease. J Heart Lung Transplant 1992;11:S111–19.
27. DiSesa VJ. Cardiac xenotransplantation. Ann Thorac Surg 1997;64:1858–65.
28. Lawson JH, Platt JL. Molecular barriers to xenotransplantation. Transplantation 1996;62:303–10.
29. Leech SH, Mather PJ, Eisen HJ, et al. Donor-specific HLA antibodies after transplantation are associated with deterioration in cardiac function. Clin Transplantation 1996;10:639–45.
30. Cherry R, Nielsen H, Reed E, et al. Vascular (humoral) rejection in human cardiac allograft biopsies: Relation to circulating anti-HLA antibodies. J Heart Lung Transplant 1992;11:24–30.

31. Moraes JR, Stastny P. Human endothelial cell antigens: molecular independency from HLA expression in blood monocytes. Transplant Proc 1977;9:605–7.
32. Paul LC, Van Es LA, Van Rood JJ, et al. Accelerated rejection of a renal allograft associated with pretransplantation antibodies directed against donor antigens on endothelium and monocytes. N Engl J Med 1979;301:1258–60.
33. Cerilli J, Brasile L, Galouzis T, et al. The vascular endothelial cell antigen system. Transplantation 1985;39:286–9.
34. Haisch C, Brasile L, Galouzis T, et al. The importance of the vascular endothelial cell antigen system in non-HLA identical renal transplants. Transplant Proc 1985;17:128.
35. Baldwin WM, Claas FHJ, Van Es LA, et al. Distribution of endothelial-monocyte and HLA antigens on renal vascular endothelium. Transplant Proc 1981;13:103–7.
36. Cerilli J, Bay W, Brasile L. The significance of the monocyte crossmatch in recipients of living-related HLA identical kidney grafts. Hum Immunol 1983;7:45–50.
37. Brasile L, Zerbe T, Rabin B, et al. Identification of the antibody to vascular endothelial cells in patients undergoing cardiac transplantation. Transplantation 1985;40:672–5.
38. Trento A, Hardesty RL, Griffith BP, et al. Role of the antibody to vascular endothelial cells in hyperacute rejection in patients undergoing cardiac transplantation. J Thorac Cardiovasc Surg 1988;95:37–41.
39. O'Connell JB, Renlund DG, Hammond EH, et al. Sensitization to OKT3 monoclonal antibody in heart transplantation: correlation with early allograft loss. J Heart Lung Transplant 1991;10:217–22.
40. Hammond EH, Yowell RL, Greenwood J, et al. Prevention of adverse clinical outcome by monitoring of cardiac transplant patients for murine monoclonal CD3 antibody (OKT3) sensitization. Transplantation 1993;55:1061–3.
41. Hammond EH, Watson FS, Bristow MR, et al. Fibrinoid necrosis of a temporal artery complicating the treatment of refractory cardiac allograft rejection with murine monoclonal CD3 antibody (OKT3). J Heart Transplant 1990;9:236–8.
42. Hillebrand G, Dendorfer U, Feucht HE, et al. Vascular rejection episodes reduce success in renal graft outcome after therapy with BMA 031. Transplant Proc 1991;23:1092–3.
43. Kemnitz J, Restrepo-Specht I, Haverich A, et al. Acute humoral rejection: a new entity in the histopathology of heart transplantation (Letter). J Heart Transplant 1990;9:447–8.
44. Hammond EH. Reply (Letter). J Heart Transplant 1990;9:448–9.
45. Mihatsh MJ, Theil G, Spichtin HP, et al. Morphologic findings in kidney transplants after treatment with cyclosporine. Transplant Proc 1983;15:2821–35.
46. Sommer BG, Innes JT, Whitehurst RM, et al. Cyclosporine-associated renal arteriopathy resulting in loss of allograft function. Am J Surg 1985;149:756–64.
47. Demetris AJ, Lasky S, Van Thiel DH, et al. Pathology of hepatic transplantation. A review of 62 adult allograft recipients immunosuppressed with a cyclosporine/steroid combination. Am J Pathol 1985;118:151–8.
48. Shulman H, Striker G, Deeg HJ, et al. Nephrotoxicity of cyclosporine A after allogeneic marrow transplantation: glomerular thrombosis and tubular injury. N Engl J Med 1981;305:1392–5.
49. Bergstrand A, Bohman SO, Farnsworth A, et al. Renal histopathology and kidney transplant recipients immunosuppressed with cyclosporin A: results of an international workshop. Clin Nephrol 1985;24:107–19.
50. Wilczek HE, Groth CG, Bohman SO. Effect of reduced cyclosporin dosage on long-term renal allograft histology. Transpl Int 1992;5:65–70.
51. Van Saase JLCM, Van der Woude FK, Thorogood J, et al. The relation between acute vascular and interstitial renal allograft rejection and subsequent chronic rejection. Transplantation 1995;59:1280–85.
52. Ballardie FW, Winearls CG, Evans DJ, et al. Cyclosporine for steroid-resistant acute rejection of renal cadaver grafts. Transplantation 1986;41:537–9.
53. Crowson MC, Berisa F, McGonigle RJS, et al. Selective conversion from azathioprine to cyclosporine for steroid-resistant rejection in renal transplants: an alternative therapy. Nephrol Dial Transplant 1989;4:129–32.
54. Thomas PP, Jacob CK, Kirubakaran MG, et al. Cyclosporine in the treatment of acute vascular rejection of renal allografts. Transplantation 1990;50:521–2.
55. Brunt EM. Pathology of transplanted organs. In: Flye MW. Principles of organ transplantation. Philadelphia: Saunders, 1989:105.
56. Delaney VB, Campbell WG, Nasr SA, et al. Efficacy of OKT3 monoclonal antibody therapy in steroid-resistant, predominantly vascular acute rejection. Transplantation 1988;45:743–8.
57. Schroeder TJ, Weiss MA, Smith RD, et al. The efficacy of OKT3 in vascular rejection. Transplantation 1991;51:312–15.
58. Ballester M, Obrador D, Carrio I, et al. Reversal of rejection-induced coronary vasculitis detected

early after heart transplantation with increased immunosuppression. J Heart Transplant 1989; 8:413–17.
59. Cupps TR, Edgar LC, Fauci AS. Suppression of human B lymphocyte function by cyclophosphamide. J Immunol 1982;128:2453–7.
60. Zhu LP, Cupps TR, Whalen G, et al. Selective effects of cyclophosphamide therapy on activation, proliferation, and differentiation of human B cells. J Clin Invest 1987;79:1082–90.
61. Wagoner LE, Taylor DO, Olsen SL, et al. Cyclophosphamide in cardiac transplant recipients with frequent rejection: a six-year retrospective review. Clin Transplantation 1996;10:437–43.
62. Taylor DO, Bristow MR, O'Connell JB, et al. A prospective, randomized comparison of cyclophosphamide and azathioprine for early rejection prophylaxis after cardiac transplantation. Transplantation 1994;58:645–9.
63. Franco A, Anaya F, Niembro E, et al. Plasma exchange in the treatment of vascular rejection. Relationship between histological changes and therapeutic response. Transplant Proc 1987;19:3661–3.
64. Grandtnerova B, Javorsky P, Kolacny J, et al. Treatment of acute humoral rejection in kidney transplantation with plasmapheresis. Transplant Proc 1995;27:934–5.
65. Aichberger C, Nussbaumer W, Rosmanith P, et al. Plasmapheresis for the treatment of acute vascular rejection in renal transplantation. Transplant Proc 1997;29:169–70.
66. Sakellariou G, Paschalidou E, Tsobanelis T, et al. The role of plasma exchange in renal transplantation. Transplant Proc 1985;17:2779–82.
67. Fassbinder W, Scheuermann EH, Hanke P, et al. Improved graft prognosis by treatment of steroid-resistant rejections with rabbit antithymocyte globulin and/or plasmapheresis. Transplant Proc 1985;17:2769–72.
68. Salmela KT, von Willebrand EO, Kyllonen LEJ, et al. Acute vascular rejection in renal transplantation-diagnosis and outcome. Transplantation 1992;54:858–62.
69. Allen NH, Dyer P, Geoghegan T, Harris K, et al. Plasma exchange in acute renal allograft rejection. Transplantation 1983;35:425–8.
70. Partanen J, Nieminen MS, Krogerus L, et al. Heart transplant rejection treated with plasmapheresis. J Heart Lung Transplant 1992;11:301–5.
71. Catalan M, Llorens R, Legarra JJ, et al. Plasmapheresis as therapy to resolve vascular rejection in heart transplantation with severe heart failure: "A report of one case." Transplant Proc 1998;30:176–9.
72. Berglin E, Kjellstrom C, Mantovani V, et al. Plasmapheresis as a rescue therapy to resolve cardiac rejection with vasculitis and severe heart failure. A report of five cases. Transpl Int 1995;8:382–7.
72a. Grauhan O, Knosalla C, Ewert R, et al. Plasmapheresis and cyclosphosphamide in the treatment of humoral rejection after heart transplantation. J Heart Lung Transplant 2001;20:316–21.
73. Pretagostini R, Berloco P, Poli L, et al. Immunoadsorption with protein A in humoral rejection of kidney transplants. ASAIO Journal 1996;42:M645–8.
74. Olivari MT, May CB, Johnson NA, et al. Treatment of acute vascular rejection with immunoadsorption. Circulation 1994;90:II-70–3.
75. Wasik M, Stepien-Sopniewska B, Lagodzinski Z, et al. Effects of FK506 and cyclosporine on human T and B lymphoproliferative responses. Immunopharmacology 1990;20:57–61.
76. Stevens C, Lempert N, Freed BM. The effects of immunosuppressive agents on in vitro production of human immunoglobulins. Transplantation 1991;51:1240–4.
77. Woodle ES, Perdrizet GA, So SKS, et al. FK 506 rescue therapy for hepatic allograft rejection: Experience with an aggressive approach. Clin Transplantation 1995;9:45–52.
78. Eberhard OK, Kliem V, Oldhafer K, et al. How best to use tacrolimus (FK506) for treatment of steroid- and OKT3-resistant rejection after renal transplantation. Transplantation 1996;61:1345–9.
79. Woodle ES, Spargo B, Ruebe M, et al. Treatment of acute glomerular rejection with FK 506. Clin Transplantation 1996;10:266–70.
80. Jordan ML, Shapiro R, Vivas CA, et al. FK506 "rescue" for resistant rejection of renal allografts under primary cyclosporine immunosuppression. Transplantation 1994;57:860–5.
81. Woodle ES, Phelan DL, Saffitz JE, et al. FK506-reversal of humorally mediated cardiac allograft rejection in the presence of preformed anti-class I antibody. Transplantation 1993;56:1271–5.
82. Morris RE, Hoyt EG, Murphy MP, et al. Mycophenolic acid morpholinoethylester (RS-61443) is a new immunosuppressant that prevents and halts heart allograft rejection by selective inhibition of T and B cell purine synthesis. Transplant Proc 1990;22:1659–62.
83. Fujino Y, Kawamura T, Hullett DA, et al. Evaluation of cyclosporine, mycophenolate mofetil, and brequinar sodium combination therapy on hamster-to-rat cardiac xenotransplantation. Transplantation 1994;57:41–6.
84. O'Hair DP, McManus RP, Komorowski R. Inhibition of chronic vascular rejection in primate cardiac xenografts using mycophenolate mofetil. Ann Thorac Surg 1994;58:1311–5.
85. Allison AC, Kowalski WJ, Muller CJ, et al. Mycophenolic acid and brequinar, inhibitors of purine

and pyrimidine synthesis, blocks the glycosylation of adhesion molecules. Transplant Proc 1993;25(3 Suppl 2):67–70.

86. Qiao JH, Ruan XM, Trento A, et al. Expression of cell adhesion molecules in human cardiac allograft rejection. J Heart Lung Transplant 1992;11:920–5.
87. Sadahiro M, McDonald TO, Allen MD. Reduction in cellular and vascular rejection by blocking leukocyte adhesion molecule receptors. Am J Pathol 1993;142:675–83.
88. Ahsan N, Holman MJ, Katz DA, et al. Successful reversal of acute vascular rejection in a renal allograft with combined mycophenolate mofetil and tacrolimus as primary immunotherapy. Clin Transplantation 1997;11:94–7.
89. Lafferty ME, Lang S, McGregor E, et al. Treatment of severe acute vascular rejection in a renal allograft with mycophenolate mofetil and high dose steroids. Scott Med J 1997;42:79–80.
90. Morikawa K, Oseko F, Morikawa S. The suppressive effect of deoxyspergualin on the differentiation of human B cell lymphocytes maturing into immunoglobulin-producing cells. Transplantation 1992;54:526–31.
91. Fujii H, Takada T, Nemoto K, et al. Deoxyspergualin directly suppresses antibody formation in vivo and in vitro. J Antibiot 1990;43:213–19.
92. Walter P, Bernhard U, Seitz G, et al. Xenogeneic heart transplantation with 15-deoxyspergualin. Prolongation of graft survival. Transplant Proc 1987;19:3993–4.
93. Suzuki Seiichi, Nishimori H, Ohdan H, et al. Prolongation of cardiac xenograft survival in a hamster-to-rat combination by recipient treatment with deoxymethylspergualin. Transplantation 1993;56:1257–60.
94. Marchman W, Araneda D, DeMasi R, et al. Prolongation of xenograft survival after combination therapy with 15-deoxyspergualin and total-lymphoid irradiation in the hamster-to-rat cardiac xenograft model. Transplantation 1992;53:30–4.
95. Tanabe K, Takahashi K, Nemoto K, et al. Effect of deoxyspergualin on vascular rejection in canine kidney transplantation. J Urol 1994;152:562–6.
96. Gannedahl G, Ohlman S, Persson U, et al. Rejection associated with early appearance of donor-reactive antibodies after kidney transplantation treated with plasmapheresis and administration of 15-deoxyspergualin. Transplant Int 1992;5:189–92.
97. DiSalvo TG, Narula J, Cosimi AB, et al. Actinomycin D is an effective adjunctive immunosuppressive agent in recurrent cardiac allograft rejection. J Heart Lung Transplant 1995;14:955–62.
98. Jagetia R, Small Jr. W, Stuart FP, et al. Local Graft Irradiation after failure of modern immunosuppression in acute cellular and vascular graft rejection. Int J Radiation Oncology Biol Phys 1996;36:907–11.
99. Labarrere CA, Pitts D, Halbrook H, et al. Natural anticoagulant pathways in normal and transplanted human hearts. J Heart Lung Transplant 1992;11:342–7.
100. Rose EA, Smith CR, Petrossian GA, et al. Humoral immune responses after cardiac transplantation: correlation with fatal rejection and graft atherosclerosis. Surgery 1989;106:203–8.
101. Hess ML, Hastillo A, Mohanakumar T, et al. Accelerated atherosclerosis in cardiac transplantation: role of cytotoxic B-cell antibodies and hyperlipidemia. Circulation 1983:68(suppl II):II-94–101.

Section 3. Newer Diagnostic Tools for the Management of Cardiac Allograft Rejection

13. EVOLUTION OF NONINVASIVE TESTING FOR THE DETECTION OF CARDIAC ALLOGRAFT REJECTION

Rohit Srivastava, MBBS, MD,
and Jeffrey D. Hosenpud, M.D.
The Division of Cardiovascular Medicine, Medical College of Wisconsin Milwaukee, Wisconsin USA

INTRODUCTION

Early detection and treatment of allograft rejection remains the most crucial aspect of transplant management, given the high mortality in patients with acute rejection associated with allograft dysfunction. Even twenty-five years after its introduction by Caves and associates,[1] endomyocardial biopsy still remains the most reliable and frequent technique to assess allograft rejection. Unfortunately, this early diagnosis requires up to 20 biopsies per patient within the first year after cardiac transplantation. Aside from its obvious costs, there is patient discomfort and potential risk form the multiple invasive procedures. Moreover, endomyocardial biopsy may not predict the occurrence of clinically significant acute allograft rejection in a small number of patients. Accordingly, the search for new and noninvasive techniques for the diagnosis of cardiac allograft rejection has continued to receive much interest.

What is required for a perfect screening test is not dissimilar to any ideal screening test. It should be easy to administer repetitively, should be noninvasive, have a low cost, and most importantly, it should have a high sensitivity. The need for specificity varies with the implications for further diagnosis. In the diagnosis of cardiac allograft rejection, the screening test should be nearly 100% sensitive, given the potentially fatal implications of missing acute rejection. Even if the specificity were only 50%, this would result in a decrement of one half of the biopsies performed on a routine basis. In other words, it is critical for the test to have a high negative predictive value. A high positive predictive value is desirable but not essential.

Four general approaches have been investigated as possible screening tests for cardiac allograft rejection: electrocardiography, cardiac functional assessment, biochemical/ immunologic assays and myocardial imaging.

ELECTROCARDIOGRAPHY

In the early days of cardiac transplantation, a decline in the R wave amplitude obtained from the surface 12-lead electrocardiogram correlated with graft rejection. This has been postulated to be due to myocardial edema, necrosis and lymphocytic infiltrate. With the advent of cyclosporine, this technique was no longer valid: the rejection process demonstrated less diffuse edema,[2,3,4] and the electrocardiographic changes were not consistent and did not correlate with the rejection process.

Intramyocardial electrocardiogram was first reported in 1984 as an index of irreversible myocardial ischemic injury.[5] This technique was later used to noninvasively diagnose cardiac allograft rejection.[6] Several investigators have assessed the utility of intramyocardial electrocardiogram (IMEG) in detection of cardiac allograft rejection in animal models.[6–12] Pirolo and associates[9] used a canine model of intrathoracic heterotopic cardiac transplantation and used four unipolar intramyocardial leads. They recorded unipolar peak to peak amplitude (UPPA) from each lead. Significant correlation was found between the quantitative rejection score and decline in UPPA. Sensitivity and specificity was 91% and 84% when UPPA data was used from all four leads and 94% and 91% when UPPA data was used from the two left ventricular leads. The same group[13] used prospective UPPA surveillance in detecting rejection of heterotopic canine cardiac allografts occurring despite triple drug immunosuppression. Intramyocardial unipolar electrodes implanted in the native heart and the graft were connected to subcutaneously implanted telemetric pacemakers. A fall in normalized UPPA to less than 85% of baseline was used as an indication for endomyocardial biopsy. Sensitivity and specificity for detecting histologic rejection were 88% and 91%, respectively. Everett and associates[12] used a canine orthotopic model of cardiac transplant and found that UPPA had a sensitivity and specificity of 100% in detecting allograft rejection. Avitall and associates,[7] who used a bipolar ring electrode for recording of the IMEG, found a correlation between alterations of the IMEG amplitude and the histologic findings of severe but not moderate rejection in endomyocardial biopsy specimens. They also found higher grades of rejection in the atria than the ventricles as well as significant prolongation of intra-atrial conduction but not intra-ventricular conduction.

Enthusiasm led to clinical trials in Europe. Warnecke and associates,[14] prospectively used the telemetry function of a dual chamber pacemaker system to obtain continuous overnight recordings of intramyocardial electrocardiogram. An amplitude decrease of more than 8% below the individual range of variability was considered as an indicator of rejection. The time interval (Te) between maximal posterior wall contraction and the point of peak posterior wall retraction velocity was derived from digitized M-mode echocardiogram. This echocardiographic parameter was used as an additional indicator of rejection associated left ventricular dysfunction. Routine endomyocardial biopsies were performed for patient safety but the results were undisclosed to the transplantation team. Detection and management of rejection episodes was carried out using the noninvasive tests. IMEG showed a negative predictive value of 100% with no false negative results. Echocardiography yielded a negative predictive value of 96.9%. The authors concluded that 90% of the endomyocardial biopsies could be avoided using these noninvasive techniques. Mueller and associates[15] from the same center reported the results of this trans-telephonic follow-up method in over 1000 patients over a period of 8 years. Routine endomyocardial biopsy was abolished and resulted in 75% reduction in the number of biopsies. Death caused by unrecognized acute rejection was less than 0.4%. False positive reduction in IMEG amplitude was caused most often by infection (usually CMV). Disadvantages include (1) the varying distance between anode and cathode of the unipolar lead configuration, which leads to variability of the QRS amplitude, (2) the scarring process around the electrodes in the long-term course, and (3) the necessity of implantation of a device for telemetric data transfer. Auer and associates[16] used an implanted VVI pacemaker with a lead having a fractal surface (to eliminate polarization artifact secondary to pacing) to assess the association between rejection and signal averaged spontaneous QRS amplitude (QRSA) as well as paced ventricular evoked response depolarization amplitude (VERDA). They found significant reduction in both parameters with grade 2 and 3 rejection. VERDA had a sensitivity of 100% and a specificity of 77%. QRSA had a sensitivity of 91% and specificity of 77%. Combination of both parameters yielded the best sensitivity of 100% and specificity of 80%. The same group[17] also demonstrated significant improvement in the parameters with successful treatment of the episodes of rejection. Wahlers and associates[18] studied the intramyocardial electrocardiogram derived from an implanted pacemaker in 13 patients with orthotopic heart transplantation and found a high diurnal variability (up to 30% in individual patients) in the voltage of the intramyocardial electrocardiogram. There was significant variability with exercise as well and they did not find correlation between moderate/ severe rejection and intramyocardial voltage. They however, did not use resting states or comparable times of the day as used by the other investigators.

Signal-averaged electrocardiogram has also been studied as a means of detecting rejection. One study[19] compared histologic rejection in 25 patients with signal averaged electrocardiogram obtained within 24 hours of the endomyocardial biopsy—218 endomyocardial biopsy specimens were compared with 277 signal-averaged electrocardiograms. They found significant decreases in peak and root-mean-square voltages of both filtered and unfiltered QRS complexes, as well as the total spectral area. The root-mean-square voltage of the 70-Hz high pass filtered QRS complex was found to be the most reproducible and the most accurate variable in detecting rejection. The optimal rejection criterion was defined as an 11% decrease in voltage between two consecutive recordings. It provided 88% sensitivity and 78% specificity. Morocutti and associates[20] compared the presence of late potentials derived from signal-averaged electrocardiograms to the histologic presence of clinically relevant rejection. They found a sensitivity of 69%, specificity of 71% and negative predictive value of 93%.

Some necropsy studies of transplanted dogs have shown that histologic lesions of rejection are more severe in the atrial tissue and the atrio-ventricular conduction tissue as compared with the ventricular myocardium.[7,21] Babuty and associates studied high resolution electrocardiography in a rat model of heterotopic heart transplant.[22] In the allogeneic group they found an early and progressive increase of the duration of the P wave and the PQ interval associated with rejection. No such change was found in the syngeneic group. The sensitivity and specificity of an increase in P wave duration ≥20% was found to be 100%. The results of these studies are summarized in Table 1.

Table 1. Electrocardiographic indecies used in the diagnosis of rejection

Author	Study	Parameter studied	Sensitivity	Specificity	Reference
Pirolo et al.	Animal	UPPA 4 lead, retrospective	91%	84%	9
		UPPA 2 lead	94%	91%	
Pirolo et al.	Animal	UPPA, prospective	88%	91%	13
Everett et al.	Animal	UPPA	100%	100%	12
Babuty et al.	Animal	$\uparrow$ in p wave duration	100%	100%	22
Warnecke et al.	Human	$\downarrow$ in QRS voltage (IMEG telemetry)	94%	95%	14
Auer et al.	Human	QRS amplitude, spontaneous	91%	77%	16
		Paced ventricular QRS amplitude	100%	77%	
		Combined	100%	80%	
Lacroix et al.	Human	Signal averaged ECG	88%	78%	19
Morocutti et al.	Human	Late potentials	69%	71%	20

CARDIAC FUNCTIONAL ASSESSMENT

Early studies of echocardiographic correlates of acute allograft rejection focused on the changes in ventricular morphology rather than physiology. In the pre-cyclosporine era, increases in left ventricular (LV) mass and wall thickness, measured by M-mode echocardiography, were reported during episodes of acute rejection.[23,24] In a more recent study in patients treated with cyclosporine based immunosuppression, Gill and associates[25] found no correlation between changes in left ventricular wall thickness, mass and dimension with moderate and severe cellular rejection. However, marked changes were noticed in patients with vascular (humoral) rejection. These patients demonstrated a significant increase in left ventricular mass, wall thickness and dimension. They also found a decrease in fractional shortening and increased incidence of hemodynamic compromise with vascular rejection (50% vs. 11% for vascular and cellular rejection, respectively).

It has long been appreciated that systolic function as assessed by ejection phase indexes is neither sensitive nor specific for allograft rejection.[26,27] This has lead to several studies investigating the use of diastolic indexes of left ventricular function as potentially more sensitive in this diagnosis (see Chapter 14). Paulsen and associates[27] first demonstrated that echocardiographic-derived indexes of diastolic function were abnormal in patients with acute allograft rejection. They reported a decrease in LV lengthening rate and posterior wall thinning rate consistent with significant diastolic dysfunction. Dawkins and associates[28] applied echocardiography and phonocardiography to examine the correlation of isovolumic relaxation time (IVRT) with acute cardiac rejection in patients treated with cyclosporine. A 10% decrease in IVRT was 87% sensitive and 90% specific for diagnosis of moderate cardiac rejection. Desruennes and associates[29] found a sensitivity and specificity of 60% and 87%, respectively for the detection of rejection using a criterion of 20% decrease in IVRT. However, Forster and associates[30] found sensitivity and specificity of 56% and 79% in serially obtained IVRT measurements and concluded that IVRT is not a reliable enough non-invasive test to detect and treat acute rejection clinically.

Table 2. Cardiac functional indices used in the diagnosis of rejection

Author	Parameter studied	Sensitivity	Specificity	Reference
Dawkins et al.	Isovolumic relaxation time (IVRT)	87%	90%	28
Desruennes et al.	IVRT	60%	87%	29
Forster et al.	IVRT	56%	79%	30
Warnecke et al.	Te*	65%	94%	14
Desruennes et al.	Mitral pressure half time (PHT)	87%	87%	33
Fauchier et al.	Mitral PHT	36%	72%	35
Novitzky et al.	Radionuclide ventriculography	85%	96%	41
Angermann et al.	Echocardiographic back scatter	83–92%	85–90%	44

* Te: Time between maximum posterior wall contraction and point of peak posterior wall retraction.

Valantine and associates[31] have described changes in Doppler indexes of left ventricular diastolic function in patients with heart transplant (see Chapter 14). In the early post-transplant period and acute rejection there is the development of restrictive LV physiology characterized by increased peak early (E) mitral flow velocity, increased rapid deceleration, decreased flow velocity during atrial contraction and a short isovolumic relaxation time. They also reported that during the 6 weeks after cardiac transplant, there is a gradual increase in the pressure half-time and IVRT and a decrease in E velocity. This is consistent with decreased LV diastolic pressure and improved diastolic function.[32] Desruennes and associates[33] also studied the effect of mild and moderate rejection on the Doppler indices of left ventricular diastolic function and reported significant decrease of mitral pressure half-time during episodes of mild rejection. This normalized after 5 days of treatment with prednisone. During moderate rejection they found significant decrease in both the isovolumic relaxation time as well as pressure half time. These parameters also normalized after successful treatment for the rejection episode. Decrease in pressure half-time by 20% yielded sensitivity and specificity of 87%. However, Mannaerts and associates[34] have indicated that pulsed-wave mitral Doppler could not allow the diagnosis of moderate rejection due to wide overlap of measurements in individual patients. Fauchier and associates[35] found that the only variable that showed a significant decrease was the percentage of variation of pressure half-time compared to the last examination with negative endomyocardial biopsy. Moreover, Valantine et al.[36] and others[37] have reported late "restrictive" physiology without histological rejection after cardiac transplantation. Additional factors such as donor-recipient size matching may play an important role in the diastolic properties of the allograft.[38,39] Radionuclide ventriculography based assessment of left ventricular diastolic function has also yielded similar results as echocardiography.[40,41] Imaging and characterization of the myocardium to diagnose rejection have been attempted using a variety of techniques, including echocardiographic tissue characterization,[42] and backscatter analysis[43,44] Angermann and associates[44] used unprocessed RF signals and compared two-dimensional integrated backscatter with histologically diagnosed rejection. They found sensitivities of 83–92% and specificity of 85–90%. Based on the available data (Table 2), one must therefore conclude that functional indexes by themselves are unlikely to provide the sensitivity required for rejection screening in asymptomatic patients.

BIOCHEMICAL/ IMMUNOLOGIC ASSAYS

Another area of interest has attempted to directly assay for increases in alloimmunologic activity. The earliest study reported by Copeland and associates[45] involved the measurement of urinary polyamines that reflected increased cellular proliferation or degeneration. Sensitivity and specificity was 85% and 88%, respectively. The same group[46] found elevated prolactin levels to correlate with histologic rejection. Consistent elevation of prolactin levels was seen several days before every primary positive biopsy, but this increase was not always observed prior to recurrent rejection. Sensitivity of prolactin level to predict all primary positive biopsies was 100% and specificity was 88%. Other markers of activation of the alloimmune response which have been studied are neopterine[47] and β_2-microglobulin.[48] These biochemical markers suffer from lack of specificity since they are elevated in conditions such as viral infections and insufficient increase in the presence of cyclosporine (reduced renal clearance of polyamines).

With the further understanding of immunologic activation, lymphocyte subsets, and activation markers, several groups have investigated the possibility that cyoimmunological monitoring may be useful in detection of acute rejection. In one study[49] acute rejection episodes were associated with increase in the number of "activated" lymphocytes. A sensitivity of 94% and a specificity of 68% was found. Seventy-two percent of the false-positive results were due to viral infections, particularly cytomegalovirus. Other studies have found usefulness only until the first episode of rejection and with unacceptably low sensitivity[50] or increase in cytoimmunological values only in the first 30 days after transplantation.[51] Monitoring of transferrin receptor-positive circulating lymphocytes has also been studied in the diagnosis of acute rejection. These receptors are known to increase on the surface of lymphocytes after either antigenic or mitogenic stimulation. The Richmond group[52] monitored recipients for the presence of circulating transferrin receptors by flow cytometry using a murine antitransferrin monoclonal antibody. During the pre-rejection and rejection period, they found a significant increase in the percentage of transferrin receptor positive cells in the peripheral blood. Successful treatment resulted in decrease in the percentage. Persistence of the level after treatment predicted recurrent rejection in 80% of these patients. Other markers (Table 3) utilized include interleukin-2 (IL-2) receptor positive T4 cells[53] (sensitivity 73%, specificity 97% in the

Table 3. Biochemical/Immunologic indecies used in the diagnosis of rejection

Author	Parameter studied	Sensitivity	Specificity	Reference
Copeland et al.	Urinary polyamines	85%	88%	45
Copeland et al.	Prolactin (for first positive biopsy)	100%	88%	46
May et al.	Activated lymphocytes	94%	68%	49
Miller et al.	Interleukin-2 receptor positive T4 cells	78%	97%	53
Loertscher et al.	Combination of early & late activation antigens	38%	52%	54

first 5 weeks post-transplant; sensitivity of 25%, thereafter) and a combination of early (IL-2R, transferrin) and late (PTA1, alpha 1 integrin VLA-1) activation antigens[54] (sensitivity 38%, specificity 52%). One potential problem with these approaches, however, is that what is occurring in the periphery may not accurately reflect immunologic activity in the allograft.

MYOCARDIAL IMAGING

ECG-gated magnetic resonance imaging (MRI) has been also studied experimentally and clinically for the detection of cardiac allograft rejection (see Chapter 15). Allograft rejection is associated with tissue inflammation, edema, and necrosis, all of which may contribute to an increase in T2 relaxation. Animal studies found a correlation between rejection and T2 relaxation time.[55] Wisenberg and associates[56] studied the usefulness of MRI in 25 patients after recent heart transplantation. In the 19 patients imaged within 24 days after transplantation, all, including one which showed biopsy evidence of rejection, had increased T1 and T2 values as compared with normal volunteers and patients who had undergone non-transplant cardiac surgery. In patients with non-rejecting transplants who were imaged more than 25 days after transplant, the T1 and T2 values had decreased to control values. However, in those grafts with rejection, T1 and T2 values were both elevated. 14/15 (93%) of late rejection events (>25 days following surgery) were correctly identified on the basis of increase in T1 and T2 values to more than 2 standard deviations above normal. Only 1 of the 28 studies of non-rejecting grafts had elevated T1 and T2 values indicating good specificity. These results show that MRI is not useful in the detection of rejection in the early period after transplantation but may be a useful technique after the first 1 month to screen for rejection.

Since the development of anti-myosin monoclonal antibody[57] there have been a number of studies demonstrating its usefulness in the diagnosis of myocardial infarction, myocarditis and cardiac allograft rejection (see Chapter 20). The antibody or its Fab fragment has been found to bind to myocytes in which the sarcolemma is no longer intact and when labeled with ^{111}Indium have provided an excellent means to diagnose myocardial damage. Ballester and associates[58] in their initial experience of 53 studies in 21 patients found that an abnormal antimyosin heart/lung uptake ratio (greater than 1.55) yielded a sensitivity of 95% for the diagnosis of clinically relevant rejection requiring treatment. As might be anticipated, specificity was low (29%). In a follow-up study of patients by the same group, at least 1 year after cardiac transplantation,[59] a negative scan assured the absence of rejection requiring treatment (sensitivity 100%, specificity 33%). Schutz and associates[61] also used the ^{111}Indium monoclonal antimyosin antibody in the detection of cardiac allograft rejection. They found a sensitivity of 91% with a heart/lung uptake ratio of >1.6. A heart/lung uptake ratio of <1.6 correlated with a negative endomyocardial biopsy in 98% of the cases. Serial echocardiography (fractional shortening, ventricular wall thickness), however, showed deterioration in only 64% of patients with a positive endomyocardial biopsy. False negative antimyosin scans were found in two patients with anti-murine antibody, presumed to be due to OKT3 therapy. Follow up studies done in one third of the patients revealed decrease of the heart/lung uptake ratio to <1.6 after treatment after rejection. De Nardo and associates[62] studied the antimyosin

Table 4. Myocardial Imaging techniques used in the diagnosis of rejection

Author	Parameter studied	Sensitivity	Specificity	Reference
Wisenberg et al.	MRI	93%	96%	56
Ballester et al.	Antimyosin scan	95%	29%	58
Ballester et al.	Antimyosin scan	100%	33%	59
Schutz et al.	Antimyosin scan	91%		61
De Nardo et al.	Antimyosin scan	100%	36%	62

antibody for the detection of rejection. 19/30 studies were negative and none of these were false negative. Eleven of the 30 positive scans revealed mild rejection in 2 cases, moderate rejection in 2 cases, myocyte necrosis due to ischemic injury in 6 cases and possibly cytotoxic damage in 1 case. They concluded that in the presence of negative finding from antimyosin scintigraphy, it might be possible to avoid endomyocardial biopsy. A positive scan however, mandates histologic confirmation.

Increased expression of MHC class II antigens occur during the process of rejection. In a recent studies using dog and mouse models of heterotopic cardiac transplantation, McGhie and associates[63] and Isobe and associates[64] used ^{111}In-labeled monoclonal antibody against MHC class II antigens (see Chapter 19). Uptake of this antibody increased over baseline in animals that demonstrated progressively worsening allograft rejection, whereas no significant change was seen in those, which did not demonstrate progressively worsening rejection. There was significant increase in uptake as the histologic grade of rejection worsened from mild to severe. Histologic evidence of mild, moderate and severe MHC II expression correlated with significantly increasing antibody uptake. If confirmed by clinical studies, this interesting finding may have direct clinical implication. The results of these studies are summarized in Table 4.

CONCLUSION

Endomyocardial biopsy is less than perfect as a screening tool for rejection surveillance. It is associated with a number of drawbacks including its invasiveness, potential for serious complications and high cost. In addition, there is a small incidence of false negative biopsy findings due to the patchy nature of the acute rejection process or the occurrence of vascular rejection. Nonetheless, the use of this technique for surveillance and monitoring the efficacy of therapy has been associated with exceedingly low rates of rejection leading to serious graft dysfunction. Its application has, therefore, to a large extent, been very relevant clinically. This fact is coupled with the fact that despite the large number of non-invasive tests that have been developed for the diagnosis of acute rejection, none has been proven unequivocally to provide a reliable enough measure to be applied clinically. All show abnormalities in the early period after transplantation, which preclude their use in that period, but serial studies later on may be useful. Some, like telemetrically monitored changes in intramyocardial electrocardiogram and ^{111}In labeled antimyosin monoclonal antibody uptake have shown promise, but large clinical trials from a number of centers are still needed to prove their effectiveness in prospective screening.

BIBLIOGRAPHY

1. Caves PK, Stinson EB, Billingham ME, Rider AK, Shumway NE. Diagnosis of human cardiac allograft rejection by serial cardiac biopsy. J Thor Cardiovasc Surg 1973;66:461–466.
2. Irwin ED, Bianco RW, Clack R, Grehan J, Slovut DP, Nakhleh R, Bolman RM 3d, Shumway SJ. Use of epicardial electrocardiograms for detecting cardiac allograft rejection. Ann Thorac Surg 1992; 54:669–675.
3. Valentino VA, Ventura HO, Abi SF, Van MC, Price HL. The signal-averaged electrocardiogram in cardiac transplantation. A noninvasive marker of acute allograft rejection. Transplantation 1992; 53:124–127.
4. Grace AA, Newell SA, Cary NR, Scott JP, Large SR, Wallwork J, Schofield PM. Diagnosis of early cardiac transplant rejection by fall in evoked T wave amplitude measured using an externalized QT driven rate responsive pacemaker. Pacing Clin Electrophysiol 1991;14(6):1024–1031.
5. Lofland G, German L, Ross M. The local unipolar depolarization complex: a quantitative electrophysiologic index of irreversible myocardial ischemic injury. Surg Forum 1984;35:269.
6. Rosenbloom M, Laschinger JC, Saffitz JE, Cox JL, Bolman M, Branham BH. Noninvasive detection of cardiac allograft rejection by analysis of unipolar peak-to-peak amplitude of intramyocardial electrograms. Ann Thorac Surg 1989;47:407–411.
7. Avitall B, Payne DD, Connolly RJ, Levine HJ, Dawson PJ, Isner JM, Salem DN, Cleveland RJ. Heterotopic heart transplantation: electrophysiologic changes during acute rejection. J Heart Transplant 1988;7(3):176–182.
8. Koike K, Hesslein PS, Dasmahapatra HK, Wilson GJ, Finlay CD, David SL, Kielmanowicz S, Coles JG. Telemetric detection of cardiac allograft rejection. Correlation of electrophysiological, histological, and biochemical changes during unmodified rejection. Circulation 1988;78(3 Pt 2):I106–I112.
9. Pirolo JS, Tweddell JS, Brunt EM, Pyo R, Shuman TS, Cox JL, Ferguson TB. Influence of activation origin, lead number, and lead configuration on the noninvasive electrophysiologic detection of cardiac allograft rejection. Circulation 1991;84(5 Suppl):III344–III354.
10. Irwin ED, Bianco RW, Clack R, Grehan J, Slovut DP, Nakhleh R, Bolman RM 3d, Shumway SJ. Use of epicardial electrocardiograms for detecting cardiac allograft rejection. Ann Thorac Surg 1992;54(4):669–674.
11. Grauhan O, Warnecke H, Muller J, Knosalla C, Cohnert T, Voss A, Hetzer R. Intramyocardial electrogram recordings for diagnosis and therapy monitoring of cardiac allograft rejection. Eur J Cardiothorac Surg 1993;7(9):489–494.
12. Everett JE, Palmer MN, Jessurun J, Shumway SJ. Noninvasive diagnosis of cardiac allograft rejection in an orthotopic canine model. Ann Thorac Surg 1996;62:1337–1341.
13. Pirolo JS, Shuman TS, Brunt EM, Liptay MJ, Cox JL, Ferguson TB. Noninvasive detection of cardiac allograft rejection by prospective telemetric monitoring. J Thorac Cardiovasc Surg 1992;103:969–979.
14. Wernecke H, Mueller J, Cohnert T, Hummel M, Spiegelsberger S, Siniawski K, Lieback E, Hetzer R. Clinical heart transplantation without routine endomyocardial biopsy. J Heart Lung Transplant 1992;11:1093–1102.
15. Mueller J, Hetzer R. Invited commentary. Ann Thorac Surg 1996;62:1337–1341.
16. Auer T, Schreier G, Hutten H, Tscheliessnigg KH, Allmayr T, Grasser B, Iberer F, Wasler A, Petutschnigg B, Muller H, et al. Intramyocardial electrograms for the monitoring of allograft rejection after heart transplantation using spontaneous and paced beats. Transplant Proc 1995; 27(5):2621–2624.
17. Grasser B, Schreier G, Iberer F, Wasler A, Petutschnigg B, Muller H, Prenner G, Hipmair G, Hutten H, Schaldach M, Tscheliessnigg KH. Noninvasive monitoring of rejection therapy based on intramyocardial electrograms after orthotopic heart transplantation. Transplant Proc 1996;28(6):3276–3277.
18. Wahlers T, Haverich A, Schafers HJ, Fieguth HG, Frimpong-Boateng K, Herrmann G, Borst HG. The intramyocardial electrogram: a reliable marker of allograft rejection in orthotopic heart transplantation? Transplant Proc 1987;19(1 Pt 2):1059.
19. Lacroix D, Kacet S, Savard P, Molin F, Dagano J, Pol A, Lekieffre J. Signal averaged electrocardiography and detection of heart transplant rejection. J Am Coll Cardiol 1992;19:553–558.
20. Morocutti G, Chiara AD, Proclemer A, Fontanelli A, Bernardi G, Morocutti A, Earle K, Albanese MC, Feruglio GA. Signal-averaged electrocardiography and doppler echocardiographic study in predicting acute rejection in heart transplantation. J Heart Lung Transplant 1995;14:1065–1072.
21. Bieber CD, Stinson EB, Shumway NE. Pathology of the conduction system in cardiac rejection. Circulation 1969;39:567–575.
22. Babuty D, Aupart M, Machet C, Rouchet S, Cosnay P, Garnier D. Detection of acute cardiac allo-

graft rejection with high-resolution electrocardiography: Experimental study in rats. J Heart Lung Transplant 1996;15:1120–1129.
23. Popp RL, Schroeder JS, Stinson EB, Shumway NE, Harrison DC. Ultrasonic studies for the early detection of acute cardiac rejection. Transplantation 1971;11:543–550.
24. Sagar KB, Hastillo A, Wolfgang TC, Lower RR, Hess ML. Left ventricular mass by M-mode echocardiography in cardiac transplant patients and acute rejection. Circulation 1981;64(suppl II):II-216–220.
25. Gill EA, Borrego C, Bray BE, Renlund DG, Hammond EH, Gilbert EM. Left ventricular mass increases during cardiac allograft vascular rejection. J Am Coll Cardiol 1995;25(4):922–926.
26. Stinson EB, Techklenberg PL, Hollingsworth JF, Jones KW, Sloane R, Rahmoeller G. Changes in left ventricular mechanical and hemodynamic function during acute rejection of orthotopically transplanted hearts in dogs. J Thorac Cardiovasc Surg 1974;68:783–791.
27. Paulsen W, Magid N, Sagar K, Hastillo A, Wolfgang TC, Lower RR, Hess ML. Left ventricular function of heart allografts during acute rejection: An echocardiographic assessment. J Heart Transplant 1985;4:525–529.
28. Dawkins KD, Oldershaw PJ, Billingham ME. Changes in diastolic function as a non-invasive marker of cardiac allograft rejection. Heart Transplant 1984;3:286–294.
29. Desruennes M, Corcos T, Cabrol A, Gandjbakhch I, Pavie A, Leger P, Eugene M, Bors V, Cabrol C. Doppler echocardiography for the diagnosis for the diagnosis of acute allograft rejection. J Am Coll Cardiol 1988;12:63.
30. Forster T, Mcghie J, Rijsterborgh H, Meeter K, Balk A, Essed C, Roelandt J. Does the measurement of left ventricular isovolumic relaxation time allow early prediction of cardiac allograft rejection. Acta Cardiologica 1992;Vol XLVII (5):459–471.
31. Valantine HA, Appleton CP, Hatle LK, Hunt SA, Billingham ME, Shumway NE, Stinson EB, Popp RL. A hemodynamic and Doppler echocardiographic study of ventricular function in long-term cardiac allograft recipients. Etiology and prognosis of restrictive-constrictive physiology. Circulation 1989;79(1):66–75.
32. St. Goar FG, Gibbons R, Schnittger I, Valantine HA, Popp L. Left ventricular diastolic function: Doppler echocardiographic changes soon after cardiac transplantation. Circulation 1990;82:872–878.
33. Desruennes M, Solis E, Cabrol A, Leger P, Corcos T, Gandjbakhch I, Pavie A, Cabrol C. Doppler echocardiography: An excellent noninvasive method for the detection of acute cardiac allograft rejection. Transpl Proc 1989;21(4):3634–3638.
34. Mannaerts HF, Simoons ML, Balk AH, Tijssen J, van der Borden SG, Zondervan PE, Mochtar B, Wiemar W, Roelandt JR. Pulsed-wave transmitral doppler do not diagnose moderate acute rejection after heart transplantation. J Heart Lung Transplant 1993;12:411–421.
35. Fauchier L, Sirinelli A, Aupart M, Babuty D, Marchand M, Pottier JM. Performances of doppler echocardiography for diagnosis of acute, mild, or moderate cardiac allograft rejection. Transpl Proc 1997;29:2442–2445.
36. Valantine HA, Appleton CP, Hatle LK, Hunt SA, Billingham ME, Shumway SE, Stinson EB, Popp RL. A hemodynamic and doppler echocardiographic study of ventricular function in long-term cardiac allograft recipients: Etiology and prognosis of restrictive-constrictive physiology. Circulation 1989;79:66–75.
37. Young JB, Leon CA, Short HD, Noon GP, Lawrence EC, Whisennand HH, Pratt CM, Goodman DA, Weilbaecher D, Quinones MA, DeBakey ME. Evolution of hemodynamics after orthotopic heart and heart-lung transplantation: Early restrictive pattern persisting in occult fashion. J Heart Transplant 1987;6:34–43.
38. Hausdorf G, Banner NR, Mitchell A, Khaghani A, Martin M, Yacoub M, Diastolic function after cardiac and heart-lung transplant. Br Heart J 1989;62:123–132.
39. Hosenpud JD, Pantely GA, Morton MJ, Norman DJ, Cobanoglu AM, Starr A. Relation between recipient:donor body size match and hemodynamics three months after heart transplantation. J Heart Transplant 1989;8:241–243.
40. Tatum JL, Thompson JA, Prasad U, Burke TS, Quint RI. Radionuclide detection of abnormal ventricular filling patterns in rejecting human allografts. Clin Nucl Med 1989;14:175–178.
41. Novitzky D, Cooper DK, Boniaszczuk J. Prediction of acute cardiac rejection by changes in left ventricular volumes. J Heart Transplant 1988;7(6):453–455.
42. Wear KA, Schnittger I, Director BA, Dawkins KD, Haverich A, Billingham ME, Jamieson SW, Popp RL. Ultrasonic characterization of acute cardiac rejection from temporal evolution of echocardiograms. J Heart Transplant 1986;5:425–429.
43. Masuyama T, Valantine HA, Gibbons R, Schnittger I, Popp RL. Serial measurement of integrated ultrasonic backscatter in human cardiac allografts for the recognition of acute rejection. Circulation 1990;81:829–839.
44. Angermann CE, Nassau K, Stempfle HU, Kruger TM, Drewello R, Junge R, Uberfuhr P, Weiß M,

Theisen K. Recognition of acute cardiac allograft rejection from serial integrated backscatter analyses in human orthotopic heart transplant recipients: comparison with conventional echocardiography. Circulation 1997;95:140–150.
45. Carrier M, Russell DH, Davis TP, Emery RW, Copeland JG. Urinary polyamines as markers of cardiac allograft rejection: A clinical evaluation. J Thorac Cardivasc Surg 1988;96:806–810.
46. Carrier M, Emery RW, Wild-Mobley J, Perrotta NJ, Russell DH, Copeland JG. Prolactin as a marker of rejection in human heart transplantation. Transpl Proc 1987;XIX(4):3442–3443.
47. Margreiter R, Fuchs D, Hausen A, Huber C, Reibnegger G, Spielberger M, Wachter H. Neopterin as a new biochemical marker for diagnosis of allograft rejection. Experience based upon evaluation of 100 consecutive cases. Transplantation 1983;36(6):650–653.
48. Havel M, Laczkovics A, Muller MM, et al. Fruherkennung von Absto<b>ungskrisen mit nichtivasiven immunologischen Parametern bei herztransplantierten Patienten. In: Helmer F, Horcher E, eds. Kongressbericht der 26. Tagg. Wein: Osterr. Gesell. Chirurgie, 1985;120.
49. May RM, Cooper DKC, Du Toit ED, Reichart B. Cytoimmunological monitoring after heart and heart-lung transplantation. J Heart Transplant 1990;9:133–135.
50. Wijngaard PLJ, van der Meulen A, Schuurman HJ, Meyling G, Heyn A, Borleffs JCC, Jambroes G. Cytoimmunologic monitoring for the diagnosis of acute rejection after heart transplantation. Transpl Proc 1989;21(1):2521–2522.
51. Jutte NHPM, Daane R, van der Bemd JMG, Hop WCJ, Essed CE, Simoons ML, Bos E, Weimar W. Cytoimmunological monitoring to detect rejection after heart transplantation. Transpl Proc 1989; 21(1):2519–2520.
52. Hoshinaga K, Mohanakumar T, Pascoe EA, Szentpetery S, Lee HM, Lower RR. Expression of transferrin receptors on lymphocytes: its correlation with T-helper/T-suppressor cytotoxic ratio and rejection in heart transplant recipients. J Heart Transplant 1988;7(3):198–204.
53. Roodman ST, Miller LW, Tsai CC. Role of interleukin 2 receptors in immunologic monitoring following cardiac transplantation. Transplantation 1988;45(6):1050–1056.
54. Loertscher R, Forbes RD, Halabi G, Lavery P, Quinn T. Expression of early and late activation markers on peripheral blood T lymphocytes does not reliably reflect immune events in transplanted hearts. Clin Transplant 1994 Jun;8(3 Pt 1):230–238.
55. Nishimura T, Sada M, Sasaki H, Yutani C, Fujita T, Amemiya H, Kozuka T, Akutsu T, Manabe H. Assessment of severity of cardiac rejection in heterotopic heart transplantation using indium-111 antimyosin and magnetic resonance imaging. Cardiovasc Res 1988;22(2):108–112.
56. Wisenberg G, Pflugfelder PW, Kostuk WJ, McKenzie FN, Prato FS. Diagnostic applicability of magnetic resonance imaging in assessing human cardiac allograft rejection. Am J Cardiol 1987 1;60(1):130–136.
57. Khaw BA, Fallon Jt, Beller GA, Haber E. Specificity of localization of myosin-specific antibody fragments in experimental myocardial infarction. Histologic, histochemical, autoradiographic, and scintigraphic studies. Circulation 1979;60:1527–1531.
58. Ballester-Rodes M, Carrio-Gasset I, Abadal-Berini L, Obrador-Mayol D, Berna-Roqueta L, Caralps-Riera JM. Patterns of evolution of myocyte damage after human heart transplantation detected by indium-111 monoclonal antimyosin. Am J Cardiol 1988;62:623–627.
59. Ballester M, Obrador D, Carrio I, Auge JM, Moya C, Pons-Llado G, Caralps-Riera JM. Indium-111-monoclonal antimyosin antibody studies after the first year of heart transplantation. Circulation 1990;82:2100–2108.
60. Ballester M, Obrador D, Carrio I, Moya C, Auge JM, Bordes R, Marti V, Bosch I, Berna-Roqueta L, Estorch M, Pons-Llado G, Camara ML, Padro JM, Aris A, Caralps-Riera JM. Early postoperative reduction of monoclonal antimyosin antibody uptake is associated with absent rejection-related complications after heart transplantation. Circulation 1992;85:61–68.
61. Schutz A, Frotsch S, Kugler C, Anthuber M, Sudoff F, Wenke K, Spes C, Angermann C, Gokel JM, Kemkes BM. Indium-111 monoclonal antimyosin for the diagnosis of cardiac rejection. Transpl Proc 1990;22(4):1464–1465.
62. De Nardo D, Scibilia G, Macchiarelli AG, Cassisi A, Tonelli E, Papalia U, Gallo P, Antolini M, Pitucco G, Reale A, et al. The role of indium-111 antimyosin (Fab) imaging as a noninvasive surveillance method of human heart transplant rejection. J Heart Transplant 1989;8(5):407–412.
63. McGhie AI, Radovancevic B, Capek P, Moore WH, Kasi L, Lamki L, Clubb FJ Jr, Frazier OH, Willerson JT. Major histocompatibility complex class II antigen expression in rejecting cardiac allografts: detection using in vivo imaging with radiolabeled monoclonal antibody. Circulation 1997;96(5): 1605–1611.
64. Isobe M, Narula J, Strauss HW, Khaw BA, Haber E. Imaging the rejected heart. In vivo detection of MHC class II antigen induction. Circulation 1992;85:738–746.

14. ECHOCARDIOGRAPHIC DIAGNOSIS OF ACUTE ALLOGRAFT REJECTION

Nadia Giannetti, MD

Hannah A. Valantine, MD
Division of Cardiovascular Medicine, Stanford University, Stanford, California

The "gold-standard" for detection of allograft rejection is the right ventricular endomyocardial biopsy, sampled on a regular basis particularly during the first year after transplantation. Individual patients routinely have more than 10 biopsies in the first year alone. Endomyocardial biopsies are expensive, time-consuming and not 100% sensitive since sampling error may occur. These limitations have created a need for developing an inexpensive, non-invasive methods to assess the entire allograft for rejection and to follow its response to therapy.

NORMAL ANATOMIC ECHOCARDIOGRAPHIC CHARACTERISTICS OF THE TRANSPLANTED HEART

Atrial Findings

The traditional surgical procedure for the orthotopically transplanted heart involves a biatrial anastamosis. On M-mode echocardiographic recordings, left atrial dimensions appear enlarged compared to the non-transplanted heart. Recipient and donor atrial contractions are dissociated which alters the appearance of mitral valve and posterior wall movement.[1] Beat-to-beat variations in mitral valve motion are readily apparent. These are due to the timing of the recipient atrial contraction relative to the donor atrial cardiac cycle. Recipient atrial contraction occurring in late systole causes premature opening of the mitral valve, while simultaneous recipient and donor contractions in late diastole will augment mitral valve motion due to atrial systole (Figure 1).

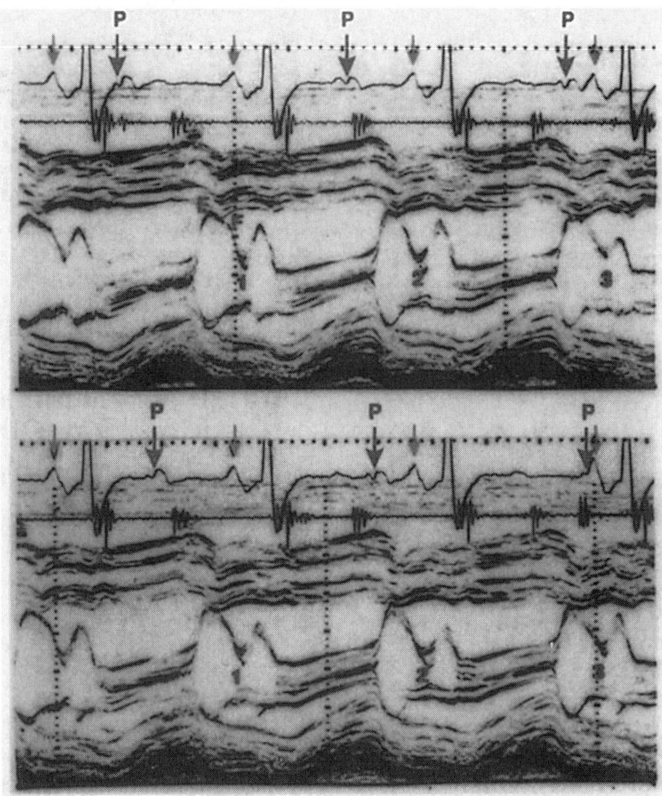

Figure 1. Influence of recipient atrial contraction on mitral leaflet motion. Upper panel: Simultaneous phonocardiogram and M-mode mitral valve echocardiogram showing the influence of recipient atrial contraction (long arrows labeled P) on mitral valve motion. Recipient atrial contraction in late systole (beat 2) is associated with a steeper E–F slope than in early systole (beat 1) or diastole (beat 3). Recipient atrial contraction in early diastole gives a decrease in amplitude of the a-wave (beat 3). Lower panel: Simultaneous contractions of donor (short arrows) and recipient atria result in increased amplitude of the a-wave in beat 3 compared with beat 2 and with beat 3 of the upper panel.

Two-dimensional echocardiography allows for a more detailed visualization of the structure and function of the orthotopically transplanted cardiac allograft. The most characteristic finding is that of "double atria" due to the biatrial anastamoses that is best visualized in the apical 4-chamber view. Anastamosis of recipient atrial remnants with donor atria serves as a potential site for thrombus formation and results in biatrial enlargement. The recipient atrial remnant retains its electrical and mechanical function, but because electrical activity is dissociated from that of the donor atrium, overall atrial function is abnormal.[2]

A newer surgical technique involves bicaval anastamoses. In hearts transplanted using this technique, the donor left atrium is sewn to a recipient pulmonary venous cuff and separate SVC and IVC anastamoses are substituted for the single right atrial anastamosis. This allows maintenance of atrial shape, the preservation of sinus node function, and improved AV valvular competence.[3] On echocardiography, the "double atria" appearance is not present.

Ventricular Findings

The left ventricle as seen in M-mode can have a variable septal motion relative to the posterior wall. Most commonly, there is abnormal septal motion with decreased net posterior motion of the left-sided septal endocardium, or true paradoxical septal motion. There is also diminished septal thickening during contraction as opposed to normal or exaggerated systolic posterior wall thickening.[4] Left ventricular cavity dimensions and percent fractional shortening are normal. Left ventricular posterior wall thickness and mass are increased compared to normal controls.[4] The transplanted heart may have abnormal rates of posterior wall motion during diastole consistent with impaired relaxation.[5]

On two-dimensional echocardiographic images, the left ventricle retains its normal cavity dimension while contractility varies from patient to patient. Most commonly, left ventricular contractility is at the upper limit of normal, which may be related to cardiac denervation and increased circulating catecholamines.[6,7] Left ventricular hypertrophy is also frequently found, although some studies have reported normal left ventricular mass in stable heart transplant patients beyond one year after transplantation.[8]

Reported incidences of left ventricular segmental wall motion abnormalities in the cardiac allograft vary. One study did not observe segmental wall motion abnormalities in a cohort of heart transplant patients studied beyond one year after heart transplantation.[8] Conversely, in the Stanford experience, segmental wall motion abnormalities are frequently observed in both early and long-term patients. Wall motion abnormalities that are seen during the first 24 months are usually not associated with epicardial coronary artery stenosis. In long-term patients, these segmental abnormalities are believed to reflect microvascular coronary artery disease which is not apparent by angiography.

Early after transplantation right ventricular dimensions are usually within normal limits. One report of transplanted hearts in clinically well recipients documented that right ventricular wall thickness and cavity size were significantly increased compared to normal subjects.[4] End-systolic and end-diastolic right ventricular short-axis dimensions and areas were increased compared to normal control subjects. However, the change in right ventricular fractional area was not significantly different from normal. Patients who have significant pulmonary hypertension during the preoperative or perioperative period often have transient or prolonged right ventricular dilatation.

Pericardial Findings

A pericardial effusion is often found early after heart transplantation.[9] This is usually small, located posteriorly and laterally and is rarely associated with hemodynamic compromise. A small pericardial effusion can rapidly become organized, evolving into a pattern of pericardial thickening which is often seen posteriorly during visualization of the left ventricular cavity. These "normal variants" in pericardial appearances of the transplanted heart contrast with the occasional finding of increasing pericardial effusion and/or signs of pericardial constriction[10] (see below).

NORMAL DOPPLER ECHOCARDIOGRAPHIC CHARACTERISTICS OF THE TRANSPLANTED HEART

Doppler echocardiography has been used as a non-invasive parameter to monitor cardiac allograft function. Key measurements include isovolumic relaxation time and the patterns of blood flow across atrioventricular valves and in the pulmonary and hepatic veins. Because a group of characteristic findings have been described as suggesting acute rejection, it is important to understand the important baseline parameters. These include left ventricular isovolumic relaxation time (time from aortic valve closure to mitral valve opening), peak early mitral flow velocity (peak of E-wave), and mitral valve pressure half-time (the time required for peak left atrial/ left ventricular pressure to decline by one-half) (Table 1) (Figure 2, see color plates section, back of book).

The parameters of left ventricular diastolic function assessed are isovolumic relaxation time, measured from aortic valve closure (confirmed by phonocardiogram) to the onset of transmitral flow; peak E-wave velocity, and mitral valve pressure half-time. Doppler values are calculated from an average of 10 consecutive beats after exclusion of cycles in which recipient atrial contraction occurred between late systole and mitral valve opening. The decision to omit such beats is based upon previous observation that recipient atrial contractions occurring in late systole significantly shorten the measurement of left ventricular isovolumic relaxation time and pressure half-time and increase E-wave velocity, most likely due to increase in left atrial pressure.[1] All measurements are obtained using an automated software program, and the mean value for each diastolic index is computed. The group mean and standard deviation of all variables are calculated. Reproducibility of Doppler measurements are determined from calculations of the mean square differences between paired measurements. Intra- and inter-observer correlation coefficients have

Table 1. Left Ventricular Filling Dynamics in Normal Subjects

Left Ventricular Inflow	<50 years	≥50 years
Peak E (cm/sec)	72 ± 14	62 ± 14
Peak A (cm/sec)	40 ± 10	59 ± 14
E:A	1.9 ± 0.6	1.1 ± 0.3
DT (msec)	179 ± 20	210 ± 36
IVRT (msec)	76 ± 11	90 ± 17

DT = deceleration time.
IVRT = isovolumic relaxation time.
(From Klein AL, Cohen GI. Doppler echocardiagraphic assessment of constrictive pericarditis, cardiac amyloidosis, and cardiac tamponade. Cleve Clin J Med 59;281, 1992).

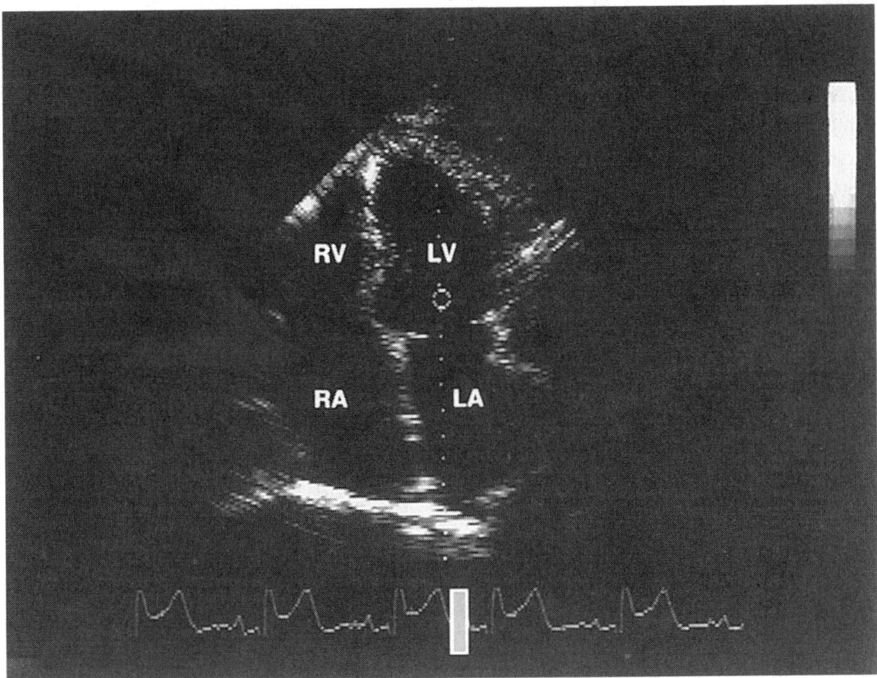

Figure 2. Methods for obtaining the diastolic indices. A) This shows the apical four-chamber view and the positioning of the pulsed Doppler sample volume (denoted by the white circle) at the tip of the mitral leaflet so as to obtain optimal perpendicular orientation with respect to mitral valve flow for recording of maximum velocities across the mitral valve. Sample volume is also positioned so as to obtain the signal of aortic valve closure. LV = left ventricle, LA = left atrium, RV = right ventricle, RA = right atrium.

previously been defined as 0.85 and 0.95 respectively for measurements of left ventricular isovolumic relaxation time and pressure half-time.[11]

Immediately after heart transplantation, the left ventricular isovolumic relaxation time and pressure half-time are usually shortened as would be found in restrictive cardiomyopathy. Isovolumic relaxation time and pressure half-time subsequently increase, reaching a plateau at six weeks.[12] These alternations are likely a reflection of improvement in diastolic function as the allograft recovers from early ischemic injury. After the initial 6 week period, the left ventricular isovolumic relaxation time and pressure half-time are prolonged compared to normals. This suggests persisting relaxation abnormalities even in the presence of normal filling pressures.[13] Despite normal filling pressures, relaxation abnormalities may be present and can be unmasked by a volume load challenge.[14] Irrespective of the time following transplantation, the mitral flow velocity at the time of atrial contraction is usually diminished compared to normal subjects or recipients of heart/lung transplants.[15]

Doppler echocardiography can also assess venous return to the heart in order to indirectly study diastolic function. Blood flow in the hepatic veins and superior vena cava are used to assess right ventricular diastolic function, while patterns of blood flow in the pulmonary veins can aid in evaluating left ventricular diastolic function. Venous flow is typically biphasic. In middle-aged adults with native hearts, the systolic time velocity integral is greater than the diastolic time velocity integral. The opposite is seen in the non-rejecting cardiac allograft, where diastolic venous flow exceeds systolic venous flow by a ratio of 1.5 : 1. Further loss of systolic filling may represent an early manifestation of diastolic dysfunction in the allograft. Extreme dysfunction is manifest by prominent systolic flow reversal and diastolic flow reversal at donor atrial contraction.[16]

THE TRANSPLANTED HEART DURING ACUTE ALLOGRAFT REJECTION

Acute rejection is histologically characterized by varying degrees of myocardial mononuclear cell infiltration and edema in the perivascular space and the interstitial myocardium. These changes result in increased stiffness of the myocardium which results in impaired ventricular filling properties and diastolic dysfunction.[17] "Rejection" when used in this chapter will refer to cellular rather than humoral rejection.

Changes most frequently described in association with acute rejection relate to a) left ventricular systolic and diastolic function; b) left ventricular mass; c) pericardial effusion; and d) myocardial echogenicity (Table 2).

Echocardiographic Changes in Left Ventricular Systolic Function Associated with Acute Rejection

In adult patients on cyclosporine-based maintenance immunosuppression, left ventricular systolic function deteriorates relatively late during the process of acute cellular rejection. Several studies have shown a lack of significant change in systolic function during episodes of moderate or even moderately severe acute cellular rejection.[18–22] However, humoral rejection in adult patients is often manifest by a decline in percent fractional shortening, particularly when accompanied by increased left ventricular mass.[23] Furthermore, patients who have a decline in systolic function with associated hemodynamic compromise have an unfavorable long-term prognosis even if their biopsies fail to reveal any evidence for cellular rejection.[24] A decline in systolic function during the first year should always raise the possibility of acute rejection and warrants prompt endomyocardial biopsy. If the biopsy fails to show at least moderate rejection, the possibility of acute humoral rejection should be entertained. In

Table 2. Echocardiographic Changes in Acute Rejection

1) Increase in left ventricular mass >10%
2) Decrease in left ventricular systolic function >10%
3) Increase in myocardial texture
4) New or increased pericardial effusion

the absence of facilities for histologic confirmation of humoral rejection, empiric treatment is often instituted and therapeutic response monitored by echocardiographic study of left ventricular function.[25] In a patient presenting with a decreased systolic function beyond one year after transplantation, the possibility of transplant coronary artery disease should be considered if a biopsy fails to demonstrate rejection. Preliminary reports suggest that the presence of intimal thickening by intracoronary ultrasound imaging is of particular prognostic significance in this setting.[26]

In pediatric recipients, a decline in percent fractional shortening has been shown to be predictive of acute cellular rejection.[27] These results were obtained in children whose immunosuppressive regimen did not include corticosteroids.[28] Conversely, in a recent prospective study of 32 pediatric patients, Neuberger et al. assessed left ventricular systolic function and stress-velocity relation of corrected velocity of circumferential fiber shortening to wall stress. They found no significant correlation between either of these contractile parameters and biopsy proven rejection.[29]

Therefore, adult studies suggest that impairment in systolic function remains insensitive for detecting acute allograft rejection; data from pediatric studies are limited but yield similar findings.

Echocardiographic Changes in Left Ventricular Diastolic Function During Acute Rejection

The use of echocardiography to assess cardiac physiology in native human hearts has been validated by comparison with hemodynamic and radionuclide studies.[30] Reproducible measurements of left ventricular filling and emptying rates, using standard digitizing methods, can be obtained as well as rates of myocardial thinning and thickening. In the transplanted heart, parameters of left ventricular systolic and diastolic function were initially investigated by Paulsen et al.[19] Acute rejection was associated with decreased left ventricular lengthening rate and posterior wall thinning, consistent with diastolic dysfunction. Dodd et al. have reported on multiple parameters obtained from the digitized M-mode echocardiographic recordings obtained during the three months following transplantation.[31] The parameters found to be significantly different between rejecting (ISHLT grade greater than or equal to 2) and non-rejecting patients were: LVEDV (59.8 ± 5.6 vs. $89.0 \pm 6.8\,mm^2$); left ventricular filling velocity (52.3 ± 3.6 vs. 72.2 ± 4.5 dD/dt, mm/sec); maximum velocity left ventricle posterior wall normalized for chamber size at the time of maximal velocity (8.8 ± 1.1 vs. 13.7 ± 1.1 1/sec); and velocity of left ventricular posterior wall thinning (21.5 ± 3.2 vs. 33.4 ± 2.6 mm/sec). However, no single parameter was significantly sensitive to be useful clinically because of considerable overlap between non-rejecting and rejecting hearts.

Changes in Left Ventricular Mass Associated with Acute Rejection

Acute rejection in adult[32-32] and pediatric[27,35] heart transplantation has been associated with an increase in left ventricular mass by M-mode and 2-D echocardiography. In the pre-cyclosporine era, an increase in posterior left ventricular wall thickness was correlated with acute rejection.[33] In a larger study also pre-cyclosporine, Sagar et al. documented an increase in left ventricular mass during rejection using M-mode echocardiography.[36] During 19 consecutive episodes of acute rejection, a doubling in left ventricular mass was reported in all patients; there was only one false positive result.

Despite this, multiple studies using cyclosporine-based immunosuppressive therapy have failed to show an increase in left ventricular mass with rejection.[28,29,31,37] Gill et al. looked more specifically at histologic type of allograft rejection in 41 patients and correlated histopathology with changes in left ventricular mass.[23] They found no increase in left ventricular mass in moderate or severe *cellular* (ISHLT grade 3 or 4) allograft rejection. However, when analyzing specifically *humoral* (vascular) allograft rejection, they demonstrated an echocardiographic mean increase in left ventricular mass (from 109 ± 17 to 151 ± 17 g) and left ventricular wall thickness (from 1.3 ± 0.1 to 1.6 ± 0.1 cm) during the rejection episode. Using two-dimensional echocardiography, Dubroff and colleagues reported an increase in left ventricular mass during allograft cellular rejection.[38] Subgroup analysis revealed substantial variation in the measurement of left ventricular mass determined by echocardiography.[39] Hence, although changes in left ventricular mass do occur with rejection, the magnitude of these changes is quite variable and often falls within the variability of the measurement. These limitations have prevented the use of left ventricular mass as a single parameter for routine rejection surveillance.

Pericardial Effusion as Marker of Acute Rejection

A small pericardial effusion occurs in up to 40% of transplant recipients during the first 3 months after surgery.[40] A sudden increase in the size, or the appearance of a new effusion, is often an indicator of acute rejection.[9] Observational studies indicate that frequently the concurrent endomyocardial biopsy is negative, but the subsequent biopsy often demonstrates rejection that requires a more protracted course of anti-rejection therapy to achieve complete resolution.[41] These observations suggest that the immune response may be directed at the epicardial surface of the heart, a concept that is supported by the finding of a marked epicardial lymphocytic infiltrate at autopsy examination.[9] Clearly, the development of a new effusion or the unexplained increase in a small to moderate pericardial effusion is an indication for enhanced rejection surveillance and/or treatment.

Ultrasound Tissue Characterization in Acute Cardiac Transplant Rejection

Alterations in echogenicity (myocardial texture) of the myocardium in various pathological states have been previously reported.[42] Prominent myocardial texture can sometimes be observed on two-dimensional echocardiography during acute rejection, but its qualitative assessment alone is too unreliable for accurate diagnosis of acute rejection. Different approaches to measure changes in echogenicity have been sought, all with the hypothesis that acute rejection results in measurable alterations in acoustic properties. Prior to the use of cyclosporine, significant tissue edema was associated with acute rejection and prominent changes in acoustic properties were observed. The changes in echogenicity that occur during acute rejection in patients treated with cyclosporine are more subtle. Investigators have postulated that alterations in local elasticity and density, as well as changes in fiber architecture, geometry, orientation, and contractile performance,[43] are sufficient to affect myocardial texture to alter the acoustic properties of tissue.

Several different techniques have been employed in the assessment of acute cardiac rejection include analysis of the video-processed signal[44] and measurements of integrated backscatter, using either cyclic variation[45] or time-averaged integrated backscatter.[46]

Dawkins et al.[47] studied the intensity of the echocardiographic myocardial ultrasound signal, expressed as median pixel intensity, during acute unmodified rejection in a canine model. They found a progressive increase in the pixel intensity correlated well with histologic severity of rejection. Masuyama et al.[45] utilized cyclic variation of integrated ultrasonic backscatter to study the changes in decibels (dB) that occur in 11 cyclosporine-treated patients during rejection. The magnitude of the cyclic variation of integrated ultrasonic backscatter from the septum and posterior wall decreased, with moderate (cellular infiltrate with myocyte necrosis) to severe (myocyte necrosis with hemorrhage) rejection from 4.2 ± 2.1 to 2.9 ± 1.8 dB and from 6.7 ± 1.2 to 5.1 ± 1.4 dB, respectively. Reduced magnitude of the variation in integrated backscatter in the posterior wall of $\leq$1.5 dB was seen in 12 out of 14 episodes of acute rejection. Using that level as a criterion of rejection, sensitivity, specificity and accuracy of the integrated backscatter measure were 86%, 85% and 85%, respectively. In the septum, reduced magnitude of the variation in integrated backscatter of 1.0 dB as a criterion of rejection had a sensitivity, specificity and accuracy of the integrated backscatter measure of 83%, 71% and 76%, respectively. There was no significant difference in integrated ultrasonic backscatter between normal controls and non-rejecting transplant patients without myocardial hypertrophy. However, in a group of 8 heart transplant patients with significant cardiac hypertrophy there was a lower integrated ultrasonic backscatter of the septum at baseline compared to those without hypertrophy. Overall, the diagnostic reliability of integrated backscatter is substantially diminished in patients with myocardial hypertrophy.

More recently, Angermann et al. followed 52 transplant patients with serial endomyocardial biopsies, conventional echocardiograms and parasternal long-axis radiofrequency signals for determination of posterior wall and septal end-diastolic two dimensional integrated backscatter.[48] They found that increases in end-diastolic posterior wall and septal two-dimensional integrated backscatter provided reliable identification not only of moderate and severe acute rejection but also of mild acute rejection. More importantly, assessment of severity of acute rejection was also possible because two-dimensional integrated backscatter was greater in acute rejection when myocyte damage was present. Using posterior wall measurments, the sensitivity for detecting grade $\leq$1B rejection was 88% and for detecting grade $\leq$3A rejection was 92%. Specificities were 89% and 90%, respectively. Unfortunately, the imaging and processing system that was used in this study is not yet commercially available.

Looking specifically at the pediatric population, Gotteiner et al. reported that measures of myocardial homogeneity decreased during moderate rejection. In 22 patients, they identified 96% of first rejection episodes, 93% of moderate and severe episodes and 69% of all rejection episodes.[49]

Therefore, although several studies suggest that statistically significant alterations occur in acoustic properties during acute rejection, the wide individual variability precludes the use of a single measurement in a given patient as a definite criteria for rejection. Serial measurements where each individual serves as his/her own control appear to be most useful. Another limitation in applying ultrasound tissue characterization for rejection surveillance is the variability in time to normalization of acoustic properties after a rejection episode. Also, there may be difficulty in detecting mild, and possibly moderate, acute rejection with current techniques.

Doppler Echocardiographic Assessment of Diastolic Function for Monitoring Acute Rejection

Changes in the mitral inflow velocity signal correlate well with hemodynamic parameters of left ventricular function, thus providing non-invasive markers of left ventricular diastolic function for serial monitoring of patients.[50–52] Among the parameters most frequently studied are left ventricular isovolumic relaxation time, mitral valve pressure half-time, and peak mitral valve early flow velocity (E-wave). Doppler echocardiographic indices during acute rejection are consistent with restrictive physiology. Therefore, there is an increase in mitral inflow velocity, a decrease in isovolumetric relaxation time and a decrease in pressure half-time. These indices have been shown to correlate with biopsy proven cellular rejection[13,19,22,53–57] (Table 3). Although the overall sensitivity and specificity described in published studies exceeds 80%, these findings are not universally reported by all investigators. For example, a recent study including 23 patients by Fauchier et al. found Doppler left ventricular filling parameters to be of limited value for the diagnosis of mild or moderate rejection.[37] Compared to baseline, the only Doppler echocardiographic parameter with a significant difference during acute allograft rejection was pressure half-time. Even this finding had a low sensitivity (36%) and specificity (72%). Similarly, Wilensky at al. attempted to correlate Doppler echocardiographic findings with transplant rejection severity looking at pressure half-time, deceleration time and peak diastolic velocity of the mitral valve in 23 consecutive cardiac transplant patients.[21] They found a non-significant decrease in pressure half-time in patients with moder-

Table 3. Doppler Changes in Acute Rejection

Impairment of diastolic function
a) Decrease in pressure half-time >15%
b) Decrease in isovolumic relaxation time >15%
c) Increase in $M_1 > 20\%$

M^1 = peak mitral valve early flow velocity

ate transplant rejection. Other Doppler parameters were not found to correlate with rejection. The reason for the discrepancy between studies is unclear but may be partly related to the small number of patients with moderate to severe rejection and therefore an inadequate number of patients to reach statistically significant results.

Diagnosis of Left Ventricular Diastolic Dysfunction Due to Acute Rejection

As detailed studies have described a wide inter-subject variability in diastolic indexes, it is of utmost importance that each patient serve as his/her own control.[50] A change from baseline indices in any given patient can establish the Doppler diagnosis of left ventricular diastolic dysfunction. Stable "baseline" values are defined as "two consecutive measurements that do not change beyond the threshold of expected variations of the method."[11] Prior studies have defined the threshold for statistically significant change in left ventricular isovolumic relaxation time and pressure half-time to be 15% and for mitral E-wave velocity to be 20%. Thus, severity of diastolic dysfunction can be graded as mild, moderate, or severe, according to the associated decrease in either left ventricular isovolumic relaxation time or pressure half-time (mild if decrease was 15–19%, moderate if 20–39%, and severe if ≤40%) compared to stable baseline data of that patient (Figure 3A and 3B). An increase in mitral E-wave flow velocity in the presence of stable isovolumic relaxation time and pressure half-time measurements is not regarded as indicative of diastolic dysfunction, owing to the propensity for this parameter to be influenced by heart rate. In the rare event of left ventricular isovolumic relaxation time and pressure half-time changing in opposite directions, an increase 20% in mitral E-wave velocity is used as an indicator of left ventricular diastolic dysfunction. Such an observation occurs if aortic valve closure is early due to diminished stroke volume, causing prolongation of isovolumic relaxation time, while pressure half-time shortens due to restrictive left ventricular physiology.

New Doppler Echocardiographic Methods for Monitoring Acute Rejection

A recent study by Boyd et al. applied a new Doppler echocardiographic measurement of left ventricular diastolic function and correlated this parameter with endomyocardial biopsy rejection scores in 23 cardiac transplant patients.[58] Biopsy samples were graded using the Texas Heart Institute Score for rejection.[59] Patients were classified as no or minimal rejection (score 0–1) or moderate rejection (score 4–5). The new technique uses the left ventricular inflow atrial contraction, A wave, and the left ventricular outflow A wave reversal (Ar) which is calculated 1 cm below the aortic valve (Figure 4). The A-Ar interval is a measure of the transmission time of the A-velocity within the left ventricle and is related to left ventricular stiffness. This echocardiographic method has been validated in native hearts by Pai et al.[60] Boyd et al. reported a significant reduction in A-Ar interval between patients with no or minimal rejection (mean A-Ar interval of 68.5 msec) compared to patients with moderate rejection (mean A-Ar interval of 36.7 msec). An inverse relationship was

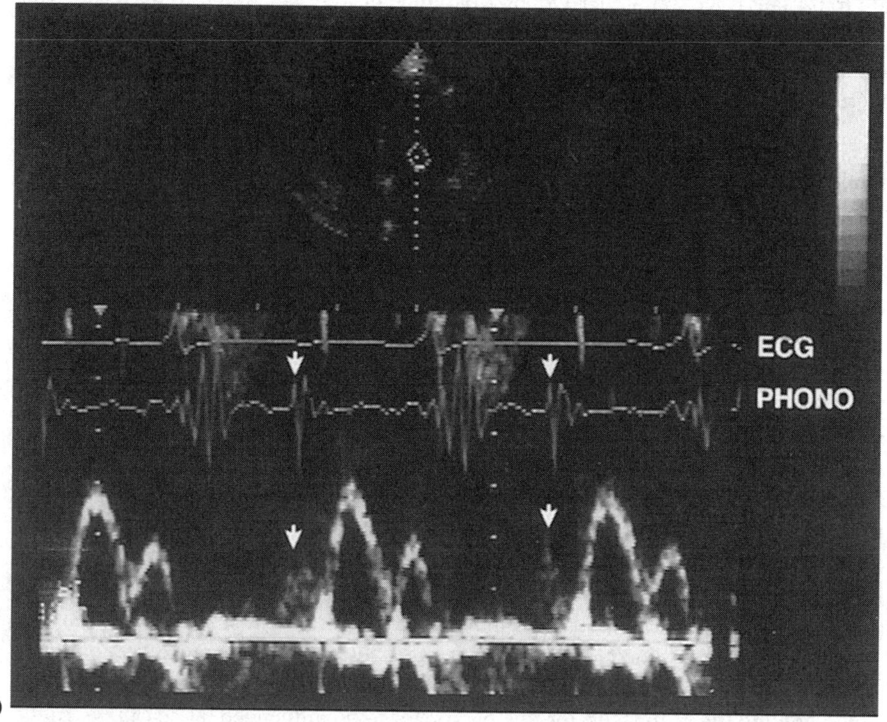

(a)

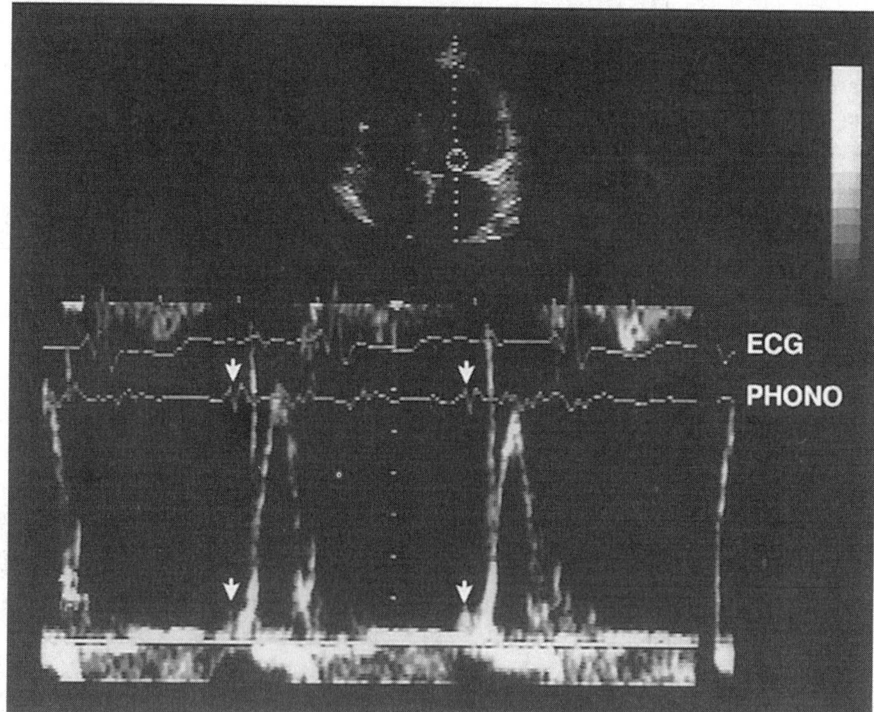

(b)

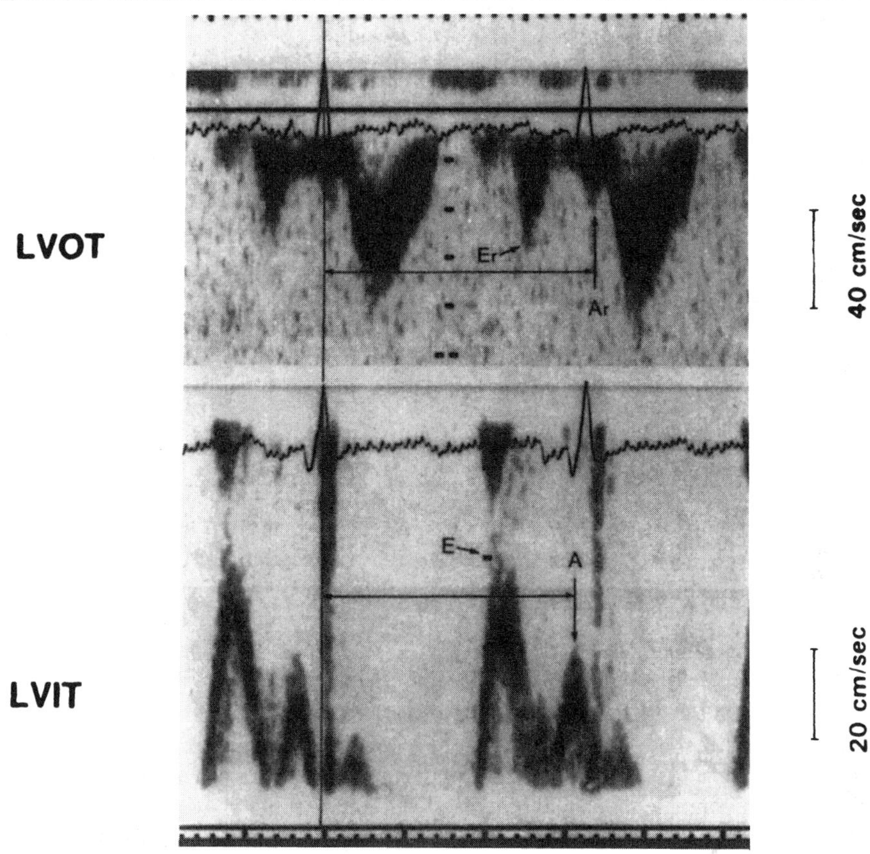

Figure 4. Method of alignment of LVOT and LVIT pulse wave Doppler velocity recording for measurement of A-Ar. The A-Ar interval is a measure of the transmission time of the A-velocity within the left ventricle and is related to the left ventricular stiffness. LVIT = left ventricular outflow tract, LVIT = left ventricular inflow tract. (*Reproduced with permission of S.Y.N. Boyd, MD.*)

Figure 3. Changes in the diastolic indices during acute rejection measured from the pulsed Doppler mitral flow velocity curve. A) Recordings were obtained from a patient when right ventricular endomyocardial biopsy showed no evidence of rejection. The upper image is a four-chamber view indicating positioning of the pulsed Doppler sample volume. Below this image is the simultaneous recording of the electrocardiogram (ECG), phonocardiogram (PHONO), and the mitral flow velocity curve. The arrows indicate aortic valve closure, which can be seen in the pulsed Doppler recording and confirmed as aortic valve closure by the first high-intensity signal on the phonocardiogram. The calibration marks at the top are at 200 msec intervals. Velocity calibration is at 0.2 M/sec intervals. IVRT = 101 msec, pressure half-time = 36 msec, and peak early mitral flow velocity = 0.6 M/sec. B) Recorded from the same patient as Figure 3A when endomyocardial biopsy showed acute rejection (ISHLT grade 3B). Upper panel shows positioning of the pulsed Doppler sample volume at the tip of the mitral leaflets; lower panel shows simultaneous recording of electrocardiogram (ECG), phonocardiogram (PHONO), and mitral flow velocity curve. Note that, in comparison to Figure 3A, IVRT and pressure half-time have shortened, and peak early mitral flow velocity has increased. IVRT = 60 msec, and pressure half-time = 24 msec. Peak early mitral flow velocity = 1.1 M/sec.

identified between biopsy rejection scores and A-Ar intervals presumably reflecting changes in diastolic compliance.

More recently, Puleo et al. used Doppler tissue imaging for detection of allograft rejection. This ultrasound modality is capable of selectively measuring the low-velocity, high-amplitude signals in the range of moving myocardium, while filtering out the high-velocity, low-amplitude signals in the range of moving blood cells. It can be used to quantify myocardial relaxation and contraction velocities. Their results showed that the peak relaxation velocity in nonrejecting allograft recipients was 0.21 m/sec ± 0.01. During moderate allograft rejection, peak relaxation velocities decreased to 0.14 m/sec ± 0.01 and increased to 0.23 m/sec ± 0.01 after successful treatment. Using a cutoff less than 0.16 m/sec, the sensitivity of peak myocardial relaxation velocities for detection of rejection was 76%. The specificity and negative predictive values were 88% and 92%, respectively.[61] Additional studies of this technique appear warranted.

COMBINED ECHOCARDIOGRAPHIC PARAMETERS FOR SCREENING AND DIAGNOSING ACUTE ALLOGRAFT REJECTION

Although echocardiography can identify several morphologic and functional changes associated with acute rejection, imperfect sensitivity for any one parameter prevents its use as the primary modality of rejection surveillance. Clustering of multiple echocardiographic parameters has been suggested as an approach to enhance the sensitivity of echocardiography without sacrificing specificity.[31] Dodd et al. have developed a computer-driven algorithm which incorporates changes in left ventricular mass, volume and function to detect rejection.[31] This study involved both a retrospective model derivation set and a prospective validation data set. Quantitative analyses of two-dimensional guided M-mode echocardiograms of the left ventricle were performed using a digitized computer-assisted measurement format. Left ventricular minor axis dimension, inter-ventricular septum thickness, and posterior wall thickness were measured. Left ventricular chamber volume was calculated from left ventricular minor axis dimension according to the relationship: LVEDV = (LVED/10) and expressed as the percent of normal predicted for body surface area. Systolic function was estimated from left ventricular shortening fraction, interventricular septal thickening, and left ventricular posterior wall thickening. Left ventricular diastolic function was obtained from the filling velocity of ventricular cavity; the maximum velocity of posterior wall thinning normalized for chamber size at the time of maximum velocity (Max Vel LVPW/LVD); and the average velocity of left ventricular posterior wall thinning. When comparing rejection grades (no/mild versus moderate/severe) echocardiographic measurements were significantly different for left ventricular end-diastolic volume, filling velocity, maximum velocity left ventricular posterior wall, and velocity of left ventricular posterior wall thinning. However, no single measurement was adequately sensitive to be useful clinically due to considerable overlap between normal/mild and moderate/severe groups. To determine whether multiple M-mode parameters would be more sensitive to discriminate moderate/severe rejection, parameters that were significantly different between these grade of rejection were assigned a score of 1 or 2, depending on the level of significance of the difference and on the scatter of data. Indices of systolic function and mass were also assigned a score, and a scoring algorithm developed. In the retrospective arm, the ECHO score for patients with no/mild rejection on biopsy was 2.32 ± 1.96 versus 5.95 ± 1.56 in patients with moderate/severe rejection; ROC analysis suggested that a threshold score of 4 would be associated with 100% sensitivity and 84% specificity. In the prospective arm, the sample size was too small (N = 9) to draw any meaningful conclusions.

Ciliberto et al. have investigated an extensive combination of echocardiographic criteria for detection of rejection.[62] In 130 patients, 1400 serial echocardiograms recorded within 24 hours of endomyocardial biopsy were analyzed for previously reported markers of acute rejection including: 1) increasing wall thickness >4 mm (interventricular septum plus left ventricular posterior wall); 2) increased myocardial echogenicity; 3) appearance or increase in pericardial effusion; 4) >20 ms decrease in pressure half-time; 5) >20 ms decrease left ventricular isovolumic relaxation time; and 6) >10% decreasing left ventricular ejection fraction. The number and distribution of echocardiographic criteria were significantly related to the biopsy grade, the presence of one or more echocardiographic criteria being highly specific (96%) for rejection of all grades. Of the echocardiographic false positives, 40% occurred as a consequence of viral myocarditis or pericarditis, or in patients with accelerated coronary artery disease. In contrast, the sensitivity of ≤1 criteria for detection of mild or moderate rejection was 60% and 80%, respectively. The following sensitivities were observed: reduced pressure half-time 44%, increased wall thickness 40%, increased echogenicity 40%, pericardial effusion 28%, decreased isovolumetric relaxation time 28% and decreased ejection fraction less than 5%. All false negatives findings were associated with biopsies showing only one focus of myocyte necrosis (i.e. focal moderate rejection). When the cases of mild rejection were analyzed for outcome related to evolution of rejection, it was apparent that poor sensitivity was mainly due to low sensitivity for patients whose biopsy grade did not warrant anti-rejection treatment. Thus, the sensitivity of two or more echocardiographic criteria for diagnosis of mild rejection requiring treatment (diffuse multifocal lymphocyte infiltrate or clinically significant) was 70%. Analysis of evolution of rejection in 46 patients with mild untreated rejection revealed that patients with two or more echocardiographic criteria at onset had a more aggressive course and were more likely to require subsequent treatment. Following anti-rejection therapy, changes in echocardiographic criteria paralleled evolution of rejection grade, suggesting that the echocardiographic response during the initial two weeks of therapy was predictive of outcome. Thus, patients with a benign course showed an improved echocardiographic picture as early as the first week after treatment. In contrast, those with an unfavorable course had a further worsening in echocardiographic criteria during the initial week, and only a slight improvement after two weeks. The investigators concluded that poor sensitivity of echocardiography for detection of mild rejection precludes its replacement of the endomyocardial biopsy for rejection surveillance.

Similarly, Pellicelli et al. recently evaluated 40 patients using a multiparametric evaluation of echocardiographic indexes (M-mode and Doppler).[57] Doppler echocardiography had excellent specificity but insufficient sensitivity for the diagnosis of

TIMING OF DIAGNOSTIC MODALITIES POST-CARDIAC TRANSPLANTATION

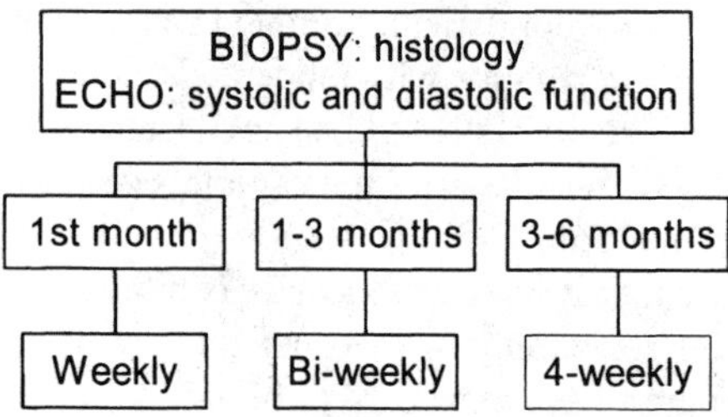

Figure 5. Simplified flow chart of the timing of diagnostic studies in the first 6 months post-cardiac transplantation done at Stanford in the patient with no complications and no evidence of rejection. When these studies are abnormal, further evaluation may be needed but a simple algorithm is problematic due to the need to consider both allograft function and biopsy findings, the possibility of humoral as well as cellular rejection, and variation in the criteria used for grading and treating rejection.

Table 4. Limitations of Doppler Indices for Acute Rejection

1) Simultaneous alteration in heart rate and loading condition
2) Recipient and donor atria 2-Pwaves
3) Inter-subject variation
4) Inter-study variation
5) "Restrictive physiology" *early* after transplantation
6) Persisting occult restrictive physiology
7) Acute rejection superimposed on chronically impaired diastolic function
8) Measurement of respiratory variation in mitral and tricuspid valve flow velocities limited by dissociated donor and recipient atrial contraction

acute allograft rejection. When combined with M-mode posterior wall thickness, the sensitivity improved.

It is now recognized by most transplant centers that mild rejection does not generally require anti-rejection treatment since at least 50% will resolve spontaneously.[63] Thus, application of combined echocardiographic criteria for detection of rejection which requires treatment has the potential to reduce the number of surveillance endomyocardial biopsies. The timetable used at our institution for performing echocardiography and other surveillance tests is outlined in Figure 5.

LIMITATIONS OF ECHOCARDIOGRAPHY

The application of Doppler indices of diastolic function to monitor rejection in heart transplant recipients makes several assumptions, the most important being the fundamental hypothesis that the acute development of a pattern characteristic of restrictive left ventricular physiology is due primarily to the effects of acute rejection, and less likely to changes in heart rate and loading conditions which are independent of acute rejection (Table 4). This assumption seems reasonable, since there appears to be little correlation between development of restrictive left ventricular physiology by Doppler criteria with evidence for fluid retention or heart rate increase when patients are serially studied.[53]

Further limitations unique to the transplant heart which could impact on left ventricular physiology must be considered. The first is the unique physiology imposed by the anatomy of the orthotopically transplanted heart, in which variable proportions of recipient atria are anastomosed to donor atria. These atrial remnants retain both electrical and mechanical function, and have been shown to contribute significantly to parameters of systolic and diastolic function, whether determined by hemodynamic or echocardiographic criteria. In the early experience of Doppler echocardiographic studies in heart transplant patients, it was demonstrated that the timing of recipient atrial contraction could significantly affect the Doppler indices of diastolic function, emphasizing the importance of selecting appropriate cardiac cycles for serial monitoring in patients.[3] As might be anticipated, recipient atrial contraction occurring in late systole increases atrial pressure, causing earlier mitral valve opening and shortening of the isovolumic relaxation time. Earlier mitral valve opening at a steeper point in the ventricular pressure decline results in a greater instantaneous left atrial/left ventricular pressure gradient on mitral valve opening, which might explain the higher peak early mitral flow velocity. Likewise, higher mitral valve opening pressure due to recipient atrial contraction could account for rapid deceleration of antigrade transmitral flow velocity, and a shortened left ventricular pressure half-time. Thus, if cycles are not standardized for measurements in serial studies, there is potential for measurements of beats which are affected by late systolic recipient atrial contraction, and others in which recipient atrial contraction occurred in early systole or diastole, giving rise to averaged values which do not differ from study to study. These "averaged" results would be expected to correlate poorly with histopathologic findings.[64] Without the application of specific methods to exclude beats in which recipient atrial contraction occurred in late systole, any interpretation of differences between serial measurements must be guarded. In patients with chronic atrial fibrillation or who require pacing post-transplantation, these non-invasive echo measures are not applicable.

The inter-subject and inter-study variation seen in the mitral flow velocity curve is another potential limitation. Frequently, only one component of the mitral flow velocity curve can be seen in diastole, corresponding to early diastolic filling, with absence of atrial contribution to the flow velocity signal. Occasionally, the early diastolic velocity signal is lost, and only the velocity at atrial contraction is apparent. It is thus crucial to distinguish between the signal of early diastolic flow versus that of atrial contraction for any interpretation of changes between studies and between patients.

Further, during the initial few weeks after transplantation, indices of diastolic function are often quite abnormal as a consequence of ischemic rather than immunologic injury. The mitral flow velocity pattern typically seen in the initial postoperative period is characterized by a shortened isovolumic relaxation time and pressure half-time, and a high mitral E-wave velocity. During the ensuing six weeks there was a gradual increase in pressure half-time and isovolumic relaxation time, and decrease in E, consistent with decrease in left ventricular diastolic pressures and improved diastolic function.[12] Clearly, making a diagnosis of diastolic dysfunction due to acute rejection poses a major challenge in this setting. Thus, failure of recovery of diastolic function during the initial weeks post-transplantation, even in the absence of further shortening of left ventricular isovolumic relaxation time or pressure half-time, should suggest diastolic dysfunction due to rejection.

The inter-subject variation in diastolic indices may relate to variable recovery of left ventricular function following mechanical, pharmacologic, or ischemic injury during the transplant procedure. Alternatively, persistent diastolic dysfunction can occur as a consequence of incomplete resolution of the immunologic events that impact upon cardiac function. Furthermore, chronic mild rejection, which is not treated in most transplant centers, may occur concurrently with significant impairment in cardiac function, as reported by Yeoh et al.[65] Thus in the presence of chronically impaired diastolic function, irrespective of its cause, relatively small changes in diastolic indices may go unrecognized as significant indicators of immunologic injury.

A final important limitation is that many of these non-invasive echocardiographic studies are time-consuming. They also require dedicated personnel and close attention to detail. This feature may limit their use in many centers.

SUMMARY OF UTILIZATION OF ECHOCARDIOGRAPHY AS A SCREENING AND DIAGNOSTIC TOOL

Use of echocardiography as a screening tool requires close to 100% sensitivity in order to not miss clinically relevant rejection requiring therapy. If this is possible, only patients with echocardiograms suggestive of rejection would then proceed to right ventricular endomyocardial biopsies in order to confirm the diagnosis of rejection. This strategy would eliminate the majority of surveillance biopsies. In echocardiographic studies, the echocardiograghic findings are compared to endomyocardial biopsy findings, the gold-standard for diagnosis of rejection, which in themselves are not 100% sensitive. This renders the accuracy of the non-invasive test more difficult to evaluate.

Reviewing Dodd's retrospective data[31] using combined parameters, there appears to be sufficient sensitivity for detecting rejection requiring therapy. Unfortunately, prospective validation of this approach and its effects in patient outcomes is still required. In contrast, Ciliberto's[62] data showed a very high specificity but only modest sensitivity suggesting that although the diagnosis of rejection can almost certainly be confirmed, too many patients with rejection would not be detected. Therefore, at the present time, screening for rejection with echocardiography appears promising but unproved.

To date, no study has compared the use of echocardiography alone versus right ventricular biopsy results for detection, diagnosis and follow-up of allograft rejection. Therefore, no conclusion as to its utility as a stand-alone test can be reached.

FUTURE DIRECTIONS

A recent study done by Gopal et al. compared the accuracy of one, two and three dimensional echocardiography to determine left ventricular mass.[66] They analyzed 28 patients awaiting cardiac transplantation and performed conventional and freehand 3-dimensional echocardiography.[66] At the time of cardiac transplantation, the explanted hearts were trimmed of non-myocardial tissue and weighed. Echocardiographic mass was compared to true mass by linear regression. They found the correlation coefficient to be 0.992 for 3-D echo, 0.905 for 2-D echo and 0.721 for the M-mode "Penn-cube" method. They concluded that the accuracy of 3-D echo was superior to conventional echo. Using this methodology, we are currently involved in a study using 3-D echo to assess for left ventricular mass in acute cardiac allograft rejection.

Other Doppler parameters for evaluation of diastolic functions which are not currently used in the assessment of acute rejection may be useful. Such parameters include venous inflow. In non-transplanted hearts, Doppler assessment of pulmonary venous flow serves as an important adjunct in the evaluation of left ventricular diastolic dysfunction. Limited reports from studies of superior vena cava flows during acute rejection suggests that inflow to the right heart does change with acute rejection.[18] Other modalities to assess diastolic function, such as acoustic quantification or automated border detection, with analysis of diastolic filling patterns, may prove to be valuable. Future developments in this area will be facilitated by advancements in ultrasound technology which allow for more accurate measurements of each of the individual echocardiographic parameters which have been associated with rejection. Paralleling these technologic advancements will be the need for prospective collection of data to create sufficiently large databases required for computer modeling, using multiple parameters to determine which combinations adequately predict acute rejection. Of crucial importance for advancement of non-invasive diagnosis of acute rejection is improvement upon the current histologic diagnosis of rejection which focuses on only one part of the alloimmune response. An improved understanding of the role of cytokines and microvascular injury as the mediators of allograft dysfunction could impact significantly on the clinical application of non-invasive measures of allograft function for rejection surveillance.

REFERENCES

1. Valantine HA, Appleton CA, Hatle L, Hunt SA, Stinson EB, Popp RL: Influence of recipient atrial contraction on left ventricular filling dynamics of the transplanted heart assessed by Doppler echocardiography. Am J Cardiol 59:1159–63, 1987.
2. Angermann CE, Spes CH, Tammen A, Stempfle HU, Schutz A, Kemkes BM, Theisen K: Anatomic characteristics and valvular function of the transplanted heart: Transthoracic versus transesophageal echocardiographic findings. J Heart Transplant 9:331–8, 1990.
3. McCarthy PM, Smith JA, Siegel LC, Engstrom RH, Fitzgerald DC, Sarris GE, Stinson EB: Chapter 3, Cardiac Transplant Admission, Anesthesia, and Operative Procedures. In: Smith JA, McCarthy PM, Sarris GE, Stinson EB, Reitz BA. The Stanford Manual of Cardiopulmonary Transplantation. Futura Publishing Company, Armonk, New York, 1996.
4. Gorcsan II J, Snow FR, Paulsen W, Arrowood JA, Thompson JA, Nixon JV: Echocardiographic profile of the transplanted human heart in clinically well recipients. J Heart Lung Transplant 11:80–9, 1992.
5. Valantine HA, Oldershaw PJ, Fowler MB, Gibson DG, Hatle L, Hunt, SA, Billingham ME, Stinson EB, Popp RL: Changes in Doppler and M-mode echocardiographic indices of left ventricular function during acute cardiac allograft rejection. Br Heart J 57:86, 1987.
6. McGiffin C, Karp RB, Logic JR, Tauxe WN, Cegallos R: Results of radionuclide assessment of cardiac function following transplantation of the heart. Ann Thorac Surg 37:382–6, 1984.

7. Schuler S, Thomas D, Thebken M, Frei U, Wagner T, Warnecke H, Hetzer R: Endocrine response to exercise in cardiac transplant patients. Transplant Proc XIX:2506–9, 1987.
8. Tischler MD, Lee RT, Plappert T, Mudge GH, S MS, Parker JD: Serial assessment of left ventricular function and mass after orthotopic heart transplantation: A 4-year longitudinal study. J Am Coll Cardiol 19:60–6, 1992.
9. Valantine HA, Hunt SA, Billingham ME, Stinson EB, Popp RL: Increasing pericardial effusion in cardiac transplant recipients. Circulation 79:603–9, 1989.
10. Valantine HA, Appleton CA, Hatle LK, Hunt SA, Billingham ME, Shumway NE, Stinson EB, Popp RL: A hemodynamic and Doppler echocardiographic study of ventricular function in long-term cardiac allograft recipients: Etiology and prognosis of restrictive-constrictive physiology. Circulation 79:66–75, 1989.
11. Valantine HA, Hatle LK, Appleton CP, Gibbons R, Popp RL: Variability of Doppler echocardiographic indices of left ventricular filling in transplant recipients and normal subjects. J Am Soc Echocardiogr 3:276–84, 1990.
12. St. Goar FG, Gibbons R, Schnittger I, Valantine HA, Popp L: Left ventricular diastolic function: Doppler echocardiographic changes soon after cardiac transplantation. Circulation 82:872–8, 1990.
13. Valantine HA, Fowler MB, Hunt SA, Naasz C, Hatle LK, Billingham ME, Stinson EB, Popp RL: Changes in Doppler echocardiographic indices of left ventricular function as potential markers of acute cardiac rejection. Circulation 76(suppl V):V86–V92, 1987.
14. Young JB, Leon CA, Short HD II, et al: Evolution of hemodynamics after orthotopic heart and heart/lung transplantation: Early restrictive patterns persisting in occult fashion. J Heart Transplant 6:34–43, 1987.
15. Parry G, Malbut K, Dark JH, Bexton RS: Differences in left ventricular filling patterns in heart and heart-lung transplant recipients as assessed by Doppler echocardiography of transmitral flow. J Heart Lung Transplant 11:875–7, 1992.
16. Simmonds MB, Lythall DA, Slorach C, Ilsley CDJ, Mitchell AG, Yacoub MH: Doppler examination of superior vena caval flow for the detection of acute cardiac rejection. Circulation 86(suppl II): II-259–II-266, 1992.
17. Caves PK, Stinson EB, Billingham ME, et al: Diagnosis of human allograft rejection by serial cardiac biopsy. J Thorac Cardiovasc Surg 66:461–6, 1973.
18. Sagar KB, Hastillo A, Wolfgang TC, Lower RR, Hess ML: Left ventricular mass by M-mode echocardiography in cardiac transplant patients and acute rejection. Circulation 64(suppl II):216–20, 1981.
19. Paulsen W, Magid N, Sagar K, Hastillo A, Wolfgang TC, Lower RR, Hess ML: Left ventricular function of heart allografts during acute rejection: An echocardiographic assessment. J Heart Transplant 4:525–9, 1985.
20. Dawkins KD, Oldershaw PJ, Billingham ME, Hunt SA, Oyer PE, Jamieson SW, Popp RL, Stinson EB, Shumway NE: Changes in diastolic function as a non-invasive marker of cardiac allograft rejection. Heart Transplant 3:286–94, 1984.
21. Wilensky RL, Bourdillon PDV, O'Donnell JA, Sharp SM, Armstrong WF, Fineberg NS, Himes V, Waller BF: Restrictive hemodynamic patterns after cardiac transplantation: Relationship to histological signs of rejection. Am Heart J 122:1079–87, 1991.
22. Amende I, Simon R, Seegers A, et al: Diastolic dysfunction during acute cardiac allograft rejection. Circulation 81(suppl III):III-60–III-70, 1990.
23. Gill EA, Borrego C, Bray BE, Renlund DG, Hammond EH, Gilbert EM: Left ventricular mass increases during cardiac allograft vascular rejection. J Am Coll Cardiol 25:922–6, 1995.
24. McNamara D, DiSalvo T, Mathier M, Vlahakes G, Southern J, Semigran M, Dec GW: Biopsy negative left ventricular dysfunction after cardiac transplantation: Outcome and role of enhanced immunosuppression. J Heart Lung Transplant 14(no. 1, pt. 2):S46, 1995.
25. Czerska B, Hobbs RE, James KB, Bott-Silverman C, Rincon G, McCarthy PM, Ratliff NV, Stewart RW: Clinical manifestation of acute vascular rejection in cardiac transplant recipients. J Heart Lung Transplant 14(no. 1, pt. 2):S46, 1995.
26. Wiedermann JG, Drusin R, Levin H, Schwartz A, Apfelbaum M: Unexplained heart failure in cardiac transplant recipients: Intracoronary ultrasound identifies two distinct subgroups. J Am Coll Cardiol (special issue):334A, 1995.
27. Boucek MM, Mathis CM, Boucek Jr. RJ, Hodgkin DD, Kanakriyeh MS, McCormack J, Gundry SR, Bailey LL: Prospective evaluation of echocardiography for primary rejection surveillance after infant heart transplantation: Comparison with endomyocardial biopsy. J Heart Lung Transplant 13:66–73, 1994.
28. Harada K, Reller MD, Shiota T, Marcella CP, Sahn DJ: Echocardiographic indexes of rejection in pediatric cardiac transplant recipients managed without maintenance steroid immunosuppresion. Am J Card 79:693–6, 1997.
29. Neuberger S, Vincent R, Doelling N, Sullivan K, Honeycutt S, Kantor KR, Fyfe D: Comparison of

quantitative echocardiography with endomyocardial biopsy to define myocardial rejection in pediatric patients after cardiac transplantation. Am J Cardiol 79:447–50, 1997.

30. Upton MT, Gibson DG, Brown DJ: Echocardiographic assessment of abnormal left ventricular relaxation in man. Br Heart J 38:1001–9, 1976.
31. Dodd DA, Brady LD, Carden KA, Frist WH, Boucek MM, Boucek Jr. RJ: Pattern of echocardiographic abnormalities with acute cardiac allograft rejection in adults: correlation with endomyocardial biopsy. J Heart Lung Transplant 12:1009–18, 1993.
32. Mastropolo R, Clark MB, Spotnitz HM, et al: Variation in LV mass in cyclosporine-treated humans after cardiac transplantation: Determination by two-dimensional echocardiography. Surg Forum 35:371–3, 1985.
33. Popp RL, Schroeder JS, Stinson EB, Shumway NE, Harrison DE: Ultrasonic studies for the early detection of acute cardiac rejection. Transplantation 11:543–50, 1971.
34. Stempfle HU, Strom C, Spes C, Uberfuhr P, Kruger TM, Reichart B, Theisen K, Angermann CE: Intramyocardial electrograms for monitoring allograft rejection after heart transplantation. Transp Pro 27:1981–2, 1995.
35. Boucek MM: Echocardiographic evaluation in pediatric heart transplantation: A platinum standard? J Heart Lung Transplant 10:842–4, 1991.
36. Sagar KB, Hastillo A, Wolfgang TC, Lower RR, Hess ML: Left ventricular mass by M-mode echocardiography in cardiac transplant patients and acute rejection. Circulation 64(suppl II):216–20, 1981.
37. Fauchier L, Sirinelli A, Aupart M, Babuty D, Marchand M, Pottier JM: Performances of doppler echocardiography for diagnosis of acute mild, or moderate cardiac allograft rejection. Transp Pro 29:2442–5, 1997.
38. Dubroff JM, Clark MB, Wong CYH, et al: Changes in left ventricular mass associated with the onset of acute rejection after cardiac transplantation. Heart Transplant 3:105–9, 1984.
39. Clark MB, Spotnitz HM, Dubroff JM, et al: Acute rejection after cardiac transplantation: Detection by two-dimensional echocardiography. Surg Forum 34:248–50, 1983.
40. Vanderberg BF, Mohanty PK, Craddock KJ, et al: Clinical significance of pericardial effusion after heart transplantation. J Heart Transplant 7:128–34, 1988.
41. Cilberto GR, Anjos MC, Gronda E, et al: Significance of pericardial effusion after heart transplantation. Am J Cardiol 76:297–300, 1995.
42. Popp RL: Recent experience with ultrasonic tissue characterization. Am J Cardiol 69: 112H–116H, 1992.
43. Skorton DJ, Miller JG, Wichline SA, Barzullai B, Collins SM, Perez JE: Ultrasonic characterization of cardiovascular tissue. In: Marcus ML, Schelbert HR, Skorton DJ, Wolt GL (eds). Cardiac Imaging. Philadelphia: Saunders, 1991, pp. 538–56.
44. Stempfle H-U, Angermann CE, Kraml P, Schutz A, Kemkes BM, Theisen K: Serial changes during acute cardiac allograft rejection: Quantitative ultrasound tissue analysis versus myocardial histologic findings. J Am Coll Cardiol 22:310–17, 1993.
45. Masuyama T, Valantine HA, Gibbons R, Schnittger I, Popp RL: Serial measurement of integrated backscatter in human cardiac allografts for the recognition of acute rejection. Circulation 81:829–39, 1990.
46. Angermann CE, Nassau K, Drewello R, Kruger TM, Junge R, Uberfuhr P, Stempfle H-U: Time averaged myocardial integrated backscatter measurements allow to identify and estimate severity of acute allograft rejection after transplantation in man. Circulation 90:I-326, 1994.
47. Dawkins K, Haverich A, Salim A, Billingham ME, Jamieson SW, Gibson DG: Detection of acute cardiac rejection using color echocardiography. Circulation 72(suppl II):III-207, 1985.
48. Angermann CE, Nassau K, Stempfle HU, Kruger TM, Drewello R, Junge R, Uberfuhr P, Weib M, Theisen K: Recognition of acute cardaic allograft rejection from serial integrated backscatter analyses in human orthotopic heart transplant recipients. Circulation 95:140–50, 1997.
49. Gotteiner NL, Vonesh MJ, Crawford SE, Burns WR, Duffy E, Zales VR, McPherson DD: Myocardial acoustics in pediatric allograft rejection. J Heart Lung Transplant 15:596–604, 1996.
50. Appleton CP, Hatle LK, Popp RL: Demonstration of restrictive ventricular physiology by Doppler echocardiography. J Am Coll Cardiol 11:757–68, 1988.
51. Rokey R, Kuo LC, Zoghbi WA, Limacher MC, Auinones MA: Determination of parameters of left ventricular diastolic filling with pulsed Doppler echocardiography: Comparison with angiography. Circulation 71:543, 1985.
52. Spirito P, Maron BJ, Bonow RO: Noninvasive assessment of left ventricular diastolic function: Comparative analysis of Doppler echocardiographic and radionuclide angiographic techniques. J Am Coll Cardiol 7:518, 1986.
53. Valantine HA, Fowler M, Hatle L, Hunt S, Billingham ME, Stinson EB, Popp RL: Doppler echocardiographic indices of diastolic function as markers of acute cardiac rejection. Transplant Proc 19:2556–9, 1987.

54. Valantine HA, Yeoh TK, Gibbons R, McCarthy P, Stinson EB, Billingham ME, Popp RL: Sensitivity and specificity of diastolic indexes for rejection and surveillance: temporal correlation with endomyocardial biopsy. J Heart Lung Transplant 10:757–65, 1991.
55. Desruennes M, Corcos T, Cabrol A, Gandjbakhch I, Pavie A, Leger P, Eugene M, Bors V, Cabrol C: Doppler echocardiography for the diagnosis of acute allograft rejection. J Am Coll Cardiol 12: 63–70, 1988.
56. Furniss SS, Murray A, Hunter S, Dougenis V, McGregor CG: Value of echocardiographic determination of isovolumic relaxation time in the detection of heart transplant rejection. J Heart Lung Transplant 10:557–61, 1991.
57. Pellicelli AM, Cosial JB, Ferranti E, Gomez A, Borgia MC: Alteration of left ventricular filling evaluated by doppler echocardiography as a potential marker of acute rejection in orthotopic heart transplant: Angiology, The Journal of Vasc Dis 47:35–41, 1996.
58. Boyd SYN, Mego DM, Khan NA, Rubal BJ, Gilbert TM: Doppler echocardiography in cardiac transplant patients: Allograft rejection and its relationship to diastolic function. J Am Soc Echocardiogr 10:526–31, 1997.
59. McAllister HA, Schnee MJM, Radovancevic B, Frazier OH: Transplantation. A system for grading allograft rejection. Texas Heart Institute J 13:1–3, 1986.
60. Pai RG, Suzuki M, Heywood T, Ferry DR, Shah PM: Mitral A velocity wave transit time to the outflow tract as a measure of left ventricular diastolic stiffness. Hemodynamic correlations in patients with coronary artery disease. Circulation 89:553–7, 1994.
61. Puleo JA, Aranda JM, Weston MW, Cintron G, French M, Clark L, Fontanet HL: Noninvasive detection of allograft rejection in heart transplant recipients by use of Doppler tissue imaging. J Heart Lung Transplantation 17:176–84, 1998.
62. Ciliberto GR, Mascarello M, Gronda E, Bonacina E, Anjos MC, Danzi G, Colombo P, Frigerio M, Alberti A, DeVita C: Acute rejection after heart transplantation: Noninvasive echocardiographic evaluation. J Am Coll Cardiol 23:1156–60, 1994.
63. Rizeq MN, Masek MA, Billingham ME: Acute rejection: Significance of elapsed time after transplantation. J Heart Lung Transplant 13:862–8, 1994.
64. Forster T, McGhie J, Rijsterborgh H, et al: Can we assess the changes of ventricular filling resulting from acute allograft rejection with Doppler echocardiography? J Heart Transplant 7:430–4, 1988.
65. Yeoh T-K, Frist WH, Eastburn TE, Atkinson J: Clinical significance of mild rejection of the cardiac allograft. Circulation 86(suppl II):II-267–II-271, 1992.
66. Gopal AS, Schnellbaecher MJ, Shen Z, Akinboboye OO, Sapin PM, King DL: Freehand three-dimensional echocardiography for measurement of left ventricular mass: in vivo anatomic validation using explanted human hearts. J Am Coll Cardiol 30:802–10, 1997.

15. THE USE OF MAGNETIC RESONANCE IMAGING IN CARDIAC TRANSPLANTATION REJECTION

Todd M. Koelling M.D.
Division of Cardiology University of Michigan Medical Center
Ann Arbor, MI

Several attempts have been made to monitor cardiac allograft rejection using noninvasive imaging modalities. Previous efforts to employ noninvasive imaging to follow transplant recipients for signs of rejection have included echocardiography,[1] antimyosin scintigraphy,[2] anti-vascular adhesion molecule scintigraphy,[3] and radio-labeled lymphocyte scintigraphy.[4] Each method has shown to detect clinical or experimental allograft rejection, but evidence of adequate sensitivity and specificity exists to supplant endomyocardial biopsy has been lacking.

Since the mid 1980's several investigators have reported on the possibility of diagnosing rejection by magnetic resonance imaging (MRI) techniques. Owing to the versatility of the field, the approaches to the MRI assessment of rejection have varied (Table 1). The precision of left and right ventricular measurements made using MRI may allow physicians the ability to follow changes in chamber size, wall thickness, and left ventricular mass that occur with episodes of rejection. An additional strength of MRI lies in its potential to define tissue characteristics through the assessment of magnetic relaxation properties. Many investigators have previously focused their interest on magnetic resonance spectroscopy (MRS) for the diagnosis of cardiac rejection utilizing its ability to accurately detect decreases in energy-rich phosphates (phosphocreatine, PCr, and adenosine-triphosphate, ATP) and increased in inorganic phosphates (Pi) or phosphomonoester (PME).[5–7] Other potential uses of magnetic resonance include the assessment of myocardial flow reserve, coronary flow velocity and coronary flow velocity reserve, all of which have been shown to exhibit abnormalities during acute rejection.

The potential application of magnetic resonance imaging to the clinical diagnosis of cardiac allograft rejection is currently unrealized. The ability of this modality to provide anatomy, tissue characterization, quantitative myocardial perfusion, and chemical composition in a single examination makes MRI a leading methodology for the future noninvasive assessment of transplant recipients (Table 1).

Table 1. Application of magnetic resonance to the assessment of cardiac allograft rejection. Methods that have been studied have varied from analysis of anatomic changes to changes in tissue relaxation properties, perfusion characteristics, and chemical composition

- Wall thickness
- Left Ventricular Mass
- T1 Relaxation Time
- T2 Relaxation Time
- Myocardial Perfusion Imaging
- ^{31}Phosphorous Spectroscopy
- ^{23}Sodium Spectroscopy
- Plasma Proton Spectroscopy

ANATOMIC INFORMATION

Magnetic resonance imaging has replaced left ventriculography as the "gold standard" for the assessment of ventricular function. Left ventriculography was previously considered to be the preferred method to measure ventricular function, but clearly has the limitation of being an invasive test requiring the dangers of arterial catheterization as well as potentially nephrotoxic contrast agents. Additionally, left ventriculography is limited by providing only planar images of a three dimensional structure. Radionuclide angiography supplies information about both left and right ventricular function, but requires use of radioactive contrast agents. This modality is also limited by its planar characteristics, and includes inherent inaccuracies caused by chamber overlap, signal averaging, and background activity subtraction. Echocardiography benefits by being the most readily available tool for cardiologists, and by providing information about cardiac anatomy as well as function. However, as a quantitative tool, echocardiography is limited by the acoustic windows provided by the patient which can hinder image quality to the point that functional assessment is based on the viewers general sense of the heart rather than a true quantitative measurement.

Echocardiography has been studied as a method to detect the development of myocardial edema leading to thickening of myocardial walls (See Chapter 14).[1,8] Increased wall thickness, myocardial echogenicity, pericardial effusion, shorter pressure half-time, isovolumetric relaxation time and a decrease in left ventricular ejection fraction were studied as markers of rejection by Ciliberto et al.[1] The distribution of echocardiographic markers revealed highly significant differences between histologic graded moderate rejection, mild rejection and no rejection and between untreated and treated rejection episodes. Specificity was 98.6% if two of the markers for rejection were present, but sensitivity was good (80%) for only moderate rejection because of the large number of false negatives in untreated patients with mild rejection. Poor sensitivity to mild rejection indicates that serial echocardiography cannot replace endomyocardial biopsy in the early diagnosis of acute rejection. Additionally, studies performed by Gill et al. showed that changes in left ventricular mass are noted by echocardiography during vascular rejection, but not necessarily during cellular rejection.[8]

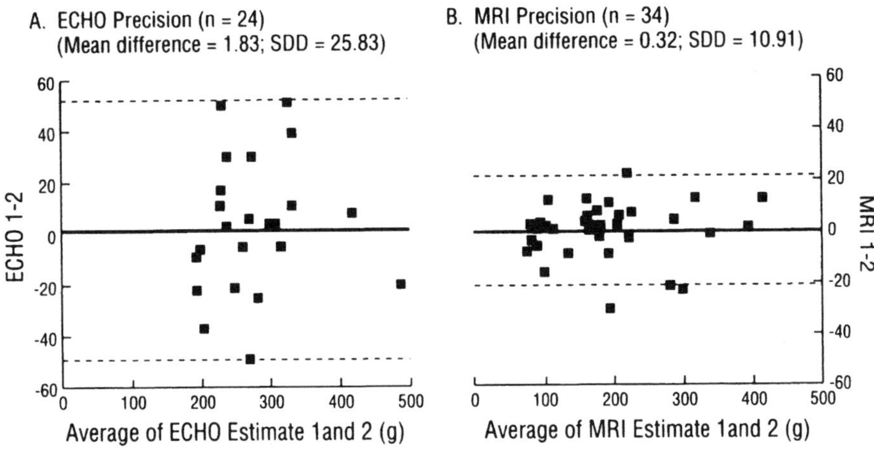

Figure 1. Less variability is translated into greater precision. In this graph, the precision of left ventricular mass estimates by MRI is shown to be improved over two-fold from those provided by echocardiography (ECHO). Reproduced with permission of the authors, Bottini, P. B., A. A. Carr, L. M. Prisant, F. W. Flickinger, J. D. Allison, and J. S. Gottdiener. "Magnetic Resonance Imaging Compared to Echocardiography to Assess Left Ventricular Mass in the Hypertensive Patient." *American Journal of Hypertension* 8, no. 3 (1995): 221–8.

Magnetic resonance imaging provides high-resolution images of the cardiovascular system and is capable of rapid and precise measurement of left ventricular mass[9–12] Because the images are not limited by anatomic windows, as is the case with echocardiography, magnetic resonance images of the left and right ventricles can be used to measure volumes of cardiac chambers, and indices of systolic function can be calculated. Assessment of changes in left ventricular mass are facilitated as the precision of the MRI measurement is over twice that observed for echocardiography (Figure 1).[12]

Revel et al. showed in six human transplant recipients that MRI could be used to measure wall thickness in several areas of the left ventricle and right ventricle.[13] They found that patients with biopsies showing ISHLT Grade 1 or 2 rejection had significantly thicker myocardial walls than in normal volunteers, non-rejecting transplant recipients, or after treatment with immunosuppression. Furthermore, Wisenberg et al. showed in 28 transplant recipients that right ventricular thickness (6 ± 2 mm vs 3 ± 1 mm) intraventricular septal thickness (18 ± 3 mm vs 12 ± 2 mm) and left ventricular free wall thickness (20 ± 3 mm vs 13 ± 2 mm) were significantly higher during episodes of rejection (defined as a cellular infiltrate associated with myocytolysis) than when biopsies showed no rejection (Table 2).[14] These studies illustrate that MRI is capable of taking advantage of the observations made by investigators using echocardiography and can provide precise anatomical measurements which may prove clinically useful in the serial evaluation of transplant recipients.

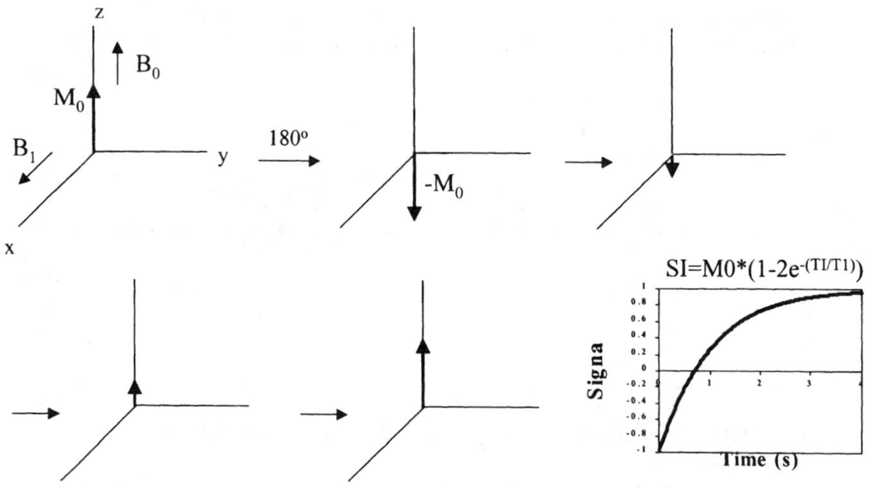

Figure 2. Longitudinal relaxation in the B_0 field is described by the relaxation constant T_1. T_1 can be measured by performing an inversion recovery pulse sequence employing a 180° pulse. As the time to imaging, TI, is delayed further and further after the inversion pulse, the overall magnetization in the B_0 field becomes closer to the fully relaxed state, M_0. The signal intensity will increase as the imaging time increases, obeying the equation: $SI = M0*(1 - 2e^{-(TI/T1)})$.

Table 2. In a study of 28 cardiac transplantation recipients, right ventricular, left ventricular, and intraventricular septum thickness was found to be significantly elevated during times of acute rejection (* $p < 0.05$) From Wisenberg, G., P. W. Pflugfelder, W. J. Kostuk, F. N. McKenzie, and F. S. Prato. "Diagnostic Applicability of Magnetic Resonance Imaging in Assessing Human Cardiac Allograft Rejection." *American Journal of Cardiology* 60, no. 1 (1987): 130–6

		Wall thickness measurements		
	n	Right Ventricle	Intra-ventricular Septum	Left Ventricle
Non-rejecting transplants	28	3 ± 1	12 ± 2	13 ± 2
Rejecting transplants	15	6 ± 2*	18 ± 3*	20 ± 3*

T1 AND T2 RELAXATION CONSTANTS

Besides anatomic and morphologic information provided by magnetic resonance imaging, tissue characterization is possible by measuring T1 and T2 relaxation times and spin density.[15] T1 relaxation is defined by the rate of longitudinal relaxation of protons in the magnetic field (Figure 2). T2, on the other hand, is related to the rate at which proton spins fall out of phase (Figure 3). Increases of both of the relaxation times correlate with an increase in the water content of the tissue.[15] Since cardiac rejection is associated with myocyte edema and swelling, assessment of relaxation time may provide a sensitive measure of rejection. Increases in T2 may also occur with focal hemorrhage and myocyte necrosis.

Huber et al. described a study of twenty-five Lewis-Brown Norway rat hearts transplanted into Lewis recipients, and compared them to 25 Lewis rat isograft

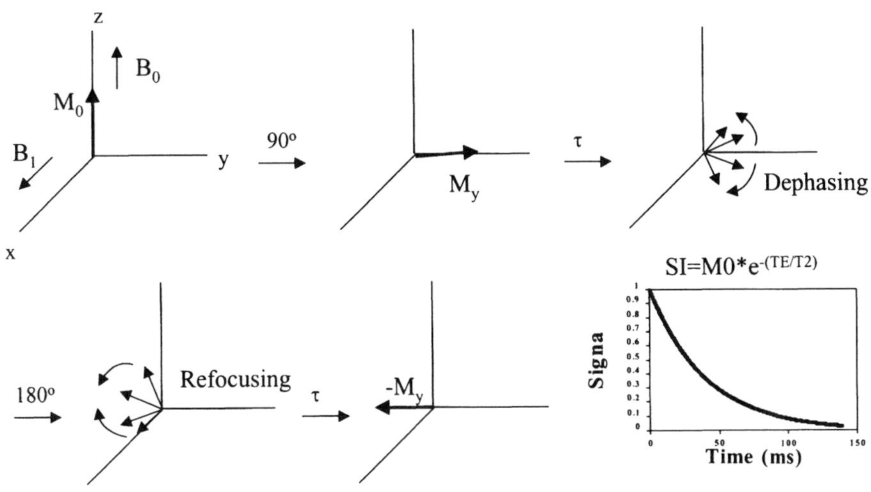

Figure 3. T_2 is the time constant that describes the way spins dephase after being focused by a 90° excitation pulse. Signal is maximal immediately after the excitation pulse, and degrades with time as spins fall out of phase and net magnetization in the transverse plane approaches zero. The magnetization after any echo time, TE, is described by the equation: $SI = M0{*}e^{-(TE/T2)}$.

Table 3. MRI results of T2 relaxation time according to degree of rejection using the Stanford classification. (* $p < 0.05$ compared to rejection grade 0). From Walpoth, B. H., F. Lazeyras, A. Tschopp, T. Schaffner, U. Althaus, M. Billingham, and R. Morris. "Assessment of Cardiac Rejection and Immunosuppression by Magnetic Resonance Imaging and Spectroscopy." *Transplantation Proceedings* 27, no. 3 (1995): 2088–91

Rejection Grade	T2
0	55 ± 9.2
1	58 ± 17
2	65 ± 22
3	78 ± 19*

controls.[16] Prolongation of T1 and T2 relaxation times were demonstrated in the non-immunosupressed allograft animals. However, treatment of an additional 21 allograft animals with cyclosporine showed no significant changes in T1 and T2 compared with controls. Walpoth et al. studied a similar rat transplantation model where the degree of immunosuppression was varied and compared T2 relaxation time to histologic rejection grade.[17] Their findings demonstrated a consistent increase in T2 with increasing rejection grade (Table 3), however, only grade 3 was significantly different than grade 0 at the $p < 0.05$ level.

Aherne et al. studied heterotopic cardiac transplantation in nine immunosuppressed (cyclosporine 25 mg/kg/day and prednisone 1 mg/kg/day) dogs and compared them to six dogs that were transplanted but did not receive immunosuppression.[18] Untreated allografts showed a significant increase ($p < 0.01$) in T2

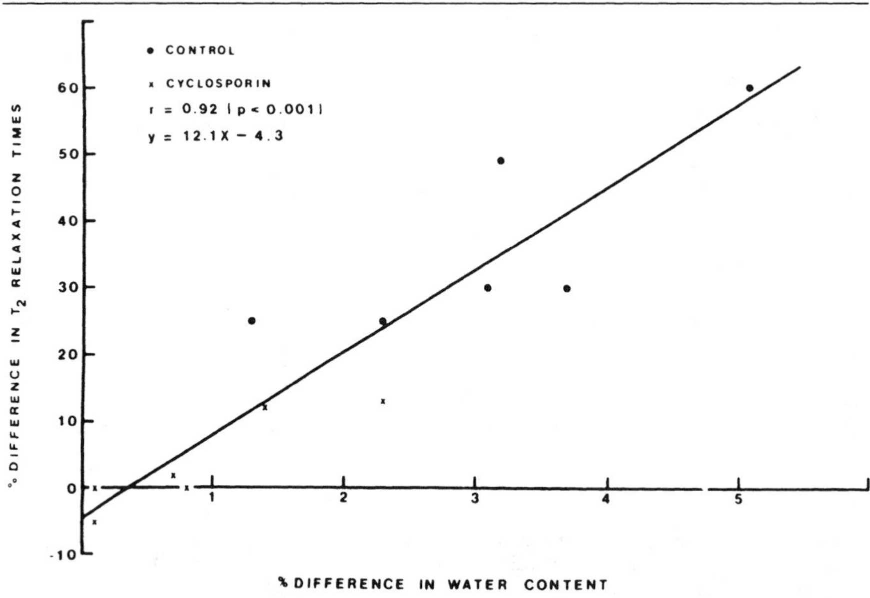

Figure 4. Correlation between percent difference in T2 relaxation times (transplanted hearts minus native hearts) and percent difference in water content (transplanted hearts minus native hearts). Reproduced with permission of the authors, Aherne, T., D. Tscholakoff, W. Finkbeiner, U. Sechtem, N. Derugin, E. Yee, and C. B. Higgins. "Magnetic Resonance Imaging of Cardiac Transplants: the Evaluation of Rejection of Cardiac Allografts With and Without Immunosuppression." *Circulation* 74, no. 1 (1986): 145–56.

relaxation time (T2 = 66 ± 8 ms) compared with values observed in the native hearts (T2 = 44 ± 6 ms) as early as one week after transplantation. There was no significant difference in T1, T2, or intensity values in 7 cyclosporine-treated animals; however, T2 relaxation times and signal intensity increased in 2 of the transplanted hearts simultaneously with development of histologic evidence of rejection. There was a significant correlation between histologic grading of severity of rejection and T2 relaxation times of the cardiac transplant (r = 0.72). There was also a significant linear relationship between *in vivo* T2 values and difference in percent water content in the allograft and pretransplant native heart ($r = 0.92$, $p < 0.001$) (Figure 4).

Wisenberg et al. applied this strategy to the assessment of human cardiac allograft rejection.[14] Twenty-five patients were studied on a 0.15-Tesla system. In the 19 transplant patients imaged within 24 days of graft implantation, all showed evidence of increased T1 and T2 values, regardless of the result of the biopsy, consistent with a healing ischemic process. However, when patients were examined more than 25 days after surgery, the T1 and T2 values were found to be normal in patients without rejection, and elevated in those grafts with rejection (defined as presence of a cellular infiltrate with myocytolysis). Fourteen of 15 late rejection events were correctly identified on the basis of increases in T1 and T2. Only 1 of 28 images of nonrejecting grafts was incorrectly identified as indicating rejection on the basis of prolonged T1 and T2 values (Table 4). More recently, Marie et al. have confirmed that myocardial T2 values (>56 msec) can identify most episodes of moderate (1 SWLT grade 22) rejection in heart transplant recipients.[14a]

Table 4. In a study of 28 cardiac transplantation recipients, T1 and T2 relaxation times were found to be significantly elevated during times of acute rejection (* $p < 0.05$.) From Wisenberg, G., P. W. Pflugfelder, W. J. Kostuk, F. N. McKenzie, and F. S. Prato. "Diagnostic Applicability of Magnetic Resonance Imaging in Assessing Human Cardiac Allograft Rejection." *American Journal of Cardiology* 60, no. 1 (1987): 130–6

	n	T1	T2
Non-rejecting transplants	28	360 ± 21	36 ± 5
Rejecting transplants	15	497 ± 30*	62 ± 6*

Criticism of the use of T2 relaxation time to monitor heart transplantation recipients has focused on the low specificity of the measurement. Because the technique is sensitive to changes in the water content of the myocytes, other conditions such as ischemia, capillary leakage, and infection could lead to similar increases in T2 relaxation time.[10,19,20] If validated in larger clinical studies, the MRI T2 surveillance may offer transplant recipients a non-invasive alternative to routine endomyocardial biopsy.

MYOCARDIAL AND CORONARY FLOW

Acute rejection has been previously described to cause alterations of vascular endothelial function.[21] Chan et al. described a study of 16 transplant patients where they measured myocardial blood flow using positron emission tomography. Patients with acute moderate rejection (defined by the Billingham criteria) were found to have an elevated resting blood flow (1.7 +/– 0.3 mL/min/g) but blunted hyperemic blood flow (2.5 +/– 0.9 mL/min/g) compared with patients without rejection (0.9 +/– 0.2 mL/min/g and 3.9 +/– 0.7 mL/min/g, respectfully). The resting myocardial blood flow values were shown to decline to 1.2 +/– 0.3 mL/min/g ($P < .001$) while the hyperemic blood flows increased to 3.9 +/– 1.1 mL/min/g ($P < .001$) after augmentation of immunosuppression.

The results of the study by Chan et al. suggest a potential role for serial non-invasive flow measurements to guide immunosuppressive therapy. Because of the limited access to cyclotrons, and because of its prohibitive expense, broad applicability of positron emission tomography is now unrealistic. Intracoronary flow can be measured with good precision using intravascular Doppler, however, these studies are more invasive than endomyocardial biopsy and may be associated with more serious complications. Nuclear perfusion scanning requires the injection of radiotracers, and would expose the patients to unacceptable risk with frequent testing. Echocardiographic assessment of myocardial blood flow is possible using sonicated micro-bubble preparations.[22] Precise quantification of perfusion in humans, however, has not been validated using this method.

Recent progress in the development of magnetic resonance imaging sequences for the quantification of coronary and myocardial blood flow has been demonstrated. Hundley et al. reported on the used of phase velocity mapping to quantify blood flow

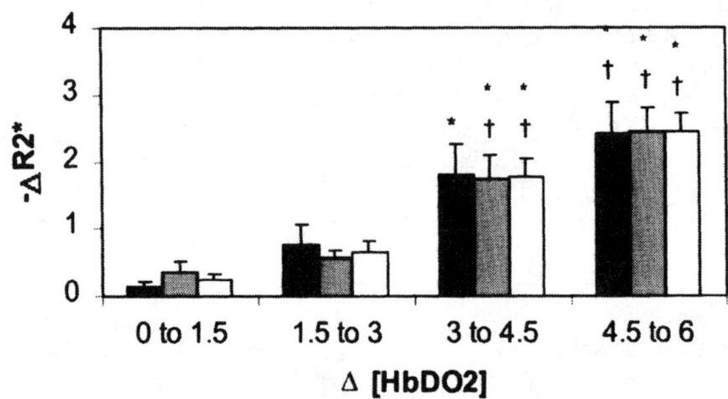

Figure 5. Quartiles of changes in coronary sinus deoxyhemoglobin concentration and changes in relaxation rate ($-\Delta R_2$*) for all studies. Septal wall (white bars), lateral wall (striped bars), and the average of the septum, anterior and lateral walls (black bars) are depicted. Deoxyhemoglobin concentrations (0 to 1.5 (n = 15), 1.5 to 3 (n = 11), 3 to 4.5 (n = 10), and 4.5 to 6 (n = 17)) are given as g/dl. *$p < 0.05$ vs. 0 to 1.5. †$p < 0.05$ vs. 1.5 to 3. Used with permission of the authors, Koelling, T. M., B. P. Poncelet, C. J. Schmidt, P. Ledden, K. K. Kwong, T. G. Reese, T. J. Brady, H. L. Kantor, and R. M. Weisskoff. "Gradient-Echo EPI BOLD T2* Contras: Changes With Varying Doses of Adenosine and Correlation With Coronary Venous Oxygen Saturation in Swine. (Abstract)." *International Society of Magnetic Resonance in Medicine* Scientific Proceedings (1997).

in the left anterior descending artery.[23] These investigators compared coronary flow measurements using phase velocity mapping to those obtained using intravascular Doppler ultrasound in twelve patients. A strong agreement was found between the two techniques, where $r = 0.89$. This group of investigators, and others, have shown stronger correlations with measurements made in dogs (presumably due to improved respiratory gating in the sedated animal), where $r = 0.94 - 0.95$. [24,25]

Other efforts using magnetic resonance imaging to quantify blood flow have focused on flow in the myocardial bed. Most efforts have included the use of injectable contrast agents, such as Gd-DTPA.[26–28] Recently, Jerosch-Herold et al. described a method of using the image time-course data after injection of Gd-DTPA to quantify flow in myocardium. These investigators compared the MRI measurement to Doppler flow wire measurements in eight patients with microvascular angina and showed an excellent correlation in myocardial flow reserve, where $r = 0.97$.[28]

Because of the potential variability of myocardial blood flow measurements using venous contrast injections in patients with low flow states and/or valvular regurgitation, additional studies have been performed leading to the development of methods taking advantage of "intrinsic contrast". Changes in blood deoxyhemoglobin content can alter tissue gradient echo magnetic resonance imaging signal intensity through this susceptibility contrast,[29] and are termed "blood oxygen level dependent", or "BOLD" contrast. Gradient echo EPI (echo planar imaging) imaging has been shown to effectively demonstrate areas of myocardium that are served by a stenotic coronary,[30] and more recently has shown promise as a method of measuring myocardial flow reserve.[31] Koelling et al. showed in a swine model with intravenous adenosine infusions that the changes in signal intensity in gradient echo images correlate with changes in coronary sinus oxygen saturation (Figure 5). Using a modification of the Fick equation, these investigators also showed that the

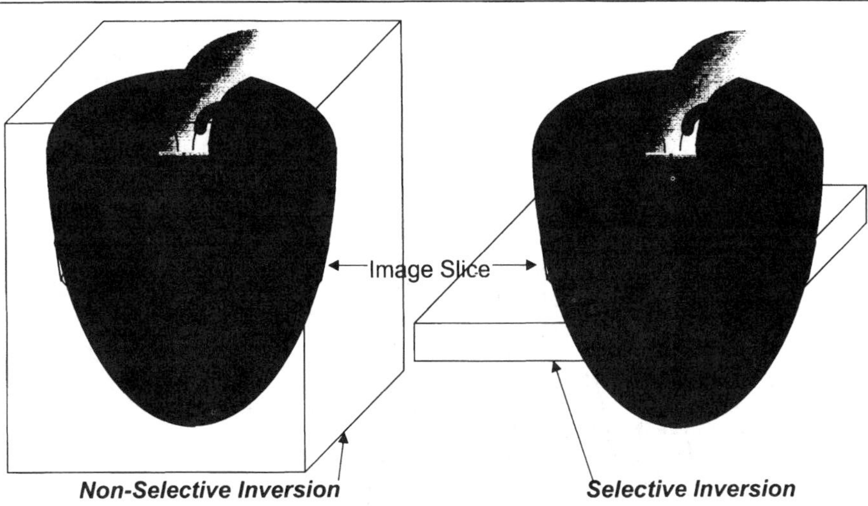

Figure 6. Depiction of the inversion recovery volumes used in flow-sensitive alternating inversion recovery (FAIR) imaging of the heart. The inversion pulse is applied to the entire heart during end systole of one heart beat. The spin echo EPI image is then acquired one or two heart beats later, again at end-systole. All tissues, including blood flowing into the imaging slice is treated with the non-selective inversion pulse. The selective inversion pulse affects only the imaging slice, and the blood flowing into the slice is not inverted, causing the image signal intensity to be higher in this image. Images of higher flow states will therefore show higher signal intensity.

technique had a good correlation with myocardial flow reserve. Application of gradient echo BOLD contrast to the transplant population, to date, has not been done.

Perhaps a more promising use of intrinsic contrast to measure myocardial flow using magnetic resonance is one employing a "flow-sensitive alternating inversion recovery", or "FAIR", sequence. The FAIR method employs two types of single-shot EPI images. One image is taken after the application of an pulse of radiofrequency energy designed to flip the spins in the entire field, and a second image is taken after a radiofrequency pulse that flips only the spins in the area of tissue to be imaged (Figure 6). These two types of images are acquired in alternating fashion, and later used to calculate a value for flow rate in the tissue. This technique has been widely used to measure blood flow in the brain,[32] and very recently has been shown to be feasible in the heart.[33] Poncelet et al. showed that the FAIR method agrees well ($r = 0.82$) with radioactive microsphere measurements in swine studied at various flow states. Although the slope of the line describing the relationship between microsphere flow and MR FAIR flow was found to be 0.93, rather than 1.0, further refinements in this technique are expected that should provide for the robustness that will be needed to apply this to the cardiac transplant population.

HIGH ENERGY PHOSPHATE SPECTROSCOPY

Magnetic resonance spectroscopy offers the opportunity of assessment of the chemical composition of the myocardium, including molecules that represent the

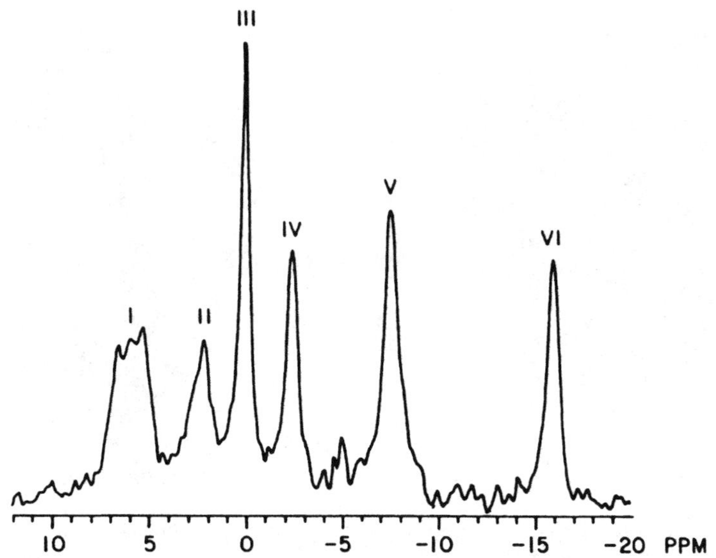

Figure 7. Representative ^{31}P spectrum from a transplanted heart one hour after reperfusion. Peak designations are: I, inorganic phosphate plus phosphomonoester; II, phosphodiester; III, phosphocreatine; IV, gamma ATP; V, alpha ATP; and VI, beta ATP. Reproduced with permission of the authors, Fraser, C. D. Jr, V. P. Chacko, W. E. Jacobus, R. L. Soulen, G. M. Hutchins, B. A. Reitz, and W. A. Baumgartner. "Metabolic Changes Preceding Functional and Morphologic Indices of Rejection in Heterotopic Cardiac Allografts. A 31P Nuclear Magnetic Resonance Study." *Transplantation* 46, no. 3 (1988): 346–51.

energetic state of the tissue. Native adenosine triphosphate (ATP), the body's fundamental unit of energy, and phosphocreatine (PCr), a reservoir of substrate for this energy, can be measured in the heart with ^{31}P magnetic resonance spectroscopy (Figure 7). Imaging using magnetic resonance is best done with a focus on the spins of the hydrogen nucleus, the most abundant substance in the body. However, with adaptations of the same equipment, magnetic resonance experiments of other nuclei can be performed, albeit with a signal-to-noise ratio per unit tissue volume per unit time of only $1–2 \times 10^{-5}$ of that seen with hydrogen, or proton, spectra.[34]

Because the heart consumes more energy per unit mass than any other organ in the body, there has been considerable interest in the application of ^{31}P MR to cardiac diseases. When oxygen supply to the heart is limited, as may occur in patients with acute rejection and abnormalities with augmentation of flow,[21] excess PCr may be consumed to replenish ATP by means of the creatine kinase reaction:

PCr + adenosine diphosphate (ADP) $\leftrightarrow$ ATP + creatine

This depletion of PCr results in a transient reduction in the PCr/ATP ratio. The ratio of PCr or ATP to inorganic phosphate (Pi) may further decline as:

ATP $\rightarrow$ ADP + Pi + energy

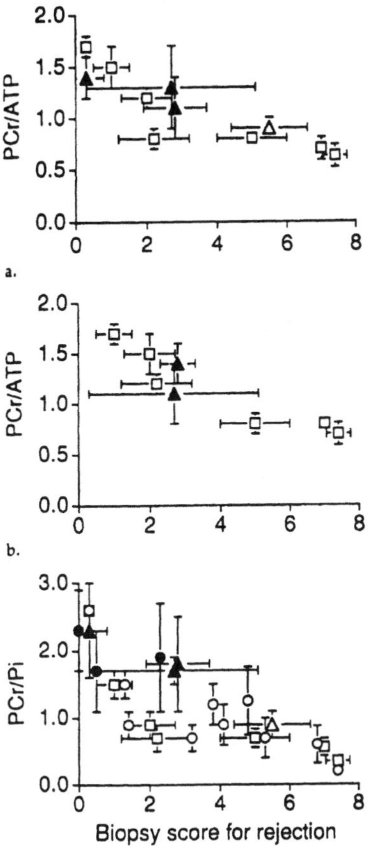

Figure 8. Myocardial PCr/ATP ratio as a function of severity of hitologic rejection assessed with Billingham criteria in endomyocardial biopsy specimens acquired (a) on the day of the P-31 MR study and (b) on the day following the MR examination or the next biopsy following the day of the MR examination. (c) The myocardial PCr/Pi ratio as a function of the biopsy score on the day of the MR study. Data are mean ± standard deviation from groups of seven to 10 immunosuppressed (filled symbols) and nonimmunosuppressed dogs with heterotopic allografts from Fraser et al. (squares [Fraser, 1988]; circles, [Fraser, 1989]; triangles, [Fraser, 1990]). Correlation coefficients for nonimmunosuppressed data are r = 0.87, 0.92, and 0.77 for a, b, and c respectively. Reproduced with permission of the authors, Bottomlcy, P. A. "MR Spectroscopy of the Human Heart: the Status and the Challenges. [Review] [103 Refs]." *Radiology* 191, no. 3 (1994): 593–612.

Chronic reductions in PCr have been reported in myocardial biopsy specimens from patients with dilated cardiomyopathy.[35] Initial animal studies of cardiac transplantation were encouraging for the use of ^{31}P spectroscopy to assess for allograft rejection, however more recent studies have revealed limitations.[5] Comparison of PCr/ATP ratio and PCr/Pi ratio with severity of histologic rejection by Fraser et al. reveals a good correlation in studies performed in immunosuppressed and non-immunosuppressed dogs (Figure 8).[5,36,37] However, the plots demostrate possible difficulties in using the method to discriminate between various degrees of rejection due to significant overlap of values.

Herfkens et al. studied eight transplant recipients on 14 occasions.[6] They reported a gradual increase in myocardial Pi level in hearts classified histologically as having no rejection through mild, mild to moderate, and moderate rejection. PCr levels were also lower in rejection hearts than in nonrejecting hearts, although the data showed little change in PCr level in progressing from mild to moderate rejection.

Evanochko et al. reported that myocardial PCr/ATP ratio was normal in five patients with mild rejection (1.81 ± 0.06), and low in three of four patients with moderate rejection (1.13 ± 0.17) compared with six healthy control subjects (1.76 ± 0.11).[7] A third human study reported by Wolfe et al. showed that the PCr/ATP ratio was lower in patients with mild rejection (1.16 ± 0.1) than in patients with no rejection (1.45 ± 0.09), but PCr/ATP did not distiguish between patients with mild and moderate (1.29 ± 0.13) rejection.[38] Finally, Bottomley et al. reported on 14 transplant recipients studied using MRS, showing that patients with mild and moderate rejection had lower PCr/ATP ratios than control subjects. The patients with mild and moderate rejection did not differ significantly from each other, thereby calling into question the ^{31}P MRS ability to identify clinically significant rejection.[39] This group reported further that if the myocardial PCr/ATP ratios had been used to indicate rejection of severity sufficient to warrant intervention (Billingham biopsy scores of ≥ 4), the ^{31}P MR results and decision based on the histologic evaluations would concur in only about 60%–70% of examinations.

The decision to treat patients with cardiac allograft rejection is most often based on the evidence for myocyte necrosis rather than edema or lymphocytic infiltration. Myocytes that have undergone necrosis do not have functioning mitochondria, and as a result have very little stores of ATP. This would result in a lack of correlation between PCr/ATP and moderate/severe rejection. The discrepancy between PCr/ATP ratio and histologic rejection grade could, in theory, be ameliorated through simultaneous quantification of Pi. Pi levels should increase when cells undergo necrosis. However, reliability of spectral quantification of Pi is hampered due to scatter of the signal caused by contamination with DPG.[40] Further study is warranted before ^{31}P MRS can be routinely applied to the noninvasive evaluation of cardiac allograft rejection.

SODIUM SPECTROSCOPY

In humans, healthy myocytes maintain an intracellular sodium concentration of about 5–10 nM versus 150 nM extracellularly. Animal models have shown that the intracellular sodium concentration rises reliably with cell damage caused by ischemia.[41] In light of evidence suggesting that parenchymal injury in allograft rejection may be linked to ischemia (or cell damage, as well) Waldrop et al. studied the feasibility to detect changes in ^{23}Na MRS in transplanted syngeneic and non-immunosuppressed allogeneic rats.[42] They found that the ^{23}Na MRS signal from the syngeneic grafts held steady or decreased during the thirty days post transplantation, while the signal in the allogeneic grafts rose with time following transplantation, becoming significantly elevated above that from syngeneic grafts (Figure 9).

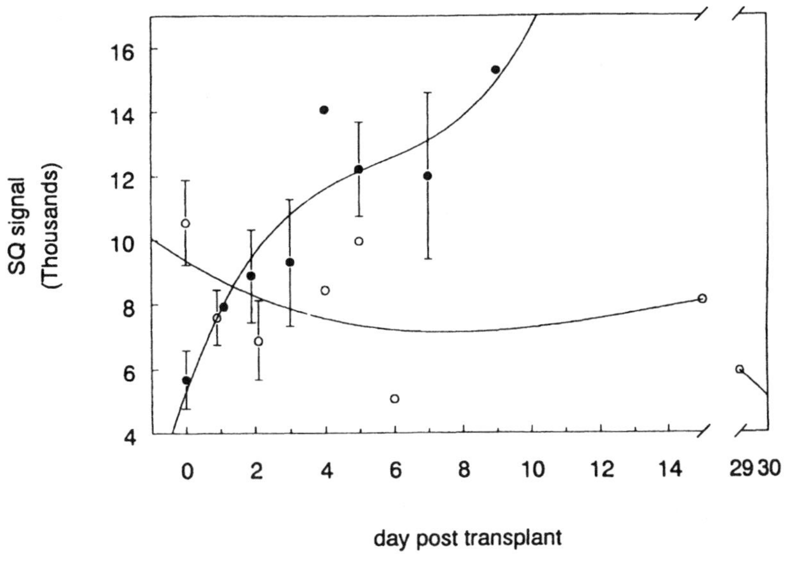

Figure 9. Scatter plots showing ^{23}Na MRS data for all grafts studied, on all days examined. Each point is displayed as an average number (±SD) for all animals studied on that particular day post transplant as described in the text. A third degree polynomial line was fit to the pooled allogeneic and syngeneic data. The allogeneic data are displayed as closed symbols and the syngeneic data as open symbols. Data points offset around the x coordinate are done so for clarity and are not intended to show fractional days. Reproduced with permission of the authors, Waldrop, S. M., D. Z. Alexander, R. Lowry, K. J. Winn, T. C. Pearson, and I. Constantinidis. "Analysis of Allogeneic and Syngeneic Rat Heart Transplants Using 23Na Magnetic Resonance Spectroscopy." *Biochemical & Biophysical Research Communications* 223, no. 2 (1996): 379–83.

The cause of the change in ^{23}Na MRS signal has not been fully elucidated, but may arise from a variety of sources. First of all, ischemia can cause dysfunction of sodium transport ion channels, and if cell death results, a loss of cell membrane integrity. Secondly, lymphocytic infiltration may be expected to lead to interstitial edema, and, simply by enlargement of the extracellular space, cause ^{23}Na MRS signal to rise. And finally, given that this particular study was performed comparing syngeneic and allogeneic transplants, the change in signal may have been caused by differences in the intravascular space represented by incompatibility of blood types. Further studies, including those in humans, are needed to determine if ^{23}Na MRS may have a role in the evaluation of cardiac allograft rejection.

PLASMA PROTON SPECTROSCOPY

While most attention for the use of nuclear magnetic resonance in transplantation has been directed at the direct characterization of the myocardium, some investigators have shown interest in plasma lipoproteins and their changes with varying immune states. It appears that different normal plasma lipoproteins variably suppress *in vitro* immune responses, and their biologically active constituents can alter after

Table 5. Evaluation of the accuracy of plasma ^{1}H lipoprotein TLW test for detection of cardiac allograft rejection. A TLW value greater than 62 Hz, or a TLW/TLW at day 8 ratio of greater than 1.15 were selected to be the threshold values indicative of cardiac allograft rejection. From Eugene, M., L. Le Moyec, J. de Certaines, M. Desruennes, E. Le Rumeur, J. B. Fraysse, and C. Cabrol. "Lipoproteins in Heart Transplantation: Proton Magnetic Resonance Spectroscopy of Plasma." *Magnetic Resonance in Medicine* 18, no. 1 (1991): 93–101

	N	TLW (Hz)	TLW/TLW D8
Control Group	32	69.2 ± 5.8	—
Group 1—Pre-Transplant	46	68.2 ± 8.9	1.27 ± 0.18
Group 2—D8 after Transplant	46	53.6 ± 5.1	1
Group 3—No Rejection	213	52.3 ± 8.3	0.97 ± 0.13
Group 4—Rejection	105	65.6 ± 7.9	1.24 ± 0.14

transplantation.[43] Initial observations to this effect were made in the field of oncology. Using nuclear magnetic resonance, the half-height width of the methyl and methylene resonances arising from lipoproteins can be measured. The sum of the two linewidths, or total linewidth (TLW), is used to assess the changes in plasma concentration of lipoproteins.

Eugene et al. reported a study of 410 measurements performed in 46 cardiac transplant recipients.[43] Results of nuclear magnetic resonance from serum samples were then compared to results on endomyocardial biopsy performed on the same day. Biopsy specimens were assessed according to the grading system of Billingham (I light, II mild, III moderate, IV severe). Data for the nuclear magnetic resonance experiment was expressed as the TLW as well as TLW/TLW D8, an index of the TLW value to the value obtained at day 8 after transplantation. Grouping of samples based on the result of biopsies showed that patients with any evidence of rejection (grades I–IV), RP(+), had a significantly higher TLW and TLW/TLW D8 compared with samples with no rejection process (Table 5). Further analysis to determine critical cut-off values for the measurements determined that the TLW value of 62 Hz had a sensitivity of 71% and a specificity of 90% for the detection of rejection (Table 6). A TLW/TLW D8 ratio of 1.15 was somewhat better with a sensitivity of 80% and a specificity of 95%.

More recently, Le Floch et al. reported on their use of proton MRS to predict future rejection episodes in eighteen patients monitored for 16 months after cardiac transplantation.[44] These investigators found that none of the patients with $TLW_{8/0}$ (the ratio of the total linewidth measurement on day 8 after transplant to the day of the transplant) less than 0.8 had more than 2 episodes of rejection (ISHLT Grade 2 or higher) over the follow-up period (492 ± 269 days) (Table 7). In contrast, five of six patients with $TLW_{8/0}$ greater than 0.8 had three or more rejection episodes during the follow-up period. The authors suggested that the linkage between plasma lipoprotein concentration and future episodes of rejection exists because of the dependence of cyclosporine transport and subsequent cyclosporine levels on plasma lipid concentrations. They hypothesized that if the plasma lipoprotein level fell in the first eight days after transplant, then, for the remainder of the transplant, cyclosporine would be expected to have a better immunosuppressive effect because it would not be bound to plasma lipoproteins.

Table 6. Evaluation of the accuracy of plasma ^{1}H lipoprotein TLW test for detection of cardiac allograft rejection. A TLW value greater than 62 Hz, or a TLW/TLW at day 8 ratio of greater than 1.15 were selected to be the threshold values indicative of cardiac allograft rejection. From Eugene, M., L. Le Moyec, J. de Certaines, M. Desruennes, E. Le Rumeur, J. B. Fraysse, and C. Cabrol. "Lipoproteins in Heart Transplantation: Proton Magnetic Resonance Spectroscopy of Plasma." *Magnetic Resonance in Medicine* 18, no. 1 (1991): 93–101

	Criterion for the test	
	TLW	TLW/TLW D8
Critical Value	62 Hz	1.15
Sensitivity	71%	80%
Specificity	90%	95%
Positive Predictive value	78%	90%
Negative Predictive value	86%	91%
Prevalence	33%	33%

Table 7. NMR detection of early response to initial immunosuppressive treatment as a prognosis factor. A $TLW_{8/0}$ ratio of less than 0.8 predicted all patients who had no rejection processes during the follow-up period, 492 ± 269 days. Alternatively, a $TLW_{8/0}$ ratio of greater than 0.8 predicted all patients with more than three rejection processes. From Le Floch, M., M. P. Ramee, B. LeLong, G. Leray, M. Kerbaol, and J. D. de Certaines. "Proton Magnetic Resonance Spectroscopy of Blood Plasma in Heart Transplant Recipients Treated With Cyclosporine: an Early Prognosis Test of Long-Term Graft Tolerance." *Journal of Heart & Lung Transplantation* 16, no. 4 (1997): 381–6

		$TLW_{8/0}$	
	No.	>0.8	<0.8
0 Rejection Processes	6	0	6
1–2 Rejection Processes	7	1	6
≥3 Rejection Processes	5	5	0

Questions that remain to be answered include a determination of the applicability of TLW to discern varying grades of rejection. The results of Eugene et al. lumped the biopsy results from five separate grades (0 through IV) into two groups. The ability to distinguish mild, moderate and severe grades of rejection will be critical for the future of this noninvasive method.

SUMMARY

The current standard for the diagnosis of cardiac allograft rejection remains the endomyocardial biopsy. Clinical utility of a noninvasive diagnostic method such as MRI would be to determine the point of time when biopsy should be performed and to follow the patients under treatment for acute rejection. The advantage of MR imaging over the other noninvasive methods such as two-dimensional echocardiography, computerized tomography, and thallium scintigraphy is the broad versatility of the modality. With streamlining and integration of pulse sequences, physicians may eventually be able to obtain excellent resolution of pathoanatomy showing myocardial wall thickness and left ventricular mass, direct tissue characterization with measurements of T1 and T2 relaxation times, and energy supply through the assessment of myocardial perfusion within a single examination. Further technical developments in spectroscopy of nuclei such as ^{31}P and ^{23}Na may also allow for characterization of the biochemical composition of transplant myocardium. Although magnetic resonance is not capable of sampling the myocardium for lymphocytes as might be expected of a technique that would provide a direct agreement with endomyocardial biopsy, a large amount of information that can be acquired during a single MRI exam. With additional study, MRI may ultimately play an important role in the routine, serial, noninvasive assessment of cardiac transplant recipients.

REFERENCES

1. Ciliberto GR, Mascarello M, Gronda E, Bonacina E, Anjos MC, Danzi G, et al. Acute rejection after heart transplantation: noninvasive echocardiographic evaluation. J Am Coll Cardiol 1994;23: 1156–61.
2. Hesse B, Mortensen SA, Folke M, Brodersen AK, Aldershvile J, Pettersson G. Ability of antimyosin scintigraphy monitoring to exclude acute rejection during the first year after heart transplantation. Journal of Heart & Lung Transplantation 1995;14:23–31.
3. Isobe M, Ohtani H, Yagita H, Okumura K, Strauss HW, Yazaki Y. Detection of cardiac rejection in mice by radioimmune scintigraphy using 123iodine-labeled anti-ICAM-1 monoclonal antibody. Acta Cardiol 1993;48:235–43.
4. Rubin PJ, Hartman JJ, Hasapes JP, Bakke JE, Bergmann SR. Detection of cardiac transplant rejection with 111In-labeled lymphocytes and gamma scintigraphy. Circulation 1996;94:II298–303.
5. Fraser CD Jr, Chacko VP, Jacobus WE, Soulen RL, Hutchins GM, Reitz BA, et al. Metabolic changes preceding functional and morphologic indices of rejection in heterotopic cardiac allografts. A 31P nuclear magnetic resonance study. Transplantation 1988;46:346–51.
6. Herfkens RJ, Charles HC, Negro-Vilar R, van Trigt P. In vivo phosphorus-31 NMR spectroscopy of human heart transplants (abstr). Society of Magnetic Resonance in Medicine 1988;827.
7. Evanochko WT, Bouchard A, Kirklin JK, Bourge RC, Luney D, Pohost GM. Detection of cardiac transplant rejection in patients by ^{31}P NMR spectroscopy (abstract). Society of Magnetic Resonance in Medicine 1990;246.
8. Gill EA, Borrego C, Bray BE, Renlund DG, Hammond EH, Gilbert EM. Left ventricular mass increases during cardiac allograft vascular rejection. J Am Coll Cardiol 1995;25:922–6.
9. Florentine MS, Grosskreutz CL, Chang W, Hartnett JA, Dunn VD, Ehrhardt JC, et al. Measurement of left ventricular mass in vivo using gated nuclear magnetic resonance imaging. J Am Coll Cardiol 1986;8:107–12.
10. Caputo GR, Tscholakoff D, Sechtem U, Higgins CB. Measurement of canine left ventricular mass by using MR imaging. American Journal of Roentgenology 1987;148:33–8.
11. Forbat SM, Karwatowski SP, Gatehouse PD, Firmin DN, Longmore DB, Underwood SR. Technical note: rapid measurement of left ventricular mass by spin echo magnetic resonance imaging. Br J Radiol 1994;67:86–90.
12. Bottini PB, Carr AA, Prisant LM, Flickinger FW, Allison JD, Gottdiener JS. Magnetic resonance imaging compared to echocardiography to assess left ventricular mass in the hypertensive patient. Am J Hypertens 1995;8:221–8.
13. Revel D, Chapelon C, Mathieu D, Cochet P, Ninet J, Chuzel M, et al. Magnetic resonance imaging of human orthotopic heart transplantation: correlation with endomyocardial biopsy. Journal of Heart Transplantation 1989;8:139–46.
14. Wisenberg G, Pflugfelder PW, Kostuk WJ, McKenzie FN, Prato FS. Diagnostic applicability of magnetic resonance imaging in assessing human cardiac allograft rejection. Am J Cardiol 1987;60: 130–6.

14a. Marie PY, Angioi M, Carteaux JP et al. Detection and prediction of acute heart transplant rejection with the myocardial T2 determination provided by a black-blood magnetic resonance imaging sequence. J Am Coll Cardiol 2001;37:825–831.
15. Tscholakoff D, Aherne T, Yee ES, Derugin N, Higgins CB. Cardiac transplantations in dogs: evaluation with MR. Radiology 1985;157:697–702.
16. Huber DJ, Kirkman RL, Kupiec-Weglinski JW, Araujo JL, Tilney NL, Adams DF. The detection of cardiac allograft rejection by alterations in proton NMR relaxation times. Invest Radiol 1985;20:796–802.
17. Walpoth BH, Lazeyras F, Tschopp A, Schaffner T, Althaus U, Billingham M, et al. Assessment of cardiac rejection and immunosuppression by magnetic resonance imaging and spectroscopy. Transplant Proc 1995;27:2088–91.
18. Aherne T, Tscholakoff D, Finkbeiner W, Sechtem U, Derugin N, Yee E, et al. Magnetic resonance imaging of cardiac transplants: the evaluation of rejection of cardiac allografts with and without immunosuppression. Circulation 1986;74:145–56.
19. Kurland RJ, West J, Kelley S, Shoop JD, Harris R, Carr EA Jr, et al. Magnetic resonance imaging to detect heart transplant rejection: sensitivity and specificity. Transplant Proc 1989;21:2537–43.
20. Higgins CB, Herfkens R, Lipton MJ, Sievers R, Sheldon P, Kaufman L, et al. Nuclear magnetic resonance imaging of acute myocardial infarction in dogs: alterations in magnetic relaxation times. Am J Cardiol 1983;52:184–8.
21. Chan SY, Kobashigawa J, Stevenson LW, Brownfield E, Brunken RC, Schelbert HR. Myocardial blood flow at rest and during pharmacological vasodilation in cardiac transplants during and after successful treatment of rejection. Circulation 1994;90:204–12.
22. Kaul SMD, Senior RMD MRCP, Dittrich HMD, RavalUsha BS, Khattar RMD, Lahiri AMD MRCP. Detection of coronary artery disease with myocardial contrast echocardiography: comparison with sup 99m Tc-sestamibi single-photon emission computed tomography. Circulation1997;96:785–92.
23. Hundley WG, Lange RA, Clarke GD, Meshack BM, Payne J, Landau C, et al. Assessment of coronary arterial flow and flow reserve in humans with magnetic resonance imaging. Circulation 1996;93:1502–8.
24. Clarke GD, Eckels R, Chaney C, Smith D, Dittrich J, Hundley WG, et al. Measurement of absolute epicardial coronary artery flow and flow reserve with breath-hold cine phase-contrast magnetic resonance imaging. Circulation 1995;91:2627–34.
25. Sakuma H, Saeed M, Takeda K, Wendland MF, Schwitter J, Szolar DH, et al. Quantification of coronary artery volume flow rate using fast velocity-encoded cine MR imaging. American Journal of Roentgenology 1997;168:1363–7.
26. Arteaga C, Canet E, Ovize M, Janier M, Revel D. Myocardial perfusion assessed by subsecond magnetic resonance imaging with a paramagnetic macromolecular contrast agent. Invest Radiol 1994;29 Suppl 2:S54–7.
27. Larsson HB, Fritz-Hansen T, Rostrup E, Sondergaard L, Ring P, Henriksen O. Myocardial perfusion modeling using MRI. Magn Reson Med 1996;35:716–26.
28. Jerosch-Herold M, Wilke N, Wang Y, Huang Y, Christensen B, Wilson RF, et al. MR first pass measurement of myocardial perfusion reserve in patients. (Abstract). International Society of Magnetic Resonance in Medicine 1997;22:476.
29. Atalay MK, Forder JR, Chacko VP, Kawamoto S, Zerhouni EA. Oxygenation in the rabbit myocardium: assessment with susceptibility-dependent MR imaging. Radiology 1993;189:759–64.
30. Niemi P, Poncelet BP, Kwong KK, Weisskoff RM, Rosen BR, Brady TJ, et al. Myocardial intensity changes associated with flow stimulation in blood oxygenation sensitive magnetic resonance imaging. Magn Reson Med 1996;36:78–82.
31. Koelling TM, Poncelet BP, Schmidt CJ, Ledden P, Kwong KK, Reese TG, et al. Gradient-Echo EPI BOLD T2* contrast changes with varying doses of adenosine and correlation with coronary venous oxygen saturation in swine. (Abstract). International Society of Magnetic Resonance in Medicine 1997;22:475.
32. Kwong KK, Belliveau JW, Chesler DA, Goldberg IE, Weisskoff RM, Poncelet BP, et al. Dynamic magnetic resonance imaging of human brain activity during primary sensory stimulation. Proc Natl Acad Sci U S A 1992;89:5675–9.
33. Poncelet BP, Koelling TM, Schmidt CJ, Ledden P, Kwong KK, Reese TG, et al. In vivo measurement of human myocardial tissue perfusion at rest and during hyperemia by double gated flow alternated inversion recovery EPI. Proceedings of the 5th Annual Meeting of the International Society of Magnetic Resonance in Medicine 1997;22:88.
34. Bottomley PA. Noninvasive study of high-energy phosphate metabolism in human heart by dept-resolved ^{31}P NMR spectroscopy. Science 1985;229:769–72.

35. Ingwall JS, Kramer MF, Fifer MA, et al. The creatine kinase system in normal and diseased human myocardium. N Engl J Med 1985;313:1050–4.
36. Fraser CD Jr, Chacko VP, Jacobus WE, Hutchins GM, Glickson J, Reitz BA, et al. Evidence from 31P nuclear magnetic resonance studies of cardiac allografts that early rejection is characterized by reversible biochemical changes. Transplantation 1989;48:1068–70.
37. Fraser CD Jr, Chacko VP, Jacobus WE, Mueller P, Soulen RL, Hutchins GM, et al. Early phosphorus 31 nuclear magnetic resonance bioenergetic changes potentially predict rejection in heterotopic cardiac allografts. Journal of Heart Transplantation 1990;9:197–204.
38. Wolfe CL, Caputo G, Chew W. Detection of cardiac transplant rejection by magnetic resonance imaging and spectroscopy (abstract). Society of Magnetic Resonance in Medicine 1991;574.
39. Bottomley PA, Weiss RG, Hardy CJ, Baumgartner WA. Myocardial high-energy phosphate metabolism and allograft rejection in patients with heart transplants. Radiology 1991;181:67–75.
40. Bottomley PA. MR spectroscopy of the human heart: the status and the challenges. [Review]. Radiology 1994;191:593–612.
41. Malloy CR, Buster DC, Castro MMCA, Geraldes CFGC, Jeffrey FMH, Sherry AD. Influence of global ischemia on intracellular sodium in the perfused rat heart. Magn Reson Med 1990;15:33–4.
42. Waldrop SM, Alexander DZ, Lowry R, Winn KJ, Pearson TC, Constantinidis I. Analysis of allogeneic and syngeneic rat heart transplants using 23Na magnetic resonance spectroscopy. Biochemical & Biophysical Research Communications 1996;223:379–83.
43. Eugene M, Le Moyec L, de Certaines J, Desruennes M, Le Rumeur E, Fraysse JB, et al. Lipoproteins in heart transplantation: proton magnetic resonance spectroscopy of plasma. Magn Reson Med 1991;18:93–101.
44. Le Floch M, Ramee MP, LeLong B, Leray G, Kerbaol M, de Certaines JD. Proton magnetic resonance spectroscopy of blood plasma in heart transplant recipients treated with cyclosporine: an early prognosis test of long-term graft tolerance. Journal of Heart & Lung Transplantation 1997;16: 381–6.

Section 4. Radionuclide Imaging for Surveillance of Cardiac Allograft Rejection

16. TARGETS FOR RADIONUCLIDE IMAGING OF CARDIAC ALLOGRAFT REJECTION

H. William Strauss, M.D.
Division of Nuclear Medicine, Stanford University School of Medicine, Room H0101, 300 Pasteur Drive, Stanford CA 94305

Radionuclide imaging of the myocardium can target receptor or transport systems that are present under normal or abnormal conditions.[1–6] Targeting normal systems makes abnormal tissue appear as a decrease in the signal. Conversely when abnormal states are targeted, there is minimal localization in normal tissue, but abnormalities are detected by increased tracer deposition. Table 1 summarizes some of the targets that have been utilized to detect attributes of the normal heart.

IMAGING HEART FAILURE AND TRANSPLANT REJECTION

Evaluating ventricular function is a key factor in determining the etiology of heart failure. Blood pool imaging or myocardial perfusion imaging can distinguish between systolic and diastolic etiologies of failure, differentiate regional versus global dysfunction, and define major sites of valvular regurgitation. Other markers, however, are necessary to identify processes that may be reversible causes of failure.

Cold Spot Markers

Perfusion, a major marker for ischemia and scar, is most helpful when heart failure is due to systolic dysfunction associated with atherosclerotic coronary heart disease. Under those circumstances, focal zones of decreased tracer uptake are seen. However, when the etiology is associated with diastolic dysfunction secondary to severe hypertrophy or systolic dysfunction, the regional distribution of perfusion is often normal.

Metabolic indicators have been sought to identify the etiology of heart failure. Changes in substrate utilization, particularly a reduction in the utilization of fatty acids, have been suggested as a cause of failure.[7] Recent studies identified a reduction in mRNA coding for mitochondrial beta oxidation.[8] Part of this reduction may

Table 1. Cellular targets and physiologic measurements made by selected radiopharmaceuticals—"cold spot" agents

Physiologic measurements	Radiopharmaceutical	Normal cellular function
Perfusion	Potassium-43 Thallium-201 Rubidium-82 Ammonia-N-13	Sodium-Potassium Pump
	^{99m}Technetium-Teboroxime	Cell Membrane Lipid[1]
	^{99m}Technetium-Tetrofosmin	Diffusion and intracellular binding proteins[2]
	^{99m}Technetium-Sestamibi	Diffusion and intracellular binding proteins[3]
Glucose metabolism	Fluorodeoxyglucose (^{18}FDG)	Glucose Transporter[4]
Fatty Acid Consumption	Iodophenylpentadecanoic acid (^{123}IPPA) Betamethyliodophenylpentadecanoic acid (^{123}I-BMIPP) C-11 Palmitate	Fatty Acid Transport Protein*
Norepinephrine re-uptake receptor	Monoiodobenzylguanidine (^{131}I-MIBG) Ephedrine (^{11}C-Ephedrine)	Adrenergic Receptor[5]
Cholinergic receptor	Iodo or C-11 Quinylnuclidylbenzadine	Cholinergic receptors[6]
Beta receptor	Pindolol (^{125}I hydroxybenzylpindolol)	
Calcium channel	?	
Oxidative metabolism	1 Acetate	Tricarboxylic acid cycle

be due to the increase in diffusion distance from capillary to mitochondria in hypertrophied tissue, resulting in mitochondrial hypoxia. Studies by Yonekura et al. with a modified long chain fatty acid, beta-methyliodophenylpentadecanoic acid (BMIPP) in the salt sensitive Dahl strain rat support this hypothesis.[9] Yonekura and his colleagues observed a reduction in fatty acid uptake in the endocardium of rats with hypertension, while perfusion to that region was well maintained. Subsequent studies by Shimonagata et al.[10] and Mochizuki et al.[11] confirmed this finding. Recently, a congenital deficiency of a fatty acid transport enzyme, CD36, was observed.[12] This anomaly is associated with heart failure and an absence of BMIPP uptake in the myocardium of human subjects. A partial deficiency of this enzyme is found in 0.3% of the population, and may place these patients at higher risk of myopathy.

A specific measure of mitochrondrial oxidative metabolic function is obtained with carbon-11 acetate imaging.[13] While abnormalities of acetate flux have been reported in ischemia and myopathy, recovery of acetate metabolism is a good predictor of functional recovery in the tissue.[14]

Glucose metabolism has been employed most often to identify myocardium that is viable but ischemic.[15] While this determination is very important in selecting patients with ischemic heart disease and depressed ejection fraction for revascularization, thallium redistribution imaging is almost as effective.[16] Each of these tracers evaluates the regional distribution of the radiopharmaceutical. An intriguing result was recently reported by Rechavia et al.[17] These investigators evaluated patients with cardiac tranplants with FDG imaging. They observed a 196% increase in global FDG uptake in the transplanted heart compared that of normal volunteers. These observations suggest that there may be a metabolic signature in transplantation.

In addition to metabolic abnormalities, heart failure is associated with an increase in circulating levels of catecholamines. Studies of myocardial uptake of the adrenergic receptor marker monoiodiobenzylguanidine (MIBG) in these patients demonstrate reduced retention of this agent in the myocardium.[18,19] Although this finding is interesting, it too is likely to be a secondary observation, which will change in magnitude with the severity of the heart failure.

Cholinergic receptors have not been as well studied, since the agent used to evaluate this receptor system, iodo QNB or C-11 QNB, is difficult to synthesize. However, preliminary evidence suggests that cholinergic receptor uptake is not altered in transplant rejection.

In addition to these factors, other potential targets for imaging the normal myocardium include specific receptor systems or channels expressed by the cells. This concept is particularly intriguing in light of the important role that genetic changes in the calcium channel are known to play in the development of hypertrophic myopathy. Administration of calcineurin inhibitors, such as FK506 to mice with a genetic predisposition for hypertrophic myopathy, or cyclosporine to rats with pressure overload, prevented the development of myopathy.[20] Thus far, in spite of the potential of this technique, calcium channel imaging of the myocardium has not been described. Imaging β receptors, on the other hand, has had some success.[21] A major problem with beta receptor imaging is the high expression of beta receptors in the lung, which reduces the contrast between the heart and background. Even with this problem, however, changes in receptor occupancy can be readily measured. Homcy et al. utilized dynamic imaging of relative tracer concentration in the lung when non-radiolabeled drug was administered to displace the radiolabeled compound from receptors to demonstrate this phenomena.

Hot Spot Markers

A mild reduction in the normal signal may be difficult to detect. On the other hand, some localization of a tracer that is not normally found in the myocardium is easier to detect. Table 2 summarizes the compounds that have been suggested to image the diseased myocardium.

Ischemia and hypertrophy result in a significant decrease in oxygen delivery to the cell, because of either a primary decrease in supply, or an increase in the diffusion distance between capillary and mitochondria in the hypertrophied cell. In either event, myocyte work is restricted because there is a reduced amount of ATP available. To provide the maximal amount of ATP requires oxidative metabolism, with its production of 96 ATP's from the catabolism of a single molecule of palmitate to CO_2 and H_2O. On the other hand, anaerobic metabolism can only provide 12 ATP's from a single glucose molecule when the product of catabolism is lactate. The detection of reduced oxygen tension in the cell has been successfully imaged with four different compounds, F-18 nitroimidazole, BMS 181321, BMS 197891, and HL91. These molecules are retained in tissue with reduced oxygen tension. From a mechanistic perspective, it is known that the nitroimidazole compounds are retained because a single electron reduction takes place, which, in the presence of adequate oxygen levels is rapidly reversed. In the absence of an adequate intracellular

Table 2. Abnormal cellular state, physiologic mechanism and radiopharmaceuticals for detecting selected disease states—"hot spot" markers

Abnormal cellular function	Radiopharmaceutical	Physiologic function
Hypoxia	HL91	Hypoxic trapping (PNaO moiety—trapping mechanism unknown)
	F-18 Nitroimidazole	Hypoxic trapping[22] (nitroimidazole—single electron reduction)
	BMS 181321	Hypoxic trapping[23] (nitroimidazole—single electron reduction)
	BMS 197891	Hypoxic trapping (nitroimidazole—single electron reduction)
Necrosis	Antimyosin	Fab fragment recognizing heavy chain of cardiac myosin[24]
	Glucarate	Mechanism of binding to necrotic cells unknown[25]
	Pyrophosphate	Binding to free intracellular calcium[26]
Apoptosis	Annexin V lipocortin	Binding to phosphatidylserine on cell membrane*
Rejection	Increased expression of MHC in tissue undergoing rejection	Antibodies recognizing increased expression of MHC II[27]
	Annexin V lipocortin	Rejection is associated with increased apoptosis
Myocarditis	Antimyosin	Myocyte death occurs in severe myocarditis
Vascular injury	MCP-1	Inflammation is associated with increased monocyte infiltration
	Endothelin analog	Increased expression of endothelin receptors*

concentration of oxygen (>10 torr), the single electron reduction is followed by additional reduction steps that result in an insoluble compound that is retained in the cell. Some of the most detailed work has been done with BMS 181321, where oxygen electrode studies documented retention in cells where oxygen tension is decreased to <50% of control values.

The necrosis marker antimyosin provides sufficient contrast between the diseased heart and normal tissue that, in addition to acute infarction, the agent has been successfully employed in transplant patients to identify individuals undergoing rejection.[28,29] In patients with transplant rejection myocyte death is a major outcome. Several investigators have sucessfully employed antimyosin imaging as a means of identifying cell death. At the time of cell death, myosin is exposed to the extracellular milieu. Since myosin's one of the least soluble proteins in the body, it takes a considerable interval of time to digest this protein and eliminate it completely from the site of injury. It appears that the antigen recognized by antimyosin is also retained. This allows antimyosin imaging to define an integral of cell death over some interval of time. This phenomena may account for the remarkable sensitivity of antimyosin imaging for the detection of transplant rejection. Similarly, antimyosin uptake has been used to identify patients with myocarditis.[30,31]

Necrosis, however, is an atypical cause of myocyte death in myopathy. It is now apparent that apoptosis occurs far more often.[32] A recent report by Blankenberg et al.[33] suggests that technetium-99m labeled Annexin V lipocortin, a 36 kD physiologic protein radiolabeled with technetium-99m, can be used to image the distribution of apoptosis in vivo.

Apoptosis is an orderly process that involves a well defined sequence of steps. An early change that occurs, shortly after the cell is committed to undergo programmed cell death, is found in the composition of the outer leaflet of the cell membrane. In the normal state, phosphatidylserine (PS) is actively constrained to the inner leaflet of the membrane by an energy dependent translocase enzyme system. When apoptosis is initiated by either a constituitive mechanism (release of endogenous cytochrome C from the mitochondrial membrane) or by external signaling (production of *fas* by invading lymphocytes, triggering *fas* receptor-mediated apoptosis) the translocase pump is shut down. In addition, another enzyme system, scramblase, is activated which accelerates the appearance of phosphatidylserine on the external leaflet of the membrane. Annexin V will bind to the outer leaflet of the membrane when it expresses PS because the protein has an affinity of 10^{-9} for membrane bound phosphatidylserine. Membrane expression of PS is an early change in the apoptosis cascade, occurring prior to fragmentation of DNA.

There is a growing body of evidence that apoptosis plays a major role in heart failure[34] and transplant rejection.[35] Recent studies suggest that transplant rejection can be detected with this imaging technique. Furthermore, the effect of therapy can be identified by a decrease in annexin uptake.

In addition to necrosis and apoptosis, several other cellular markers are upregulated in the presence of transplant rejection. Isobe and his colleagues demonstrated upregulation of MHC II histocompatibility antigens. When antibodies recognizing these antigens were administered to animals with experimental heart transplants, increased localization was observed in rejecting hearts. In myopathies and in transplant rejection there is an increased in inflammatory (mononuclear) cell infiltration. This increase in cell traffic has been successfully detected by external imaging of radiolabeled lymphocytes in animals with experimental transplants.[36] Rejecting hearts had fifty-fold more uptake of indium lymphocyte activity compared to the native heart. In addition, when the rejecting hearts were treated with cyclosporine and prednisone, the lymphocyte uptake was similar to the native heart, but when anti-rejection medication was withdrawn, lymphocyte uptake increased.

A disadvantage of radiolabeled lymphocyte imaging is the requirement for the radiolabeled cells to find the chemotactic signal and follow it to the source. An alternative approach would label cells that have already arrived in the tissue. This approach could be accomplished by labeling a recognized chemokine such as monocyte chemoattractant peptide, and administering this material intravenously. Cells at sites of inflammation typically upregulate their receptors for chemokines. The relatively small size of the chemokines makes them diffusible, and results in delivery of the material to sites with reduced perfusion. The relative value of the labeled chemokine approach should be a low tissue background, and relatively high concentration in target regions. This idea has been validated for granulocyte imaging using chemotactic peptides,[37] and should work for the monocyte macrophage system as well.

Another potential target for imaging the damaged heart is the vascular endothelium. Vascular endothelium is a major organ, serving as a transducer for the underlying smooth muscle. When signals are correctly translated vessels dilate or constrict on demand. When the signals are not correctly sensed, or are mis-communicated, the smooth muscle will constrict when it should dilate. Identifying these physiologic receptors, or alternatively some aspect of the damaged endothelium directly, could provide an indication about the underlying health of the endothelial system. For example, there is an increase in expression of endothelin receptors. Dinkelborg and his colleagues[38] employed a rediolabeled endothelin derivative to localize and successfully image these receptors in animals with arterial injury.

A major challenge to radionuclide imaging is the direct detection of transplant vasculopathy. This vexing problem bears some similarities to the vasculopathy of diabetes and involves cellular infiltration, subendothelial deposition of substances, and proliferation of cells. Although successful imaging of this process has not yet been achieved, it is possible that radiolabeled chemokines may provide sufficient signal and contrast for success.

In summary, potential targets for imaging can be found in the vasculature, sarcolemma, or in the intracellular milieu. These targets present a hierarchy of difficulty for imaging. Most radiopharamceuticals are administered intravenously, thus achieving a high concentration in the intravascular space, and lower concentrations with each step of diffusion. Imaging fundamental processes which occur in abnormal tissue, such as apoptosis or cellular infiltration, in addition to the phenomena of normal tissue, will offer a means for radionuclide imaging to expand its role in cardiology, defining specific stages of disease and in the selection of therapy.

REFERENCES

1. Gewirtz H. Differential myocardial washout of technetium-99m-teboroxime: mechanism and significance. J Nucl Med 1991 Oct;32(10):2009–11.
2. Platts EA, North TL, Pickett RD, Kelly JD. Mechanism of uptake of technetium-tetrofosmin. I: Uptake into isolated adult rat ventricular myocytes and subcellular localization. J Nucl Cardiol 1995 Jul–Aug;2(4):317–26.
3. Crane P, Laliberte R, Heminway S, Thoolen M, Orlandi C. Effect of mitochondrial viability and metabolism on technetium-99m-sestamibi myocardial retention. Eur J Nucl Med 1993 Jan;20(1): 20–5.
4. Krivokapich J, Huang SC, Selin CE, Phelps ME. Fluorodeoxyglucose rate constants, lumped constant, and glucose metabolic rate in rabbit heart. Am J Physiol 1987 Apr;252(4 Pt 2):H777–s87.
5. Glowniak JV, Kilty JE, Amara SG, Hoffman BJ, Turner FE. Evaluation of metaiodobenzylguanidine uptake by the norepinephrine, dopamine and serotonin transporters. J Nucl Med 1993 Jul;34(7):1140–6.
6. Bohm M, Schmidt U, Schwinger RH, Bohm S, Erdmann E. Effects of halothane on beta-adrenoceptors and M-cholinoceptors in human myocardium: radioligand binding and functional studies. J Cardiovasc Pharmacol 1993 Feb;21(2):296–304.
7. Kalff V, Hicks RJ, Hutchins G, Topol E, Schwaiger M. Use of carbon-11 acetate and dynamic positron emission tomography to assess regional myocardial oxygen consumption in patients with acute myocardial infarction receiving thrombolysis or coronary angioplasty. Am J Cardiol 1993 Mar 1;71(7):529–35.
8. Sack MN, Rader TA, Park S, Bastin J, McCune SA, Kelly DP. Fatty acid oxidation enzyme gene expression is downregulated in the failing heart. Circulation 1996 Dec 1;94(11):2837–42.
9. Yonekura Y, Brill AB, Som P, Yamamoto K, Srivastava SC, Iwai J, Elmaleh DR, Livni E, Strauss HW, Goodman MM, et al. Regional myocardial substrate uptake in hypertensive rats: a quantitative autoradiographic measurement. Science 1985 Mar 22;227(4693):1494–6.
10. Shimonagata T, Nishimura T, Uehara T, Hayashida K, Kumita S, Ohno A, Nagata S, Miyatake K. Discrepancies between myocardial perfusion and free fatty acid metabolism in patients with hypertrophic cardiomyopathy. Nucl Med Commun 1993 Nov;14(11):1005–13.
11. Mochizuki T, Tsukamoto E, Ono T, Itoh K, Kanegae K, Katoh C, Shiga T, Nakada K, Kohya T, Tamaki N. Sequential change of BMIPP uptake with age in spontaneously hypertensive rat model. Ann Nucl Med 1997 Nov;11(4):299–306.

12. Hwang EH, Taki J, Yasue S, Fujimoto M, Taniguchi M, Matsunari I, Nakajima K, Shiobara S, Ikeda T, Tonami N. Absent myocardial iodine-123-BMIPP uptake and platelet/monocyte CD36 deficiency. J Nucl Med 1998 Oct;39(10):1681–4.
13. Gropler RJ, Geltman EM, Sampathkumaran K, Perez JE, Moerlein SM, Sobel BE, Bergmann SR, Siegel BA. Functional recovery after coronary revascularization for chronic coronary artery disease is dependent on maintenance of oxidative metabolism. J Am Coll Cardiol 1992 Sep;20(3):569–77.
14. Rubin PJ, Lee DS, Davila-Roman VG, Geltman EM, Schechtman KB, Bergmann SR, Gropler RJ. Superiority of C-11 acetate compared with F-18 fluorodeoxyglucose in predicting myocardial functional recovery by positron emission tomography in patients with acute myocardial infarction. Am J Cardiol 1996 Dec 1;78(11):1230–5.
15. Tamaki N. Current status of viability assessment with positron tomography. J Nucl Cardiol 1994 Mar–Apr;1(2 Pt 2):S40–7.
16. Yamagishi H, Akioka K, Takagi M, Tanaka A, Takeuchi K, Yoshikawa J, Ochi H. Relation between the kinetics of thallium-201 in myocardial scintigraphy and myocardial metabolism in patients with acute myocardial infarction. Heart 1998 Jul;80(1):28–34.
17. Rechavia E, de SR, Kushwaha SS, Rhodes CG, Araujo LI, Jones T, et al. Enhanced myocardial 18F-2-fluoro-2-deoxyglucose uptake after orthotopic heart transplantation assessed by positron emission tomography [see comments]. J Am Coll Cardiol 1997;30:533–8.
18. Dae MW. Imaging of myocardial sympathetic innervation with metaiodobenzylguanidine. J Nucl Cardiol 1994 Mar–Apr;1(2 Pt 2):S23–30.
19. Suwa M, Otake Y, Moriguchi A, Ito T, Hirota Y, Kawamura K, et al. Iodine-123 metaiodobenzylguanidine myocardial scintigraphy for prediction of response to beta-blocker therapy in patients with dilated cardiomyopathy. Am Heart J 1997;133:353–8.
20. Sussman MA, Lim HW, Gude N, Taigen T, Olsen EN, Robbins J, Colbert MC, Gualberto A, Wieczorek DF, Molkentin JD. Prevention of cardiac hypertrophy in mice by calcineurin inhibition. Science 1998;281:1690–3.
21. Homcy CJ, Strauss HW, Kopiwoda S. Beta receptor occupancy. Assessment in the intact animal. J Clin Invest 1980 May;65(5):1111–8.
22. Caldwell JH, Revenaugh JR, Martin GV, Johnson PM, Rasey JS, Krohn KA. Comparison of fluorine-18-fluorodeoxyglucose and tritiated fluoromisonidazole uptake during low-flow ischemia. J Nucl Med 1995 Sep;36(9):1633–8.
23. Okada RD, Nguyen KN, Strauss HW, Johnson G. 3rd Effects of low flow and hypoxia on myocardial retention of technetium-99m BMS181321. Eur J Nucl Med 1996 Apr;23(4):443–7.
24. Khaw BA, Scott J, Fallon JT, Cahill SL, Haber E, Homcy C. Myocardial injury: quantitation by cell sorting initiated with antimyosin fluorescent spheres. Science 1982 Sep 10;217(4564):1050–3.
25. Ohtani H, Callahan RJ, Khaw BA, Fishman AJ, Wilkinson RA, Strauss HW. Comparison of technetium-99m-glucarate and thallium-201 for the identification of acute myocardial infarction in rats. J Nucl Med 1992 Nov;33(11):1988–93.
26. Buja LM, Tofe AJ, Parkey RW, Francis MD, Lewis SE, Kulkarni PV, Bonte FJ, Willerson JT. Effect of EHDP on calcium accumulation and technetium-99m pyrophosphate uptake in experimental myocardial infarction. Circulation 1981 Nov;64(5):1012–7.
27. Isobe M, Narula J, Southern JF, Strauss HW, Khaw BA, Haber E. Imaging the rejecting heart. In vivo detection of major histocompatibility complex class II antigen induction. Circulation 1992 Feb;85(2):738–46.
28. Ballester M, Bordes R, Tazelaar HD, Carrio I, Marrugat J, Narula J, Billingham ME. Evaluation of biopsy classification for rejection: relation to detection of myocardial damage by monoclonal antimyosin antibody imaging. J Am Coll Cardiol 1998 May;31(6):1357–61.
29. Ballester M, Obrador D, Carrio I, Moya C, Auge JM, Bordes R, Marti V, Bosch I, Berna-Roqueta L, Estorch M, et al. Early postoperative reduction of monoclonal antimyosin antibody uptake is associated with absent rejection-related complications after heart transplantation. Circulation 1992 Jan;85(1):61–8.
30. Narula J, Southern JF, Dec GW, Palacios IF, Newell JB, Fallon JT, Strauss HW, Khaw BA, Yasuda T. Antimyosin uptake and myofibrillarlysis in dilated cardiomyopathy. J Nucl Cardiol 1995 Nov–Dec;2(6):470–7.
31. Narula J, Khaw BA, Dec GW, Palacios IF, Newell JB, Southern JF, Fallon JT, Strauss HW, Haber E, Yasuda T. Diagnostic accuracy of antimyosin scintigraphy in suspected myocarditis. J Nucl Cardiol 1996 Sep–Oct;3(5):371–81.
32. Narula J, Haider N, Virmani R, DiSalvo TG, Kolodgie FD, Hajjar RJ, Schmidt U, Semigran MJ, Dec GW, Khaw BA. Apoptosis in myocytes in end-stage heart failure. N Engl J Med 1996 Oct 17;335(16):1182–9.
33. Blankenberg FG, Katsikis PD, Tait JF, Davis RE, Naumovski L, Ohtsuki K, Kopiwoda S, Abrams MJ, Darkes M, Robbins RC, Maecker HT, Strauss HW. In vivo detection and imaging of phos-

phatidylserine expression during programmed cell death. Proc Natl Acad Sci USA, Vol. 95, pp. 6349–6354, May 1998 Medical Sciences.
34. Goussev A, Sharov VG, Shimoyama H, Tanimura M, Lesch M, Goldstein S, et al. Effects of ACE inhibition on cardiomyocyte apoptosis in dogs with heart failure. Am J Physiol 1998;275:H626–31.
35. Blankenberg F, Ohtsuki K, Tait J, Berry G, Davis E, Vriens P, Stoot J, Hoyt G, Robbins R, Kopiwoda S, Strauss HW. Effect of cyclosporine therapy on apoptosis in experimental heart transplants. J Nucl Med 1998;39:160P.
36. Eisen HJ, Eisenberg SB, Saffitz JE, Bolman RM, Sobel BE, Bergmann SR. Noninvasive detection of rejection of transplanted hearts with indium-111-labeled lymphocytes. Circulation 1987;75:868–76.
37. Fischman AJ, Pike MC, Kroon D, Fuccello AJ, Rexinger D, ten Kate C, Wilkinson R, Rubin RH, Strauss HW. Imaging focal sites of bacterial infection in rats with indium 111 labeled chemotactic peptide analogs. J Nucl Med 1991 Mar;32(3):483–91.
38. Dinkelborg LM, Duda SH, Hanke H, Tepe G, Hilger CS, Semmler W. Molecular imaging of atherosclerosis using a technetium-99m-labeled endothelin derivative. J Nucl Med 1998 Oct;39(10): 1819–22.

17. DETECTION OF APOPTOSIS FOR THE NONINVASIVE DIAGNOSIS OF CARDIAC ALLOGRAFT REJECTION

Francis G. Blankenberg, MD,
Jagat Narula MD, PhD, Johnathan F. Tait MD, PhD,
Robert C. Robbins MD and H. William Strauss, MD
Stanford University Medical Center,
Stanford, California 94305

An important feature of transplant rejection is the immune mediated death of graft myocytes and host mononuclear cells invading the graft. In this instance, a major cause of cell death is apoptosis as mentioned in previous chapters. This stereotyped form of cell death is associated with the expression of phosphatidylserine (PS) on the surface of the apoptotic cell (most likely as a signaling mechanism to adjacent cells and phagocytes). A physiologic protein, annexin V, binds with nanomolar affinity to cell membrane bound PS, and likely plays an important role in the cell-cell signaling and local inhibition of apoptotic cell death. We describe the animal model work and the initial clinical imaging potential of radiolabeled annexin V imaging.

MOLECULAR BASIS FOR IMAGING REJECTION WITH ANNEXIN V

A novel imaging approach for the detection of acute rejection was suggested by special staining for apoptotic cell death in regions of mononuclear infiltrates present with in the interstium of rejecting cardiac allografts.[1,2,3,4,5,6,7,8,9] These infiltrates are associated with myocyte programmed (apoptotic) cell death and drop out.[10,11] Blankenberg et al. took advantage of the observation of selective annexin V binding to apoptotic cells to develop an in-vivo imaging technique to identify sites of apoptosis.[12]

Annexin V belongs to a family of endogenous proteins which share the common property of calcium dependent binding to membrane bound phosphatidylserine.[13] At least 20 different annexins have been identified, of which 10 have been described in mammals.[14] Annexin V (MW 36.000, 319 amino acids), initially purified from human placenta[15,16] belongs to this family of proteins. Annexin V is ubiquitously distributed in most cells of the body including myocytes, endothelial and mononuclear cells and fibroblasts. Circulating levels of annexin V average 1.7 ng/mL in healthy individuals and increase approximately ten-fold with acute disease such as myocardial infarction.[17] The physiology of annexin V is unclear at this time but it may play significant roles in membrane permeability to calcium and the inhibition of pro-apoptotic signals from protein kinase C and phospholipase A_2. In some cell lines annexin V inhibits apoptosis by increasing intracellular calcium ion concentrations.[18] In heart failure annexin V is upregulated and is translocated from the cell to the interstium suggesting that it has a role interstitial fibrosis and myocardial remodeling.[19]

Early studies demonstrated anticoagulant properties of annexin. To identify the source of its anti-coagulant properties, Tait et al.[20,21] investigated the binding of annexin to phosphatidylserine present in the membrane of lipid vesicles, while Dachary-Prigrent et al.[22] demonstrated binding to activated platelets (which express high levels phosphatidylserine on their surface). These observations encouraged Tait and colleagues to radioiodinate annexin V and test the ability of this agent to identify thrombus in rabbits and pigs.[23.24] Using a crush injury to produce the thrombus, a thrombus to blood ratio of 14 was found with in-vitro counting. Tait et al. also labeled annexin V with ^{99m}Tc using a diamide dimercatptide N_2S_2 chelate for imaging studies in this model. A clot to adjacent tissue ratio of 3.9 was found in the tomographic images. These observations led to clinical studies in patients with atrial fibrillation, where, unfortunately, atrial thrombus was very difficult to identify reliably.[24]

In parallel with these studies on clot imaging, Koopman et al. and Boersma et al. were evaluating annexin V labeled with fluorescein isothiocynate (FITC) as a marker for apoptosis in flow cytometry studies.[25,26] Cells undergoing apoptosis selectively redistribute phosphatidylserine, a anionic phospholipid actively restricted to the inner leaflet of the plasma lipid bilayer by a complex interaction of energy-requiring enzymes in normal cells, to the outer leaflet of the cell membrane.[27,28] Annexin V has a high affinity for phosphatidylserine bound to cell membranes ($k_d = 10^{-10}$ M). About 8 annexin molecules bind to each exposed phosphatidylserine head group. Because there are several hundred thousand to several million binding sites per cell during apoptosis FITC-labeled annexin V provides a striking signal at flow cytometry.[29] Annexin-V is highly specific, binding only to anionic phospholipids such as PS but not to neutral or cationic phospholipids. The ability of annexin-V to bind PS is strictly calcium dependent and completely reversible.

The selective exposure of phosphatidylserine on the cell surface is also one of the earliest morphologic changes in the apoptotic cascade. PS expression occurs immediately following activation of the caspase family of proteases.[30] PS exposed on cell surface appears to the principle signal for the phagocytosis and clearance of cells undergoing apoptosis.[31]

Exposure of PS occurs well before DNA fragmentation is apparent, the terminal event of programmed cell death.[32] FITC-labeled annexin V is currently one of the gold standards for the flow cytometric assay of apoptotic cell death.[33] Using another form of labeled protein, biotinylated-annexin V, investigators have also detected apoptosis during embryonic development in situ.[34]

EXPERIMENTAL VALIDATION OF APOPTOSIS IMAGING WITH ANNEXIN V

Following intravenous injection, physiologic localization of the annexin-^{99m}Tc coupled material occurs primarily in the kidneys, with less localization in the liver and spleen. There is occasional localization in the thymus, especially of younger animals. Tissue with significant apoptosis, such as the liver stimulated to undergo apoptosis by administration of Fas antibody to activate hepatic Fas receptors, or rejecting cardiac transplants in experimental animals, achieve imageable concentrations of ^{99m}Tc annexin in these organs within 60 minutes of intravenous administration.

Detection of Fas Antibody Induced Apoptosis

Fas receptors are physiologically expressed on many cells. The liver has an unusually high concentration of Fas receptors. Rapid induction of massive hepatic apoptosis has been demonstrated following administration of an antibody that bound to Fas receptor in similar fashion to Fas ligand. To determine if ^{99m}Tc Annexin imaging could detect this process studies were performed in normal mice and in genetically altered knockout lpr mice that do not express Fas receptors.[35] In the normal (wild type) mice hepatic annexin concentration increased by threefold within two hours of antibody administration, while there was no increase in the lpr animals.

Apoptosis in Cardiac Transplantation

Since apoptosis significantly contributes to myocardial damage in cardiac allograft rejection, the potential utility of ^{99m}TcAnnexin imaging for the detection of transplant rejection was tested in rats with heterotopic heart transplants (Figure 1).[36] The animals were imaged serially for the first 10 days after transplantation. In addition to in-vivo imaging the native transplanted hearts were subjected to ex-vivo organ counting and histologic analysis. The transplanted heart developed marked uptake on day 4. At that time histologic evidence of apoptosis was present, but minimal, and routine histologic evidence of rejection was absent. Over the succeeding days, staining for apoptotic cells became increasingly positive, as did conventional histologic evidence of apoptosis. To determine how long that signal might remain if therapy were administered to minimize graft rejection, therapy was started with cyclosporine after day 4. Within 2 days the scan became negative (Figure 1). Vriens et al.[36] demonstrated the utility of ^{99m}Tc annexin V imaging in heterotopic cardiac transplants in rats with different grades of rejection as shown in Figure 1. The images demonstrated striking localization of technetium-99m annexin V in the rejecting heart, beginning 3 days after transplantation at a time when TUNEL staining was minimally abnormal. Not only did annexin V imaging detect the onset of rejection

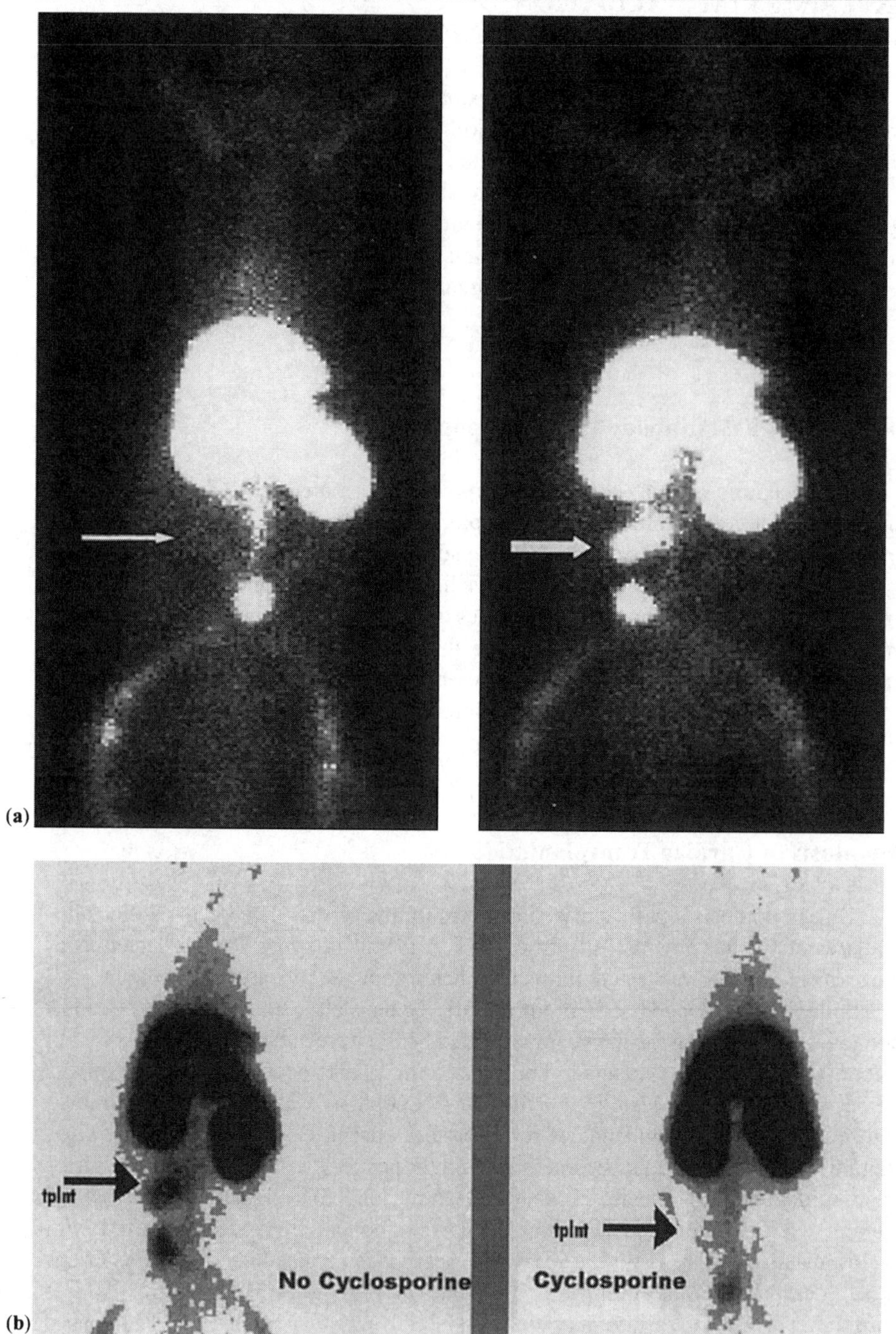
(a)
(b)
tplnt
No Cyclosporine
tplnt
Cyclosporine

earlier than TUNEL staining, it was also able to demonstrate cessation of apoptosis when the animals were treated with cyclosporine. In a similar experimental model, Kown et al.[37] demonstrated the value of zinc chloride, an inhibitor of caspase-3 activation, as a means of suppressing transplant rejection.

In other experimental models, annexin V imaging has been successful at identifying apoptosis associated with hypoxic injury in the neonatal brain,[38] and acute organ transplant rejection of lung,[39] and liver.[40]

RADIONUCLIDE IMAGING OF APOPTOSIS FOR NONINVASIVE CLINICAL DETECTION OF ACUTE ALLOGRAFT REJECTION

The in-vitro observations and experimental studies detailed above led to the testing of radiolabeled annexin V as clinical marker for apoptosis. Clinical phase I trials of are being conducted to examine apoptosis as seen by radiolabeled annexin V imaging during cancer therapy of tumors of the neck and chest[41] and in the course of acute myocardial infarction.[42,43] In experimental studies Palojoki et al.[44] demonstrated >100 fold increase in apoptosis by TUNEL staining 1 day after acute infarction and remained elevated for several weeks. These observations serve as the basis for further human trials.

Another phase II multicenter clinical trial is underway to determine the potential clinical utility of 99mTc annexin imaging for the detection of significant rejection in cardiac transplant recipients. In the largest of these initial clinical trials, Narula et al.[45] studied a series of 14 consecutive patients (ages 41 to 68 years; M:F 12:2) who had undergone heart transplantation within the one year of scintigraphic study using technetium-99m labeled annexinV (Theseus Imaging Corporation, Cambridge, MA). SPECT images were obtained at 2–3 hours after the injection of radiotracer. Processing of the SPECT images was performed initially as "chest tomographic" transaxial, coronal, and sagittal slices in order to characterize any cardiac activity within the chest. Once these were defined, "cardiac tomographic" slices in the short, vertical long, and horizontal long axes were reconstructed using filtered back-projection. A positive study was identified when myocardial uptake was seen in the chest SPECT images and, more importantly, in the cardiac SPECT images if both myocardium and LV cavity were identified during reconstruction. A negative study was otherwise identified, specifically when activity was seen within the cardiac

Figure 1. *Demonstration of the feasibility of noninvasive detection of apoptosis in an experimental cardiac allograft rejection model.* (A) Scintigraphic images of a rat recorded in the anterior view following intravenous injection of technium-99m radiolabeled annexin V. Images were recorded one hour following intravenous injection at one day (left) and 4 days (right) following heterotopic heart transplantation to the abdomen. Physiological uptake is seen in the skeleton, urinary bladder, kidneys and liver. The region of the transplanted heart, indicated by the arrow, has minimal uptake one day after surgery, and more intense uptake at the early phase of rejection at four days. (B) Anterior view scintigraphic images of ^{99m}Tc labeled Annexin V in the same rat. Left panel depicts the radioannexin uptake four days after heterotopic heart transplantation in the abdomen, at a time when histology suggested mild to moderate rejection. The arrow delineates the transplanted heart (tplnt). Right panel depicts the same animal after 10 days of cyclosporine therapy. The arrow points to the same region. The lack of radioannexin uptake correlates with histologic evidence of decreased rejection.

blood pool, or by absence of tracer in the cardiac region. Right ventricular EMB was performed within 4 days of imaging; in 9 patients the biopsy was performed within 24 hours of imaging. EMB specimens were interpreted for the evidence of transplant rejection and apoptosis by TUNEL staining (positive in the later stages of apoptosis) and activation of caspase-3. Caspase-3 is present in cells just prior to expression of PS, the binding site for annexin V.

Planar images in anterior and left anterior oblique views one hour after annexin V injection revealed presence of blood pool in all patients due to the slower clearance of radiolabeled annexin V in humans ($t_{1/2} \cong 15$ minutes) as compared with animal studies with N_2S_2 labeled annexin V ($t_{1/2} \cong 3–7$ minutes). Analysis of SPECT images demonstrated no uptake of annexin V in 9 of the 14 patients. EMB in these 9 patients were unremarkable and interpreted as ISHLT grade 0-1A/4. Lack of immunohistochemical evidence of caspase-3 upregulation in EMB confirmed the absence of significant apoptosis and hence allograft rejection in myocardium.

The remaining patients demonstrated variable degrees of ^{99m}Tc-annexin V uptake in the left ventricular myocardium (Figure 2). Reconstruction of the SPECT images as myocardial perfusion scans revealed predominantly non-diffuse and regional uptake in 3 patients and diffuse global uptake in patients. The right ventricular EMB specimens in the 3 patients with non-diffuse annexin-V uptake demonstrated ISHLT grade 2/4 rejection; 2 of these 3 patients also demonstrated intense caspase-3 staining in scattered myocytes, endothelial and interstitial cells. On the other hand, 2 of the 5 patients with positive annexin scans demonstrated diffuse global uptake of radiolabeled annexin V in the myocardium. EMB from these two patients revealed ISHLT grade 3A/4 rejection and severe vascular rejection, respectively. TUNEL-positive nuclei were seen within myocytes, and endothelial cells, with corresponding caspase-3 upregulation and activation. The caspase-3 staining was particularly intense and was observed in almost every endothelial cells in the patient with acute vascular rejection.

Overall, this preliminary patient series demonstrated that patients without histologic evidence of rejection had a negative scan. Similarly, patients with a positive scan had histologically-verified transplant rejection of ISHLT grade 2/4 or higher. Caspase-3 upregulation in the patients with positive annexin-V scan confirmed the specificity of noninvasive detection of apoptotic process. Histologic evidence of apoptosis was observed in both myocytes and non-myocytic cells.

Strauss et al.[46] studied 10 patients, eight males and two females, mean age 56.3 ± 4.2 years, within one year of transplant. Renal and liver uptake of annexin V observed by ROI analysis of the whole body images two hours after injection were 18% and 14% of whole body activity, respectively. The renal activity in patients at two hours was significantly lower than the average value of 40% noted in animal studies using HYNIC-labeled material.[12] At 24 hours whole body images demonstrated minimal renal or liver activity, however, there was a marked amount of tracer excreted in the biliary/GI tract, a known feature of the clearance of the N_2S_2 agent.[46]

These patients demonstrated significantly milder degrees of acute rejection as seen by EMB as compared with Narula's series. Eight patients had ISHLT grade of acute rejection of 1A or less, while there was only one patient with Grade 2 and another with Grade 3A. No patient in this series demonstrated the diffuse or regional uptake of annexin V. Foci of intense uptake (2 or more) were seen in the right ven-

Short Axis

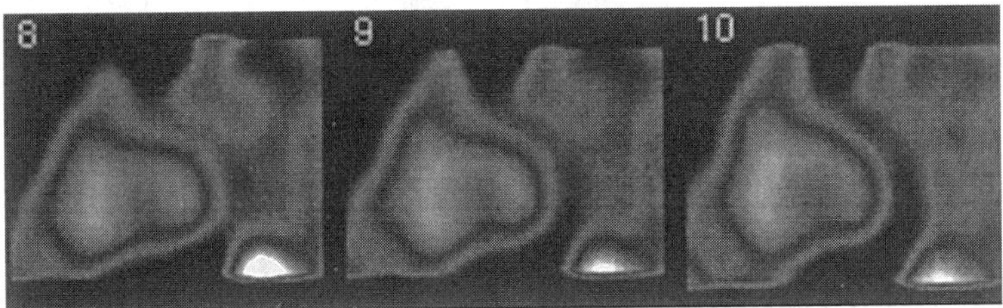

Vertical Long Axis

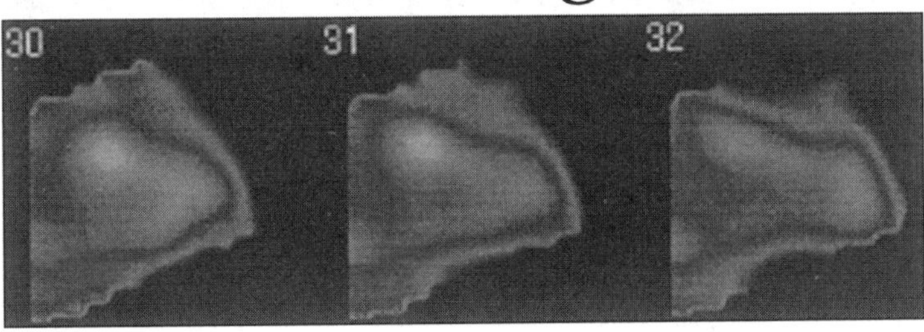

Horizontal Long Axis

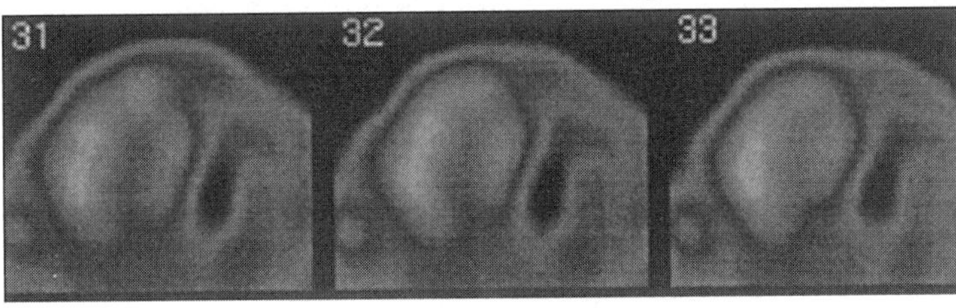

Figure 2. *Noninvasive detection of apoptosis with ^{99m}Tc-AnnexinV imaging in clinical heart transplant rejection.* SPECT imaging was performed 3H after intravenous injection of radiolabeled annexin V in a cardiac allograft recipient. Tomographic images are displayed in short axis (A), vertical long axis (B), and horizontal long axis (C). A diffuse uptake of radiotracer is evident in whole myocardium suggestive of apoptotic process. Endomyocardial biopsy performed within 48H of imaging revealed severe vascular rejection and an evidence of significant endothelial and occasional myocytic apoptosis.

tricular myocardium and right atrium in six of the seven patients with 1A or greater rejection. One of these patients with Grade 1A failed to show any foci of abnormally increased annexin V uptake. In the three patients without histologic evidence of rejection, two revealed complete absence of annexin V uptake while one demonstrated two foci of increased uptake within the right ventricle. These results revealed two striking findings, a) that annexin V uptake maybe overly sensitive with respect to EMB results particularly with lower (subclinical) grades of rejection and b) that apoptosis present in cardiac transplant rejection, particularly in its early stages is truly multifocal.

Analysis of these studies reveals that mild rejection (not requiring therapy) demonstrated small foci of increased uptake within the myocardium as opposed to moderate/severe rejection which was associated with regional or diffuse increased myocardial uptake. These observations of the multiple locations of apoptosis throughout the rejecting myocardium seems to parallel the multifocal as opposed to diffuse nature of mononuclear cell infiltrates and myocyte drop out seen pathologically.[47] In order for annexin V imaging to be useful clinically certain issues need to be addressed, namely, a) standard methods to interpret and quantify annexin V uptake in the heart need to be established, b) definitive identification of the myocardium for correlation with the radionuclide images (using either transmission maps or a myocardial perfusion marker such as thallium-201 to record dual tracer studies) and c) more sophisticated histologic analyses with new more specific markers of cell death such as caspase-3 immunostaining which reflect the earlier stages of rejection.

REFERENCES

1. Seino K, Kayagaki N, Bashuda H, Okumura K, Yagita H. Contribution of Fas ligand to cardiac allograft rejection. *Int Immuno* 1996;8:1347–1354.
2. Laguens RP, Cabeza Meckert PM, San Martino J, Perrone S, Favaloro R. Identification of programmed cell death (apoptosis) in situ by means of specific labeling of nuclear DNA fragments in heart biopsy samples during acute rejection episodes. *J Heart Lung Transplant* 1996;15:911–918.
3. Jollow KC, Sundstrom JB, Gravanis MB, Kanter K, Herskowitz A, Ansari AA. Apoptosis of mononuclear cell infiltrates in cardiac allograft biopsy specimens questions studies of biopsy-cultured cells. *Transplantation* 1997;63:1482–1489.
4. Matiba B, Mariani SM, Krammer PH. The CD95 System and the death of a lymphocyte. *Immunology* 1997;9:59–68.
5. Bergese SD, Klenotic SM, Wakely ME, Sedmak DD, Orosz CG. Apoptosis in murine cardiac grafts. *Transplantation* 1997;63:320–325.
6. Schultz M, Schuurman HJ, Joergensen J, et al. Acute rejection of vascular heart allografts by perforin deficient mice. *Eur J Immunol* 1995;25:474–480.
7. Larsen CP, Alexander DZ, Henrix R, Ritchie S, Pearson TC. Fas-mediated cytotoxicity. *Transplantation* 1995;60:221–224.
8. Nagata S, Golstein P. The Fas death factor. *Science* 1995;267:1449–1456.
9. Thompson BC. Apoptosis in the pathogenesis and treatment of disease. *Science* 1995;267:1456–1462.
10. Kageyama Y, Li X-K, Suzuki S, Suzuki H, Suzuki K, Kazui T, Harada Y. Apoptosis is involved in acute cardiac allograft rejection in rats. *Annuals of Thoracic Surgery* 1998;65:1604–1609.
11. Szaboles MJ, Ravalli S, Mihanov O, Sciacca RR, Michler RE, Cannon PJ. Apoptosis and increased expression of inducible nitric oxide synthase in human allograft rejection. *Transplantation* 1998;65:804–812.
12. Blankenberg FG, Katsikis PD, Tait JF, Davis RE, Naumovski L, Ohtsuki K, Kopiwoda S, Abrams MJ, Darkes M, Robbins RC, Maecker HT, Strauss HW. In vivo detection and imaging of phosphatidylserine expression during programmed cell death. *Proc Natl Acad Sci USA*, 95:6349–6354, May 1998 Medical Sciences.
13. Romisch J, Paques EP. Annexins: Calcium binding proteins of multifunctional importance? *Med Microbiol Immunol* 1991;180:109–126.
14. Rand JR. Annexinopathies—a new class of diseases. *New Engl J Med* 1999;340:1035–1036 (editorial).
15. Bohn H. Placental DNA pregnancy proteins. In: Carcinoembryonic proteins. Lehman FG ed. Vol 1. 1979; pp 289–99. Elsevier, North Holland Biomedical Press.
16. Reutelingsperger C, Hornstra G, Hemker H. Isolation and partial purification of a novel anticoagulant from arteries of human umbilical cord. *Eur J Biochem* 1985;151:625–629.

17. Kaneko N, Matsuda R, Hosoda S, et al. Measurement of plasma annexin V by ELISA in the early detection of acute myocardial infarction. *Clin Chim Acta* 1996;251:65–80.
18. Gidon-Jeangirard C, Solito E, Hofmann A, et al. Annexin V counteracts apoptosis while inducing Ca2+ influx in human lymphocytic T cells. *Biochem Biophys Res Comm* 1999;265: 709–715.
19. Trouvé P, Legot S, Belikova I, et al. Localization and quantification of cardiac annexins II, V, and VI in hypertensive guinea pigs. *Am J Physiol* 1999;276:H1159–H1166.
20. Tait JF, Gibson D, Fujikawa K. Phospholipid binding properties of human placental anticoagulant protein I, a member of the lipocortin family. *J Biol Chem* 1989;264:7944–7949.
21. Tait J, Gibson D. Phospholipid binding of annexin V: Effects of calcium and membrane phosphatidylserine content. *Arch Biochem Biophys* 1992;298:187–191.
22. Dachary-Prigent J, Freyssinet JM, Pasquet JM, Carron JC, Nurden A. Annexin V as a probe of aminophospholipid exposure and platelet membrane vesiculation: a flow cytometry study showing a role for free sulfhydryl groups. *Blood* 1993;81:2554–2565.
23. Tait JF, Cerqueira MD, Dewhurst TA, Fujikawa K, Ritchie JL, Stratton JR. Evaluation of annexin V as a platelet directed thrombus targeting agent. *Thromb Res* 1994;75:491–501.
24. Stratton et al. unpublished data.
25. Koopman G, Reutelingsperger CPM, Kuijten GAM, Keehnen RMJ, Pals ST, vanOers MHJ. Annexin V for flow cytometric detection of phosphatidylserine expression on B cells undergoing apoptosis. *Blood* 84:1415–1420.
26. Boersma AMW, Nooter K, Oostrum RG, Stoter G. Quantification of apoptotic cells with fluorescein isothiocyante labeled annexin V in Chinese hamster ovary cell cultures treated with cisplatin. *Cytometry* 1996;24:123–130.
27. van Heerde WL, de Groot PG, Reutelingsperger CPM. The complexity of the phospholipid binding protein annexin V. *Thromb and Hemostasis* 1995;73:172–179.
28. Zwaal RFA, Schroit AJ. Pathophysiologic implications of membrane phospholipid asymmetry in blood cells. *Blood* 1997;89:1121–1132.
29. Tait JF, Smith C, Wood BL. Measurement of phosphatidylserine exposure in leukocytes and platelets by whole-blood flow cytometry with annexin V. *Blood Cells, Molecules, and Diseases.* 1999;25:271–278.
30. Naito M, Nagashima K, Mashima T, Tsuruo T. Phosphatidylserine externalization is a downstream event of interleukin-1β-converting enzyme family protease activation during apoptosis. *Blood* 1997;89:2060–2066.
31. Fadok VA, Bratton DL, Rose DM, et al. A receptor for phosphatidylserine specific clearance of apoptotic cells. *Nature* 2000;405:85–90.
32. Allen TR, Hunter WJ, Agrawal DK. Morphological and biochemical characterization and analysis of apoptosis. *J Pharm Toxic Method* 1997;37:215–228.
33. van England M, Nieland LJW, Ramaekers FCS, Schutte B, Reutelingsperger CPM. Annexin V-affinity assay: a review on a apoptosis detection system based on phosphatidylserine exposure. *Cytometry* 1998;31:1–9.
34. van den Eijnde SM, Luijsterburg AJM, Boshart L, De Zeeuw CI, van Dierendonck JH, Reutelingsperger CPM, Vermeij-Keers C. In situ detection of apoptosis during embryogenesis with annexin V: from whole mount to ultrastructure. *Cytometry* 1997;29:313–320.
35. Blankenberg FG, Ohtsuki K, Strauss HW. Dying a thousand deaths. Radionuclide imaging of apoptosis. *Quart J Nucl Med* 1999;43:170–176.
36. Vriens PW, Blankenberg FG, Stoot JH, Ohtsuki K, Berry GJ, Tait HW, Strauss, Robbins RC. The use of technetium Tc 99m annexin V for in vivo imaging of apoptosis during cardiac allograft rejection. *J Thorac Cardiovasc Surg* 1998;116:844–853.
37. Kown MH, Van der Steenhoven TJ, Blankenberg FG, Hoyt G, Strauss HW, Robbins RC. Zn2+ blocks cardiac allograft apoptosis as measured by Annexin V imaging. *Circulation* 2000;102-Suppl: III-228–III-232.
38. D' Arceuil H, Rhine W, de Crespigny A, Yenari M, Tait JF, Strauss HW, Engelhorn T, Kastrup A, Moseley M, Blankenberg FG. ^{99m}Tc annexin V imaging of neonatal hypoxic brain injury. *Stroke* 2000;31:2692–2700.
39. Blankenberg FG, Robbins RC, Stoot JH, Vriens PW, Berry GJ, Tait JF, Strauss HW. Radionuclide imaging of acute lung transplant rejection with annexin V. *Chest* 2000;117:834–840.
40. Ogura Y, Krams SM, Martinez OM, Kopiwoda S, Higgins JP, Esquivel CO, Strauss HW, Tait JF, Blankenberg FG. Radiolabeled annexin V imaging: diagnosis of allograft rejection in an experimental rodent model of liver transplantation. *Radiology* 2000;214:795–800.
41. Belhocine TZ, Hustinx R, Jerusalem G, Fassotte MF, Duysinx B, Quaden C, Rigo P. 99m Tc rh-annexin V (Apomate™) as a marker of apoptosis resulting from chemotherapy: preliminary results. *J Nucl Med* 2000;41:263P (abstract).

42. Hofstra L, Liem IH, Dumont EA, Boersma HH, van Heerde WL, Doevendans PA, De Muinck E, Wellens HJ, Kemerink GJ, Reutelingsperger CP, Heidendal GA. Visualisation of cell death in vivo in patients with acute myocardial infarction. *Lancet* 2000;356:209–212.
43. Strauss HW, Narula J, Blankenberg FG. Radioimaging to identify myocardial cell death and probably injury. *Lancet* 2000;356:180–181.
44. Palojoki E, Saraste A,Eriksson A, Pulkki K, Kallajoki M, Tikkanen I, Volpio-Pulkki LM. Prolonged cardiomyocyte apoptosis in the remote myocardium is associated with left ventricular remodeling after experimental myocardial infarction. *J Am Coll Cardiol* 2000;35:Suppl A P39 (abstract).
45. Narula J, Acio ER, Fyfe B, Narula N, Samuels LE, Wood D, Fitzpatrick JM, Guerraty A, Tomaszewski JE, Snyder G, Kelly C, Blankenberg F, Strauss HW. Phase-I ^{99m}Tc-annexin-V imaging study in heart transplant rejection: can noninvasive detection of apoptosis in cardiac allografts rejection obviate the need for endomyocardial biopsy? *Circulation* 2000;102:II-769.
46. Strauss HW, Kown M, Hunt S, Robbins RS, Stafford-Cecil S, Tait JF, Blankenberg FG. Blood clearance of 99mTc N_2S_2 annexin V in human subjects. *J Nucl Med* 2000;41:149P (abstract).
47. Billingham MR, Cary NRB, Hammond ME, et al. A working formulation for the standardization of nomenclaure in the diagnosis of heart and lung rejection: heart rejection study group. *J Heart Transplant* 1990;9:587–593.

18. DETECTION OF CARDIAC ALLOGRAFT REJECTION BY NONINVASIVE IMAGING OF LYMPHOCYTE INFILTRATION

Ke Lin, MD

J. James Frost, MD, PhD
Division of Nuclear Medicine, Department of Radiology The Johns Hopkins University School of Medicine Baltimore, Maryland

The pathologic basis of acute cardiac transplant rejection is the infiltration of activated lymphocytes into the myocardium.[1] With increasing severity of allograft rejection, the perivascular lymphocytic infiltration evolves into multifocal and more diffuse infiltration. The interstitial lymphocytic aggregates are subsequently associated with myocyte damage in higher grades of rejection. The damage is the result of activated lymphocytes attacking the myocytes, and this effect may persistent after the rejection has started to resolve. In severe degrees of rejection, diffuse inflammatory process becomes more aggressive and is associated with vasculitis, interstitial hemorrhage, and edema. Therefore, the acute rejection is graded as IA, IB, II, IIIA, IIIB, and IV based on the pattern and degree of lymphocytic infiltration and the degree of inflammation within the myocardium.[1]

The infiltration of lymphocytes represents an ongoing rejection episode and the degree of infiltration is reduced after immunosuppressive treatment. Since progressively increasing lymphocytic infiltration determines the severity of rejection, radionuclide detection of magnitude of lymphocytic infiltration may provide a noninvasive basis of management of cardiac allograft recipients.

^{111}IN-LABELED LYMPHOCYTE IMAGING

Autologous lymphocytes can be labeled with a radionuclide and accumulation of these lymphocytes imaged with a gamma camera. The pioneer studies were conducted by Mckillop et al.,[2] Oluwole et al.[3] and Bergmann et al.[4] who demonstrated the feasibility of detecting acute cardiac transplant rejection in animals with ^{111}In-labeled lymphocytes. Bergmann et al.[4] studied 36 allogeneic and 14 isogeneic heterotopic cardiac transplants in rats. Allogeneic grafts accumulated autologous ^{111}In-lymphocytes, detectable scintigraphically 24 hours after intravenous injection of labeled cells. At the time of peak histologic rejection, the allogeneic grafts demonstrated 9.2 ± 4.8 times more activity than the native hearts. Autoradiography confirmed that graft radioactivity was associated with labeled lymphocytes. In contrast, isogeneic grafts showed no signs of rejection and did not accumulate radioactivity. This technique was further refined in several large animal studies by subtracting blood pool radioactivity.[5,6,7] Eisen et al.[5] evaluated 5 canine heterotopic cardiac allografts with acute rejection scintigraphically every 3 days after administration of ^{111}In-labeled autologous lymphocytes. Correction for labeled lymphocytes circulating in the blood pool, but not actively sequestered in the allografts was accomplished by administering 99mTc-labeled autologous erythrocytes and employing a validated blood-pool activity correction technique. Cardiac infiltration of labeled lymphocytes was quantified as percent indium excess (%IE), scintigraphically detectable ^{111}In in the transplant compared with that in blood, and results were compared with those of concomitantly performed endomyocardial biopsy (EMB). Scintigraphic %IE for hearts not undergoing rejection manifest histologically was 0.7 ± 0.4. Percent IE for rejecting hearts was 6.8 ± 4.0 ($P < 0.05$). Scintigraphy detected each episode of rejection detected by biopsy. Scintigraphic criteria for rejection (%IE > 2 s.d. above normal) were not evident in any study in which biopsies did not show rejection. Another study from Eisen et al.[6] showed of 16 heterotopic canine cardiac allografts, scintigraphic criteria of rejection correlated with results of biopsies indicative of rejection with a sensitivity of 94% and and a specificity 100%. The quantity of lymphocytes infiltrating the graft also correlated closely with the histological severity of rejection.[7]

In a pilot study in humans, 8 patients were studied at the time of routine biopsy an average of 4.5 months after cardiac transplantation.[8] Autologous lymphocytes were isolated and labeled with ^{111}In. Forty-eight to 72 hours later, patients underwent planar scintigraphic imaging. Myocardial accumulation of labeled lymphocytes was quantified as indium excess (IE). Two of 4 patients with biopsy grade 0 or IA rejection had no excess accumulation of labeled lymphocytes. The other two patients with biopsy grade 0 or IA had an average indium excess of 0.13 ± 0.04 (SD), which may actually have represented a true positive scintigraphic examination, since the whole myocardium was interrogated. All 4 patients with biopsy grade IB rejection had increased accumulation of labeled lymphocytes with an indium excess of 0.18 ± 0.06, P = 0.06 compared with all patients with grade 0 or IA biopsies) (see Figures 1 and 2). However, the patients with higher grades of rejection were not studied and hence the clinical utility of this technique remains questionable.

Furthermore, the complexity of direct labeling lymphocytes for image detection of acute heart rejection makes this technique impractical. The isolation and labeling of the lymphocytes with ^{111}Indium is time-consuming, taking an average of 4 to 4.5 hours. Also, it is possible that the cells will be injured during the procedure and the risk of contamination with viruses or bacteria is increased. There is a 48 to 72 hour delay in image acquisition. Finally, patients with cardiac transplants often

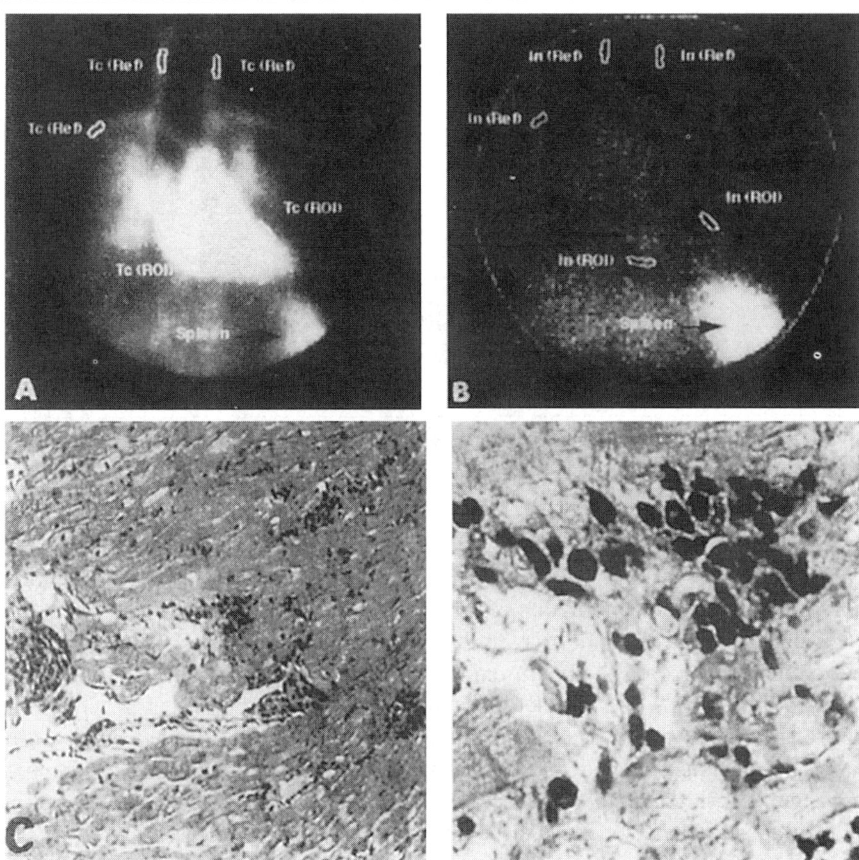

Figure 1. A, Tc-99m red blood cell image from a patient. Regions are drawn in the vasculature and over the myocardium. B, Corresponding ^{111}In-labeled lymphocytes image with the regions copied from the Tc-99m image. Quantitative analysis showed an accumulation of ^{111}In-labeled lymphocytes in the myocardial region of interest. C, Endomyocardial histological specimen from the same patient shows grade IB rejection with diffuse, perivascular, and interstitial infiltrations of large lymphocytes. Left, Low-power magnification; right, high-power magnification. (Courtesy of Dr. Steven R. Bergmann, Columbia University, New York)

have low white cell counts and lymphocytopenia and labeling an inadequate numbers of lymphocytes could lead to false-negative scintigraphic results.

SOMATOSTATIN RECEPTOR IMAGING

Somatostatin and Its Receptors

Somatostatin is a naturally occurring neuropeptide that was discovered in the hypothalamus.[9] It is a cyclic polypeptide composed of either 14 or 28 linked amino acids. It is also present in cerebral cortex, brainstem, gastrointestinal tract, and

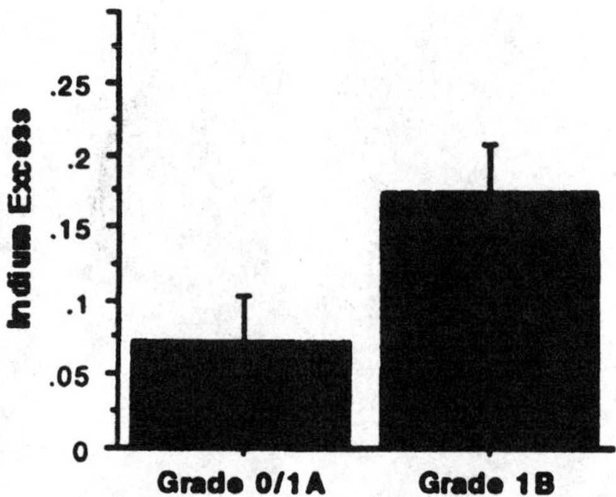

Figure 2. Indium excess by histological grade of rejection. P = 0.06 by a t test. Although the difference between the groups was of borderline statistical significance, the scintigraphic approach actually may be more sensitivity than biopsy. (By courtesy of Dr. Steven R. Bergmann, Columbia University, New York)

pancreas. The principle physiological function of somatostatin is inhibition of growth hormone release and suppression of insulin and glucagon secretion.

Somatostatin receptors have been identified on neuroendocrine cells throughout the body including the brain, pituitary, pancreas, gastraintestinal tract, adrenal medulla and thyroid.[9,10] A variety of tumors of neuroendocrine origin and some tumors of nonneuroendocrine origin express a very high level of somatostatin receptors.[11] These tumors include carcinoids, small and nonsmall cell lung carcinomas, gastrinoma, insulinoma, breast cancer, meningioma, lymphoma, etc.

Five subtypes of somatostatin receptors have been identified on human cells.[11] All subtypes are structurally related to membrane glycoproteins and mediate their effects via inhibition of adenylyl cyclase activity. The somatostatin-receptor complexes produce the following effects:[11,12] a) inhibition of secretion of hormones that are involved in tumor growth; b) antiproliferative effect on tumor cells; c) inhibition of angiogenesis; d) modulation of lymphocyte function.

Activated lymphocytes and monocytes also express a high level of somatostatin receptors.[13,14] Hiruma et al.[14] demonstrated the specific binding of ^{125}I-somatostatin of mitogen-activated human lymphocytes and human leukemic cells increased linearly with the cell numbers and was suppressed by non-iodinated somatostatin. Over 95% of the cell populations bound fluorescent somatostatin on a fluorescence-activated cell sorter and no distinct predilection was found among certain lymphocyte subpopulations and somatostatin receptor-positive cells. Scatchard analysis showed a single class (low affinity) of binding site on mitogen-activated lymphocytes and two classes (high and low affinity) of specific binding sites on leukemic cells.

Somatostatin Receptor Imaging in Tumor Detection

Somatostatin receptor imaging using ^{111}In-octreotide (an 8-amino-acid analog of somatostatin) has shown utility and cost effectiveness in management of patients with somatostatin receptor-positive tumors.[11] In addition to defining receptor status,

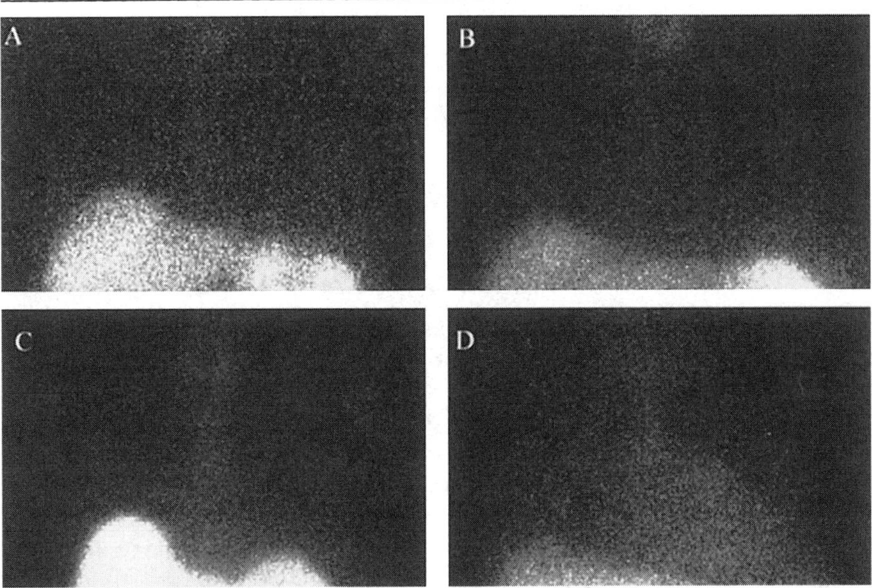

Figure 3. Anterior planar images of the chest of a normal subject 24 hrs after injection of ^{111}In-octreotide to (A) and a patient with grade II rejection (B), grade IIIA rejection (C), and grade IIIB rejection (D). Little activity is seen in the region of the heart in the normal subject. Cardiac activity (relative to lung activity) increases with the grade of rejection. The most intense tracer uptake is seen in grade IIIB rejection (D). Intense tracer activity is seen in the liver and spleen which is normal for the distribution of the ^{111}In-octreotide.

somatostatin receptor imaging is useful in tumor localization and defining tumor resectability. It also has an extremely high sensitivity (up to 100%) in detection of diseases mediated by activated lymphocytes or lymphocytes with malignant differentiation[11] such as lymphomas, Graves' ophthalmopathy,[15] Wegener's granulomatosis, and rheumatoid arthritis etc. Somatostatin analogs are effectively used for inhibition of tumor growth or control of symptoms in patients with cancer.[11,16,17] ^{111}In-octreotide and other new radioactive compounds are currently being evaluated for treatment of somatostatin receptor positive tumors and have showed promising results.[17]

Somatostatin Receptor Imaging in Detection of Acute Heart Rejection

It has been reported that activated lymphocytes express a high level of somatostatin receptors.[14] Based on this finding, we performed a pilot study on heart transplant recipients using somatostatin receptor imaging and showed increased somatostatin-receptor binding in the cardiac grafts with acute rejection.[18] In this study, 2 normal subjects and 8 cardiac transplant recipients with biopsy-proven acute rejection of grades IA to IIIB were recruited. Anterior planar images of the chest were obtained 4 hrs, 24 hrs, 48 hrs and 72 hrs after injection of ^{111}In-octreotide. All 8 patients with acute rejection showed increased tracer uptake in the cardiac graft (Figure 3 and Table 1). By using nonparametric Kendall rank order correlation

Table 1. Mean Heart/Lung uptake ratio of ^{111}In-octreotide vs rejection grade at 24 hrs after injection

Grade (No. of pts)	normal (2)	IA (1)	II (2)	IIIA (3)	IIIB (2)
H/L ratio*	1.33	1.40	1.52	1.71	2.06

* $\tau = 0.806$, $P = 0.0025$ by nonparametric Kendall rank correlation analysis.

analysis of the heart/lung (H/L) uptake ratios at a 24 hr time point, there was a positive significant correlation between the heart/lung ratio increase and the increase of rejection grade with a $\tau = 0.806$ and a $P = 0.0025$.

Grade III rejection indicates more extensive myocardial damage, is associated with increased morbidity and mortality, and needs to be treated by increasing the immunosuppression. Our results showed the mean H/L ratio was 1.47 in patients with rejection grade of II or lower while it was 1.85 in patients with grade III rejection at 24 hrs after injection ($P = 0.029$). This finding could be useful in the management of cardiac transplantation.

The revision of the 1990 working formation for cardiac allograft rejection suggests that the use of grade II classification of rejection be abandoned because it overlaps with Grades IA and IB.[19] Our results may support a new grading system that has only three grades; grade 0, low grade, and high grade rejection. In this new grading system, grade IA, IB and II are classified as low grade rejection and do not require increasing immunosuppression therapy, while grade III and grade IV are grouped into high grade rejection. The degree of ^{111}In-octreotide localization in the cardiac graft was shown to be proportional to the extent of infiltrating lymphocytes. This needs to be further confirmed in a larger patient population as well as in an *in vitro* cellular level.

Other Potential Applications of Somatostatin Receptor Imaging

The clinical potential of somatostatin receptor imaging goes beyond the detection of acute cardiac rejection. Possible future applications include detection of acute rejection in lung, heart-lung, or pancreas transplantation since similar pathologic changes are present during rejection and the ^{111}In-octreotide distribution in these organs in normal conditions is very low. Another potential application of this technique is to detect coexisting transplantation-related malignancies at an early stage.[11,20]

Because of its antiproliferative effect on lymphocytes,[12] somatostatin may be used as an immunosuppressive agent to control graft rejection. Interestingly, the somatostatin analog octreotide has shown its potential utility in treatment of chronic rejection (graft vessel disease) and in prevention of restenosis following angioplasty in patients with coronary artery disease. The mechanism of this effect seems to be through direct antiproliferative effects and down regulation of growth factors during the vascular remodeling phase.[21]

GALLIUM-67 IMAGING

Gallium-67 (^{67}Ga) has been successfully used in localization of inflammatory lesions as well as granulomatous disease.[22] The exact mechanism of ^{67}Ga localization is still not known. The first step of ^{67}Ga accumulation in inflammatory lesions is due to increased blood flow and hyperpermeability of the capillaries at sites of inflammation and infection. ^{67}Ga may then bind to lactoferrin in the extracellular space. Neutrophils, lymphocytes, and monocytes may accumulate a small fraction of ^{67}Ga.

Bochi et al.[23] studied 24 patients who were managed exclusively with EMB for routine rejection surveillance (group 1) and 10 patients (group 2) who were followed primarily with gallium 67 scintigraphy after the second week postoperation. Their results showed there was significant decrease in the use of EMB, tricuspid regurgitation, and cost in group 2 patients. The 1-year survival rate was 75% and 80% for patients managed with routine EMB and gallium-67 scintigraphy screening, respectively. In another study,[24] multiple gallium scans were performed in 15 heart transplanted children within a postoperative period of up to 50 months. Nineteen episodes of rejection were detected by clinical evaluation. Gallium was positive in 12 (6 EMB positives) and negative in 7 (2 EMB negatives). Patients with negative gallium-67 scans in sequential studies had a favorable clinical outcome. There was total agreement between gallium scans and pathology results in all patients. These results suggest that gallium-67 cardiac scintigraphy can be successfully used in the follow-up of heart transplanted patients for the evaluation of rejection. Prospective randomized studies with larger patient samples are needed to further evaluated the potential of this method of management.

SUMMARY

Myocardial infiltration of activated lymphocytes is a central feature of cardiac transplant rejection. While there is no single test that is best for the detection of acute rejection, it is feasible to detect acute rejection by quantifying myocardial accumulation of lymphocytes through direct labeling with ^{111}In of autologous lymphocytes, somatostatin receptor detection or Galium-67 localization. Functional imaging of lymphocytes and evaluation of their aggressiveness using ^{111}In-octreotide is very promising. Its advantages are: 1) low background activity; 2) it uses a native peptide so the procedure can be repeated without an adverse reaction; 3) early image acquisition is possible; and 4) it detects the ongoing process of rejection. The application of somatostatin analogs in the management of cardiac transplantation is just beginning.

REFERENCES

1. Billingham ME, Cary NRB, Hammond ME, et al. A working formulation for the standardization of nomenclature in the diagnosis of heart and lung rejection: Heart Rejection Study Group. J Heart Transplant 1990;9:587–593

2. Mckillop JH, Wallwork J, Reitz BA, et al. The use of 111-In-labeled lymphocyte imaging to evaluate graft rejection following cardiac transplantation in dogs. Eur J Nucl Med 1982;7:162–165
3. Oluwole S, Wang T, Fawaz R, Satake K, et al. Use of Indium-111 labeled cells in measurement of cellular dynamics in experimental cardiac allograft rejection. Transplantation 1981;31:51–55
4. Bergmann SR, Lerch RA, Carlson EM, et al. Detection of cardiac transplant rejection with radiolabeled lymphocytes. Circulation 1982;65:591–599
5. Eisen HJ, Rosenbloom M, Laschinger JC, et al. Detection of rejection of canine orthotopic cardiac allografts with indium-111 lymphocytes and gamma scintigraphy. J Nucl Med 1988;29:1223–1229
6. Eisen HJ, Eisenberg SB, Saffitz JE, et al. Noninvasive detection of rejection of transplanted heart with indium-111-labeled lymphocytes. Circulation 1987;75:868–876
7. Eisenberg SB, Eisen HJ, Sobel BE, et al. Sensitivity of scintigraphy with ^{111}In-lymphocytes for detection of cardiac allograft rejection. J Surg Res 1987;45:549–555
8. Rubin PJ, Hartman JJ, Hasapes JP, et al. Detection of cardiac transplant rejection with ^{111}In-labeled lymphocytes and gamma scintigraphy. Circulation 1996;94(S II):II-298–II-303
9. Reichlin S. Somatostatin (First of two parts). N Engl J Med 1983;309:1495–1501
10. Reichlin S. Somatostatin (Second of two parts). N Engl J Med 1983;309:1556–1563
11. Krenning EP, Kwekkeboom DJ, Pauwels S, Kvols LK, Reubi JC. Somatostatin Receptor Scintigraphy. Nucl Med Ann pp1–50 Freeman LM ed. Raven Press, Ltd., New York 1995
12. Payan DG, Goetzl EJ. Modulation of lymphocyte function by sensory neuropeptides. J Immunol 1985;135:783s–786s
13. Bhathena SJ, Louie J, Schechter GP, et al. Identification of human mononuclear leukocytes bearing receptors for somatostatin and glucagon. Diabetes 1981;30:127–131
14. Hiruma K, Koike T, Nakamura H, et al. Somatostatin receptors on human lymphocytes and leukemia cells. Immunology 1990;71:480–485
15. Kahaly G, Gorges R, Diaz M, et al. Indium-111-pentetreotide in Graves' disease. J Nucl Med 1997;39:533–536
16. Lamberts SWJ, Van Der Ley AJ, De Herder WW, Hofland LJ. Drug therapy: Octreotide. N Engl J Med 1996;334:246–254
17. Lin K, Nguyen BD, Ettinger DS, Chin BB. Somatostatin receptor scintigraphy and somatostatin therapy in the evaluation and treatment of malignant thymoma. Clin Nucl Med 1999;1:(in press)
18. Lin K, Po S, Kasper ED, Frost JJ. Detection of cardiac allograft rejection by somatostatin receptor imaging. J Nucl Med 1998;39(Supl):3P
19. Sumarna SK, Kennedy A, Ciulli F, Locke TJ. Revision of the 1990 working formation for cardiac allograft rejection: the Sheffield experience. Heart 1998;79:432–436
20. Taniguchi S, Cooper DKC, Chaffin JS, Zuhdi N. Primary bronchogenic carcinoma in recipients of heart transplants. Transpl Int 1997;10:312–316
21. Weckbecker G, Pally C, Raulf F, et al. The somatostatin analog octreotide as potential treatment for re-stenosis and chronic rejection. 1997;29:2599–2600
22. Bekerman C, Nayak SM. Gallium imaging In: Henkin RE et al. (eds). Nuclear Medicine, pp. 1597–1618, Mosby-Year Book, Inc., St. Louis, 1996
23. Bochi EA, Mocelin AO, Moraes AV, et al. Comparison between two strategies for rejection detection after heart transplantation: Routine endomyocardial biopsy versus gallium-67 cardiac imaging. Transpl Proc 1997;29:586–588
24. Soares J, Jr., Azeka E, Albertotti D, et al. Gallium-67 scintigraphy in children submitted to heart transplantation. J Nucl Med 1998;39(Supl):57P

19. DETECTION OF CARDIAC ALLOGRAFT REJECTION BY TARGETING EXPRESSION OF ACCESSORY MOLECULES ON CARDIAC MYOCYTES

Mitsuaki Isobe, MD
Department of Cardiovascular Medicine Tokyo Medical and Dental University Toyko, JAPAN

PATHOPHYSIOLOGY OF REJECTION AND INDUCTION OF CELL SURFACE MOLECULES

Acute cardiac allograft rejection is a complicated immune process principally mediated by T cells. T cells recognize major histocompatibility complex (MHC) antigens via direct or indirect pathways. MHC antigens also play a major role in the destruction of transplanted tissues by activated killer T cells. Since MHC antigens and minor histocompatibility antigens participate in many facets of organ rejection, they are called transplantation antigens. MHC antigens are divided into two categories, class I and class II, according to their function and structure. Normal, nucleated, nonlymphoid cells such as cardiac myocytes express low levels of MHC class I antigens and do not express detectable levels of class II antigens.[1,2] MHC class II antigens are normally expressed only on lymphoid cells and antigen-presenting cells such as macrophages, monocytes, vascular endothelial cells, and Langerhans cells in the skin. Once T cells are activated, they produce a variety of cytokines that act on cells in the vicinity. Among these cytokines, interferon γ is a potent cytokine that induces expression of MHC and other adhesion molecules not only on the antigen-presenting cells but also on non-professional antigen-presenting cells including vascular endothelial cells and cardiac myocytes[3,4] (Figure 1). Though their physiological roles in the induction process are still obscure, class II antigens are key elements in the control of the immune response to antigen, functioning in the recognition of antigen by regulatory T lymphocytes.

Correspondence to Mitsuaki Isobe, MD, Department of Cardiovascular Medicine Graduate School of Medicine, Tokyo Medical and Dental University, 1-5-45 Yushima, Bunkyo-ku, Tokyo 113-8516 JAPAN. Business phone: +81-3-5803-5951, Fax: +81-3-5803-0238, E-mail: isobemi.med3@med.tmd.ac.jp

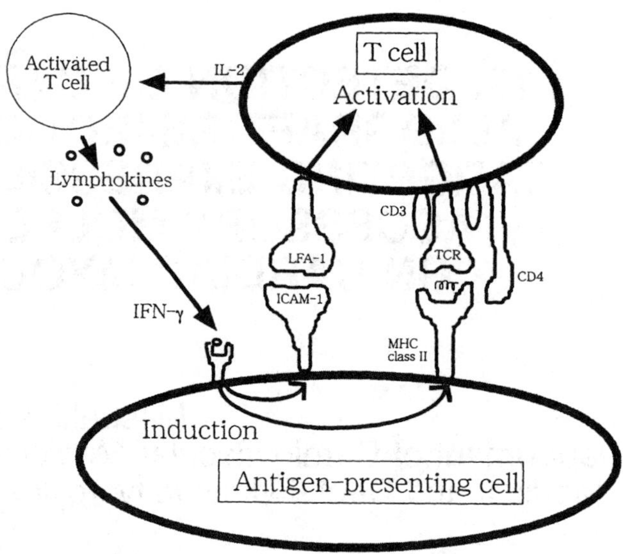

Figure 1. Activation of T cells and production of lymphokines in the process of organ rejection. Interferon (IFN)-γ promotes induction of major histocompatibility complex (MHC) antigens and adhesion molecules in association with acute rejection. ICAM = intercellular adhesion molecule, LFA = lymphocyte function-associated antigen, and TCR = T cell receptor.

Adhesion of T cells to vascular endothelium is necessary for T cell activation. The intercellular adhesion molecule (ICAM)-1 is one of the adhesion molecules that mediates T cell adhesion to antigen-presenting cells and activates T cells.[5] ICAM-1 is important in both afferent recognition and efferent cytotoxic immune responses.[6,7] Interaction of ICAM-1 and its counter receptor, lymphocyte function-associated antigen (LFA)-1, is required for optimal T cell function in vitro, including T cell-mediated lysis, mixed lymphocyte reaction, B cell help, and antigen-induced mitogenesis.[8] We have demonstrated that ICAM-1, working together with LFA-1, plays a central role in the pathophysiology of rejection.[9–11] Short-term blockade of their adhesion results in immunological tolerance to cardiac allografts in a murine model. ICAM-1 is normally expressed on vascular endothelial cells and other antigen-presenting cells.[12] It is, however, induced on a variety of cells in association with organ rejection[13–15] and other inflammatory,[16] immune,[17] and neoplastic disorders[18] (Figure 2). Therefore, ICAM-1 provides an early marker of immune activation and response.

TARGETING CELL SURFACE ANTIGENS FOR THE EARLY DETECTION OF CARDIAC ALLOGRAFT REJECTION

Both class I and class II antigens are induced during cardiac rejection.[19,20] Sell et al. reported a semiquantitative serial analysis of MHC antigen induction in six cardiac allograft recipients.[19] In all six patients, an increase in the level of MHC class II antigen expression, detected by radioimmunoassay, preceded histological evidence

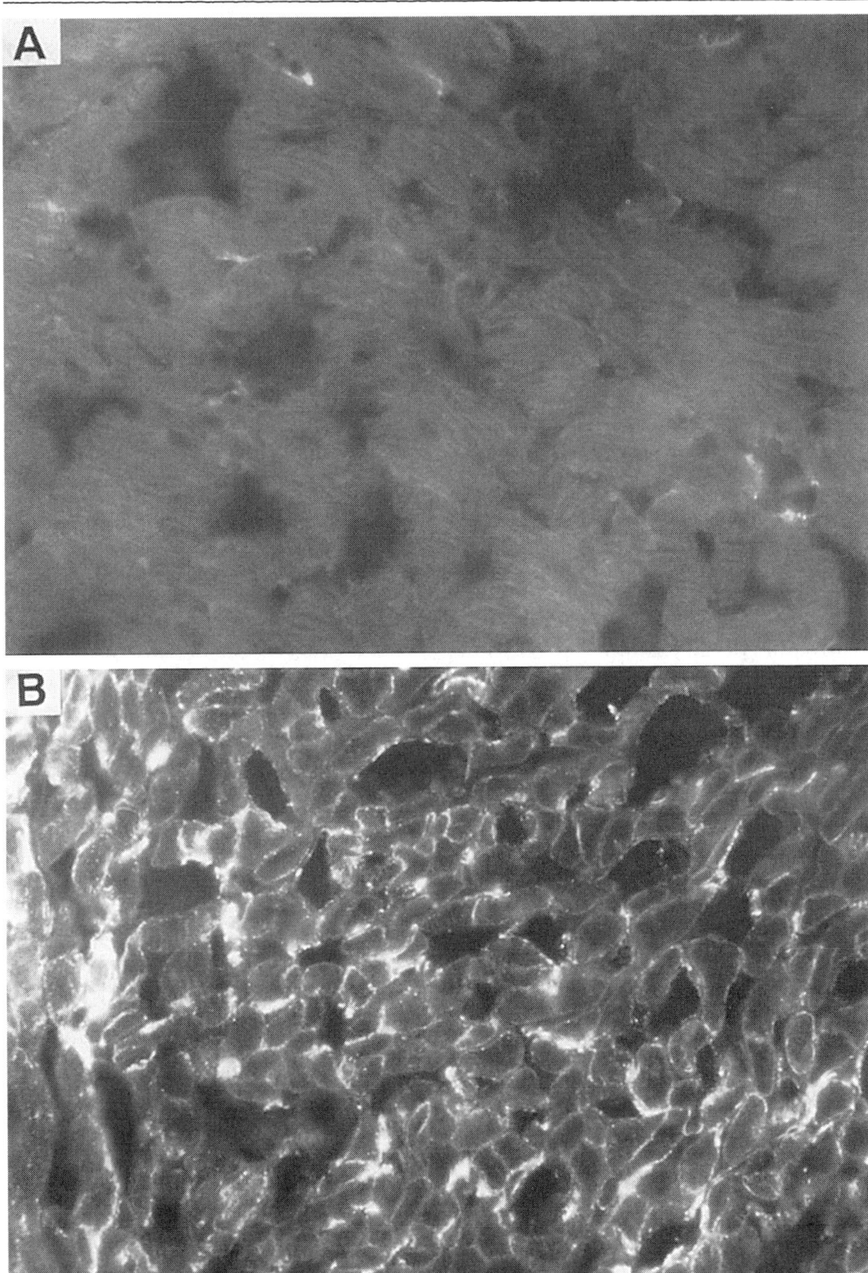

Figure 2. Immunohistochemical study for ICAM-1 in isografted (A) and allografted (B) rat hearts. Allografted heart at 6 days after transplantation showed massive induction of ICAM-1 expression on myocytes. This induction is preceded to development of myocyte necrosis.

of moderate rejection. The expression of class II antigens decreased when rejection abated. Sell et al. also showed this enhancement of MHC class II antigen expression could be normalized by immunosuppressive therapy.

The time course of ICAM-1 induction is similar to that of MHC class II antigens. Taylor et al. demonstrated increased expression of adhesion molecules, MHC class I, and DR antigen on capillary endothelium during acute rejection. ICAM-1 was induced on the myocardial membrane and intercalating discs.[21] Tanio et al. showed a strong correlation between ICAM-1 expression and the histological severity of cardiac rejection in 25 cardiac transplant patients.[22] Experimental studies in the rat heart in our laboratory revealed enhanced expression of ICAM-1 as well as MHC class II antigens on the capillary endothelium from day 4 after transplantation in parallel with the development of mononuclear cell infiltration.[23]

Clinical and experimental organ transplantation models have shown a dramatic difference in ICAM-1 and MHC class II antigen expression between normal and rejecting tissue.[19,23] Immunohistological observations have demonstrated that ICAM-1 or MHC class II antigen induction precedes the occurrence of extensive cellular infiltration. It is reasonable that these molecules could be an early marker of immune activation and response. Generally, the detection and localization of ICAM-1 or MHC class II antigens require staining of samples obtained by tissue biopsy. Noninvasive imaging of these molecular markers would facilitate diagnosis and localization of immunological and inflammatory diseases and could be used in determining therapy and intervention. We tested these hypotheses in experimental cardiac and renal allograft transplantation models.

SCINTIGRAPHIC DETECTION OF MHC CLASS II ANTIGENS

Experimental design

A murine model of abdominal heterotopic heart transplantation was employed. Allografts from C3H/He (H-2^k) donors were transplanted into BALB/c (H-2^d) recipients. C57BL/6 (H-2^b, IE^-) were also used as recipients in some experiments. Donor aorta and pulmonary artery were microvascularly anastomosed to recipient's abdominal aorta and inferior vena cava, respectively.[1,24,25] A cohort of recipient mice were treated daily with intramuscular injection of cyclosporine. Since these two strains are fully immune incompatible, donor hearts are rejected within 10 days in non-treated recipients. Anti-MHC class II antigen monoclonal antibodies[26,27] were labeled with ^{111}In using a chelating agent (DTPA).[28] Approximately 100 μCi of ^{111}In-DTPA-antibody was injected into the tail vein of the recipient mice 24 hours before scintigraphy. After scintigraphy, each mouse was sacrificed for histological examination and determination of radioactive biodistribution.

Imaging and Biodistribution of Radiolabeled Monoclonal Antibody

Regardless of the time after transplantation and the presence or absence of cyclosporine, the level of radiotracer uptake reflected the histological severity of

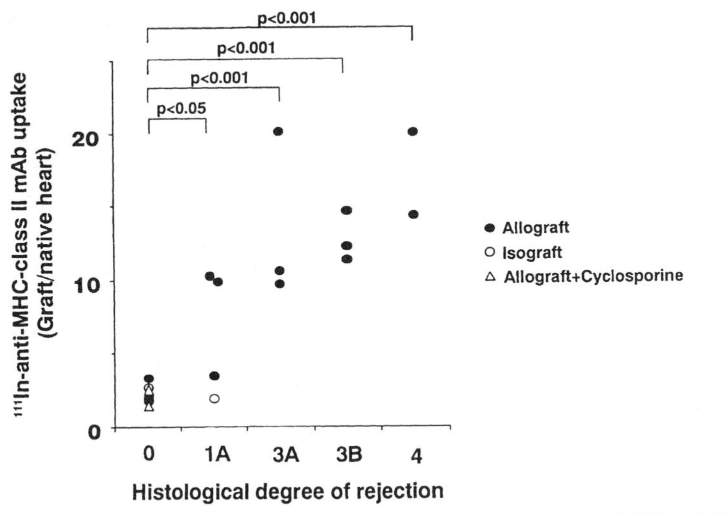

Figure 3. Comparison of graft/native heart ^{111}In-labeled anti-MHC class II monoclonal antibody (mAb) uptake versus histologic severity of rejection. Radiotracer uptake in mice with rejecting cardiac allografts is significantly greater than that in mice with nonrejecting grafts. (Reproduced with permission of the American Heart Association from *Circulation* 1992; 85, 738–746).

rejection[29] (Figure 3). The radiotracer uptake in the mice whose grafts were normal was always less than that in the mice whose grafts showed histological evidence of rejection. As shown in Figure 3, all allografts with myocyte necrosis (rejection grade > III) showed a graft to native heart ratio greater than 10, while allografts without rejection showed a ratio of less than 4. Allografts exhibiting grade IA rejection; i.e. only those with focal interstitial infiltrates but without necrosis, showed significant increases in radiotracer uptake and were clearly visible in the scintigraphic image (Figure 4A and 4B). Only heart grafts with evidence of rejection demonstrated an increase in uptake.

Specificity of Antibody Uptake

In this experiment, anti-donor and anti-recipient type MHC class II antigen monoclonal antibodies were tested to analyze the specificity of the antibody uptake. In the BALB/c (H-2^d) donor-C57BL/6 (H-2^b, IE^-) recipient combination, the rejecting heart was clearly visualized by radiolabeled anti-IE^d (donor type class II antigen) monoclonal antibody (Figure 4B). However, uptake was not detected by either radiolabeled anti-IA^k (recipient type class II antigen) monoclonal antibody (Figure 4C) or that of irrelevant specificity. Rejecting allografts were imaged only by anti-class II antibody against donor antigen but not by that against recipient antigen. These results ruled out the possibility of nonspecific accumulation of antibody in rejection sites.

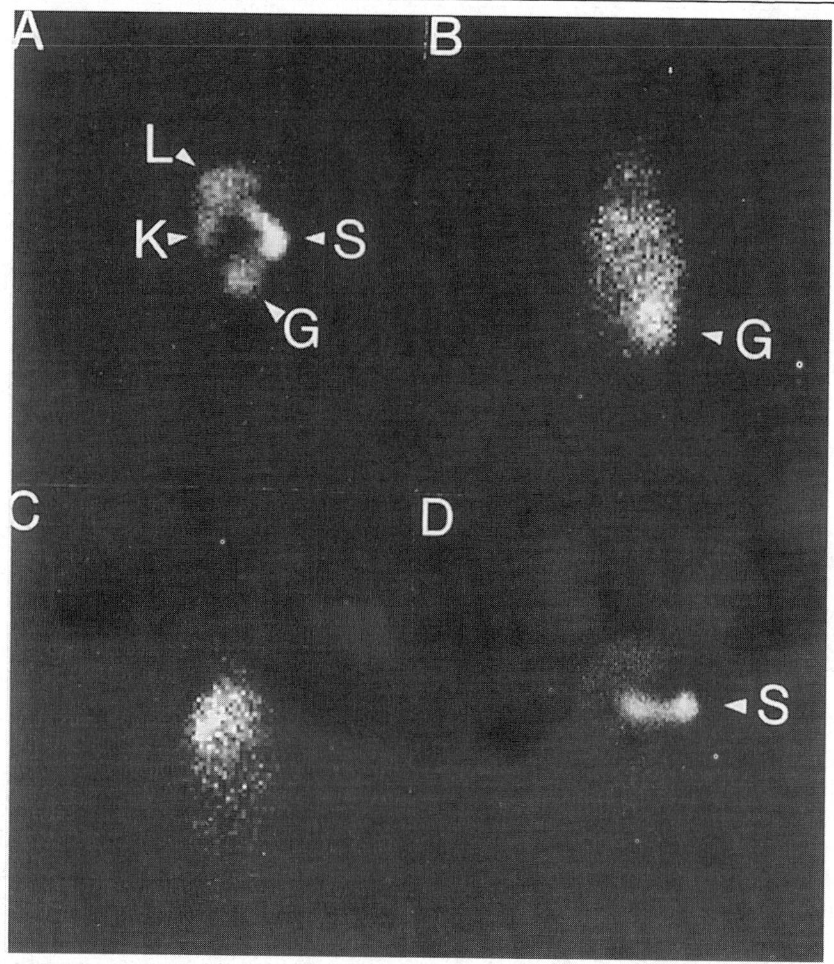

Figure 4. Scintigrams after injection of ^{111}In-labeled anti-MHC class II antigen monoclonal antibodies in mice transplanted with cardiac allografts. A: A mouse with moderately rejected cardiac allograft (grade 3A) 5 days after transplantation imaged with antibodies reactive with both donor and recipient MHC class II antigens. Rejecting allograft (G) is clearly visualized. B: A mouse with moderately rejected allograft at 7 days injected with an antibody reactive with donor class II antigen but not with recipient antigen. The rejecting allograft is clearly visualized by this antibody. C: A mouse with moderately rejected allograft 8 days after transplantation injected with an antibody reactive with recipient class II antigen but not with donor antigen. Rejected allograft is not visualized by this antibody. D: A mouse with non-rejecting cardiac allograft at 7 days treated with cyclosporine imaged with same radiotracer as the mouse shown in panel A. Non-rejecting allograft is not visualized. K = kidney, L = liver, and S = spleen. (Reproduced with permission of the American Heart Association from *Circulation* 1992; 85, 738–746).

SCINTIGRAPHY USING ANTIBODY AGAINST THE CONSTANT REGION OF MHC CLASS II ANTIGEN

MHC class II antigens are comprised of polymorphic and monomorphic determinants. Morphologically they are called variable and constant regions, respectively.

A striking feature of MHC antigen is its extensive genetic and morphological polymorphisms.[30] This design allows self-nonself discrimination in immune recognition. The polymorphic determinant is different for each individual; the monomorphic determinant is shared by all individuals. Therefore, antibodies to the variable region are donor-class II antigen specific and those to the constant region recognize both donor and recipient class II antigens. In our murine experiment, we used monoclonal antibodies against the donor-specific variable region of MHC class II antigens to demonstrate the specificity of the antibody uptake. However, from a practical point of view, the need for donor-specific monoclonal antibody may limit the utility of the scintigraphy when applied to clinical cases. Antibodies that react with monomorphic determinants of HLA class II antigens are potentially better imaging agents, since this would allow a single imaging agent to be applied to all patients irrespective of donor HLA haplotype.

This possibility was evaluated using a monoclonal antibody that reacts with the constant region of rat IA (class II) antigens.[31] DA rat hearts were transplanted into PVG recipient rats. Two monoclonal antibodies were used: Ox6, which reacts with the constant region of rat class II antigen,[32,33] and F17-23-6, which reacts with the variable region of DA class II antigen ($RT1^a$) but not with that of PVG class II antigen ($RT1^c$).[3] Monoclonal antibodies were iodinated with ^{123}I, and animal experiments were performed as described above.

Accumulation of ^{123}I labeled Ox6 well reflected the presence or absence of rejection in all cases, whether isograft or allograft, treated or untreated. The ratios of graft to blood percent injected dose per gram of wet tissue (% dose/g) in rats with grade IA and IB rejection and grade IIIA and IIIB rejection were greater than the ratios in rats with non-rejecting grafts. This ratio increased progressively with time after transplantation in rats with non-treated allografts. Rejecting allografts were identified in the scintigraphic images after injection of labeled Ox6 monoclonal antibody (Figure 5). Rats injected with ^{123}I-labeled F17-23-6 showed scintigraphic results similar to the Ox6-injected rats. The major differences seen were low background radioactivity and relatively higher radiotracer uptake in the rejected grafts. Because of this difference, the scintigraphic images of rejecting grafts were more distinct than those obtained by Ox6 monoclonal antibody injection.

These results show that scintigraphy using a monoclonal antibody against the constant region is as sensitive as that against a polymorphic determinant. Thus, this method of anti-MHC class II scintigraphy should simplify clinical application of this technique because a single radiolabeled antibody could work irrespective of patient's HLA haplotype

EFFECTS OF IMMUNOSUPPRESSION ON MHC CLASS II SCINTIGRAPHY

Because cardiac transplantation patients normally receive chronic immunosuppression therapy, the clinical relevance of this type of scintigraphy rests on whether rejecting hearts undergoing immunosuppression can be imaged by this method. In the experiments described above,[1,29,31] a cohort of mice and rats

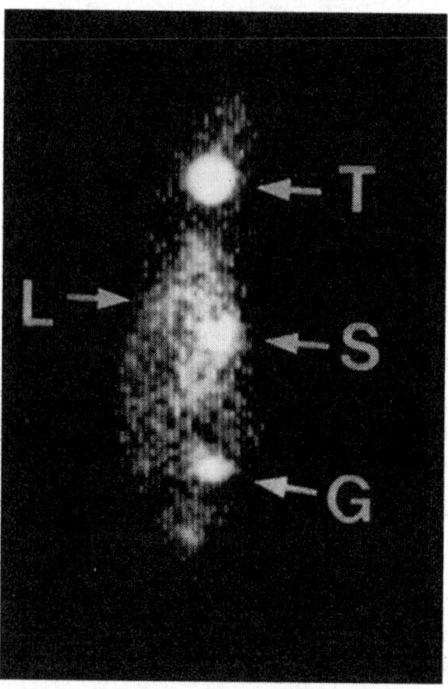

Figure 5. A scintigram after injection of ^{123}I-labeled Ox6 monoclonal antibody. Ox6 is reactive with the constant region of rat MHC class II antigens. An allografted rat without treatment 5 days after transplantation. Unequivocal accumulation of radiotracer is seen in a rejected heart (grade IB). G = graft, L = liver, S = spleen, T = thyroid. (Reproduced with permission of Mosby-Year Book Inc. from *American Heart Journal* 1994; 127: 1309–17).

were treated with calcineurin inhibitors (cyclosporine or tacrolimus). Cardiac allografts without histological evidence of rejection treated with these immunosuppressants did not show increased radiotracer uptake (Figure 4D). We recently demonstrated significant suppression of interferon-γ as well as IL-2 mRNA in cardiac allografts after treatment with tacrolimus.[34] Because induction of MHC class II antigens and adhesion molecules is almost certainly a consequence of the release of lymphokines such as interferon-γ from infiltrating leukocytes, calcineurin inhibitors are thought to suppress induction of MHC class II antigens and ICAM-1.[2,35]

In another experiment, changes in the uptake of anti-class II monoclonal antibody by immunosuppressive therapy were evaluated in mice transplanted with kidney allografts.[36] Five allografted mice imaged at 3 to 9 days after surgery showed an increase in radiotracer uptake. After 2 weeks of anti-CD3 and cyclosporine therapy, uptake was significantly reduced. After another 2 weeks of cyclosporine treatment, the ratio further decreased. Two weeks after the cessation of treatment, the uptake increased. These changes in radiotracer uptake could be identified on the scintigraphic images (Figure 6). It appears that reduction of monoclonal antibody uptake after 4 weeks of immunosuppressive therapy reflects the reduction of MHC class II antigens by immunosuppression.

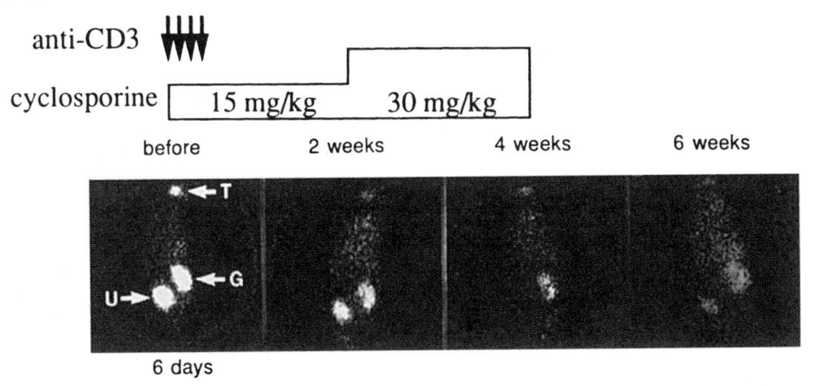

Figure 6. Serial scintigrams in a BALB/c mice transplanted with C3H/He kidney allograft before, during and after immunosuppression. The first scintigraphy was performed 6 days after transplantation. Scintigraphy was repeated every 2 weeks in the same mouse. The mouse was treated with 4-day course of anti-CD3 antibody and 4 weeks of cyclosporine starting after the initial scintigraphy. The fourth scintigraphy was obtained two weeks after the cessation of the treatment. In this mouse model of kidney transplantation, left kidney was replaced with an allograft and right kidney was left intact. Ureter of the allografted kidney was left open in the abdomen. Serial changes in the radiotracer uptake in the transplanted kidney reflect development of rejection and effects of immunosuppressants. G = grafted kidney, T = thyroid, and U = urine. (Reproduced with permission of Springer-Verlag from *Transplant International* 1993; 6:263–269).

EVALUATING CARDIAC ALLOGRAFT REJECTION BY SIMULTANEOUS SCINTIGRAPHY FOR MYOCYTE NECROSIS AND MHC CLASS II EXPRESSION

The induction of MHC antigen preceding moderate rejection is one of the initial events in the immune rejection process. In human cardiac rejection, increased expression of HLA-DR antigen determined by radioimmunoassay of biopsied samples is observed in myocytes prior to development of histologically identifiable myocyte necrosis.[19] Reports from our[1] and other institutes[27,38] have shown that anti-myosin scintigraphy is useful in detecting myocyte necrosis and can be utilized for diagnosing moderate cardiac rejection. Therefore, we hypothesized that dual scintigraphy using anti-myosin and anti-MHC class II antigen monoclonal antibodies labeled with different isotopes would allow detection of early rejection just before myocyte necrosis.

Mice with abdominal heart transplants were studied to determine the validity of our hypothesis.[39] Mice were injected intravenously with 100 μCi each of ^{123}I labeled anti-myosin and ^{111}In labeled anti-MHC class II monoclonal antibody and were sacrificed for gamma counting from 2 to 9 days after transplantation. Uptake of ^{111}In-labeled anti-MHC class II monoclonal antibody increased from the fourth day after transplantation, however, that of ^{123}I-labeled anti-myosin monoclonal antibody appeared only 9 days after transplantation (Table 1). The difference between MHC class II antigen induction and development of myocyte necrosis could be identified by gamma counting after simultaneous injection of two radiotracers.

Table 1. Uptake of ^{123}I anti-myosin and ^{111}In anti-MHC class II monoclonal antibodies after simultaneous administration of the two radiotracers. (Reproduced with permission from *Acta Cardiologica* 1996; 51:515–520)

Mouse no.	Days after transplantation	^{123}I antimyosin*	^{111}In anti-MHC class II*	Histology
1	3	1.3	1.4	0
2	4	2.0	12.0	1A
3	6	1.8	12.8	1A
4	7	1.8	8.1	1B
5	9	4.3	10.2	3A

* Ratio of graft to native heart radioactivity measured by gamma counting of excised organs.

Because of the spill of gamma emission of ^{111}In in the window of ^{123}I, we could not perform imaging in this experiment. To overcome this problem, appropriate radioisotopes such as ^{131}I and ^{99m}Tc that allow clear separation of uptake should be investigated to visualize this difference in uptake

ICAM-1 SCINTIGRAPHY

The detection of ICAM-1 induction should be able to provide an early and specific marker of immune activation associated with acute rejection. This hypothesis was tested using heterotopic cardiac transplantation models.[23,40] DA rat hearts were transplanted into PVG recipient rats. Anti-rat ICAM-1 monoclonal antibody was labeled with ^{111}In using DTPA. This radiotracer was injected 1 day prior to data acquisition.

Rejecting allografts without treatment showed increased radiotracer uptake and could be identified on the images as early as 5 days after transplantation[23] (Figure 7), and uptake accelerated with time after transplantation. In contrast, non-rejecting cardiac allografts and isografts did not show specific uptake as late as 12 days after transplantation. Mildly rejecting allografts, with mononuclear cell infiltration but without significant myocyte necrosis, could be identified scintigraphically, and the level of radiotracer uptake reflected the histological severity of rejection (Figure 8). All allografts with mild, moderate, or severe rejection showed intense and unequivocal accumulation of radiotracer. The allografted rats treated with tacrolimus did not show a significant increase in uptake as late as 22 days after transplantation.

This accumulation of radiotracer in allografted hearts was not nonspecific, since accumulation of ^{111}In-labeled monoclonal antibody of isotype-matched irrelevant specificity was not detected in the rejecting allografts. However, higher accumulations of this radiotracer were noted in the lungs and liver in normal rats as well as in the rats with rejecting hearts. This uptake could be partly due to specific antigen recognition and could cause high background uptake when this type of scintigraphy is applied to clinical orthotopic cardiac transplantation.

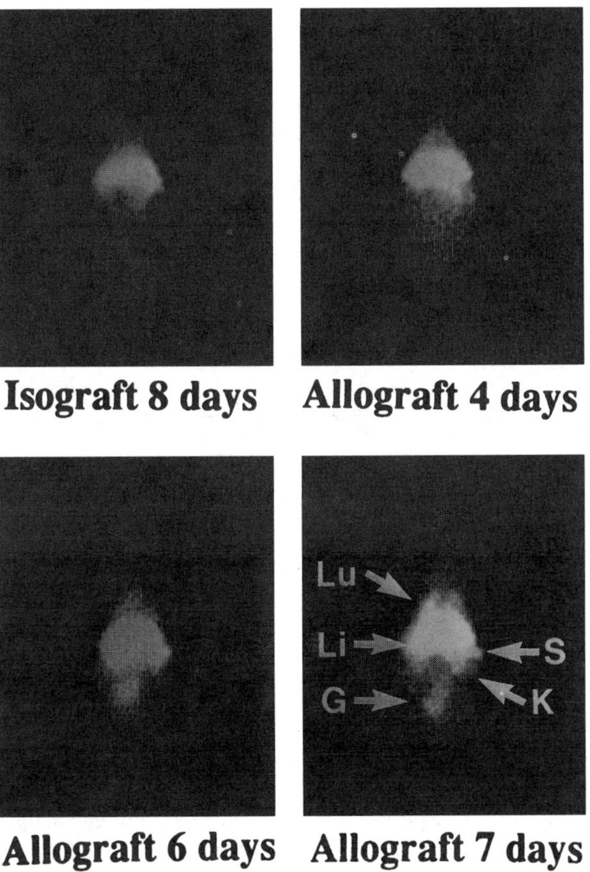

Figure 7. Scintigrams after injection of ^{111}In-anti-ICAM-1 monoclonal antibody in rats with cardiac allografts. An isograft (top, left) or nonrejected allograft 4 days after transplantation (grade 0 rejection) is not imaged (top, right). Rejecting allografts (G) at day 6 (bottom, left) (grade 1A), and day 7 (bottom right) (grade 4) are clearly visualized in the scintigrams (arrows). L = kidney, Li = liver; Lu = lung, and S = spleen.

CLINICAL RELEVANCE OF ACCESSORY MOLECULE DETECTION

We demonstrated that the induced MHC class II antigens and ICAM-1 resulting from cardiac rejection can be visualized *in vivo* by radioimmunoscintigraphy. Anti-ICAM-1 monoclonal antibody or antibodies to the constant region of MHC class II antigens can be applied to the imaging of rejection irrespective of donor haplotype. This noninvasive method is sensitive for detecting early rejection and could allow quantitative assessment of rejection. The possibility of staging cardiac rejection[39] and imaging kidney rejection[37] has also been shown. Since the induction of class II antigens and ICAM-1 occurs not only in the rejecting heart but also in the rejecting kidney,[13,14] liver,[41] and pancreas,[42] this scintigraphic method is potentially useful in detecting rejection in these organs.

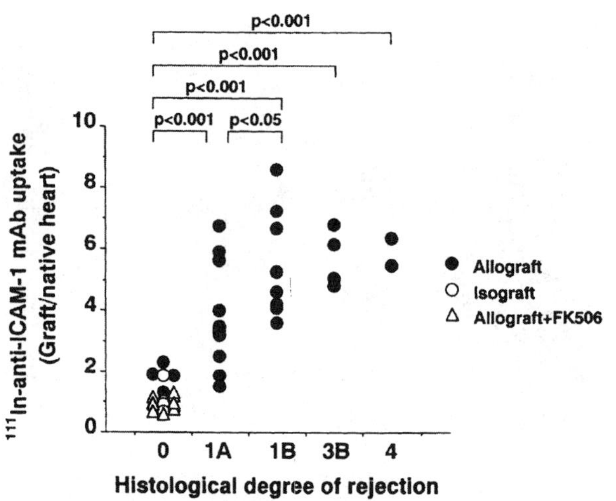

Figure 8. Comparisons of graft/native heart ^{111}In-anti-ICAM-1 monoclonal antibody uptake versus histologic severity of rejection. Radiotracer uptake in allografts with grades 1A, 1B, 3B and 4 rejection is significantly greater than that in rats with nonrejecting grafts. (Reproduced with permission of the American College of Cardiology from *Journal of the American College of Cardiology* 1995, 26: 793–799).

There are several problems inherent to this type of scintigraphy. It is possible that infection and ischemic myocyte damage could cause induction of ICAM-1 and MHC class II antigens. Differentiation between these complications after transplantation and cardiac rejection using this technology may prove difficult. Differences in distribution of the normal expression of MHC class II antigens between rodents and large animals including humans must also be considered. The vascular endothelium normally expresses certain amounts of MHC class II antigens in large animals but not in mice.[43] Since 1B rejections are not usually treated clinically, this method of scintigraphy may be too sensitive in this respect. However, reliable noninvasive clinical tests for detecting early rejection would be beneficial. Because none of the cardiac allografts without histological evidence of rejection in our series of animal experiments showed increased radiotracer uptake, the frequency of endomyocardial biopsy could be reduced with this scintigraphic method.

REFERENCES

1. Isobe M, Haber E, Khaw BA. Early detection of rejection and assessment of cyclosporine therapy by indium-111 antimyosin imaging in mouse heart allografts. *Circulation.* 1991;84:1246–1255.
2. Koene RAP, de Waal RMW, Bogman MJJT. Variable expression of major histocompatibility antigens: Role in transplantation immunology. *Kidney Int.* 1986;30:1–8.
3. Milton AD, Fabre JW. Massive induction of donor-type class I and class II major histocompatibility complex antigens in rejecting cardiac allografts in the rat. *J Exp Med.* 1985;161:98–112.
4. Skoskiewicz MJ, Colvin RB, Schneeberger EE, Russell PS. Widespread and selective induction of major histocompatibility complex-determined antigens in vivo by γ interferon. *J Exp Med.* 1985;162:1645–1664.
5. Dustin ML, Rothlein R, Bhan AK, Dinarello CA, Springer TA. Induction by IL 1 and interferon-

gamma: tissue distribution, biochemistry, and function of a natural adherence molecule (ICAM-1). *J Immunol.* 1986;137:245–254.

6. Makgoba MW, Sanders ME, Ginther LG, Gugel EA, Dustin ML, Springer TA, Shaw S. Functional evidence that intercellular adhesion molecule-1 (ICAM-1) is a ligand for LFA-1-dependent adhesion in T cell-mediated cytotoxicity. *Eur J Immunol.* 1988;18:637–640.
7. Springer TA. Adhesion receptors of the immune system. *Nature.* 1990;346:425–433.
8. Makgoba MW, Sanders ME, Shaw S. The CD2-LFA-3 and LFA-1-ICAM pathways: relevance to T-cell recognition. *Immunol Today.* 1989;10:417–422.
9. Isobe M, Yagita H, Okumura K, Ihara A. Specific acceptance of cardiac allograft after treatment with anti-ICAM-1 and anti-LFA-1. *Science.* 1992;255:1125–1127.
10. Isobe M, Ihara A. Tolerance induction against cardiac allograft by anti-ICAM-1 and anti-LFA-1 treatment: T cells respond to in vitro allostimulation. *Transplant Proc.* 1993;25:1079–1080.
11. Isobe M, Suzuki J, Yamazaki S, Horie S, Okubo Y, Sekiguchi M. Assessment of tolerance induction to cardiac allograft by anti-ICAM-1 and anti-LFA-1 monoclonal antibodies. *J Heart Lung Transplant.* 1997;16:1149–1156.
12. Pober JS, Gimbrone Jr MA, Lapierre LA, Mendrick DL, Fiers W, Rothlein R, Springer TA. Overlapping patterns of activation of human endothelial cells by interleukin 1, tumor necrosis factor and immune interferon. *J Immunol.* 1986;137:1893–1896.
13. Cosimi AB, Conti D, Delmonico FL, Preffer FI, Wee S, Rothlein R, Faanes R, Colvin RB. In vivo effects of monoclonal antibody to ICAM-1 (CD54) in nonhuman primates with renal allografts. *J Immunol.* 1990;144:4604–4612.
14. Nakai K, Taylor F, Isobe M. Time course and localization of intercellular adhesion molecule-1 induction in kidney allograft in mice. *Transplant Proc.* 1994;26:349–353.
15. Faull RJ, Russ G. Tubular expression of intercellular adhesion molecule-1 during renal allograft rejection. *Transplantation.* 1989;48:226–230.
16. Wegner CD, Gundel RH, Reilly P, Haynes N, Letts LG, Rothlein R. Intercellular adhesion molecule-1 (ICAM-1) in the pathogenesis of asthma. *Science.* 1990;247:456–459.
17. Hale LP, Martin ME, McCollum DE, Nunley JA, Springer TA, Singer KH, Haynes BF. Immunohistologic analysis of the distribution of cell adhesion molecules within the inflammatory synovial microenvironment. *Arthritis Rheum.* 1989;32:22–30.
18. Johnson JP, Stade BG, Holzmann B, Schwable W, Riethmuller G. De novo expression of intercellular-adhesion molecule 1 in melanoma correlates with increased risk of metastasis. *Proc Natl Acad Sci USA.* 1989;86:641–644.
19. Sell KW, Tadros T, Wang YC, Hertzler G, Knopf WD, Murphy DA, Ahmed-Ansari A. Studies of major histocompatibility complex class I/II expression on sequential human heart biopsy specimens after transplantation. *J Heart Transplant.* 1988;7:407–418.
20. Carlquist JF, Hammond ME, Yowell RL, O'Connell JB, Anderson JL. Correlation between class II antigen (DR) expression and interleukin-2-induced lymphocyte proliferation during acute cardiac allograft rejection. *Transplantation.* 1990;50:582–588.
21. Taylor PM, Rose ML, Yacoub MH, Pigott R. Induction of vascular adhesion molecules during rejection of human cardiac allografts. *Transplantation.* 1992;54:451–457.
22. Tanio JW, Basu CB, Albelda SM, Eisen HJ. Differential expression of the cell adhesion molecules ICAM-1, VCAM-1, and E-selectin in normal and posttransplantation myocardium. Cell adhesion molecule expression in human cardiac allografts. *Circulation.* 1994;89:1760–1768.
23. Ohtani H, Strauss HW, Southern JF, Miyasaka M, Tamatani T, Sekiguchi M, Isobe M. Intercellular adhesion molecule-1 induction: a sensitive and quantitative marker for cardiac allograft rejection. *J Am Coll Cardiol.* 1995;26:793–799.
24. Corry RJ, Winn HJ, Russell PS. Primary vascularized allografts of heart in mice. *Transplantation.* 1973;16:343–350.
25. Ono K, Lindsey ES. Improved technique of heart transplantation in rats. *J Thorac Cardiovasc Surg.* 1969;57:225–229.
26. Oi VT, Jones PP, Goding JW, Herzenberg LA, Herzenberg LA. Properties of monoclonal antibodies to mouse Ig allotypes, H-2, and Ia antigens. *Cur Top Microbiol Immunol.* 1978;81:115–120.
27. Ozato K, Mayer N, Sachs DH. Hybridoma cell lines secreting monoclonal antibodies to mouse H-2 and Ia antigens. *J Immunol.* 1980;124:533–540.
28. Khaw BA, Mattis JA, Melincoff G, Strauss HW, Gold HK, Haber E. Monoclonal antibody to cardiac myosin: imaging of experimental myocardial infarction. *Hybridoma.* 1984;3:11–23.
29. Isobe M, Narula J, Strauss HW, Khaw BA, Haber E. Imaging the rejecting heart: In vivo detection of MHC class II antigen induction. *Circulation.* 1992;85:738–746.
30. Peterson PA, Rask L. Genes and antigens of the HLA-D Region, in Solheim BG, Moeller E, Ferrone S (ed): HLA class II antigens. A comprehensive review of structure and function. Berlin, Springer-Verlag, pp 1–13.

31. Isobe M, Southern JF, Yazaki Y. Scintigraphic detection of early cardiac rejection by 123I-labeled monoclonal antibody directed against monomorphic determinant of MHC class II antigens. *Am Heart J.* 1994;127:1309–1317.
32. Barclay AN, Mayrhofer G. Bone marrow origin of Ia-positive cells in the medulla rat thymus. *J Exp Med.* 1981;153:1666–1671.
33. Barclay AN. The localization of populations of lymphocytes defined by monoclonal antibodies in rat lymphoid tissues. *Immunology.* 1981;42:593–600.
34. Isobe M, Suzuki J, Yamazaki S, Horie S, Okubo Y, Maemura K, Yazaki Y, Sekiguchi M. Regulation by differential development of Th1 and Th2 cells to peripheral tolerance to cardiac allograft induced by blocking ICAM-1 and LFA-1. *Circulation.* 1997;96:2247–2253.
35. Nelson PA, Kawamura A, Akselband Y, Peattie DA, Aldape RA, Harding MW. Effects of immunosuppressive drugs on cytokine gene transcription studied by message amplification phenotyping (mapping) polymerase chain reaction. *Transplant Proc.* 1991;23:2867–2869.
36. Isobe M. Scintigraphic imaging of MHC class II antigen induction in mouse kidney allografts: a new approach to noninvasive detection of early rejection. *Transplant Int.* 1993;6:263–269.
37. Allen MD, Tsuboi H, Togo T, Eary JF, Gordon D, Thomas R, Reichenbach DD. Detection of cardiac allograft rejection and myocyte necrosis by monoclonal antibody to cardiac myosin. *Transplantation.* 1989;48:923–928.
38. Johnson LL, Cannon PJ. Antimyosin imaging in cardiac transplant rejection. *Circulation.* 1991;84(3 Suppl):I273–I279.
39. Isobe M, Sekiguchi M. Staging of cardiac rejection by simultaneous administration of 123I-antimyosin and ^{111}In-anti MHC class II antibodies. *Acta Cardiologica.* 1996;51:515–520.
40. Isobe M, Ohtani H, Yagita H, Okumura K, Strauss HW, Yazaki Y. Detection of cardiac rejection in mice by radioimmune scintigraphy using ^{123}iodine-labeled anti-ICAM-1 monoclonal antibody. *Acta Cardiologica.* 1993;48:235–243.
41. Adams DH, Hubscher SG, Shaw J, Rothlein R, Neuberger JM. Intercellular adhesion molecule 1 on liver allografts during rejection. *Lancet.* 1989;2:1122–1125.
42. Steiniger B, Klempnauer J, Wonigeit K. Altered distribution of class I and class II MHC antigens during acute pancreas allograft rejection in the rat. *Transplantation.* 1985;40:234–239.
43. Pescovitz M, Thistlethwaite JJ, Auchincloss HJ, Ilsars ST, Sharp TG, Terrill R, Sachs DH. Effects of class II antigen matching on renal allograft survival in miniature swine. *J Exp Med.* 1984; 160:1495–1508.

20. ALGORITHMS FOR MANAGEMENT OF HEART TRANSPLANT REJECTION BASED ON SURVEILLANCE OF MYOCARDIAL DAMAGE BY ANTIMYOSIN ANTIBODY IMAGING

Manel Ballester MD*,
Ignasi Carrió† MD, Jagat Narula MD, PhD‡
*Department of Cardiology, Lleida University Lleida, Spain; †Department of Nuclear Medicine Hospital de Sant Pau, Barcelona, Spain
‡Heart Failure/Transplantation Center, Hahnemann University Hospital, Philadelphia, Pennsylvania

Endomyocardial biopsy remains the only reliable diagnostic tool to detect acute allograft rejection (see Chapters 9,13)[1–2]. Biopsies are performed serially after transplantation, especially during the initial months. Immunosuppressive treatment is augmented when myocyte damage is detected by biopsy. Biopsy-based patient management is widely used and has been associated with very good long-term survival.[3] However, there are significant limitations of endomyocardial biopsy. These include high procedural cost, a small but definite morbidity, and dwindling yield in obtaining adequate myocardial samples after the first year of transplantation. In addition, sampling error of the biopsy to detect acute rejection remains a major problem since myocardial expression of acute rejection is not a diffuse but rather a patchy. Rarely, patients who die of acute rejection demonstrate foci of myocardial damage and inflammation which can be seen surrounded by large areas of apparently intact myocardium.[4,5]

Noninvasive assessment of myocardial damage is possible by imaging with radiolabeled monoclonal antimyosin antibodies that bind specifically to the heavy chain of cardiac myosin. When injected intravenously, myocardial uptake of these highly specific antibodies only occurs in irreversibly necrotic myocytes that have lost the integrity of their sarcolemma and have exposed their intracellular myosin.[6,7] Evaluation using this antibody technique allows detection of focal and diffuse muscle cell damage throughout the myocardium.[8–14] Detection of diffuse myocardial necrosis secondary to rejection through uptake of ^{111}In-labeled monoclonal antimyosin antibodies has been reported by several groups[15–22] and may be the most sensitive noninvasive means to identify myocardial necrosis associated with cardiac allograft rejection.[23]

NONINVASIVE DETECTION OF MYOCARDIAL NECROSIS WITH ANTIMYOSIN IMAGING

The hallmark of cellular viability is cell membrane integrity. The concept of using antimyosin antibodies to delineate myocardial necrosis in vivo was based on the fact that normal myocardial cells with intact sarcolemma would not allow antimyosin antibodies to be internalized into the cytosol, where the homologous antigen cardiac myosin exists as natural and major component of the contractile myofibrils. When lesions develop in the sarcolemmal membrane of the myocytes due to different insults, such as ischemic, infective or inflammatory injury, the normally inaccessible intracellular myosin, a highly insoluble protein, becomes exposed to the extracellular milieu. If antimyosin antibodies were present at that time in the extracellular milieu, and if the antibodies were appropriately radiolabeled, then the regions of cell membrane disruption could be scintigraphically visualized as the regions of accumulation of the antimyosin antibodies.

This concept was first demonstrated in a study by Khaw and coworkers[6] using neonatal murine myocytes in primary culture incubated with antimyosin antibody linked covalently to 1 μm diameter polystyrene beads. In this study, normal myocytes with intact cell membranes did not accumulate the antimyosin beads whereas the necrotic myocytes with sarcolemmal disruption aggregated antimyosin beads at the lesion sites. To develop this concept for in vivo imaging, the specificity of antimyosin antibody for the necrotic myocardium was assessed in a canine experimental model of myocardial infarction.[24] A mixture of iodine-125 labeled antimyosin antibody and iodine-131 labeled control immunoglobulin was administered by coronary delivery into dogs with experimental myocardial infarction. After 24 hours of circulation and clearance of the injected materials, the hearts were harvested and uptake of both radiolabeled immunoglobulin species was assessed by gamma scintillation counting. Antimyosin antibody localized in the necrotic myocardial regions with a target to non-taget ratio of 32 : 1 at the center of the necrotic area.

Since visualization of the necrotic area by gamma imaging was the desired outcome of this method, experiments were undertaken using indium-111 labeled antimyosin Fab and were compared with indium-111 labeled nonspecific Fab fragments. The necrotic region was not visualized with nonspecific antibody even five hours after antibody administration, whereas antimyosin enabled visualization of the necrotic areas as early as one to two hours after intravenous administration in the reperfused infarcts. Subsequent experiments revealed that in addition to specificity, a high affinity was equally important for in vivo imaging of necrotic myocardium. Fab fragment of two monoclonal antimyosin antibodies, one with an apparent affinity of $0.5\text{–}1 \times 10^7$ L/mol and the other with a higher apparent affinity of $0.5\text{–}1 \times 10^9$ L/mol were radiolabeled with indium-111 by the identical procedure and administered into dogs with reperfused experimental myocardial infarction. Gamma images acquired at five hours for each monoclonal antibody were obtained.[25] The antibody uptake ratios in regions of interest over the infarct zone and myocardial blood pool area were determined by computer planimetry of the five hour images. The high affinity antimyosin Fab demonstrated ratios of 1.48 ± 0.14 and 1.59 ± 0.20 when radiolabeled with indium or iodine, respectively. However, the uptake ratio with low affinity antimyosin 3H3 Fab was only 0.85 ± 0.11, which did not differ that of a nonspecific control monoclonal antibody. These preclinical studies demonstrated that antimyosin antibody is specific for delineation of acute myocardial necrosis, and that a high affinity antimyosin antibody is required for in vivo visualization of the necrotic regions of the myocardium.

The time interval between tracer administration and effective visualization of the target necrotic myocardial region has been a major concern in potential clinical applicability of the technique. In reperfused canine models, the experimental myocardial infarcts could be visualized relatively soon after the administration of antimyosin Fab, although visualization of nonreperfused infarcts took a longer time. The delay in imaging accrues from the long circulation half-life of antibody that precludes development of optimum target-to-background ratio early after its administration. Therefore, a genetically engineered sFv of the monoclonal antimyosin antibody was developed in an attempt to reduce the residence time of antibody in blood.[26] The antimyosin sFv labeled with technetium-99m enabled earlier visualization of acute reperfused canine myocardial infarcts. However, sFv, a protein with a molecular weight of approximately 20,000 d, may not be able to rapidly localize in sufficiently high concentration in non-reperfused infarcts. Despite this delay in the development of diagnostic images, antimyosin Fab could still reach the infarct center in the myocardium in the non-reperfused infarct model.[27] To address the issue of regional myocardial perfusion versus myocardial antibody uptake, thallium-201 was used as a regional perfusion indicator. When comparing the thallium-201 distribution and antimyosin Fab uptake at 24 hours after intravenous administration, an inverse correlation was found.[27] Maximal antimyosin uptake occurred in regions of maximal regional perfusion deficit as reflected by decrease in thallium activity. The mechanism of localization may be due to the presence of residual blood flow, collateral circulation, venous retroperfusion and diffusion directly from the ventricular cavity. It has to be taken into account that the existing methods of blood flow determination can only detect regional blood flow within 10–20% with confidence.

Some considerations regarding molecule dimensions are relevant to understand myocardial antimyosin Fab uptake. Despite the larger size of antimyosin Fab (30,000 d) relative to sFv, it is still small enough to enter myocytes with sarcolemmal lesions smaller than 80 Å in diameter.[12] For example, lesions caused by complement-complex lysis are approximately 100 Å in diameter and those caused by T cell cytolysis have a diameter of 160 Å. Although the size of antimyosin Fab is approximately 65 × 35 Å, Fab fragments interact directly with its binding site that permits a Fab molecule to interact with an antigen that is smaller than 80 Å, and probably smaller than 50 Å. It is interesting to note that conventional histology cannot demonstrate these lesions until the sarcolemma has become disrupted. Even ultrastuctural examination may not be able to resolve such lesions. For instance, a lesion of 100 Å diameter at 4000× magnification would appear to be approximately 0.003 mm in size on the electron photomicrograph, which would be seen as normal sarcolemma. Since antimyosin Fab can enter the myocardial lesions smaller than 50 Å and its high affinity provides almost instantaneous antigen-antibody binding, the development of high enough contrast between target and background depends mostly on the access rate of the antibody into the target and the clearance rate of the antibody from the background.[12]

ANTIMYOSIN SCINTIGRAPHY FOR DETECTION OF CARDIOVASCULAR DISORDERS WITH MULTIFOCAL OR DIFFUSE MYOCARDIAL NECROSIS

The experiments that demonstrated the concept and feasibility of gamma imaging of myocardial necrosis with antimyosin antibodies were performed using a infarction model which produced focal myocardial necrosis. However, multifocal or diffuse myocardial necrosis is a common pathological substrate in several cardiac disorders such as cardiac transplant rejection and idiopathic or secondary forms of myocarditis. Systemic disorders, such as lupus, pheocromocytoma and polymyositis, also involve the heart. The underlying cardiac pathology may include diffuse myocyte necrosis with or without interstitial infiltration. Various cardiotoxic drugs may also result in diffuse myocardial necrosis. Since antimyosin antibody can reliably identify regions of myocardial necrosis, antimyosin scintigraphy should offer an effective noninvasive diagnostic aid in these disorders.

In Coxsackie B virus,[28] encephalomyocarditis[29,30] and other virus-induced experimental models of myocarditis, diffuse myocardial antimyosin uptake corresponding to diffuse myocardial damage has been observed as early as three days after viral infection. These experiments showed that the heart-to-blood activity ratio per gram reached a maximum level from day 10 to 17, when histological lesions were most extensive and prominent. The heart-to-blood ratios decreased rapidly thereafter as cellular injury decreased and fibrosis became evident.[30] Autoradiographic studies performed concurrently revealed specific antimyosin uptake in the necrotic myocardium.[28] Functional assessment performed during the experiments demonstrated that impairment of the cardiac function in the acute stages of experimental myocarditis correlated significantly with both the severity of myocardial necrosis and the intensity of radiolabeled antimyosin uptake.[29] Diffuse antimyosin uptake in the myocardium has also been demonstrated in an autoimmune myocarditis model developed by immunizing inbred rats with homologous heart homogenates.[31]

The first use of antimyosin antibody imaging for the detection of acute experimental heart transplant rejection was described by Khaw and colleagues in 1981.[32] A follow-up study involved heterotopic transplantation of B10D2 murine hearts to B6AF1 recipients. Antimyosin scintigraphy imaging performed 2 to 15 days after transplantation demonstrated unequivocal intense accumulation of indium labeled antimyosin in rejecting hearts.[33] Acute rejection was confirmed histologically in these experiments by the presence of myocyte necrosis and cellular infiltration. Using a canine model, Addonizio and coworkers[34] demonstrated antimyosin uptake in intrathoracic heterotopic heart allografts undergoing acute rejection. A subset of allografted animals treated with cyclosporine did not show antimyosin localization. When immunosuppression was withdrawn and the grafts were allowed to undergo rejection, the scans in these animals became strongly positive with enhanced myocardial antimyosin uptake. In this study, histopathological examination confirmed the scintigraphic findings of acute rejection.

Active myocarditis may produce heart failure and acute dilated cardiomyopathy. This causal relationship has been well established for certain viral infections.[35–37] It is known that a small percentage of these acute cases may subsequently evolve into a chronic form of dilated cardiomyopathy. The exact percentage of cases of idiopathic dilated cardiomyopathy that results from a previous bout of acute myocarditis or caused by an ongoing inflammatory process is uncertain. To address this problem, Dec and coworkers[38] studied 74 patients with dilated cardiomyopathy, and a global left ventricular ejection fraction less than 45%. The majority of the patients included in the study had heart failure of less than 12 months of duration. Five of these patients had had a previous episode of biopsy-verified myocarditis and then a second episode of heart failure, which suggested reactivation of their disease. Indium-111 antimyosin scans performed in these patients demonstrated positive myocardial antimyosin uptake in 53% of the cases. Of the 39 patients who were antimyosin positive, 11 had histologically verified myocarditis, but 28 patients showed no evidence of myocarditis on biopsy. Using right ventricular histologic findings as the indicator of the presence or absence of myocarditis based on the Dallas histologic criteria, the sensitivity of antimyosin imaging for detecting myocarditis was 85%, and the predictive value of a normal scan was 94%. However, the specificity was only 54%.

This study highlighted that a negative antimyosin scan enables one to reliably predict a negative biopsy for myocardial damage, but a positive scan may be associated with either a positive or a negative biopsy. The paradox to be resolved is whether the discordant results in the foregoing study represented false positive antimyosin scans or whether the antimyosin scan was actually more accurate than the biopsy for detecting diffuse myocardial damage, which might explain the observed low specificity in this disease. It is interesting to note that quantitative analysis of antimyosin uptake calculated as heart to lung ratios in scan positive and biopsy positive patients, as well as in scan positive but biopsy negative patients, has been reported to be similar, suggesting a probable identical underlying pathologic process.[39] Furthermore, Dec et al.[38] observed a higher likelihood and a greater degree of improvement in left ventricular function in patients with abnormal antimyosin scans, regardless of biopsy results. Because spontaneous improvement in cardiac function is a recognized feature of active myocarditis, it seems likely that a subset of discordant antimyosin scan-positive patients with functional improvement had myocarditis, which the right ventricular biopsy failed to detect. Similarly, it has been also shown in patients with dilated cardiomyopathies, that antimyosin scintigraphy may identify sarcolemmal breaches in myofibrillarlytic myocytes, which are small enough to admit antimyosin Fab molecules, but not large enough to result in histologically identifiable necrosis.[12] Narula et al.,[40] have also reported on the utility of antimyosin scans in the assessment of myocarditis that can occasionally present clinically as acute myocardial infarction.

Structural cardiac abnormalities are integral components of many systemic disorders.[41] Cardiac involvement may manifest as electrocardiographic abnormalities, arrythmias, or congestive heart failure. The potential utility of antimyosin scintigraphy for assessing diffuse myocardial necrosis in these conditions is suggested by reports on positive antimyosin scans in Lyme disease,[42] rheumatic fever,[43] and pheochromocytoma.[44]

Drug-induced cardiotoxicity provides an excellent model to assess diffuse myocardial damage over time. Drug and drug metabolite stimulated reactive oxygen metabolism produce histologic damage in the myocytes. Antimyosin studies in patients with adryamicin cardiotoxicity demonstrate that anthracycline-induced diffuse myocardial damage is seen as intense positive antimyosin uptake early in the time course of cardiotoxicity.[45,46] Furthermore, these studies corroborate the concept that antimyosin uptake preceedes appearance of other histologic or clinical criteria of myocardial injury.[45–49] More importantly, these studies show significant antimyosin uptake at intermediate cumulative dose of anthracyclines when left ventricular systolic function is still well maintained.

THE TECHNIQUE OF ANTIMYOSIN ANTIBODY IMAGING

Antimyosin scintigraphy involves adminitration of 0.5 mg of antimyosin Fab-DTPA labeled with 2 mCi of indium-111 by slow intravenous injection. Planar scans are obtained after injection of the radiolabeled antibody using a large field of view camera linked to a dedicated nuclear medicine computer and fitted with a medium energy collimator. A 20% symmetric window is centered on both peaks of indium-111 (173 and 247 KeV) and a preset acquisition time of 10 min is usually used to collect at least 500,000 counts per frame and to have sufficient counting statistics for myocardial uptake quantitation. The time interval to image patients after antibody administration is important. Diagnostic images of positive myocardial antibody uptake can be obtained a few hours after injection, but blood pool activity due to circulating antibody will still be apparent and may hamper quantitation of myocardial activity. The recommended time interval between injection and imaging is 48 hours, which allows complete clearing of circulating antibody.

One anterior and two left anterior oblique views at 40° and 70° are usually acquired. Scans are stored in 128 × 128 frames for subsequent analysis. Single photon emission computed tomography (SPECT) studies can be performed when there is sufficient antimyosin antibody uptake in the myocardium. This technique may be performed after planar imaging and may allow better delineation of regional myocardial uptake after reconstruction of tomograms. Images are acquired over 360° on 64 × 64 matrix frames. Tomograms of the heart along the three main axis are then reconstructed by filtered backprojection.

A quantitative method delineates a region of interest on the heart and regions on the lungs on the anterior view of the thorax.[49] A heart-to-lung ratio is obtained dividing average counts per pixel in the heart by average counts per pixel in the lungs. A cutoff point of >1.55 (2 standard deviation greater than normal value, 1.46 ± 0.04) has been used to define abnormal studies.[50–53] The intraobserver variability of this technique has been shown to be less than 3% while the interobserver variability is less than 6%.[49]

NONINVASIVE DETECTION OF MYOCARDIAL DAMAGE IN CARDIAC ALLOGRAFT REJECTION

We have recently reported a correlation between antimyosin uptake and histologic evidence of allograft rejection in endomyocardial biopsy. Results of 247 biopsies obtained in 52 patients were compared with antimyosin scans performed at the time of biopsy.[21,54] Antimyosin scans were positive in 57 of the 60 (95%) patients showing myocardial damage (ISHLT grade 2 or higher) in their endomyocardial biopsy specimens. On the other hand, antimyosin scans were also abnormal in 32 of the 38 biopsies (84%) that demonstrated interstitial mononuclear infiltration (ISHLT grade 1A or 1B) but lacked evidence of necrosis. Scans were also positive in 92 of 149 (62%) instances with normal biopsies. Despite the high overall rate of scan positivity, the magnitude of myocardial uptake was significantly higher in the patients who had evidence of myocardial damage in their biopsy specimens (heart-to-lung ratio, HLR, 1.95 ± 0.38) compared with those who demonstrated only interstitial infiltration (HLR, 1.88 ± 0.31) or had normal biopsy (HLR, 1.78 ± 0.26) (Figure 1a). Although magnitude of antimyosin uptake increases proportionally with the histologic severity of rejection, the uptake is highly variable and no definite range of antimyosin uptake can be established that corresponds to the high likelihood of detecting histologic evidence of myocyte necrosis.

The discrepancy between biopsies without myocyte damage and the high positive rate of antimyosin imaging suggests a low specificity of scintigraphy when endomyocardial biopsy is used as a gold standard. On the other hand, if antimyosin is used as the gold standard the sensitivity of endomyocardial biopsy for the detection of myocyte damage falls below 30%.[21] The discordance in the detection of myocardial damage by antimyosin imaging and endomyocardial biopsy can be explained by two possible mechanisms. First, since rejection is a patchy process and areas of damage are often surrounded by large areas of apparently normal myocytes, biopsy sampling error becomes a distinct possibility. In acute myocarditis, which is histologically similar to rejection, the maximum sensitivity of endomyocardial biopsy has been estimated to be only 33%.[14,55–57] Second, rejection may also be associated with myocyte apoptosis may not be associated with inflammation and not detected by light microscopic examination.[58–61] In a recent study,[62] apoptosis was detected, both by immunoelectrophoresis and TUNEL staining, in explanted hearts from cardiac allograft recipients who died of rejection. Apoptosis was also identified by TUNEL staining in 22 of 40 biopsies (55%) performed after transplantation. Five of nine patients with positive antimyosin scans and no evidence of myocyte necrosis at biopsy showed apoptosis, thus providing an additional mechanism for damage which may be detected by the antimyosin scan.[62]

MYOCARDIAL DAMAGE ASSOCIATED WITH REJECTION OCCURS AS A CONTINUOUS PROCESS AND ITS RESOLUTION INDICATES TOLERANCE TO THE ALLOGRAFT

Antimyosin studies are almost always positive during the first month after transplantation and reflect myocardial damage from ischemic injury.[16] The natural course of rejection-related myocardial damage can be assessed through serial antimyosin studies. Our study demonstrated that the heart-to-lung ratio of antimyosin antibody uptake at 1–4 months, 4–11, 12–23 and >24 months gradually declined from 1.93 ± 0.3, 1.73 ± 0.23, 1.65 ± 0.22 to 1.58 ± 0.2 (Figure 1b).[21]

Analysis of sequential studies in the same patients suggests that the phenomenon of allograft rejection is a continuous process and that evolution of antimyosin

(a)

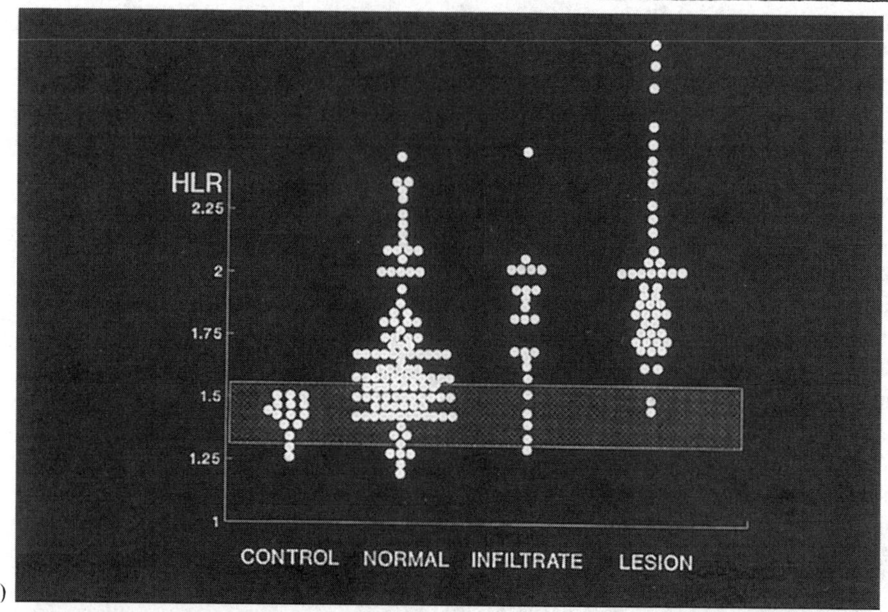

(b)

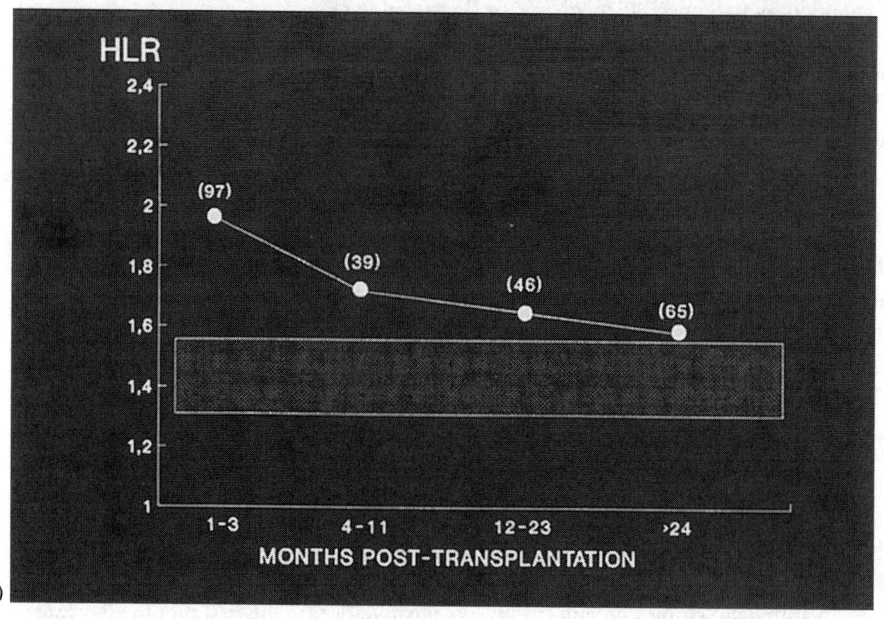

uptake may reflect net myocardial damage resulting from a baseline rejection activity and development of tolerance to graft.[63] Resolution of antimyosin uptake may represent the development of partial immunological tolerance to graft. Such an evolving trend differs substantially from the abrupt histologic evidence of acute rejection observed in endomyocardial biopsy interspersed among intervals of normal

Figure 1. Radiolabeled antimyosin antibody imaging for the detection of myocardial damage associated with cardiac allograft rejection. Antimyosin uptake was semiquantitatively calculated as a heart-to-lung ratio (HLR). Horizontal box describes normal range of antibody uptake represented as maximum of mean HLR + 2 SD detected in normal volunteers.[49] (A) Highly variable antimyosin uptake is observed in allograft recipients. The abnormal uptake occurs in almost all patients when endomyocardial biopsy demonstrated evidence of myocardial damage and interstitial infiltration. However, the abnormal uptake was also observed in 80% of patients with isolated when biopsy showed only interstitial infiltration and in 60% of patients with normal biopsy specimens. Note, that the magnitude of antimyosin uptake increases with increasing severity of histological rejection. (B) The magnitude of antimyosin antibody uptake gradually decreases after transplantation. The rate of decline, however, is highly variable and represents the development of partial tolerance in an individual patient. Persistent and complete normalization of antimyosin uptake suggests partial tolerance. This figure demonstrates results of mean antimyosin uptake in 247 studies at various intervals after transplantation.

biopsies. Furthermore, serial studies demonstrated that the resolution of antimyosin uptake *significantly varied from patient to patient* suggesting that the rate of development of tolerance to the graft is highly variable. In a series of 33 patients prospectively followed after transplantation for up to 48 months, partial tolerance to the graft (as confirmed by negative scans) was attained in 50% of patients at this time after transplantation.[21] While some patients had a negative scan as early as 2 months after transplantation, others required up to 3–4 years after the surgery. In general, once a negative scan had developed recurrent rejection was not observed in the absence of any modification of immunosuppressive therapy. The remaining half of patients showed persistent antimyosin uptake, suggesting that immunological tolerance was never attained and ongoing injury was occurring.[21]

ANTIMYOSIN UPTAKE AND REJECTION-RELATED COMPLICATIONS

Complications related to rejection are associated with intense antibody uptake. In our report of 247 patients, 238 did not suffer rejection-related complications. The remaining 9 patients developed congestive heart failure, acute infarction, accelerated vasculopathy, required retransplantation or died. Antimyosin uptake at a time of complications was lower in the former group (HLR1.74 ± 0.3) than in the latter group (HLR 2.1 ± 0.16) ($p < 0.0001$). In fact, HLR > 2.0 seemed to imply a substantial risk for the development of complications. In none of 193 studies showing HLR < 2.0 was a complication detected, whereas one or more complications were observed in 9 of the 45 studies (20%) showing HLR > 2.0. Sensitivity and specificity of HLR > 2.0 in the detection of possible complications were 100% and 80%; the positive predictive value was 16% and the negative predictive value of 100%.[21,33]

In antimyosin scans performed at 1, 2 and 3 months after transplantation, two evolving patterns of antibody uptake were detected.[21] In two-thirds of patients, a decreasing pattern was observed whereby the intensity of antibody uptake at three months was lower than the first month (Figures 2 and 3, see color plates section, back of book). In these patients no rejection-related complications were seen during the first year and a gradual decrease in the extent of myocardial damage was

(a)

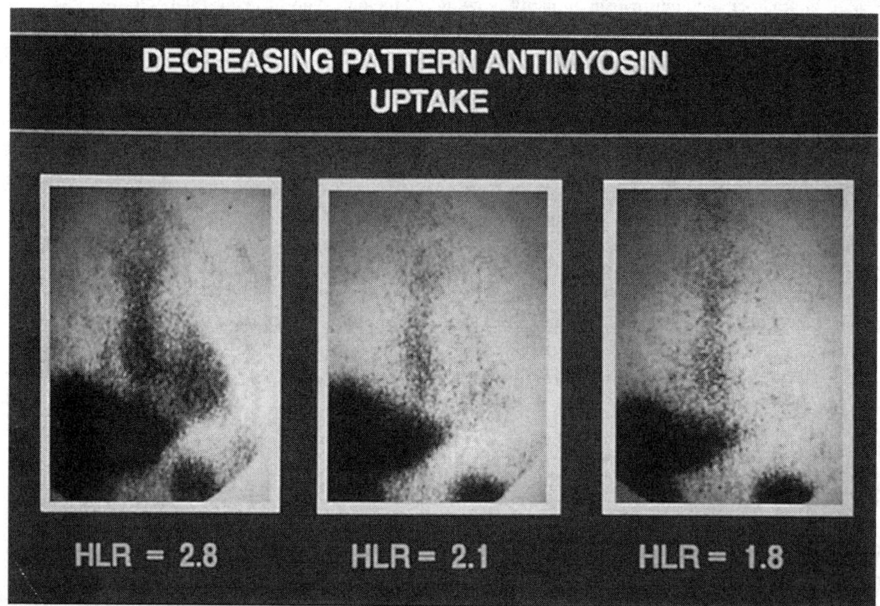

(b)

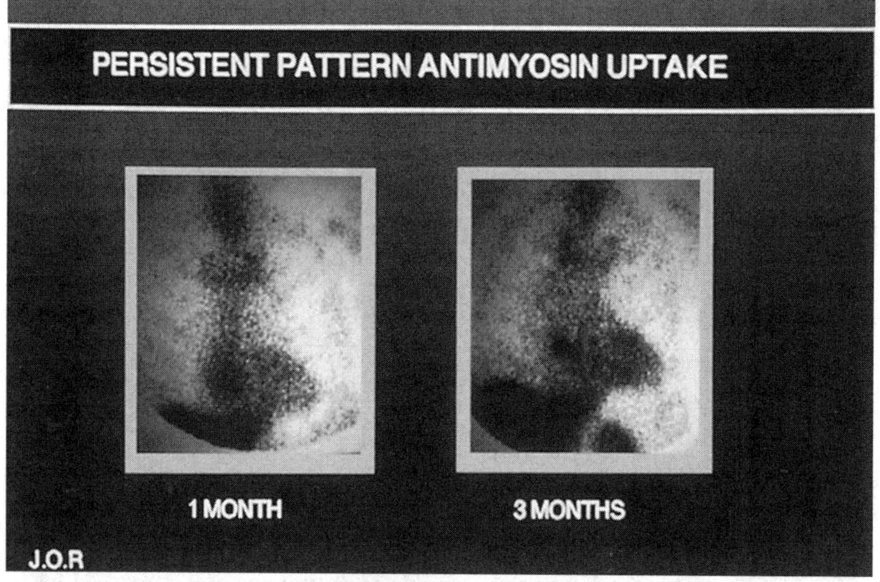

Figure 2. Serial antimyosin studies in first 3 months after transplantation. (A) Studies performed at 1, 2, and 3 months in a transplant recipient demonstrate gradual reduction in antimyosin uptake. Such decreasing pattern is suggestive of favorable prognosis and low likelihood of rejection related complications. (B) Another pattern of evolution shows persistently abnormal antimyosin uptake. Such a pattern is more often associated with transplant related complications and requires closer surveillance and more aggressive management.

observed. On the other hand, the remaining patients showed persistent uptake during the first three months (Figures 2 and 3, see color plates section, back of book). Of these, 60% patients developed complications related to rejection including heart failure, vasculopathy, retransplantation or death. It is likely that persistent myocyte damage represents an ongoing rejection activity regardless of histologic manifestations of disease in the endomyocardial biopsy. Such prognostic information provided by the evolution of scans within the first three months is not obtained from the biopsies performed during the same time. On the contrary, patients who demonstrated either a decreasing or persistence pattern showed a similar prevalence of biopsy-verified rejection; 37% and 43%, respectively.[21] Risk stratification and patient management may therefore be improved with the use of additional scintigraphic information.

MYOCARDIAL DAMAGE LATE AFTER HEART TRANSPLANTATION

We have preformed antimyosin studies in 21 patients after 1 year of transplantation who were followed for two years.[18] Of the 21 patients, 9 had normal scans, and the remaining 12 patients showed ongoing antibody uptake. Repeat biopsies were performed in all patients every 4 months during a subsequent 2-year follow-up period. These patients were treated solely on the basis of biopsy results regardless of the results of their antimyosin scans. A total of 18 rejection episodes were detected from 102 biopsies performed during follow-up (Figure 4, see color plates section, back of book). In the group of patients with normal scans, follow-up biopsies were positive for moderate rejection in only 1 occasion. Therefore, the probability of treatment for rejection based on the results of biopsies in this group was as low as 0.07 episode/per patient per year. The remaining 17 episodes occurred among patients who had showed positive antimyosin scans. In this group, the need of treatment for rejection based on the results of biopsies was 0.94 episode/per patient per year. A direct relationship was also observed between the intensity of antibody uptake and the severity of rejection activity; patients showing higher magnitude of antimyosin uptake required more frequent treatment for rejection based on the results of their biopsies.

MANAGEMENT OF PATIENTS BY ANTIMYOSIN-BASED ASSESSMENT OF MYOCARDIAL DAMAGE

The apparently higher sensitivity of monoclonal antimyosin studies when compared with biopsies raises the issue of whether antimyosin imaging can actually replace biopsy (Figure 5)?

Since myocyte damage may not necessarily represent allograft rejection *during the first few weeks after transplantation*, endomyocardial biopsies cannot be abandoned during this period. Furthermore, myocardial infections which occur early after transplantation (i.e. viral, toxoplasma) could also be associated with antimyosin uptake and may lead to inappropriate patient management.

Months After Transplantation	AM Scan Result	Recommendation
1	Likely to be intensely positive	Continue EMB-based management
2 and 3	Resolving uptake	Consider decreasing EMB frequency or Consider faster steroid taper
	Persistent uptake	↑ Endomyocardial biopsies or Consider modulation of Immunosuppressive therapy
12,24, 36,48...	No AM Uptake	Eliminate surveillance endomyocardial biopsy Baseline immunosuppression
	Positive AM Scan	Eliminate surveillance endomyocardial biopsy Oral steroid pulse

Figure 5. Suggested management of transplant recipients by surveillance for myocardial damage.

Although antimyosin uptake beyond first 4–6 weeks is felt to represent myocardial damage secondary to allograft rejection, results of single antimyosin scans should not be used to manage patients. The prevalence of antibody uptake during the first year remains high and up to 80% of patients show a positive study at this time,[16,21] which may not necessarily be accompanied by an evidence of histologic rejection. Therefore, an algorithm based solely on antimyosin results during the first year similar to that employed for biopsy detection and treatment of acute rejection (i.e. detect rejection, treat for rejection, rebiopsy the patient) would probably lead to overimmunosuppression. Further, interpretation of changes of antimyosin studies performed at very short intervals (i.e. days), may not reveal true modification of the rejection process, as antimyosin antibody may bind irreversibly to myosin exposed during earlier episodes of damage to myocytes.[65] Although a single antimyosin scan result cannot aid in the management of the allograft recipients, serial evolution of antimyosin uptake intensity in the first three months may allow optimization of immunosuppressive treatment protocols and guide the frequency of biopsy. A decreasing 3-month pattern allows either a more rapid decrement in immunosuppression, or a decrease in frequency of endomyocardial biopsies. Conversely, high persistent antimyosin uptake during this period requires closer surveillance for rejection, may warrant additional biopsies and may lead to augmented immunosuppressive therapy (Figure 5).

In contrast to the first year, subsequent repeat endomyocardial biopsies can be avoided in favor of antimyosin scintigraphy thereafter. Antimyosin studies should be performed every year[18] (Figures 4 and 5). If an antimyosin study is negative, the likelihood of detecting rejection within the next 2-year period is negligible; therefore, no additional treatment is required and baseline immunosuppression maintained. On the other hand, if antimyosin scan is positive, the annual probability for the biopsy-based detection (and treatment) of acute rejection is approximately 1 episode per patient per year. In the latter situation, patients can be routinely treated annually with oral corticosteroid pulse. The magnitude of myocardial damage or the intensity of antimyosin uptake at this stage can be used to adjust immunosuppressive management. Patients who demonstrate modest antimyosin uptake (HLR of 1.56 to 1.74) after the first year may be treated every 18 months, whereas those with intense uptake (HLR > 1.75) should receive additional steroid treatment every 9 months.[18]

The impact of discontinuation of biopsies beyond the first year using this algorithm is very favorable in terms of cost, patient comfort and allocation of catheterization resources to other non-transplant needs. In addition, it provides a rationale for long-term noninvasive risk stratification and individualized patient management.[63] Beyond the first year of transplantation, low-grade rejection may occur and not necessarily be associated with any sign of functional deterioration. Whereas it seems to be a logical assumption that rejection-related complications such as heart failure, or vascular occlusion, might be related to the smoldering rejection activity,[64] this hypothesis is yet to be proven. Solving this issue may be especially important in designing therapeutic strategies late after transplantation. If the relationship between smoldering rejection and functional deterioration is established, a more aggressive approach than the annual treatment for chronic rejection could be opportune, the aim being normalization of antimyosin uptake in the shortest period of time.

THE ROLE OF ANTIMYOSIN SCINTIGRAPHY IN EVALUATION OF CHRONIC LOW-DOSE STEROID-DEPENDENCE FOR IMMUNOSUPPRESSION

Antimyosin studies can also be used to assess the immunosuppressive properties of drugs used after transplantation. In a recent study, the role of chronic low-dose oral steroids in maintenance of partial immunological tolerance to the graft was assessed by studying patients both before and after gradual steroid withdrawal.[66] Steroids were gradually discontinued in 19 patients who had been transplanted for a mean of 57 months. These patients had developed partial tolerance to the graft and remained tolerant for a mean of 28 months as evident by persistently normal antimyosin scans. Of these 19 patients, antimyosin uptake recurred early after cessation of prednisone in 8 patients (42%), the HLR increasing from 1.42 ± 0.0 to 1.52 ± 0.13 ($p < 0.01$) (Figure 6). One year after cessation of steroids, 5 additional patients developed rejection who had not shown early recurrence of activity after steroid withdrawal. The overall results show that 13 of the 19 patients developed rejection within the first year of withdrawal, thus revealing the crucial role of chronic low-dose prednisone to maintain the tolerance to the graft. Reinstitution of steroid treatment was not always followed by disappearance of antimyosin activity, and additional oral or parenteral administration of steroid pulse treatment was required.

These results suggest that antimyosin study can be used to identify that subset of heart transplant patients who do not require long term chronic steroid immunosuppression. In order to avoid unnecessary immunosuppression and side-effects of corticosteroids, a gradual reduction in steroids can probably be attempted if normal

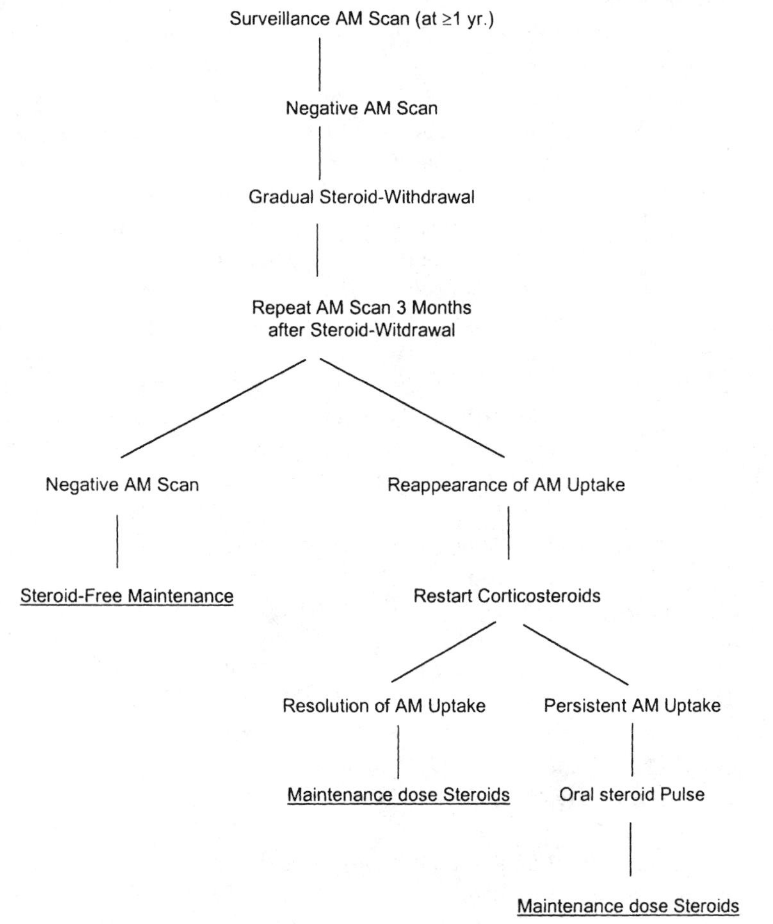

Figure 6. Safe steroid withdrawal based on antimyosin studies.

antimyosin uptake can be demonstrated during follow-up in the immediate period after drug withdrawal (Figure 6). The strategy presumes that allograft recipients who do not develop normal scans will be steroid-dependent.

CONCLUSIONS

The course of acute rejection and development of partial tolerance to graft is variable in transplant recipients and their management justifies the long-term use of diagnostic tests for the detection of acute rejection. Antimyosin imaging has demonstrated that successful management of allograft recipients can be achieved based on the pattern of antimyosin uptake during the first 3 months after transplantation. A combination of antimyosin imaging and endomyocardial biopsies performed at different stages after transplantation appear to provide a better approach to tailoring rejection treatment to meet the needs of the individual patient.

REFERENCES

1. Billingham ME, Cary NRB, Hammond ME, Kemnitz J, Marboe C, McCallister HA, Snovar DC, Winters GL, Zerbe A. A working formulation for the standardization of nomenclature in the diagnosis of heart and lng rejection: heart rejection study group. J Heart Transplant 1990;9:587–593.
2. Billingham ME. Can histopathology guide immunosuppression for cardiac allograft rejection in the light of new techniques? Transplant Proc 1997;29:35S–36S.
3. Hosenpud JD, Bennett LE, Keck B, Boucek MM, Novick R. The Registry of the International Society for heart and lung transplantation. Sixeteenth official report 2000. J Heart Lung Transplant 2000;19:909–931.
4. Goswitz JJ, Braunlin E, Kubo SH, Bolman EM III, Nakhleh RE. Pathology of heart transplantation: study of autopsied and explanted allografts with emphasis on possible biopsy findings. Clin Transplant 1992;6:450–457.
5. Billingham ME. Is acute cardiac rejection a model of myocarditis in humans?. Eur Heart J 1987;8 (Suppl):19–23.
6. Khaw BA, Scott J, Fallon JT, Cahill SL, Haber E, Homcy C. Myocardial injury: quantitation by cell sorting initiated with antimyosin fluorescent spheres. Science 1982;217:1050–1053.
7. Khaw BA, Mattis JA, Melincoff G, Strauss HW, Gold HK, Haber E. Monoclonal antibody to cardiac myosin: imaging of experimental myocardial infarction. Hybridoma 1984;3:11–23.
8. Obrador D, Ballester M, Carrió I, Bernà L, Pons G. High prevalence of ongoing myocyte damage in patients with chronic dilated cardiomyopathy. J Am Coll Cardiol 1989;13:1289–1293.
9. Obrador D, Ballester M, Carrió I, Augè JM, Moya C, Bosch I, Martí V, Bordes R. Active myocardial damage without attending inflammatory response in idiopathic dilated cardiomyopathy. J Am Coll Cardiol 1993;21:1667–1671.
10. Narula J, Khaw BA, Dec GW Jr, Palacios IF, Fallon JT, Strauss HW, Haber E, Yasuda T. Recognition of acute myocarditis masquerading as acute myocardial infarction. New Engl J Med 1992;328: 100–104.
11. Obrador D, Ballester M, Carrió I, Moya C, Bosch I, Martí V, Bernà L, Estorch M, Udina U, Marrugat J, Augè JM, Carreras F, Pons-Lladó G, Caralps JM. Presence, evolving changes, and prognostic implications of myocardial damage detected in idiopathic and alcoholic dilated cardiomyopathy by 111-In monoclonal antimyosin antibodies. Circulation 1994;89:2054–2061.
12. Narula J, Southern JF, Dec GW, Palacios IF, Newell JB, Fallon JT, Strauss HW, Khaw BA, Yasuda T. Myofibrillarlysis, antimyosin uptake and dilated cardiomyopathy. J Nucl Cardiol 1995;2:470–477.
13. Martí V, Ballester M, Udina C, et al. Evaluation of active myocardial damage in patients with major depression on long-term treatment with tricyclic antidepressant drugs. A prospective study with In-111 monoclonal antimyosin antibodies. Circulation 1995;91:1619–1623.
14. Narula J, Khaw BA, Dec GW, Newell JB, Palacios IF, Southern JF, Fallon JT, Strauss HW, Haber E, Yasuda T. Evaluation of diagnostic accuracy of antimyosin scintigraphy for the detection of myocarditis. J Nucl Cardiol 1996;3:471–481.
15. Frist W, Yasuda T, Segall G, Khaw BA, Strauss HW, Gold H, Stinson E, Oyer P, Baldwin J, Billingham M, McDougall R, Haber E. Noninvasive detection of human cardiac transplant rejection with In-111 antimyosin (Fab) imaging. Circulation 1987;76 (suppl V):81–85.
16. Ballester M, Carrió I, Abadal ML, Obrador D, Bernà L, Caralps-Riera JM. Patterns of evolution of myocyte damage after human heart transplantation detected by 111Indium monoclonal antimyosin. Am J Cardiol 1988;62 (9):623–627.
17. De Nardo D, Scibilia G, Macchiarelli AG, Cassisi A, Tonelli E, Papalia U, Gallo P, Antolini M, Pitucco G, Reale A, Caputo V, Marino B. The role of Indium-111 antimyosin (Fab) imaging as a noninvasive surveillance method of human heart transplant rejection. J Heart Transplant 1989;8:407–412.
18. Ballester M, Obrador D, Carrió I, Augé JM, Moya C, Pons-Lladó G, Caralps-Riera JM. 111In-monoclonal antimyosin antibody studies after the first year of heart transplantation: identification of risk groups for developing rejection during long-term follow-up and clinical implications. Circulation 1990;82:2100–2108.
19. Schutz A, Fritsh S, Kugler C, Anthuber M, Sudhoff F, Wenke K, Spes C, Angermann C, Gokel JM, Kemkes BM. Indium-111 monoclonal antimyosin for diagnosis of cardiac rejection. Transplant Proc 1990;22/4:1464–1465.

20. Crespo MG, Pulpón LA, Dominguez P, Chamorro JL, Argueso MJ, Padras G, Garcia M, Segovia J, Figuera D. Detection of human cardiac transplant rejection with Indium-111 monoclonal antimyosin antibody imaging. Transplant Proc 1990;22/4:1463.
21. Ballester M, Obrador D, Carrió I, Moya C, Augè JM, Bordes R, Martí V, Bosch I, Bernà L, Estorch M, Pons G, Cámara ML, Padró JM, Arís A, Caralps JM. Early postoperative reduction of monoclonal antimyosin antibody uptake is associated with absent rejection-related complications after heart transplantation. Circulation 1992;85:61–68.
22. Hesse B, Mortensen SA, Folke M, Brodersen AKS, Aldershvile J, Pettersson G. Ability of antimyosin scintigraphy monitoring to exclude acute rejection during the first year after heart transplantation. J Heart Lung Transplant 1995;14:23–31.
23. Hosenpud JD. Noninvasive diagnosis of cardiac allograft rejection. Another of many searches for the grail. Circulation 1992;85:368–371.
24. Khaw BA, Gold HK, Leinbach RC, et al. Early imaging of experimental myocardial infarction by intracoronary administration of 131I-labeled anticardiac myosin (Fab')$_2$ fragments. Circulation 1978;58:1137–1142.
25. Khaw BA, Yasuda T, Gold HK, et al. Myocardial imaging with radiolabeled antibodies. In: Spry CJF, de. Immunology and Molecular Biology of Cardiovascular Diseases. Lancaster, UK: MTP Press; 1987.
26. Nedelman MA, Shealy DJ, Boulin R, et al. Rapid infarct imaging with a technetium-99m-labeled antimyosin recombinant single chain Fv: evaluation in a canine model of acute myocardial infarction. J Nucl Med 1993;34:234–241.
27. Khaw BA, Strauss HW, Pohost GM, et al. The relationship of immediate and delayed thallium-201 distribution to localization of I125-antimyosin antibody in acute experimental infarction. Am J Cardiol 1983;51:1428–1432.
28. Rezcalla S, Kloner RA, Khaw BA, Haber E, Fallon JT, Smith FE, Khatib R. Detection of experimental myocarditis by monoclonal antimyosin antibody Fab fragments. Am Heart J 1989;117: 391–395.
29. Kishimoto C, Hung GL, Ishibashi M, Khaw BA, Kolodny GM, et al. Natural evolution of cardiac functions, cardiac pathology, and antimyosin scans in a murine myocarditis model. J Am Coll Cardiol 1991;17:821–827.
30. Matsumori A, Ohkusha T, Matoba Y, Okada I, Yasuda T, et al. Myocardial uptake of antimyosin monoclonal antibody in a murine model of viral myocarditis. Circulatin 1989;79:400–405.
31. Khaw BA, Russell PS, Roseel J, Fergusson P, Haber E. New approach to determination of heart transplant rejection by I125-antimyosin antibody and Tc99m-fibrinogen. Clin Res 1981;29:496.
32. Khaw BA, Yasuda T, Palacios I, Fallon JT, Dec GW, et al. Diagnosis of acute myocarditis with radiolabeled monoclonal antimyosin antibody: Immunoscintigraphic evaluation. In Schultheiss ed. New concepts in viral disease. Springer Verlag 1988, pp. 363–373.
33. Isobe M, Khaw BA, Haber E. Early detection of rejection and assessment of cyclosporine therapy by indium-111-antimyosin imaging in mouse heart allografts. Circulation 1991;84: 1246–1255.
34. Addonizio LJ, Michler RE, Marboe RE, Esser PE, Johnson LJ, et al. Imaging of cardiac allograft rejection in dogs using indium111-antimyosin Fab. J Am Coll Cardiol 1987;9:555–564.
35. Sainani GS, Krompotic E, Slodki SJ. Adult heart disease due to coxsackie B virus infection. Medicine (Baltimore) 1968;47:133–147.
36. Smith WG. Coxsackie B myopericarditis in adults. Am Heart J 1970;80:34–46.
37. Lerner AM, Wilson FM, Reyes MP. Enteroviruses and the heart with special emphasis on the probable role of coxsackie B viruses. Epidemiological and experimental studies. Mod Concepts Cardiovasc Dis 1975;44:7–10.
38. Dec GW, Palacios IF, Yasuda T, Fallon JT, Khaw BA, et al. Antimyosin antibody cardiac imaging: its role in the diagnosis of myocarditis. J Am Coll Cardiol 1990;16:97–104.
39. Narula J, Yasuda T, Khaw BA, Southern BA, Dec GW, et al. Antimyosin scintigraphy in detection of myocarditis: evaluation of a diagnostic methodology. J Am Coll Cardiol 1991;17:342.
40. Narula J, Khaw BA, Dec GW, Palacios IF, Southern JF, Fallon JT, et al. Recognition of acute myocarditis masquerading as acute myocardial infarction. N Engl J Med 1993;328:100–104.
41. Abelman WH, Roberts WC. Cardiomyopathy and specific heart muscle disease. In: Hurst JW ed. The Heart. New York: McGraw-Hill 1989:1313.
42. Casans I, Villar A, Almenar V, Blanes A. Lyme myocarditis diagnosed by indium-111 antimyosin scintigraphy. Eur J Nucl Med 1989;15:330–331.
43. Malhotra A, Narula J, Yasuda T, Reddy KS, Chopra P, et al. In111-antimyosin antibody imaging for diagnosis of rheumatic carditis. J Nucl Med 1990;31:841.
44. Samuels MA, Southern JF. Case records of the Massachusetts General Hospital. N Engl J Med 1988;318:970–980.

45. Estorch M, Carrió I, Berná L, et al. Indium-111 antimyosin scintigraphy after doxorubicin therapy in patients with advanced breast cancer. J Nucl Med 1990;12:1965–1970.
46. Carrió I, Estorch M, Berná L, et al. Assessment of anthracycline induced myocardial damage by quantitative indium-111 myosin specific monoclonal antibody studies. Eur J Nucl Med 1991;18:806–812.
47. Carrió I, López-Pousa L, Estorch M, et al. Detection of doxorubicin cardiotoxicity in patients with sarcomas by indium-111 antimyosin monoclonal antibody studies. J Nucl Med 1993;34:1503–1507.
48. Valdés-Olmos R, ten Bokkel-Huinink WW, ten Hoeve RF, et al. Usefulness of indium-111 antimyosin scintigraphy in confirming myocardial injury in patients with anthracycline associated left ventricular dysfunction. Ann Oncol 1994;5:617–627.
49. Carrió I, Berná Ll, Ballester M, et al. Indium-111 antimyosin scintigraphy to assess myocardial damage in patients with suspected myocarditis and heart transplant rejection. J Nucl Med 1988;29:1893–1900.
50. Pous-Llado G, Ballester M, Borras X, Carreras F, Cavrio I, Lopez-Contreras J, Roca-Cusacks A, Najula J. Myocardial cell damage in human hypertension. J Am Coll Cardiol 2000;36:2198–2203.
51. Ballester M, Obrador D, Carrió I, et al. Early post-operative reduction of monoclonal antimyosin antibody uptake is associated with absent rejection-related complications after heart transplantation. Circulation 1992;85:61–68.
52. Carrió I, Estorch M, Berná Ll, et al. Indium-111 antimyosin and iodine-123 MIBG studies in early assessment of doxorubicin cardiotoxicity. J Nucl Med 1995;36:2044–2049.
53. Obrador D, Ballester M, Carrió I, et al. Presence, evolving changes, and prognostic implications of myocardial damage detected in idiopathic and alcoholic dilated cardiomyopathy by indium-111 monoclonal antimyosin studies. Circulation 1994;89:2054–2061.
54. Ballester M, Bordes R, Tazelaar H, Carrio I, Marugat J, Narrula J, Billingham ME. Evaluation of biopsy classification for rejection: relation to detection of myocardial damage by monoclonal antimyosin antibody imaging. J Am Coll Cardiol 1998;31:1357–1361.
55. Obrador D, Bordes R, Cladellas M, Abadal ML, Ballester M, Augé JM. Detección de miocarditis mediante biopsia endomiocárdica en los candidatos a trasplante cardíaco. Rev Esp Cardiol 1987 (Supl. II);40:14–17.
56. Chow LH, Radio SJ, Sears TD, McManus BM. Insensivity of right ventricular biopsy in the diagnosis of myocarditis. J Am Coll Cardiol 1989;14:915–920.
57. Hauck AJ, Kearney DL, Edwards WD. Evaluation of postmortem endomyocardial biopsy specimens from 38 patients with lymphocytic myocarditis: implications for the role of sampling error. Mayo Clin Proc 1989;64:1235–1245.
58. Narula J, Haider N, Virmani R, DiSalvo TG, Kolodgie FD, Hajjar R, Schmidt U, Semigran MJ, Dec GW, Khaw BA. Apoptosis in end-stage heart failure. N Engl J Med 1996;335:1182–1189.
59. Narula J, Kharbanda S, Khaw BA. Apoptosis cardiac diseases. Chest 1997;112:1358–1362.
60. Narula J, Chandrashekhar Y, Dec GW. Apoptosis in heart failure: a tale of hightened expectations, unfulfilled promises and broken hearts ... Apoptosis:1998;3:309–315.
61. Dec GW, Hajjar R, Narula J. Apoptosis in the failing heart. Cardiol Clin 1998;16:691–710.
62. Puig M, Ballester M, Matias-Guiu X, Bordes R, Carrió I, Aymat MR, Marrugat J, Padró JM, Caralps JM, Narula J. Apoptosis of myocytes in cardiac allograft rejection: An addtional mechanism of myocardial damage away from foci of myocyte necrosis. J Nucl Cardiol 2000;7:132–139.
63. Ballester M, Obrador D, Carrió I, Caralps-Riera JM. 111In-monoclonal antimyosin antibody studies in the diagnosis of rejection and management of patients after heart transplantation. In: Monoclonal Antibodies in Cardiovascular Disease. Khaw BA, Narula J, Strauss WH (Eds). Lea and Febiger. Philadelphia. 1994. pp. 79–98.
64. Lamich R, Ballester M, Marti V, Brossa V, Ayurat R, Carrio I, Berna L, Camprecios M, Puig M, Estorch M, Flotats A, Bordes R, Augé JM, Dadró JM, Caralps JM, Narula J. Efficacy of augmented immunosuppressive therapy for early vasculopathy in heart transplantation. J Am Coll Cardiol 1998;32:413–419.
65. Bhattacharya S, Crawley JCW, Lahiri A. Specific binding of 99MTc-antimyosi to necrotic human myocardium: clinicopathologic correlations. Am Heart J 1991;122:857–859.
66. Moya C, Ballester M, Bernà Ll, Aymat MR, Carrió I, Altimiras J, Martí V, Tuneu L, Obrador D, Peña V, Lamich R, Padró JM, Bonal J, Narula J. Chronic low-dose steroid treatment helps in maintenance of long-term tolerance to the cardiac allografts. J Nucl Cardiol (in press).

Color Plates

The authors gratefully acknowledge Theseus Imaging Corporation, a subsidiary of North American Scientific Corporation, for their unrestricted educational grant in support of this publication.

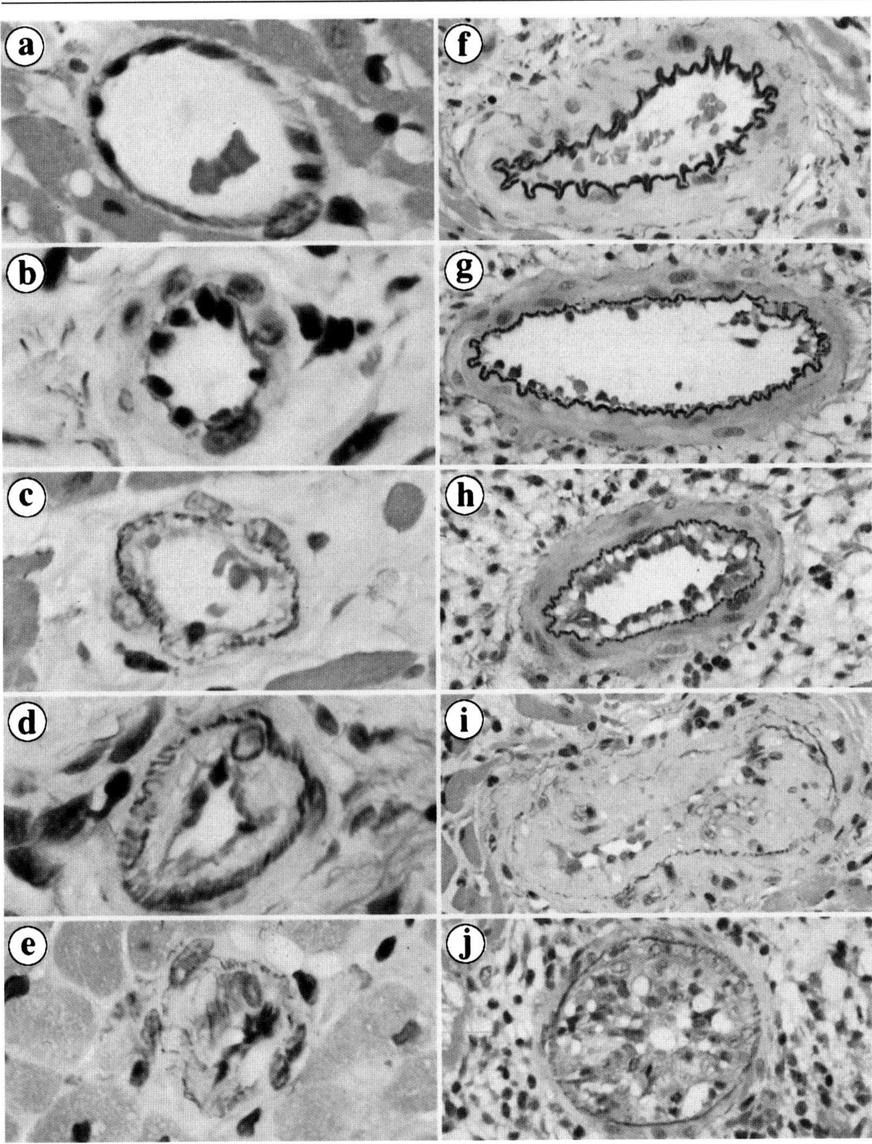

Plate 3.1. Different intensities of chronic vascular changes in cardiac allografts transplanted between two rat strains different in both MHC and non-MHC loci and immunosuppressed with cyclosporine A. Changes in intimal thickness are quantitated according to Billingham's criteria in arterioles (left panel; original magnification ×1000) and arteries (right panel; original magnification ×400): (a, f) grade 0, a normal artery with intact internal elastic lamina; (b, g) grade 1, <10% occlusion of lumen by intimal thickening and proliferation, disruption of internal elastic lamina, with some foam or vacuolated endothelial cells present; (c, h) grade 2, <50% occlusion of the lumen; (d, i) grade 3, >50% but <100% occlusion of lumen; and (e, j) grade 4, 100% occlusion of vessel lumen. Mayer's haematoxylin and eosin and Resorcin fuchsin for internal elastic lamina. (Modified from Sihvola et al., through the courtesy of the American Heart Association, Inc.)

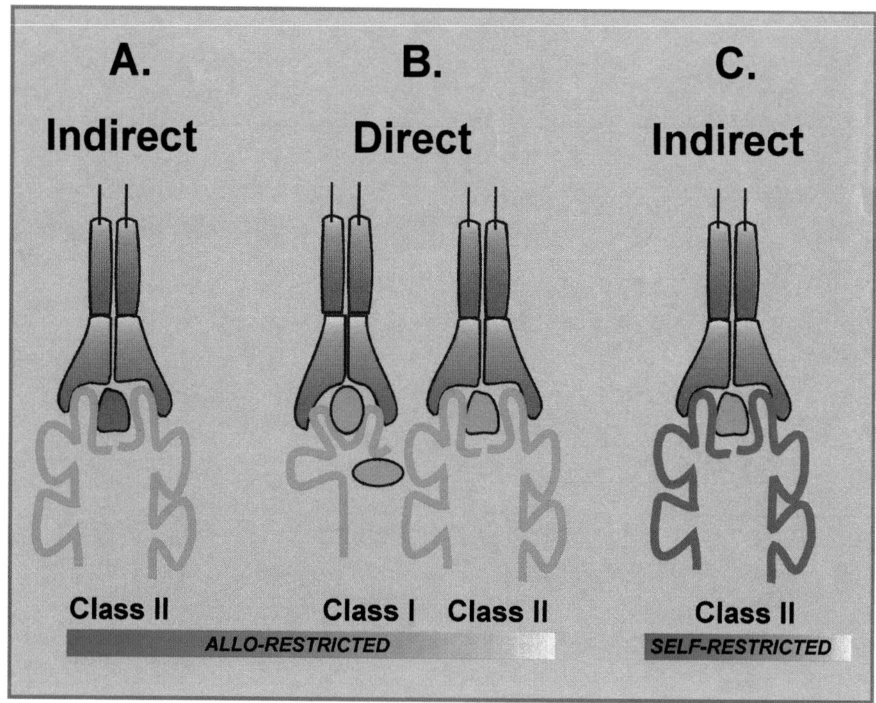

Plate 4.2. Allo-antigenic determinants recognized by the T cell receptor (TCR). T cell activation occurs by cognate interactions between the TCR and processed oligomeric peptides displayed by MHC class I/II antigens on antigen presenting cells. In the transplantation setting, antigen presentation can be either self-restricted or allo-restricted and either direct or indirect. (B) Direct presentation is always allo-restricted and involves recognition of processed donor allo-peptides presented by donor allo-MHC molecules by recipient T cells. Indirect presentation can be either allo-restricted or self-restricted. (A) Allo-restricted indirect presentation involves recognition of recipient processed self-peptides presented to the recipient self-TCR by donor allo-MHC. (C) Self-restricted indirect presentation involves recognition of processed allo-peptides presented to the recipient self-TCR by recipient's self-MHC.

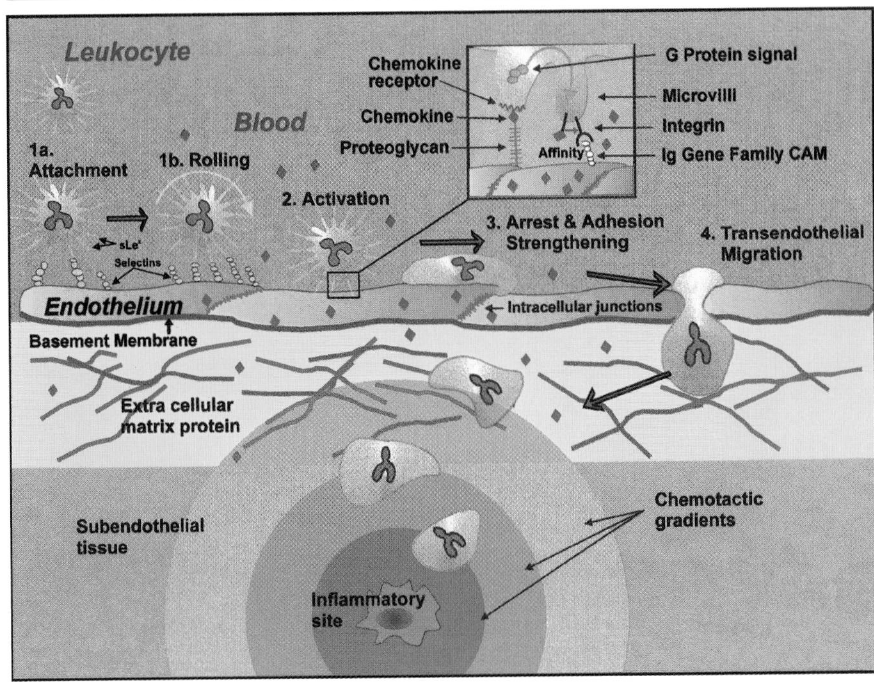

Plate 4.3. The three-step process of leukocyte trans-endothelial migration. (1a) Activated leukocytes are tethered by sialyl-Lewis x (sLe^x) determinants to selectins on endothelial cells (EC). (1b) Attachment slows the lateral motion of the leukocyte causing it to roll along the activated endothelium. (2) Chemokines posted on proteoglycans of the EC glycocalyx interact with specific chemokine receptors on the rolling leukocyte causing (G-protein mediated) activation and an increase in the affinity of leukocyte integrins for the EC Ig-like super family, CAMs (3) Interactions between high affinity leukocyte integrins and EC CAMS (e.g. ICAM-1) lead to arrest and strong adhesion of the leukocyte. (4) EC bound leukocytes expressing multiple chemokine receptors extravasate through paracellular junctions in response to chemokine gradients and navigate to focal points of tissue injury in the sub-endothelial tissues.

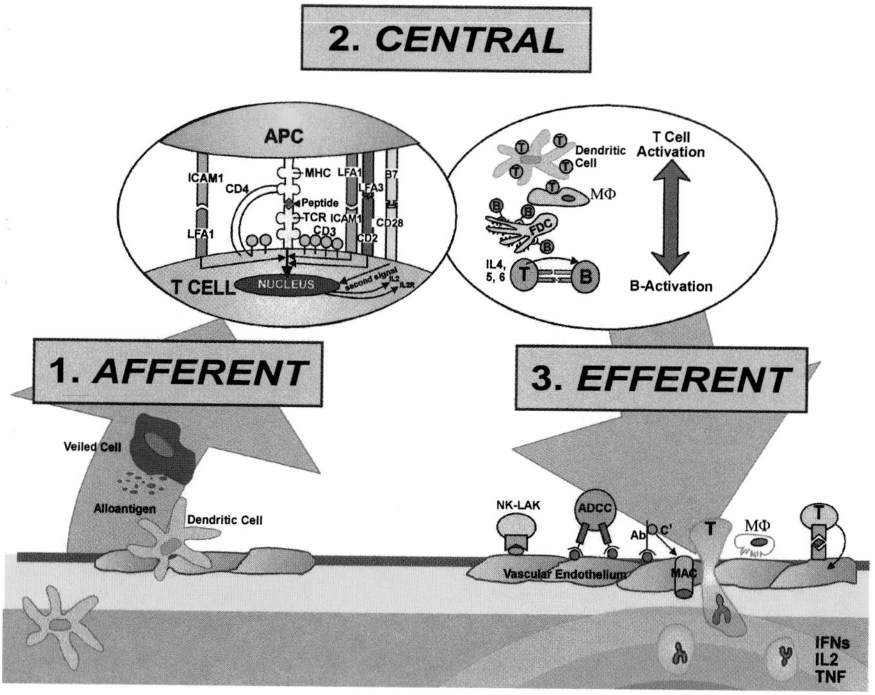

Plate 4.4. Allograft rejection is a systemic response by the immune system that involves an afferent phase, a central phase, and an efferent phase. In the afferent phase donor alloantigen is collected by tissue macrophages and resident dendritic cells (DC) of host origin to be processed into short (10–30 amino acid residues) oligomeric peptides which are presented in association with α and β chains of MHC Class II antigen on these professional antigen presenting cells (APC). As DCs acquire alloantigen, they simultaneously upregulate their expression of MHC Class II and cellular adhesion molecules (CAMs) as they migrate from their tissue sites, through the lymphatics (along with free alloantigen), to secondary lymphoid organs (spleen and draining regional lymph nodes). Passenger DC of donor origin have also been shown to migrate from organ allografts to the recipient spleen within 48 hours post transplantation. Local allosensitization is though to occur within the spleen.

In the central phase, the DCs home to specific sites within the spleen or lymph nodes where the form clusters with DC4+ T cells with specificity for the processed alloantigen. The clonally rearranged antigen receptors (TCR) on these T cells specifically associate with processed allopeptide and MHC to form a tri-molecular complex between the T cell and the APC. Alternatively, T cells may recognize donor MHC on passenger DCs directly. In either event the formation of the trimolecular complex is stabilized by interactions of CAMs on the T cell and the APC. These interactions also deliver co-stimulatory (CSM) signals that synergize with and amplify the TCR-mediated activation signal. In addition, DCs display specialized CSMs that deliver second signals necessary for the activation of naïve T cells. Activated T cells increase their synthesis of cytokines (particulary IL-2) and cytokine receptors (leading to clonal expansion of allospecific T cells) and upregulate their surface expression of CAMs. These events shape the magnitude and mode of the immune response and target T cell effetors to sites of inflammation of local graft rejection. B cells presenting alloantigen to T cells within germinal centers are also clonally expanded. Thus, alloactivation of both B and T cells occurs in the central phase.

During the efferent phase, effector T cells leave the secondary lymphoid organs and home to sites of inflammation within the allograft. Cytokine induced neoexpression of CAMs (e.g. VCAM-1, P-S, E-Selectin, and ICAM-1) on the vascular endothelium facilitates the transmigration of activated CD4+ T cells into the allograft. These DCD4+ effector T cells release lymphokines, e.g. IL-2 and INF-γ, that recruit and activate other macrophages and T cells (including CD8+CTLs) that leads to further infiltration of effector cells into the graft. In addition, cytokines (e.g. IL-1, IL-10, or IL-12) released by local APCs can also contribute to the direction of the immune response (cellular or humoral). Allograft rejection ultimately results from a variety of cytolytic events mediated by diverse combinations of CD4+ and CD8+ T cells, NK cells, macrophages and cytolytic anti-graft antibodies.

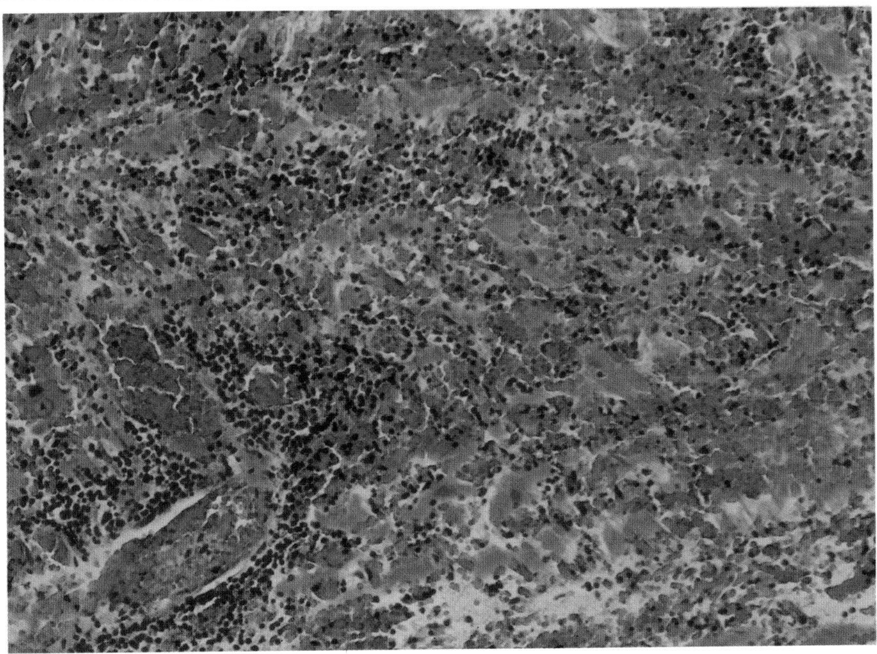

Plate 8.2. Photomicrograph of a myocardial biopsy from a hyperacutely rejected pig heart stained with hematoxylin and eosin. Interstitial hemorrhage and intravascular thrombosis is evident.

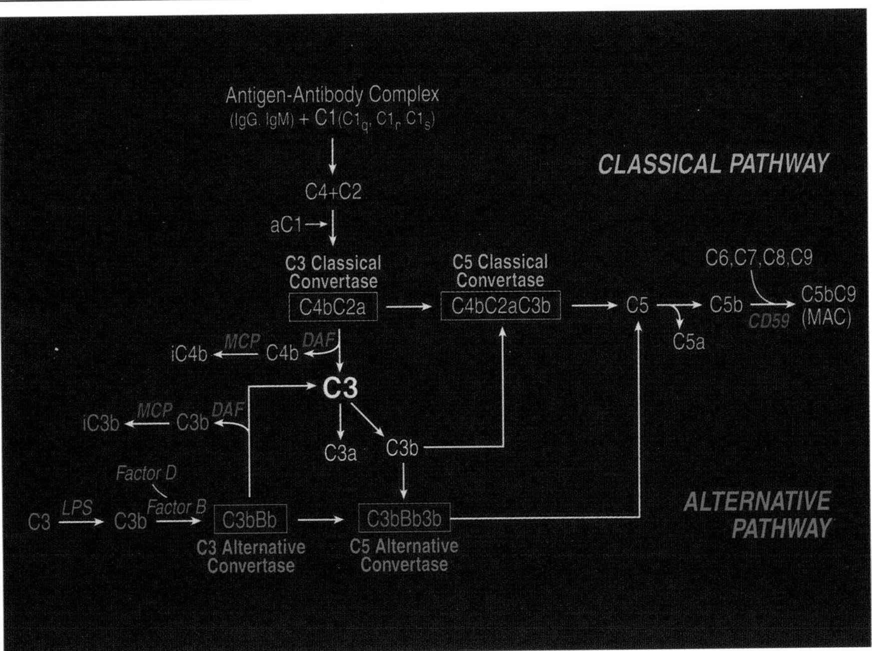

Plate 8.4. Synopsis of the complement pathways: Antigen-antibody complex triggers the initiation of the classical pathway. The alternative pathway does not require antibody for its initiation. MCP, DAF, CD59 represent regulators of complement activation, and their location denote the sites where such regulation is implemented. See text for details. Reproduced with permission from *Cellular and Molecular Immunology*, Abbas A.K., Lichtman, A.H., Pober, J. eds. W.B. Saunders Co., 1994.

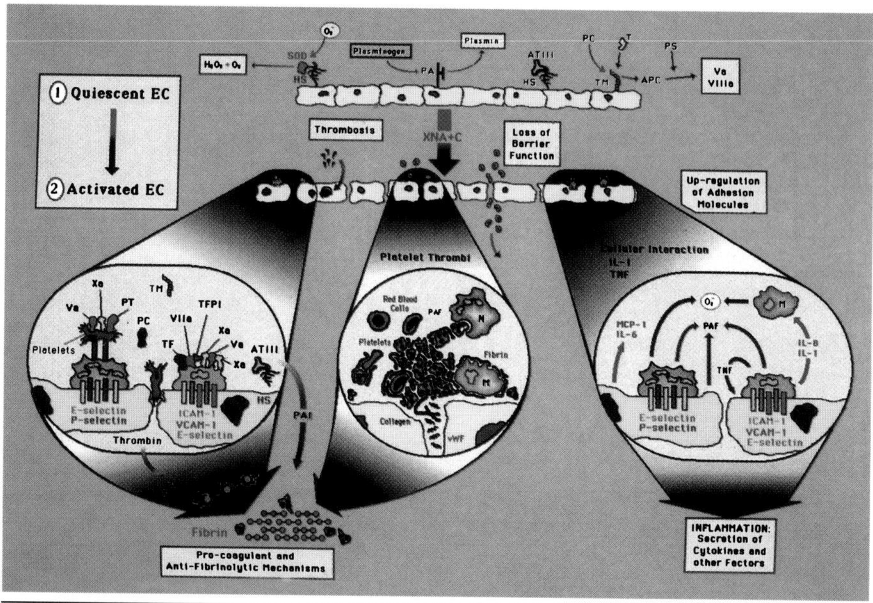

Plate 8.6. The figure presents a model of type I and type II endothelial cell activation which are the major pathophysiologic events leading to the rejection of a discordant xenograft. Quiescent endothelial cells (EC), which are tightly juxtaposed, maintain a barrier that keeps cells and proteins of blood in the intravascular space. Quiescent EC express heparan sulfate (HS) and thrombomodulin (TM) on their surface; HS binds both antithrombin III (ATIII), which functions as an anticoagulant, as well as superoxide dismutase (SOD), which breaks down superoxide (O_2^-). TM binds thrombin, leading to the generation of activated protein C (APC), which also has an anticoagulant effect. As a result of EC activation, there is a loss of vascular integrity as the EC retract from one another, resulting in hemorrhage and edema. Second, there is up-regulation and appearance on the EC surface of P selectin, E-selectin, ICAM-l, and VCAM-1, which can function as ligands to bind neutrophils, monocytes, and lymphocytes of blood. When pig EC are activated with human XNA + C, the deposition of iC3b is an important ligand for neutrophils. In addition to the ligands shown, the activated EC up-regulate class I and II antigens of the MHC. Third, the activated EC secrete IL-1, IL-6, and IL-8 as well as platelet-activating factor (PAF). IL-l is likely stimulatory to the EC in an autocrine loop, as well as function to activate monocytes. IL-8 is a chemoattractant for leukocytes and has some of the functions discussed for C5a below. PAF serves to activate neutrophils and platelets. Fourth, activated EC tip the balance from anticoagulation (promoted by quiescent EC) to procoagulation. Secreted PAF promotes the formation of platelet thrombi; loss of HS and TM results in loss of the anticoagulant mechanisms discussed for quiescent EC; secretion of plaminogen activator inhibitor (PAI.1) inhibits the naturally occurring action of plasminogen activator. Membrane vesicles break off from the activated EC containing components of the membrane attack complex (MAC, C5b-C9), which activate the prothrombinase complex leading to clotting; and the activated EC (as well as activated monocytes) produce tissue factor, perhaps the most powerful stimulus to coagulation. In addition to these events, there are others that likely impact HAR. Components of the activated complement system probably deliver a signal(s) to the EC, aiding in the full activation of the EC. In addition, C5a likely stimulates macrophages and mast cells to release TNF and/or IL-1, which can then activate EC. The cells that bind to the activated EC also participate in the inflammatory/rejection process. Neutrophils activated by C5a and PAF secrete reactive oxygen species. The production of superoxide by activated cells bound to the activated EC as well as by the EC themselves are likely major players in the overall response, perhaps primarily by activation of NF-κB; the loss of SOD aggravates these complications. Other factors produced by quiescent EC are endothelial derived relaxing factor (EDRF) (which leads not only to relaxation of the vessels but also prevents platelet thrombi), ADPases, prostacyclines, and tissue plasminogen activator. Reproduced with permission from "Xenotransplantation," Bach, F., Auchincloss, H., Robson, S.C., in *Transplantation Immunology*, Auchincloss, H., Bach, F., eds., Wiley-Liss, New York, 1995,

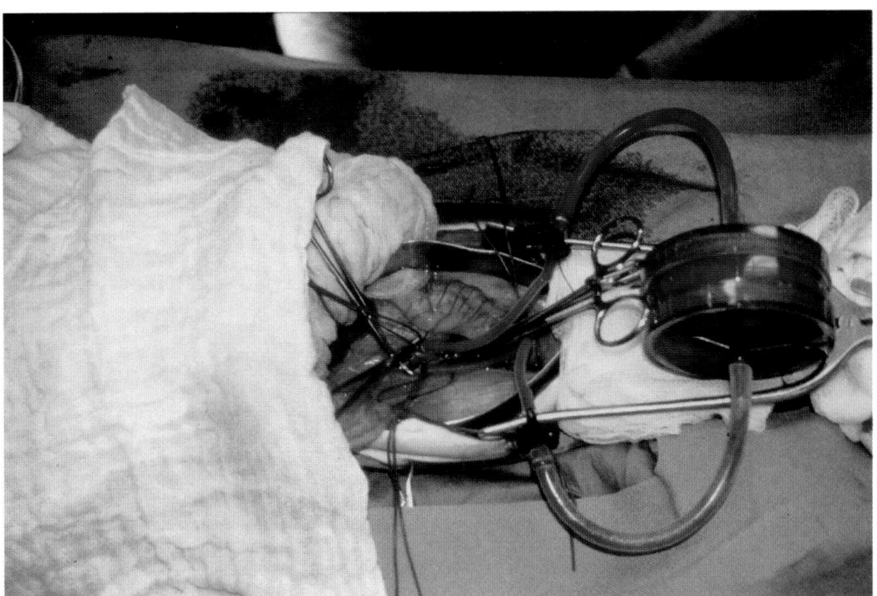

Plate 8.8. Perfusion of an α-Gal oligosaccharide immunoaffinity column with baboon blood. Blood enters the column via a cannula connected to the aorta, and it is returned to the animal by way of a cannula connected to the inferior vena cava. This technique has supplanted liver perfusion for adsorption of natural antibody in non-human primates in our laboratory.

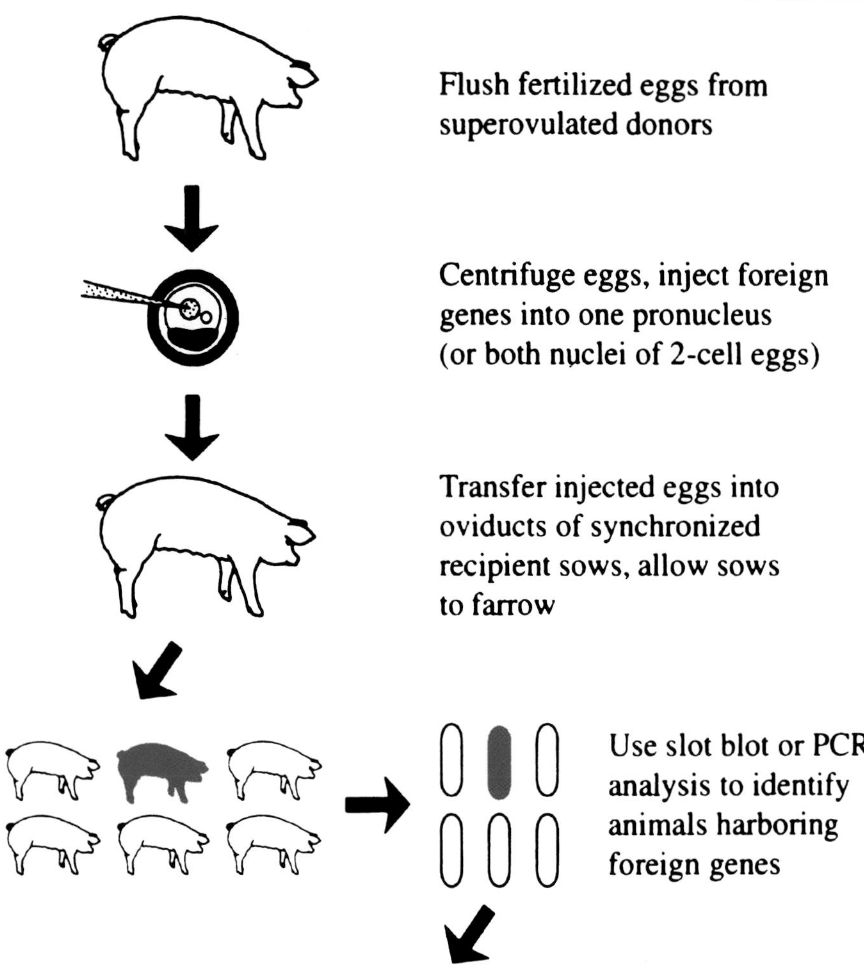

Plate 8.9. Creation of transgenic swine. **(a)** technique **(b)** photomicrograph of microinjection. Courtesy of Stem Cell Sciences, Melbourne, Australia.

(b)

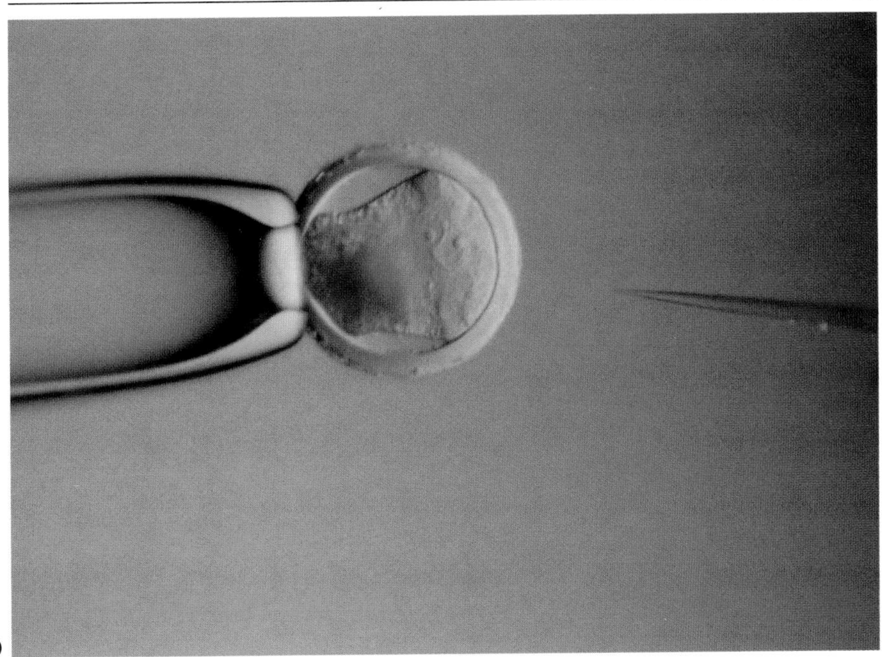

Plate 8.9. (continued)

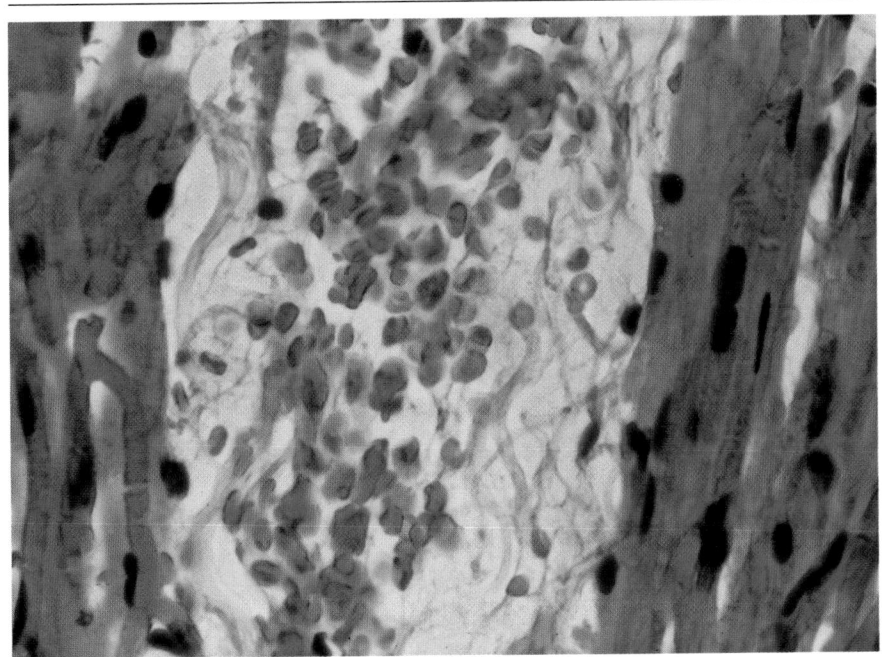

Plate 8.11. Photomicrograph of a myocardial biopsy from a pig heart undergoing delayed xenograft rejection stained with hematoxylin and eosin. Interstitial hemorrhage and intravascular thrombosis is evident.

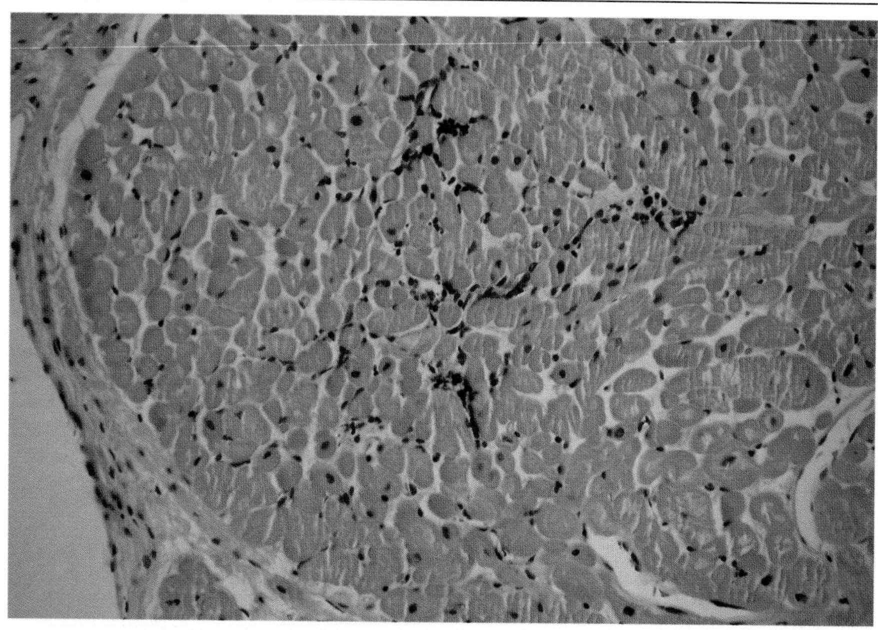

Plate 9.1. Mild rejection (ISHLT grade 1A): Minimal perivascular and interstitial infiltrate are present without myocyte disruption or separation in a "chicken wire" pattern.

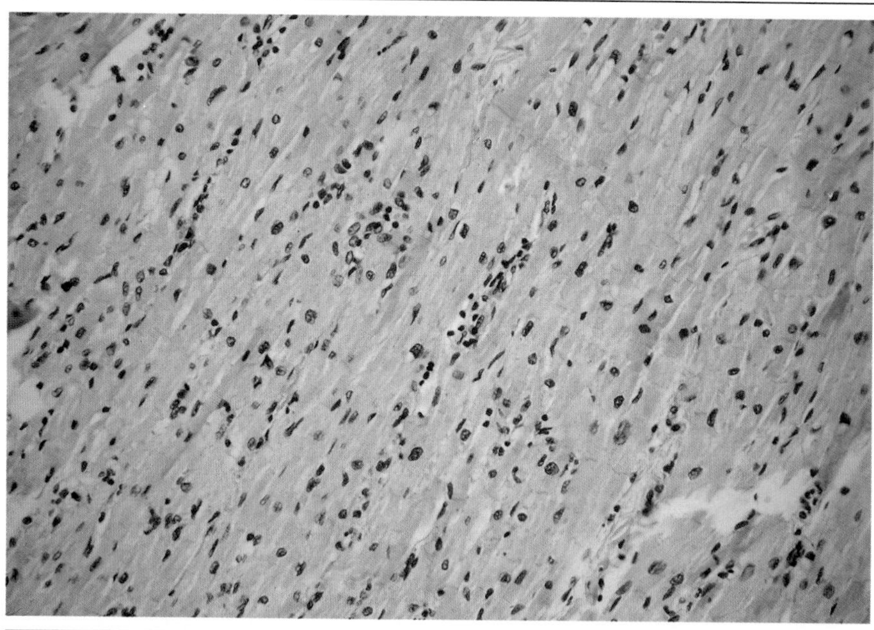

Plate 9.2. Mild rejection (ISHLT grade IB): Diffuse minimal lymhocytic infiltrates are present without myocyte separation or distortion.

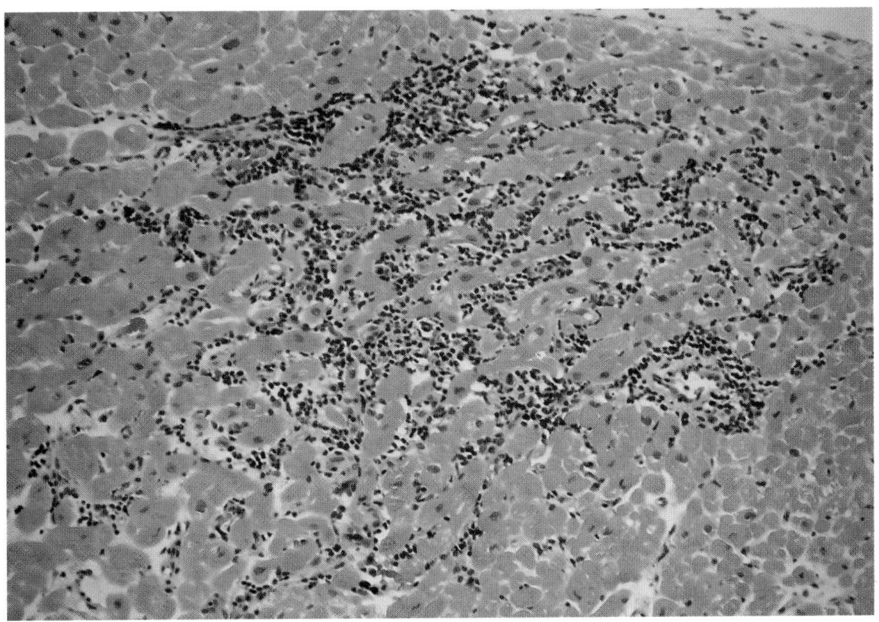

Plate 9.3. Moderate rejection (ISHLT grade 2): Single aggressive focus of activated lymphocytes is present with myocyte disruption at the periphery.

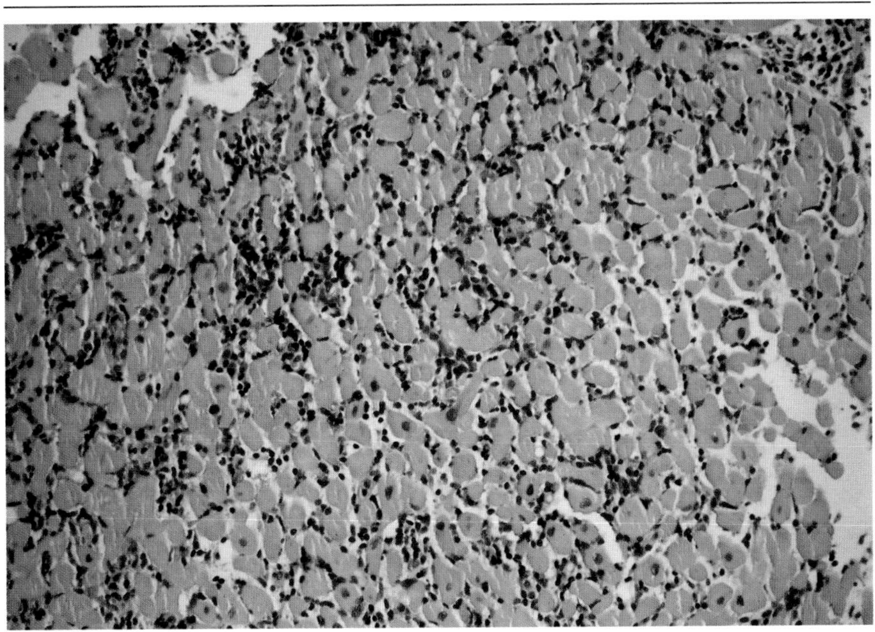

Plate 9.4. Moderate rejection (ISHLT grade 3A): Prominent interstitial lymphoid infiltrates with occasional eosinophils are associated with separation and disruption of myocytes.

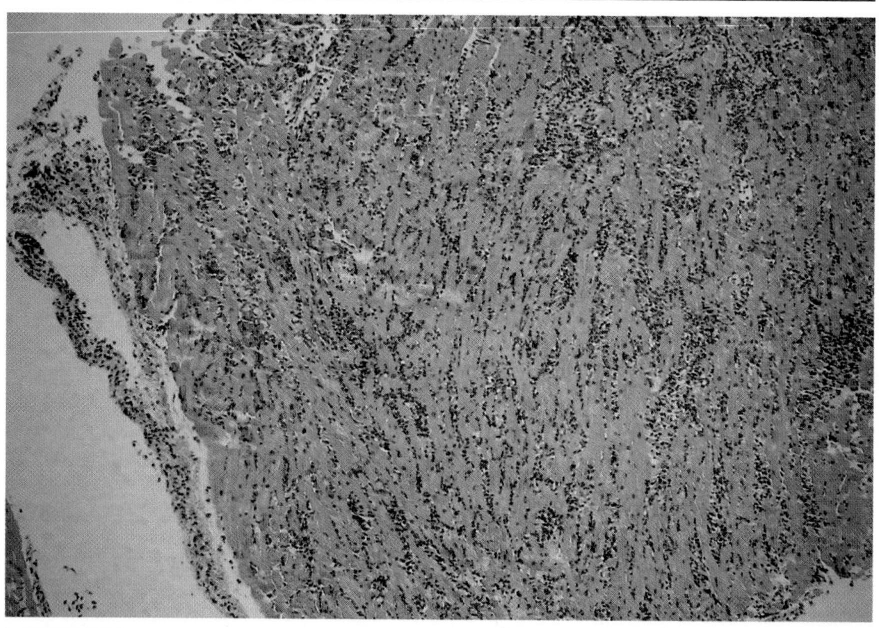

Plate 9.5. Severe rejection (ISHLT grade 3B or 4): Diffuse aggressive mixed inflammatory infiltrates are associated with interstiatial edema, hemorhage and vasculitis.

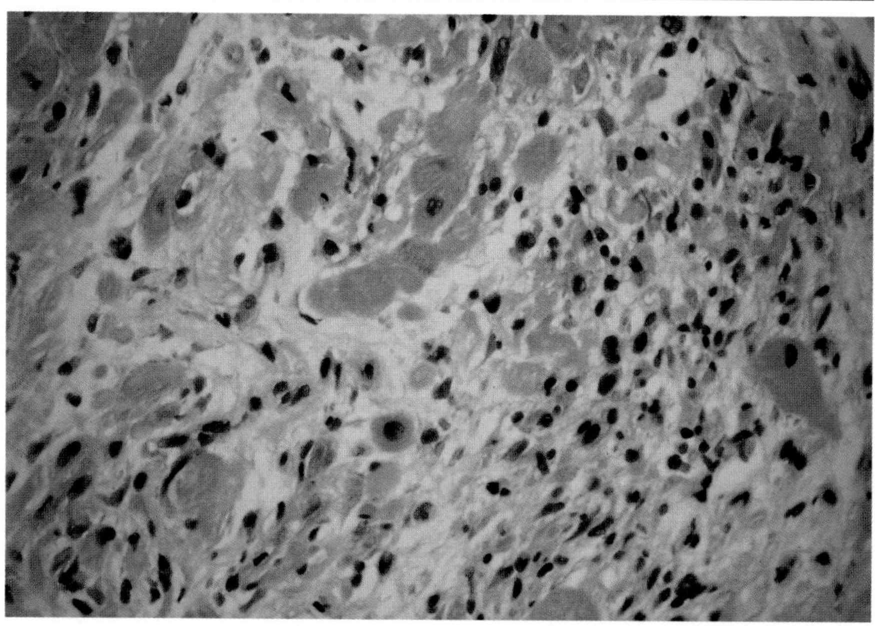

Plate 9.6. Harvesting ischemia: Biopsy taken within the first week post-transplant shows lymphoid and macrophages associated with myocyte injury.

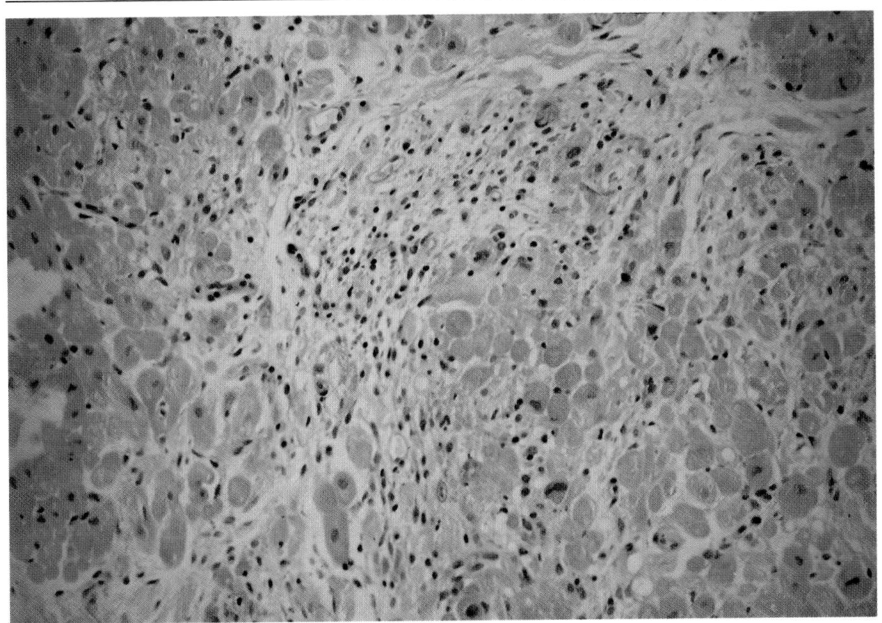

Plate 9.7. Healing ischemic injury: Focus of granulation tissue with macrophages and scant lymphocytic infiltrate.

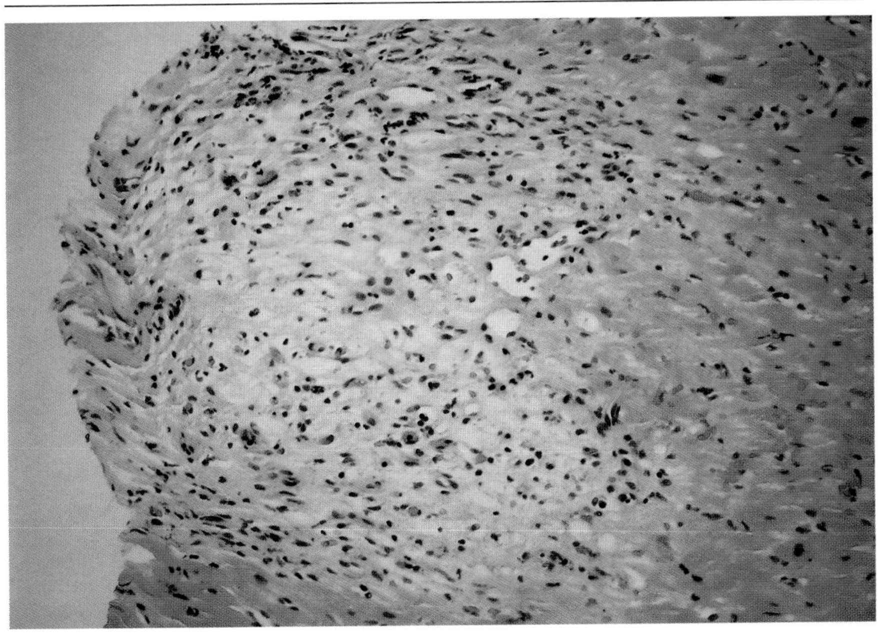

Plate 9.8. Previous biopsy site: Cup-shaped area of granulation tissue capped by thrombus is seen.

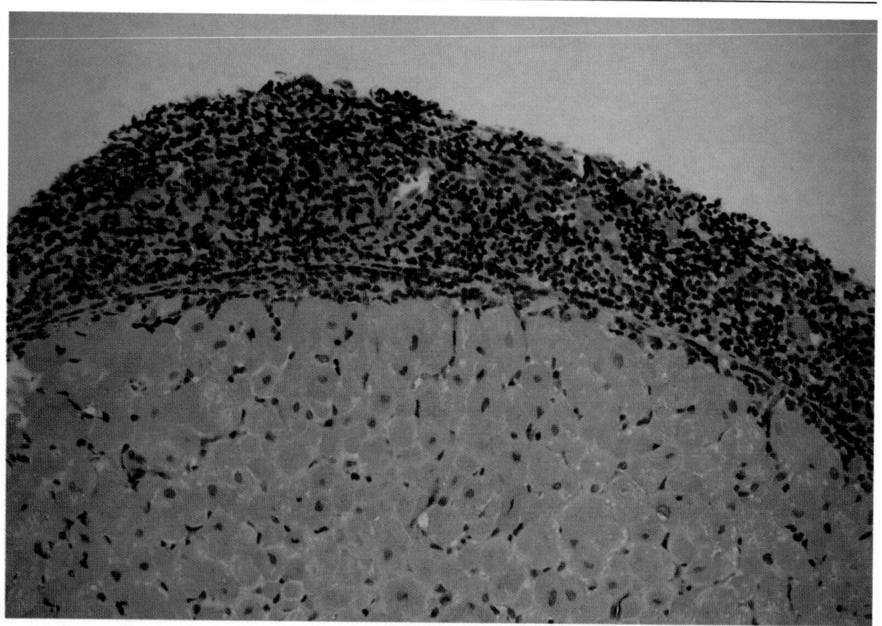

Plate 9.9. Quilty A lesion: Subendocardial collection of lymphocytes is present with a prominent capillary background.

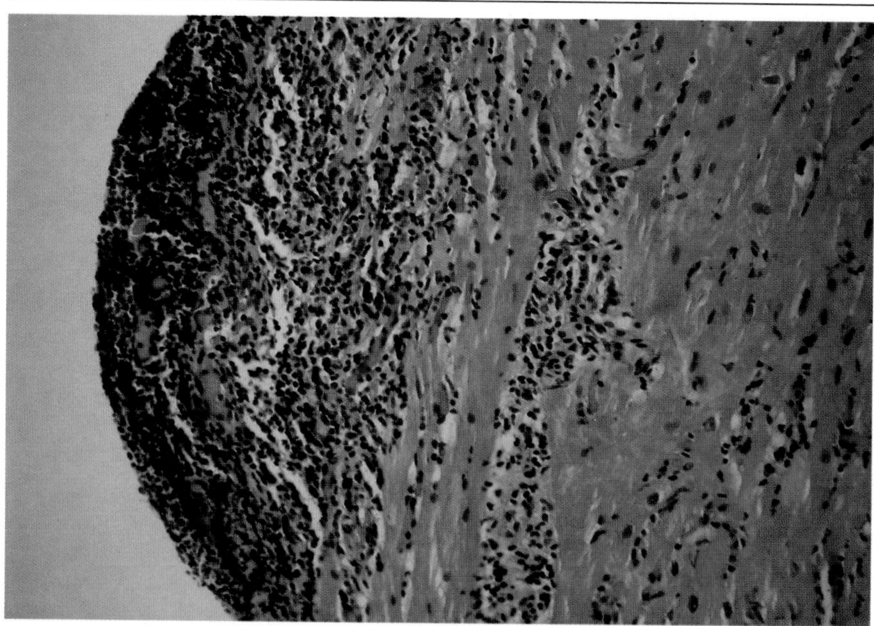

Plate 9.10. Quilty B lesion: Subendocardial collection of lymphocytes extend into the underlying myocardium.

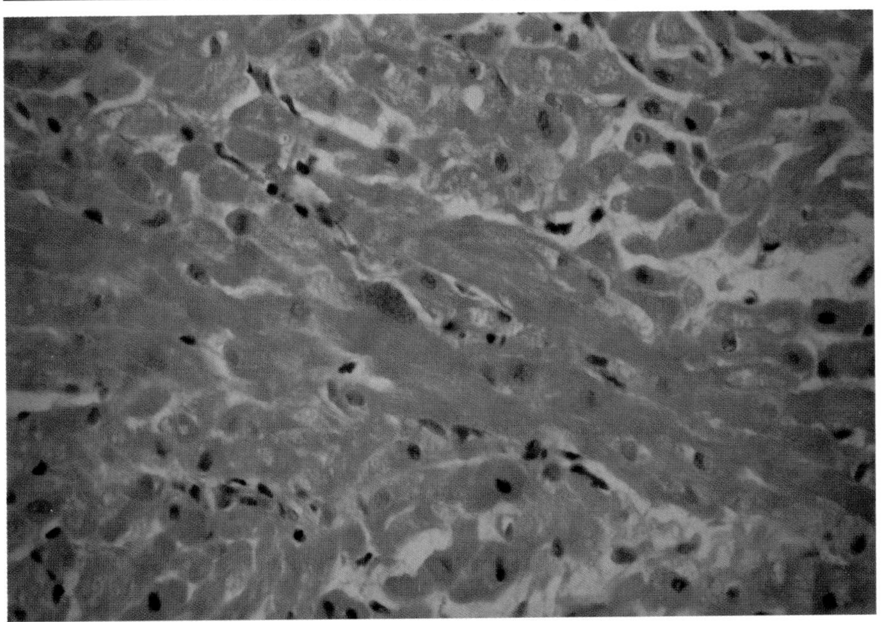

Plate 9.11. Toxoplasmosis: Encysted trophozoite of Toxoplasma is present; there is no inflammation.

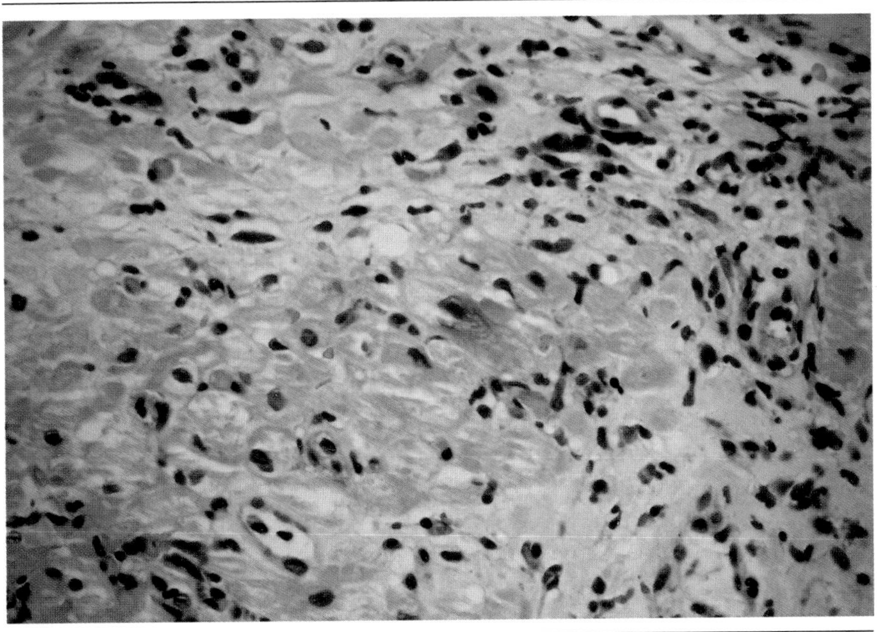

Plate 9.12. Cytomegalovirus infection: Intranuclear inclusion of cytomegalovirus is associated with a mixed inflammatory infiltrate.

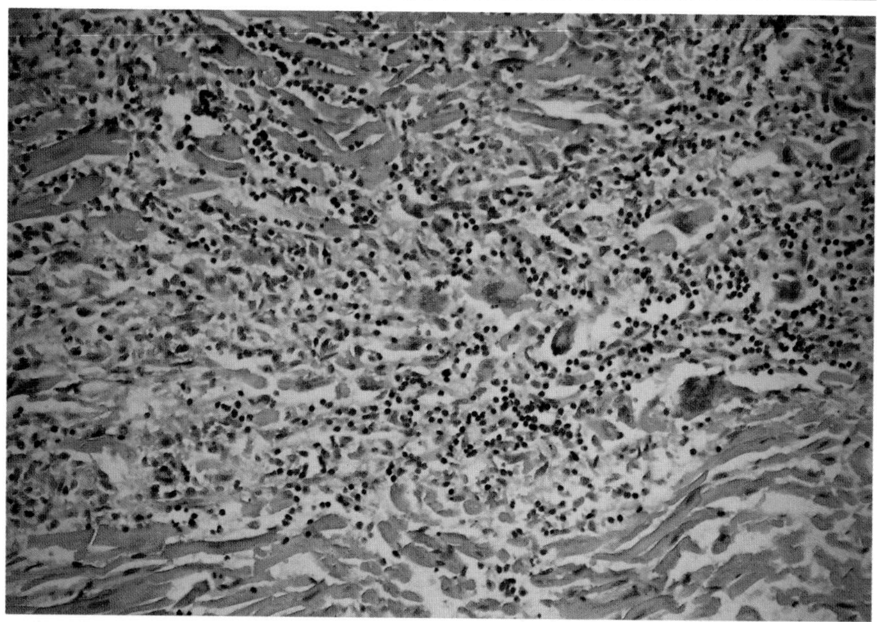

Plate 9.13. Giant cell myocarditis: Lymphoplasmocytic infiltrate with the characteristic multinucleated giant cells is associated with diffuse myocyte necrosis.

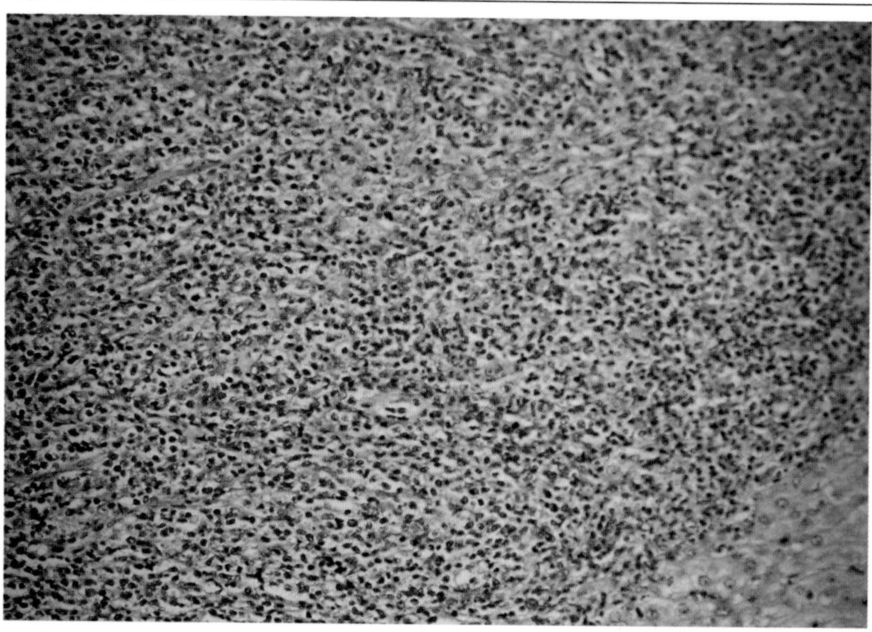

Plate 9.14. Posttransplant lymphoid proliferative disorder: Monomorphic population of atypical large lymphocytes is present in the liver of a cardiac transplant patient.

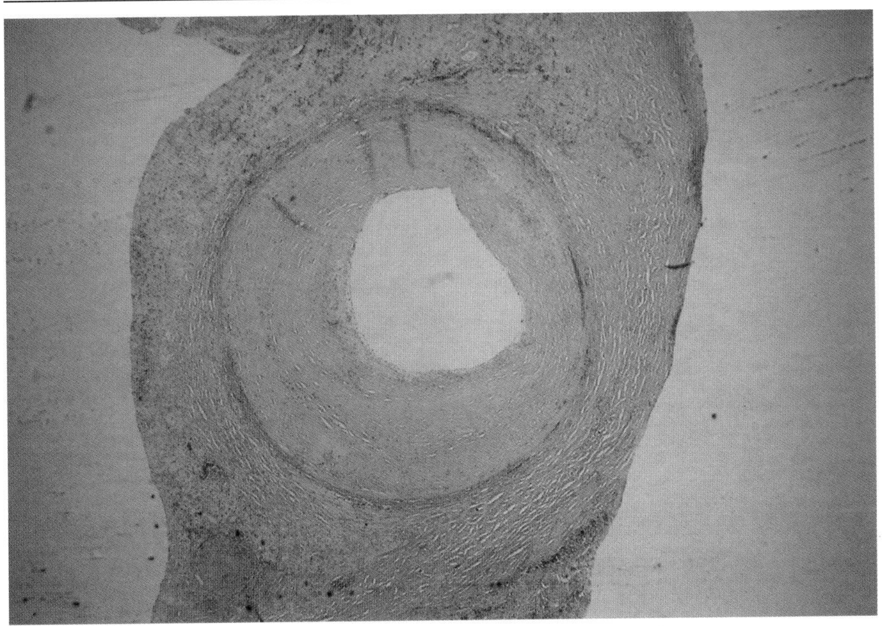

Plate 9.15. Graft vascular disease: Concentric fibrointimal proliferation characterises chronic vascular rejection.

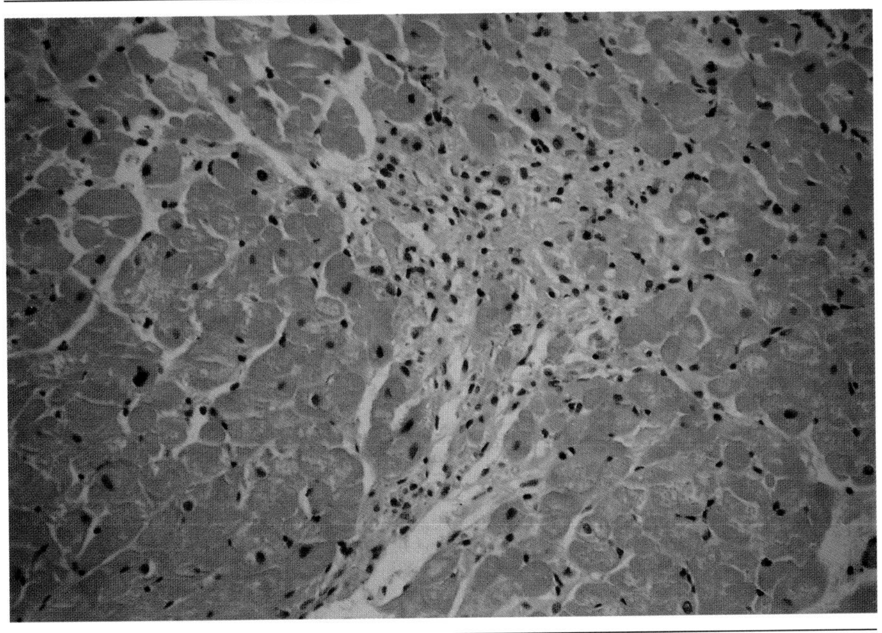

Plate 9.16. Focal ischemic injury: Well delineated focus of myocytolysis is seen in a patient with transplant associated vasculopathy.

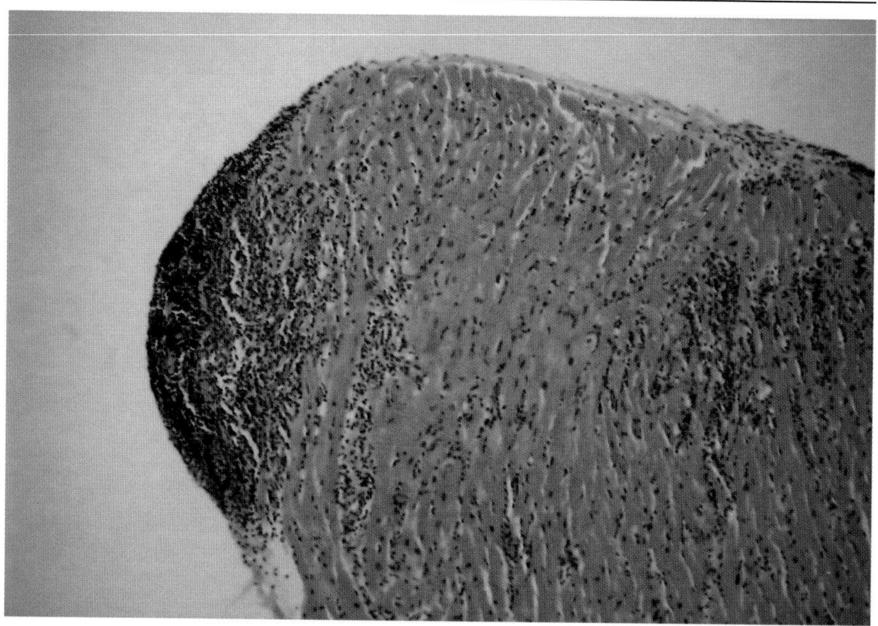

Plate 9.17. Tangentially cut Quilty B lesion: Interstitial lymphoid infiltrate seen here was in continuity with the subendocardium on deeper sections.

Plate 14.2. Methods for obtaining the diastolic indices. B) Analysis of pulsed Doppler mitral flow velocity curve using ultrasound. The upper panel shows simultaneous recording of the electrocardiogram (ECG), phonocardiogram (PHONO), and the mitral flow velocity curve. The arrows indicate aortic valve closure, which is confirmed by the first high-intensity signal on the phonocardiogram. Calibration marks at the top of the panel are at 200-msec intervals. Velocity calibration marks are at 0.2-m/sec intervals. The lower panel is a schematic representation of the mitral flow velocity curve to indicate method of measurement of diastolic indices. IVRT (A) is measured from aortic valve closure to the onset of mitral flow. Mitral valve pressure half-time is calculated from the base time (B), which is measured as the distance between the perpendicular line from the peak mitral flow velocity extended to the base line, and the line of the deceleration slope also extended to the base line. To obtain the pressure half-time, the base time is multiplied by a constant 0.29. Peak early mitral flow velocity (denoted as C in the schematic) is measured from the base line to the peak velocity recorded.

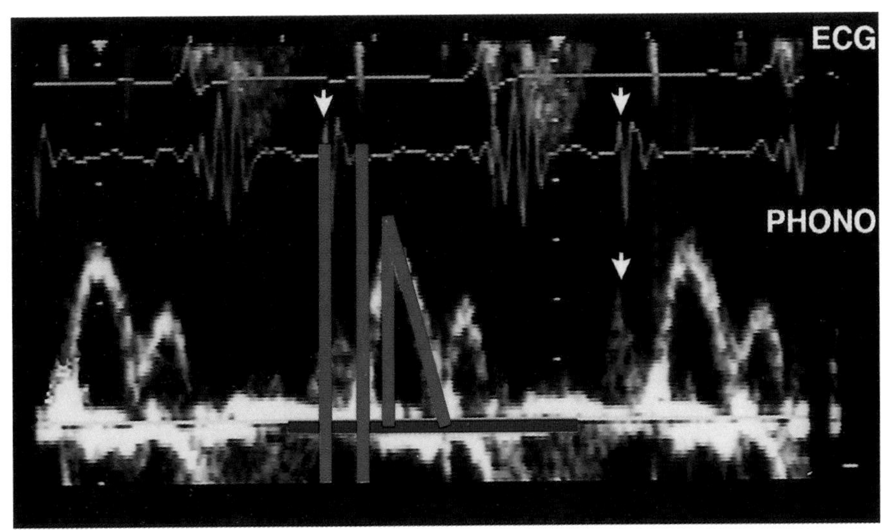
ECG
PHONO

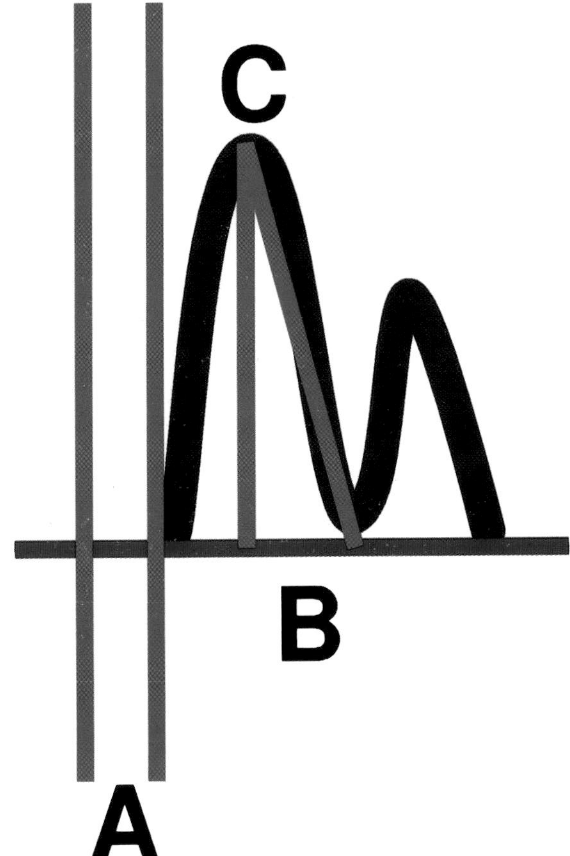
C
B
A

(a)

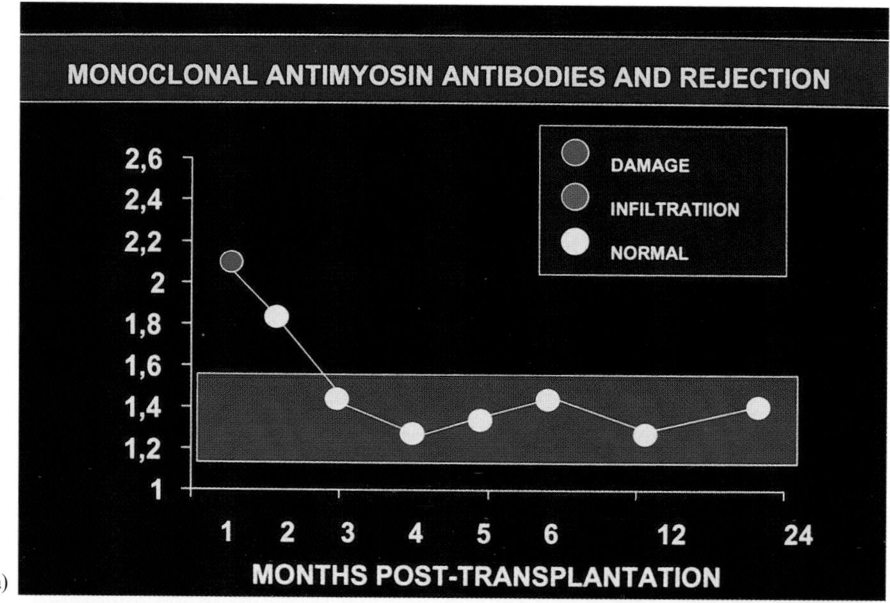

(b)

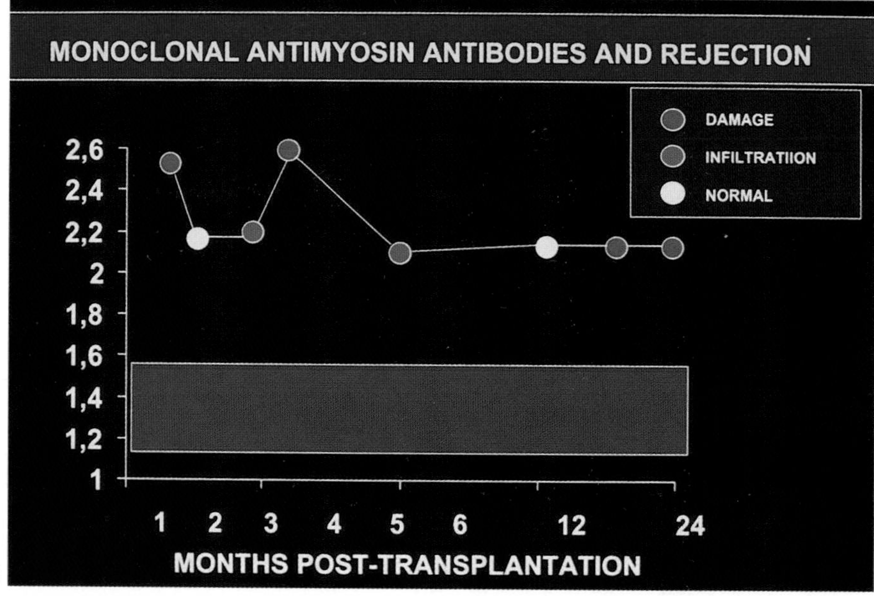

Plate 20.3. Pattern of evolution of antimyosin uptake in cardiac allograft recipients. The evolutionary patterns of two patients are illustrated here. The semiquantitative assessment of antibody uptake is compared with histologic findings obtained during concomitant endomyocardial biopsy. (A) A decreasing pattern of antimyosin uptake, similar to figure 2A, in a patient with an uneventful course. Biopsy results reconfirm a benign course. (B) A persistent antimyosin uptake pattern, similar to figure 2B, from an allograft recipient who developed severe allograft vasculopathy. Whereas antimyosin uptake remains consistently abnormal, endomyocardial biopsies fail to demonstrate a predictive role.

(a)

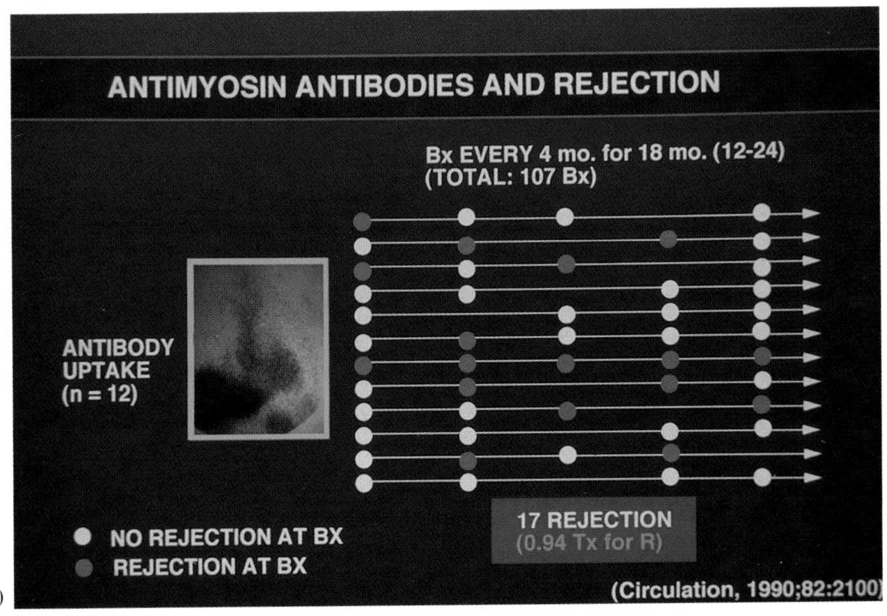

(b)

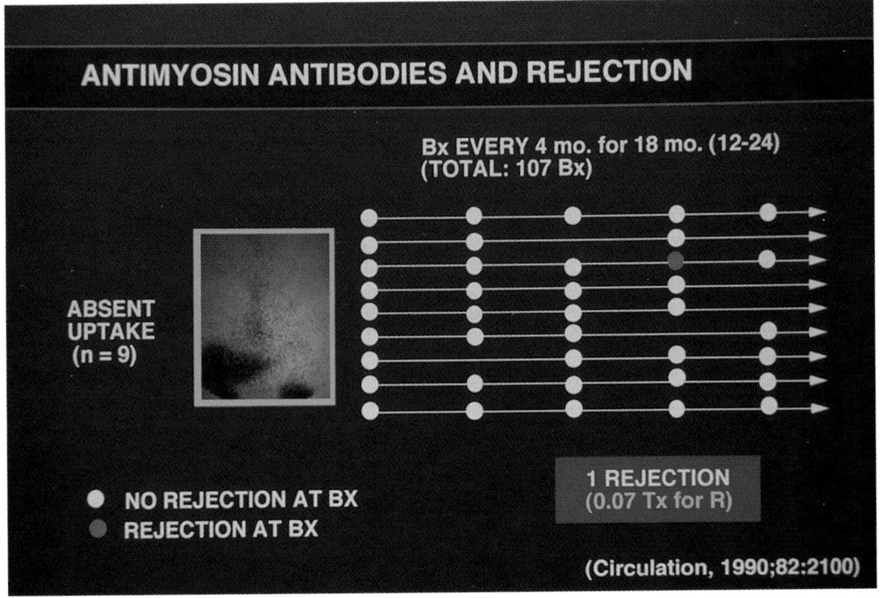

Plate 20.4. Relation of antimyosin scan findings after first year of transplantation to biopsy results. The antimyosin scans performed at the end of first year or later are compared to endomyocardial biopsies performed every 4-month. The treatment of rejection was only based solely on biopsy results. If the scan was positive at the end of the first year (A) at least one biopsy during subsequent followup demonstrated moderate rejection in the majority of patients necessitating treatment of rejection. The magnitude of antibody uptake determined the frequency of posive-biopsy results and treatment requirements (see text). (B) In case of a negative scan at the end of the first year or beyond the likelihood of biopsy evidence of moderate rejection requiring treatment was minimal.

SUBJECT INDEX

Page numbers in *italics* indicate figures. Page numbers followed by “t” indicate tables.